10th Edition

Milady's Standard Esthetics

FUNDAMENTALS

Joel Gerson

Contributing Authors

Janet D'Angelo
Shelley Lotz
Sallie Deitz

Editorial Contributors

Catherine M. Frangie
John Halal

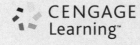
CENGAGE
Learning™

Australia • Brazil • Japan • Korea • Mexico • Singapore • Spain • United Kingdom • United States

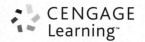

Milady's Standard Esthetics: Fundamentals, Tenth Edition
Joel Gerson, Janet D'Angelo, Sallie Deitz, Shelley Lotz, Catherine M. Frangie and John Halal

President, Milady: Dawn Gerrain

Publisher: Erin O'Connor

Acquisitions Editor: Martine Edwards

Product Manager: Jessica Burns

Editorial Assistant: Mike Spring

Director of Beauty Industry Relations: Sandra Bruce

Senior Marketing Manager: Gerard McAvey

Marketing Specialist: Erica Conley

Production Director: Wendy Troeger

Senior Content Project Manager: Nina Tucciarelli

Art Director: Joy Kocsis

For product information and technology assistance, contact us at
Professional & Career Group Customer Support, 1-800-648-7450

For permission to use material from this text or product,
submit all requests online at **cengage.com/permissions**
Further permissions questions can be e-mailed to
permissionrequest@cengage.com

Library of Congress Control Number: 2008926532

ISBN-13: 978-1-4283-1892-2

ISBN-10: 1-4283-1892-5

Delmar
5 Maxwell Drive
Clifton Park, NY 12065-2919
USA

Cengage Learning products are represented in Canada by Nelson Education, Ltd.

For your lifelong learning solutions, visit **delmar.cengage.com**

Visit our corporate website at **cengage.com**

Notice to the Reader
Publisher does not warrant or guarantee any of the products described herein or perform any independent analysis in connection with any of the product information contained herein. Publisher does not assume, and expressly disclaims, any obligation to obtain and include information other than that provided to it by the manufacturer. The reader is expressly warned to consider and adopt all safety precautions that might be indicated by the activities described herein and to avoid all potential hazards. By following the instructions contained herein, the reader willingly assumes all risks in connection with such instructions. The publisher makes no representations or warranties of any kind, including but not limited to, the warranties of fitness for particular purpose or merchantability, nor are any such representations implied with respect to the material set forth herein, and the publisher takes no responsibility with respect to such material. The publisher shall not be liable for any special, consequential, or exemplary damages resulting, in whole or part, from the readers' use of, or reliance upon, this material.

Printed in the United States of America
1 2 3 4 5 XX 10 09 08

Contents at a Glance

Contents

PART 3

SKIN SCIENCES

PART 4

ESTHETICS

PART 5

BUSINESS SKILLS

Procedures List

Preface

You are about to begin a journey into a career ripe with opportunity for success and personal satisfaction. The need for professional estheticians continues to grow in new and exciting ways, providing ample room for personal success in a variety of career paths.

As your school experience begins, consider how you will approach your course of study through attitude, study skills and habits, and perseverance, even when the going gets tough. Stay focused on your goal—to become a licensed esthetician and begin your career—and talk to your instructor should any problems arise that might prevent you from reaching it.

ENCHMARK FOR ESTHETICS EDUCATION

s *Standard Textbook for Professional Estheticians* was first published in the creation of Joel Gerson. It soon became the textbook choice of ics educators and has seen 10 revisions. Throughout this period, it onsistently been the most widely used esthetics textbook in the world. he science and business of skin care evolve, new editions of the text needed periodically, and Milady is committed to publishing the best in hetics education. With this edition, Milady marks the 30th anniversary of iblication. We have thoroughly updated the content and design of this text-ook to bring you the most valuable, effective educational resource available. To get the most out of the time you will spend studying, take a few minutes now to learn about the text and how to use it before you begin.

This 10th Edition has a new title that better reflects the content—*Milady's Standard Esthetics: Fundamentals*—and provides you with the basic informa-tion you need to pass the licensure exams for a 600-hour program. Before beginning this revision, Milady conducted extensive research to learn what needed to be changed, added, or deleted. We went to some of the top experts in the field to learn how the changing esthetics field should be reflected in the new edition of the textbook. We involved top educators in the revision process, providing firsthand knowledge of current esthetics classes. Finally, we sent the finished manuscript out for yet more reviews. What you hold in your hands is the result.

Milady's Standard Esthetics: Fundamentals 10th Edition contains compre-hensive information on many subjects, including sanitation and infection control, spa body treatments, choosing a product line, and more. In addition, a greater emphasis on personal health and well-being can be found in a new chapter entitled "Basics of Nutrition." As a part of your esthetics education, this book provides you with a valuable guide for learning the techniques you'll be performing as well as for gaining insight into how to interact with clients and even to run a business. No matter which career path you choose in the esthetics field, you'll refer to this text again and again as the foundation upon which to build your success.

In response to the suggestions of the educators and professionals who reviewed *Milady's Standard Esthetics: Fundamentals* 10th Edition and to those submitted by the students who use this text, this revision includes dramatic changes, including many new chapters.

NEW ORGANIZATION AND CHAPTERS

By learning and using the tools in this text together with your teachers' instruction, you will develop the abilities needed to build a loyal and satisfied clientele. To help you locate information more easily, the chapters are now grouped into five main parts:

> *Part 1: Orientation*—includes three chapters that cover the past, present, and future of the field of esthetics. Chapter 1, "History and Career Opportunities in Esthetics," outlines the origin of esthetics, tracing its evolution through the twenty-first century

and speculating on where it will go in the future. Chapter 2, "Your Professional Image," stresses the importance of physical hygiene and deportment and discusses how a healthy, positive attitude and strong work ethic can affect your success as an esthetician. Chapter 3, "Communicating for Success," is a veritable blueprint for using your special skills and personality to build a successful career in esthetics and to service and retain a loyal client base.

Part 2: General Sciences—includes important information that you need to know to keep you and your clients safe and healthy. Chapter 4, "Infection Control: Principles and Practice," offers the most current, vital facts about hepatitis, HIV, and other infectious viruses and bacteria and tells how to prevent them from being transmitted. Chapters 5 through 7 ("General Anatomy and Physiology," "Basics of Chemistry," and "Basics of Electricity") provide essential information that will help guide your work with clients and enable you to make decisions about treatments. Chapter 8, "Basics of Nutrition," is the final chapter in Part 2. This new chapter is vital for estheticians who seek to understand the effects of nutrition on the skin. The chapters cover nutrients, vitamins and minerals both used topically and taken internally.

Part 3: Skin Sciences—offers clear, up-to-date content on every aspect of the skin. Chapter 9, "Physiology and Histology of the Skin," includes skin anatomy and skin function, with an emphasis on the impact of good nutrition; Chapter 10, "Disorders and Diseases of the Skin," explores the many maladies of the skin, including acne, sensitive skin, and the danger of sun exposure. Chapter 11, "Skin Analysis," addresses skin types and conditions, stressing the necessity of a thorough client consultation. The foundation on which almost every retail sale is built is covered in Chapter 12, "Skin Care Products: Chemistry, Ingredients, and Selection"

Part 4: Esthetics—focuses on actual practices performed by the esthetician. Setting up the treatment room and creating the correct atmosphere for both the client and for the esthetician are covered in Chapter 13, "The Treatment Room." Chapter 14, "Basic Facials," instructs in the methods used during several types of facials and their benefits and contraindications, as well as the unique considerations and techniques of the men's facial. Chapter 15, "Facial Massage," covers the benefits of massage along with contraindications and basic movements. Chapter 16, "Facial Machines," is devoted to machines used in esthetic treatments provides instruction on the use of the steamer, galvanic, Wood's Lamp, and more; and Chapter 17, "Hair Removal," covers the critical information you'll need for these increasingly requested services. Chapter 18, "Advanced Topics and Treatments," provides an overview of body and clinical procedures used with cosmetic surgery, and the increasingly popular spa body treatments. Color theory, face shapes, and advice about selecting a product line are some of the topics addressed in Chapter 19, "The World of Makeup," which will provide a ready reference in the future with appearance-enhancement services growing in demand.

Part 5: Business Skills—contains a wealth of new information on creating financial and operational success as an esthetician. Chapter 20, "Career Planning," provides practical instruction on setting goals, preparing a resume, and preparing for an interview. Information on the skills of money management and communication is also included.

"The Skin Care Business," Chapter 21, includes valuable information on establishing your own business, as well as tips to help you recognize a successful business to join as an employee. Lastly, Chapter 22, "Selling Products and Services," stresses market-related topics including product knowledge, understanding your clients' needs, and tracking your success.

A FRESH NEW DESIGN

The changes in this 10th Edition of *Milady's Standard Esthetics: Fundamentals* go far beyond the new content and features. Over 300 new full-color illustrations and photographs enhance this book, along with a totally new text design that incorporates the most easy-to-read type and spacing. New procedure format offers clear, easy-to-understand directions and step-by-step photographs to help students visualize important techniques.

EDUCATIONAL ELEMENTS OF THIS EDITION

As a part of the extensive revision of this edition, many features have been added or reorganized to help you recognize and master key concepts and techniques.

Focus On . . .

Throughout the text are short paragraphs in the outer column that draw attention to various skills and concepts that will help you obtain your goal. The "Focus On . . ." pieces target all aspects of personal and professional development. These topics are crucial to your success as a student and as a professional.

Activity

The "Activity" boxes offer engaging and timely classroom exercises that will help you understand firsthand the concepts being explained in the text.

Did You Know?

These features provide interesting information that will enhance your understanding of what you are learning in the text, and call attention to a special point.

Regulatory Agency Alert

Laws differ from region to region, so it is important to contact state boards and provincial regulatory agencies to learn what is allowed and not allowed where you are studying. In this text you will find the "Regulatory Agency Alert" icon next to procedures or practices that are regulated differently from state to state, alerting you to refer to the laws in your region. Your instructor will provide you with contact information.

FYI

These features offer important, interesting information related to the content.

Web Resources

These features offer web addresses and references for you to check out for additional information and activities.

Chapter Glossary

The words that you will need to know in a chapter are given at the beginning, in a list of key terms. The first time a word is used and defined in the text, the word will appear in boldface. If the word is difficult to pronounce, a phonetic pronunciation appears after it in parentheses. All key terms and their definitions are included in the chapter glossary at the end of the chapter as well as in the Glossary/Index at the end of the text.

Learning Objectives

At the beginning of each chapter are the objectives for learning, which will tell you what important information you will be expected to know from the chapter. Icons placed within the chapter indicate that a learning objective has been completed.

Caution!

Some information is so critical for your safety and the safety of your clients that it deserves special attention. The text directs you to this information in the "Caution!" features found in the margins.

Here's a Tip

These helpful hints draw attention to situations that might arise or quick ways of doing things. Look for these tips in procedures and throughout the text.

Review Questions

At the end of each chapter we have included questions designed to test your understanding of the information just presented. Your instructor may ask you to write the answers to these questions as an assignment or to answer them orally in class. If you have trouble answering a question, go back to the chapter, review the material, and try again.

EXTENSIVE TEACHING/LEARNING PACKAGE

While *Milady's Standard Esthetics: Fundamentals* 10th Edition is the center of the curriculum, students and educators have a wide range of supplements to choose from. All supplements have been revised and updated to complement the new edition of the textbook, and several new supplements have been created to support this edition.

Student Supplements

All student supplements have been revised to correlate with the revision of the textbook.

Milady's Standard Esthetics: Fundamentals 10th Edition Workbook

Designed to reinforce classroom and textbook learning, the *Workbook* contains chapter-by-chapter exercises. Included are fill-in-the-blank exercises, matching exercises, short-answer questions, and labeling of illustrations, all coordinated with material from the text.

Milady's Standard Esthetics: Fundamentals 10th Edition Exam Review

The *Exam Review* contains chapter-by-chapter questions in a multiple-choice format to help students prepare for the licensure exam. While not intended to be the only form of review offered to students, it aids in overall classroom preparation. The *Exam Review* has been revised to meet the most stringent test-development guidelines. The questions in the *Exam Review* are for study purposes only and are not the exact questions students will see on the licensure exams.

Milady's Standard Esthetics: Fundamentals *Student CD-ROM*

Milady's Standard Esthetics: Fundamentals Student CD-ROM is an interactive product designed to reinforce classroom learning, stimulate the imagination, and aid in preparation for board exams. Featuring many helpful video clips and graphical animations to demonstrate practices and procedures, this exciting educational tool also contains a test bank with approximately 1,000 chapter-by-chapter or randomly accessed multiple-choice questions to help students study for the exam. Another feature is the game bank, which offers games to strengthen knowledge of terminology, and a glossary that pronounces and defines each term.

The content follows and enhances the *Milady's Standard Esthetics: Fundamentals* 10th Edition textbook. The technology of the program is designed to be interactive, allowing the learner to be surrounded or "pulled into" the content, and it tracks the student's progress through the program.

Milady's Online Licensing Preparation: Esthetics

Milady's Online Licensing Preparation: Esthetics provides students with an on-line alternative to better prepare for state board exams. One thousand multiple-choice questions, different from those in the *Exam Review*, appear with rationales for correct and incorrect choices; and the correct answer links to the portion of *Milady's Standard Esthetics: Fundamentals* 10th Edition where the information is given. Students have the flexibility to study from any computer, whether at home or at school. Because exam review preparation is available to students at any time of day or night, class time can be used for other activities, and students gain familiarity with a computerized test environment as they prepare for licensure. This product is also offered in Spanish.

Educator Supplements

Milady offers a full range of products created especially for esthetics educators to make the classroom preparation and presentation simple, effective, and enjoyable.

Course Management Guide

The *Course Management Guide* contains all the materials educators need in one package. This innovative, instructional guide is written with esthetics educators in mind and is designed to make exceptional teaching easy. With formatting that provides easy-to-use material for use in the classroom, it will transform classroom management and dramatically increase student interest and understanding. Included are comprehensive lesson plans, instructor support forms, transition guide, and the answers to the review questions in the textbook and *Milady's Standard Esthetics: Fundamentals* 10th Edition *Workbook*.

Features You Will Find on the CD-ROM Version

- Every page from the *Course Management Guide* can be printed to appear exactly like the page from the print product.
- A computerized test bank contains multiple-choice questions that instructors can use to create random tests from a single chapter or create a more comprehensive exam from all of the material in the book. In this new edition, computerized test bank questions are not the same questions as in the *Exam Review*. Answer keys are automatically created. A gradebook feature to track students' progress is also included.
- An Image Library of *all* of the photos and illustrations from *Milady's Standard Esthetics: Fundamentals* 10th Edition can be easily imported to Microsoft® PowerPoint® presentations or printed onto paper or acetate to create overheads. They can even be imported into other documents to further enhance instruction.

Microsoft® PowerPoint® presentation (Instructor Support Slides)

The PowerPoint Presentation created to accompany the *Milady's Standard Esthetics: Fundamentals* 10th Edition makes lesson plans simple yet incredibly effective. Complete with photos and art, this chapter-by-chapter CD-ROM has ready-to-use presentations that will help engage students' attention and keep their interest through its varied color schemes and styles. Instructors can use it as is or adapt it to their own classrooms by importing photos they have taken, changing the graphics, or adding slides.

SPANISH EDITION

Milady's Standard Esthetics: Fundamentals 10th Edition will also be available in Spanish. In addition, the *Workbook*, *Exam Review*, and *Online Licensing Preparation* are also available in Spanish. Each Spanish product is a page-by-page translation of the English edition.

About the Authors

JOEL GERSON

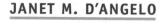

Joel Gerson, Ph.D., set the standards for esthetic skin care schools in the United States when he authored *Standard Textbook for Professional Estheticians* as the result of many years of research and experience. Before the book was published, no state offered a separate license in esthetic skin care. Since the publication of the first edition, 48 states now offer separate licenses for the practice of facial treatments and makeup.

Joel Gerson has been called the "master of skin care education" by *American Salon Magazine,* because he is a firm believer in education and enjoys sharing his knowledge with others. He has presented his dynamic and comprehensive lectures and seminars throughout the United States, Canada, Europe, and the Far East. To arrange for Joel to conduct a workshop at your school, call Milady's Career Institute at 1 (800) 998-7498, ext. 8220.

Joel's professional credentials include resident makeup artist for the House of Revlon; spokesman for Lever Brothers; vice president of Education for Christine Valmy, Inc.; facial treatment trainer to Pivot Point International Instructors; and director of skin care training for Redken Laboratories. Joel is currently serving as a technical consultant to several major manufacturers and has appeared on radio and television talk shows. His articles on facial treatments and skin care have appeared in many publications, including *Les Nouvelles Esthetiques, Dermascope, Modern Salon,* and *American Salon.* He has hosted the International Congress of Esthetics, sponsored by the American edition of *Les Nouvelles Esthetiques* and the *Dermascope Magazine* since 1993. Joel Gerson has a doctorate in Allied Health Science and holds a teaching license for Scientific Facial Treatments from the University of the State of New York. He has served as an esthetic examiner with the New York Department of State.

JANET M. D'ANGELO

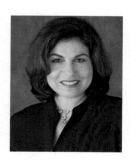

Janet M. D'Angelo, M.Ed., is founder and president of J.Angel Communications, LLC, a marketing and public relations firm specializing in the health, beauty, and wellness industry. With more than 20 years of experience developing marketing and management strategies across all segments of the skin care market, Janet is a featured speaker at trade shows and conducts seminars and workshops on a wide range of business topics.

Janet began her career in the skin care industry in 1979 as one of the first separately licensed estheticians in Massachusetts. Since then she has worked tirelessly to raise industry awareness and promote professional standards. In addition to her work on this text, Ms. D'Angelo is the author of *Spa Business Strategies: A Plan for Success* (Thomson Delmar Learning, 2006). She is also a contributing editor and author of the Business Communication Skills of *Milady's Standard Comprehensive Training for Estheticians* (Milady, 2003) and *Milady's Standard Esthetics: Advanced* (Cengage Learning, 2009). She has written numerous articles for newspaper, consumer, and trade publications and is responsible for conducting the Day Spa Association's *First Compensation & Benefits Survey*.

Ms. D'Angelo is a member of several professional organizations, including the American Marketing Association (AMA), the Day Spa Association (DSA), the International Spa Association (ISPA), and the National Coalition of Estheticians, Manufacturers, Distributors and Alliances (NCEA). She can be reached at janet@jangelcommunications.com.

SHELLEY LOTZ

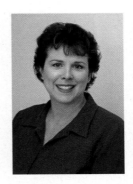

Shelley Lotz is an esthetician who has been involved in many aspects of the industry, including business management, training, marketing, retailing, writing, and consulting. She is the former owner and an instructor at the Oregon Institute of Aesthetics, an undergraduate and advanced graduate-level esthetician school. Before starting the school, she owned her own business and worked at salons and day spas. She started her career in Esthetics 20 years ago and is now a writer, consultant, and educator. She has taught community workshops and worked as a makeup artist for photographers and film/video. Lotz has a bachelor of science degree in Biology, Geography, and Communications from Southern Oregon University. Shelley has been involved with state legislative and industry changes as a member of the Oregon Department of Education curriculum committee and the Board of Cosmetology's item-writing committee. Lotz is a member of the NCEA. For her, the most rewarding part of teaching is making a difference in the student's lives. She is passionate about this exciting industry and loves sharing information through writing and education.

SALLIE DEITZ

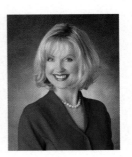

Sallie Deitz serves in education and product development with Bio Therapeutic, Inc., and the Bio Therapeutic Institute of Technology, in Seattle, Washington. Deitz has been a licensed esthetician for 25 years, and has 12 years of clinical experience. She is the author of *The Clinical Esthetician:, An Insider's Guide to Succeeding in a Medical Office*, (2004), Milady Publishing),; and *Amazing Skin:, A Girl's Guide to Naturally Beautiful Skin* (2005), Drummond Publishing Group). Sallie Deitz is a contributing author to *Milady's Standard Comprehensive Training for Estheticians* (2004), and *Milady's Standard Esthetics: Fundamentals*, 10th ed. (2009). Deitz is an editorial advisory board member for Plastic Surgery Products, in Los Angeles, California, and serves as a committee member in test development for NIC (National Interstate Council of State Boards of Cosmetology, - Esthetics Division).

CATHERINE M. FRANGIE

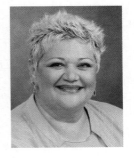

Catherine M. Frangie has been a dedicated and passionate beauty professional since 1982, when she first began her career as a licensed cosmetologist, salon owner, and beauty school instructor. Since then, Catherine has held prominent and dynamic positions throughout many facets of the professional beauty industry, including Marketing, Communications and Education vice president for a leading product company, communications director, trade magazine publisher, and textbook editor and author. In 2000 Catherine founded FrangieConsulting, a marketing and communications consulting firm catering to the exclusive and unique needs of professional beauty industry companies. FrangieConsulting has earned seven ABBIE awards (from the American Beauty Association) for its work on various national marketing campaigns.

Catherine has addressed her beauty colleagues numerous times as a guest lecturer at the International Beauty Show in New York City and in other national venues. She has personally authored more than 125 feature-length trade and consumer magazine articles and several books on beauty trends, fashion, and the business of the professional salon. Catherine holds a graduate degree in communications as well as undergraduate degrees in marketing and advertising.

JOHN HALAL

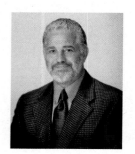

A hairstylist, licensed instructor, and president of Honors Beauty College, Inc., John Halal is an active member of the National Cosmetology Association (NCA), the Salon Association (TSA), the Beauty & Barber Supply Institute (BBSI), and the Society of Cosmetic Chemists (SCC). He serves as vice president and executive director for the American Association of Cosmetology Schools (AACS) and is the past president of the Indiana Cosmetology Educators Association (ICEA). Halal has published several books and numerous articles on hair structure and product chemistry. Halal obtained his associate's degree, with highest distinction, from Indiana University and is a member of The Golden Key National Honor Society and Alpha Sigma Lambda.

Acknowledgments

The authors and publisher wish to thank the many people who gave their time and expertise in producing this text. We also wish to thank the reviewers, who provided many insightful suggestions for improving this book. We are indebted to them.

Sheryl Baba,
Solstice Day Spa,
Massachusetts

Debbie Beatty,
Columbus Technical College,
Georgia

Carole Berube,
Massachusetts

Helen Bickmore,
Jean Paul Spa De Beaute,
New York

Felicia Brown,
Balance Day Spa,
North Carolina

Linda Burmeister,
International Dermal Institute,
California

Sarah Burns,
Caleel & Hayden,
Wisconsin

Donna Charron,
Eastern Wyoming College,
Wyoming

April J. Coleman,
Assistant Director,
Licensed Master Esthetician/Instructor, MD

Denise Fuller,
Anton Academy and International Spa Importing Specialists,
Florida

John Halal,
Honors Beauty College, Inc.
Indiana

Jean Harrity,
Refresh Institute of Esthetics,
Illinois

Patricia Heitz,
Dermatech Academy,
New York

Marsha Hemby,
North Carolina

Kathy Hernandez-McGowan,
Marinello School of Beauty,
California

Ruth Ann Holloway,
Dermal Dimensions,
Utah

Delores Hunt,
Central Florida Community College,
Florida

Kim Jarrett,
College of Hair Design,
Missouri

Tracy Johnson,
Wingate Salon & Spa,
New Hampshire

Irene Koufalis,
European Body Concepts,
Texas

Sharon MacGregor,
JcPenney Salon,
New York

Cheryl McDonald,
Solano Community College,
California

Maggie McNerney,
self-employed,
Massachusetts

Jillian Motyl,
Keiser Career College,
Florida

Elizabeth Myron,
Training Technician Consultant,
Maryland

Maria Nelson,
International Beauty School,
Oregon

Natasha Ogorodnitsky,
Florida

Sandra Peoples,
T. H. Pickens Technical Center,
Colorado

Kathy Phelps,
Moore Norman Technology Center,
Oklahoma

Amy Fields Rumley,
Merle Norman Studio Owner,
North Carolina

Alex Sokolowski,
New York

Patricia Powers Stander,
Esthetician, Instructor, and Licensed Practical Nurse,
Massachusetts

Ada Polla Tray,
Alchimie Forever LLC,
Virginia

Nancy Tomaselli,
Cerritos Community College,
California

Madeline Udod,
Career Education,
New York

Jan Walters,
Colorado School of Paramedical Esthetics,
Colorado

Shelley Lotz would like to thank the following for their assistance with Parts 3 and 4 of the text: Gretchen Facey, Crystal Koebrick, Janet Bocast, Renee Norman-Martin, Marcella Arana, Danika Blood, Kathy Lystra, Suzanne Mathis McQueen, Feather Gilmore, Serena Beach, Panos Photinos, and the students at the Oregon Institute of Aesthetics for their support and editing.

Much appreciation and thanks to Gretchen Facey, Panos Photinos, Janet Bocast, Suzanne Mathis McQueen, Marian Smith, and the students and staff at the Oregon Institute of Aesthetics for all of your support. I would not be where I am today without you.

Sallie Deitz wishes to thank the following people for their help in working on this project: Joel Gerson—Thank you for all that you have done for our industry. I still have my Gerson book (3rd ed.), well highlighted, in my office. It was a red paperback. I remember feeling a true "kinship" with you, Mr. Gerson, back so many years ago; who knew that I would actually be a part of a team bringing forth a 10th Edition?

Also many thanks to Cathy Frangie, staff of Milady/Delmar/Cengage Learning, Darla McGovern, Christopher Stacey, Maren Brown, Shelly

Lotz, Janet D'Angelo, John Halal, Bellingham ENT & Facial Plastic Surgery.

Photo Session Acknowledgments

The publisher wishes to thank Shelley Lotz for all of her time and hard work in setting up the photo shoot for the new edition. Shelley spent several days organizing the entire shoot, including finding models and locations. The photo shoot was a success due to her attention to detail and dedication.

Many thanks to the following Southern Oregon facilities and owners, who opened their doors for the photo session: Annette Draper at The Spa at Club Northwest, Grants Pass; Deb Cleland at Waterstone Spa, Ashland; Drew McDermott at Salon Isabella, Ashland; Jessica Vineyard at The Phoenix Spa, Ashland and Kate Wasserman at the Oregon Institute of Aesthetics, Talent.

Special thanks to Shelley Lotz's assistant during the photo session, Josette Fithian. Thanks to the former students, colleagues, and others who participated in the photo session—a beautiful and talented group of people.

Thanks to Rob Werfel and Alison Pazourek, photographers.

Thanks to the following models:

Tiffany Albright	Scott Draper	Shannon Peterson
Lori Allred	Kim Faeber	Demetris Photinos
Marcella Arana	Beth Forshay	Markos Photinos
Jessica Arteche	Phylicia Fratus	Zoe Photinos
Darci Baize	Joy Gosson	Jaclyn Redd
Sheana Benham	Josette Fithian	Jennifer Redd
Vanessa Blount	Amanda Kay	Allison Smith
Janet Bocast	Ashley Lawson	Julie Starrett
Tiana Bramson	Brandi Leard	Marian Szewc
Teri Burrill	Gretchen Lee	Selene Veltri
Jessica Carrico	Shelley Lotz	Kendra Wessels
Jesse Carlini	Renee Norman	Alycia Whitney
Lisa Carson	Martin	Katie Williams
Deb Cleland	Suzanne McQueen	Karen Wilson
Teresa Contreras	Wade McQueen	Chelsey Weyand
Luciene Cruz	Cory Minard	
Annette Draper	Holly Perkins	

Photo Credits:

Chapter 1—Chapter opener (beautiful brunette girl model, while make-up before shooting session): asiana, 2008; used under license from Shutterstock.com. Fig. 1–3, 1–4, and 1–5: courtesy Scherrer Photography. Fig. 1–6: Larry Hamill Photography. Fig. 1–7 (businesswoman in modern corporate interior with management team in background): © Juriah Mosin, 2008; used under license from Shutterstock.com. Fig. 1–8 (African American male working in a corporate office with intent focus on his computer screen): © Bobby Deal/ RealDealPhoto, 2008; used under license from Shutterstock. com. Fig. 1–9: courtesy of Rob Werfel Photography.

Chapter 2—Chapter opener: © Getty Images/Stockbyte Fig. 2–1 (young and smiling operator works on a laptop computer in a modern office): © Kristian Sekulic, 2008; used under license from Shutterstock.com. Fig 2–3: Larry Hamill Photography. Figs. 2–3, 2–4, 2–5, and 2–8: Paul Castle, Castle Photography. Figs. 2–6, 2–7, and 2–9: Rob Werfel Photography. Fig. 2–10 (beautiful middle eastern girl playing piano): © Galina Barskaya, 2008; used under license from Shutterstock.com. Fig. 2–11 (a session within the business concept of working outside your workplace, on the move, or at a restaurant or cafe location): © Yuri Arcurs, 2008; used under license from Shutterstock.com. Fig. 2–12 (hands typing text on the BlackBerry cell phone; isolated on white): © Igor Karon, 2008; used under license from Shutterstock.com.

Chapter 3—Chapter opener: Paul Castle Photography Fig. 3–1: Larry Hamill. Fig. 3–3 (beautiful young woman wearing workout clothes): © Varina and Jay Patel, 2008; used under license from Shutterstock.com. Figs. 3–2, 3–4, 3–6 to 3–9, 3–12: Rob Werfel. Figs. 3–10, 3–11: Paul Castle/Castle Photography.

Chapter 4—Chapter opener: (Man helping himself to a squirt of hand sanitizer, close up of bottle and hands): Svanblar, 2008; used under license from Shutterstock.com. Fig. 4–8, courtesy of the National Pediculosis Association. Fig. 4–9: Robert A. Silverman, MD, Clinical Assoc. Professor, Dept. of Pediatrics, Georgetown University. Fig. 4–11, Randall Perry. Fig. 4–12, 4–15, 4–16: Paul Castle/Castle Photography. Fig. 4–13: Courtesy of MIDMARK. Figs. 4–10, 4–14, 4–18, 4–23: Larry Hamill. Figs. 4–19 to 4–22: Rob Werfel. Fig. 4–24 (first aid kit open on a blue background): © Dana Bartekoske, 2008; used under license from Shutterstock.com.

Chapter 5—Chapter opener (anatomically correct medical model of the human body, women, muslces, and ligaments showing transparent and skeleton projected into the body): Patrick Hermans, 2008; used under license from Shutterstock.com.

Chapter 6—Chapter opener (Erlenmeyer flash and test tubes in a research laboratory): rrocio, 2008; used under license from Shutterstock.com. Fig. 6–1: Larry Hamill Artist & Photographer. Fig. 6–2 (Complete Periodic Table of the Elements, including atomic number, symbol, name, weight; arrows indicate lanthanoids and actinoids): ©Michael D. Brown, 2008; used under license from Shutterstock.com.

Chapter 7—Chapter opener (lightning in the night): Alegria, 2008; used under license from Shutterstock.com. Fig. 7–1 (lightning strike): © Scott Conrad, 2008; used under license from Shutterstock.com. Figs. 7–11, 7–12, 7–15: Larry Hamill, Artist & Photographer. Figs. 7–13 A,B: courtesy of David Suzuki, BioTherapeutic. Fig. 7–14: Rob Werfel. Fig. 7–19: courtesy of Revitalight.

Chapter 8—Chapter opener: © Getty Images Fig. 8–2: courtesy of U.S. Department of Agriculture. Fig. 8–3 (fresh vegetables, fruits, and other foodstuffs; shot in a studio): © Kiselev Andrey Valerevich, 2008; used under license from Shutterstock .com. Figs. 8–4 A,B & 8–5: courtesy of Mark Lees Skin Care, Inc. Fig. 8–6 (Caucasian mid-adult woman wearing robe and towel on deck, drinking from glass next to pool): © iofoto, 2008; used under license from Shutterstock.com. Fig. 8–7: Paul Castle, Castle Photography.

Chapter 9—Chapter opener (Face of a beautiful young woman with a puzzle collage): IKO, 2008; used under license from Shutterstock.com. Fig. 9–1: Rob Werfel. Fig. 9–9: courtesy of Godfrey F. Mix, DPM, Sacramento, CA. Fig. 9–13: adapted from Siberian Tiger Naturals, Inc., Springfield, Vermont. Fig. 9–14 (unshaven male with cigarette): © Robert Ford, 2008; used under license from Shutterstock.com. Fig. 9–16: Larry Hamill.

Chapter 10—Chapter opener (skin treatment in a beauty salon): Aleksandar-Pal Sakala, 2008; used under license from Shutterstock.com. Figs. 10–2, 10–31, 10–32: courtesy of Mark Lees Skin Care, Inc. Figs. 10–3, 10–8, 10–10, 10–21, 10–26: © 2007 Interactive Medical Media LLC; all rights reserved. Fig. 10–4: Timothy Berger, MD, Associate Clinical Professor, University of California, San Francisco. Figs. 10–7, 10–18, 10–20, courtesy of Michael J. Bond, MD. Fig. 10–9, courtesy of George Fisher, MD. Fig. 10–11: Center for Disease Control and Prevention. Fig. 10–12: reprinted with permission from the American Academy of Dermatology; all rights reserved. Fig. 10–14: courtesy of National Rosacea Society. Fig. 10–17: T. Fitzgerald, *Color Atlas & Synopsis of Clinical Dermatology*, 3rd ed. (McGraw-Hill, 1996). Figs. 10–6, 10–13, 10–16, 10–19, 10–22, 10–23, 10–24, 10–28, 10–29, Fig. 10–33, 10–34: reprinted with permission from the American Academy of Dermatology; all rights reserved. Fig. 10–25: courtesy of the Skin Cancer Foundation, http://www.skincancer.org.

Fig. 10–26, Centers for Disease Control and Prevention/Dr. Hermann. Fig. 10–27: courtesy of Rube J. Pardo, MD, Ph.D.

Chapter 11—Chapter opener (a high key portrait of woman with make-up): Phil Date, 2008; used under license from Shutterstock.com. Fig. 11–1: Paul Castle. Figs. 11–3, 11–8: Rob Werfel. Fig. 11–4, 11–8, P11–1, Table 11–1: Larry Hamill, Artist & Photographer; Fig. 11–5 (portrait of young woman expressing emotion): © MW Productions, 2008; used under license from Shutterstock.com. Fig. 11–6: courtesy of David P. Rapaport, MD, New York, NY.

Chapter 12—Chapter opener: Larry Hamill Figs. 12–1, 12–7, 12–14, 12–15, 12–18: Larry Hamill, Artist & Photographer. Figs. 12–2, 12–8 to 12–13, 12–16, 12–17, 12–18: Rob Werfel. Figs 12–6 (bottles for science): © rebvt, 2008; used under license from Shutterstock.com.

Chapter 13—Chapter opener: Alison Pazourek. Figs. 13–1, 13–3, 13–7, 13–10, 13–12, 13–16, 13–18: Rob Werfel. Figs. 13–2, 13–8, 13–9, 13–19: Paul Castle. Fig. 13–4: Alison Pazourek Fig. 13–11: Rob Werfel, Paul Castle; autoclave supplied by MIDMARK. Figs. 13–6, 13–13, 13–15, 13–17: Larry Hamill, Artist & Photographer; Fig. 13–14: Stock Studios Photography.

Chapter 14—Chapter opener: Yanik Chauvin/Touch Photography Figs. 14–1, 14–11, 14–21: Larry Hamill. Figs. 14–4 to 14–10, 14–13, 14–16, 14–17, 14–20: Rob Werfel. Figs. 14–2, 14–12, 14–14, 14–15, 14–18, 14–23, 14–24: Paul Castle. Fig. 14–19: Alison Pazourek Fig. 14–22: Michael Dzamen Photography. Fig. 14–25: reprinted with permission from the American Academy of Dermatology; all rights reserved.

Chapter 15—Chapter Opener: Getty Images. Figs. 15–1, 15–2, 15–5, 15–7, 15–11, 15–12, P15–1: Paul Castle. Figs. 15–3, 15–6, 15–8, 15–9, 15–10, 15–16, 15–17: Rob Werfel. Fig. 15–4 (professional fitness instructor/shot in workout gym): © Gabriel Moisa, 2008; used under license from Shutterstock.com. Fig. 15–13, Larry Hamill, Artist & Photographer.

Chapter 16—Chapter opener: Larry Hamill. Figs. 16–1, 16–7, 16–10, 16–11, 16–12b, 16–13a,b, 16–14, 16–15: Rob Werfel. Figs. 16–2, 16–3, 16–8, 16–18: Paul Castle. Figs. 16–4 to 16–6, 16–9, 16–16, 16–17: Larry Hamill, Artist & Photographer.

Chapter 17—Chapter opener: Getty Images. Figs. 17–5, 17–6, 17–10, 17–19: Larry Hamill, Artist & Photographer. Figs. 17–1, 17–7, 17–8, 17–11, 17–12, 17–14, 17–15: Rob Werfel. Fig. 17–13: Shelley Lotz.

Chapter 18—Chapter opener: Getty Images/Brooke Slezak Figs. 18–1, 18–8 to 18–10: Randall Perry Photography. Figs. 18–2, 18–17: Scherrer Photography. Figs. 18–4, 18–7, 18–11, 18–14, 18–15, 18–16: Rob Werfel. Figs. 18–12, 18–18: Larry Hamill. Fig. 18–5: courtesy of Leon Prete, LMT, and Barbara Prete, CE, SafeLase Institute for Cosmetic Laser Training. Figs. 18–19, 18–20: courtesy of David P. Rapaport, MD, New York, NY; Figs. 18–22, 18–23: courtesy of R. Emil Hecht, MD.

Chapter 19—Chapter Opener: Getty Images Figs. 19–1 to 19–8, 19–10 to 19–12, 19–24, 19–25, 19–36: Larry Hamill, Artist & Photographer. Fig. 19–9 (shadows on the white background): © Tim Sulov, 2008; used under license from Shutterstock.com. Fig. 19–13 (cosmetic brushes lined up on white background): © Hu Xiao Fang, 2008; used under license from Shutterstock.com. Figs. 19–23, 19–28, 19–29, 19–32, 19–37: Rob Werfel. Fig. 19–27 (woman with a special make-up): Krupetskova Alena, 2008; used under license of Shutterstock.com. Fig. 19–30 (eyes-closed bride portrait on dark background): © Flashon Studio, 2008; used under license from Shutterstock.com. Fig. 19–31A (extreme close-up and airbrush makeup): © Macro Boots, 2008; used under license from Shutterstock.com. Fig. 19–31B (geisha hiding behind straw fence): © Andrejs Pidjass, 2008; used under license from Shutterstock.com. Fig. 19–32: Fig. 19–38: courtesy of Judy Culp.

Chapter 20—Chapter opener (application for employment): Ryan R Fox, 2008; used under license from Shutterstock.com. Fig. 20–3: courtesy of Godfrey F. Mix, Sacramento, CA. Fig. 20–4: Stock Studios Photography. Fig. 20–12 (businesswoman with briefcase walking on white): © DUSAN ZIDAR, 2008; used under license from Shutterstock.com. Figs. 20–13, 20–17, 20–21: Rob Werfel. Fig. 20–15: Michael Dazman. Fig. 20–16: Paul Castle/Castle Photography. Fig. 20–18: Larry Hamill, Artist & Photographer.

Chapter 21—Chapter opener: Alison Pazourek Fig. 21–2 (two contemporary businesspeople at a meeting): © Yuri Arcurs, 2008; used under license from Shutterstock.com. Figs. 21–3, 21–4, 21–8, 21–16: Paul Castle/Castle Photography. Fig. 21–5: Getty Images. Figs. 21–1, 21–6, 21–12, 21–13, 21–14: Rob Werfel. Figs. 21–7, 21–15: Larry Hamill, Artist & Photographer. Fig. 21–9: Alison Pazourek.

Chapter 22—Chapter opener: Getty Images Figs. 22–1 to 22–4, 22–6, 22–11: Paul Castle/Castle Photography. Figs. 22–5, 22–7, 22–10: Rob Werfel. Fig. 22–8 (young and good-looking businesspeople working in a meeting room): © Zsolt Nyulaszi, 2008; used under license from Shutterstock.com.

A Message from the Author

As I sit at my desk writing this message, I find it hard to believe that it has been 30 years since I wrote my first book, the *Standard Textbook for Professional Estheticians*. Over the years the book was revised many times, and translated into many languages. *The Standard Textbook for Professional Estheticians* set the standards for teaching esthetic skin care in schools and for state board examinations in both the United States and Canada. Now, with contributions by Janet D'Angelo, Shelly Lotz, Sallie Deitz, Cathy Frangie and John Halal this 10th Edition of the book is squarely ready for the next generation of professionals. Along with the new revisions and design of the book, we have also given it a new name: *Milady's Standard Esthetics: Fundamentals* 10th Edition.

But, how did it all start? When I first began teaching facial treatments and makeup in New York City, I realized the inadequacy of educational materials available for the training of estheticians. There was no practical "how-to" book or comprehensive course of study that was both easy to understand and thorough in its contents. What was needed was a textbook providing "step-by-step" illustrations that teachers and students alike could follow with ease. With the growth of esthetic skin care in this country, our industry was in desperate need for someone to write a basic textbook that would meet the needs and standards of the American schools, their teachers, students, and state boards of cosmetology. With encouragement from Milady Publishing Company to write the book, I began the most important undertaking of my professional career. This book has been my contribution to a profession that has been extremely rewarding to me. It has literally taken me around the world as I taught the benefits of touch when combined with professional techniques and products. Having always enjoyed sharing my knowledge with others, this text has given me the opportunity to share with you, the future esthetician, cosmetician, and makeup artist, the techniques, methods, and knowledge based on my many years of experience and research. As an esthetician you will work closely with your clients. It is rewarding to know that the improvement the client sees in his or her skin has been brought about by your knowledge, skills, and personal touch as a professional esthetician. *Milady's Standard Esthetics: Fundamentals* 10th Edition will show you the way to become confident as a professional esthetician. This course of study and guidance from your instructor will help you to achieve your goals in the exciting, lucrative, and rewarding field of esthetics. I congratulate you on the profession you have chosen. Have no doubt that if your mind is set on success, if you have the feeling of concern and well-being for others, use your creative imagination, love what you are doing, and "dare to be different," then you, too, will be successful.

GOOD LUCK!
Joel Gerson, Ph.D.
New York, New York

DEDICATION

I dedicate this book to the memory of my mother, Rosella Gerson, who passed away when she was 36, and to my father, Ben Gerson, who encouraged me to continue my studies in cosmetology when I wanted to drop out of school. He said, "Finish school, and get a license, and no matter where you go, you will always be able to find work." And he was right!

ORIENTATION

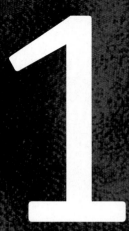

PART

1

CHAPTER **1**

HISTORY AND CAREER OPPORTUNITIES IN ESTHETICS

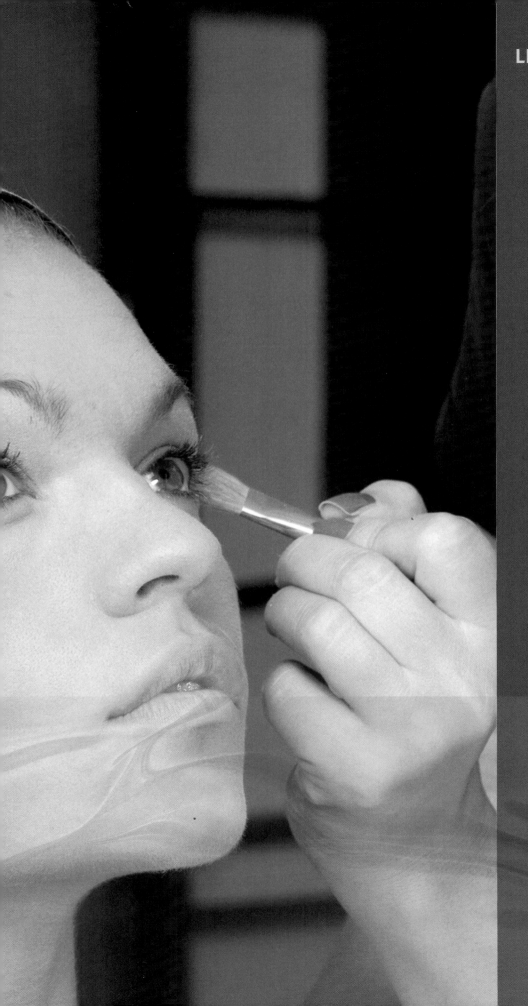

LEARNING OBJECTIVES

After completing this chapter, you will be able to:

- Describe the cosmetics and skin care practices of earlier cultures.

- Discuss the changes in skin care and grooming in the twentieth and twenty-first centuries.

- Name and describe the career options available to licensed estheticians.

- Explain the development of esthetics as a distinct, specialized profession.

Much of today's skin and body care therapies are rooted in the practices and attempts of earlier civilizations to ward off disease in order to live healthier, longer lives. The brief history outlined in this chapter will acquaint you with some of the ways men and women have tried to improve upon skin health and nature by changing and enhancing their appearance.

BRIEF HISTORY OF SKIN CARE

In early times, grooming and skin care were practiced more for self-preservation than for attractiveness. For example, an ancient African might have adorned himself with a variety of colors that would allow him to blend into his environment for hunting. During the reign of Elizabeth I, men and women would have used lead and arsenic face powder to adorn themselves because it was the social trend in the mid-1500s.

The Egyptians

The Egyptians were the first to cultivate beauty in an extravagant fashion (Figure 1–1a). They used cosmetics as part of their personal beautification habits, for religious ceremonies, and in preparing the deceased for burial. One of the earliest uses of **henna** was as an adornment in ancient Egypt for body art and on fingernails. The Egyptians placed a similar amount of importance on the animals that surrounded them. Each animal of prominence had a corresponding god or goddess that was artfully mimicked from physical characteristics, grooming, and mummification. To the early Egyptian, cleanliness was a means of protection from evil as well as from diseases.

The Hebrews

The early Hebrews had a wealth of grooming and skin care techniques. Due to their nomadic history, they adopted many techniques from other cultures. Hebrew grooming rituals were based on the principle that their bodies were gifts to be cared for. Cosmetics were primarily used for cleansing and maintenance of the skin, hair, teeth, and overall bodily health.

The Hebrews used olive and grapeseed oils to moisten and protect the skin. They prepared ointment from hyssop (an aromatic plant originally found near the Black Sea and central Asia) for cleansing, and they used cinnamon balms to keep in body heat. Myrrh and pomegranate were the Hebrews' most useful grooming and health aids. Myrrh in powder form was used to repel fleas, and in tincture form it was used for oral hygiene. Pomegranate was used as an antiseptic and was helpful in expelling intestinal worms.

The Greeks

The words *cosmetics* and *cosmetology* come from the Greek word *kosmetikos* (kos-MET-i-kos), meaning "skilled in the use of cosmetics." In ancient Greece, beauty was determined by how one looked when naked. It was the naked Grecian athlete who defined the balance between mind and body. The Greeks viewed the body as a temple. They frequently bathed in olive oil and then dusted their bodies in fine sand to regulate their body temperature and to protect themselves from the sun. They were very aware of the effects of the natural elements on the body and the aging process. They used both honey and olive oil for elemental protection and were always in search of ways to improve their health and appearance. It was this drive for perfection that made the Greeks so prominent in advancing grooming and skin care (Figure 1–1b).

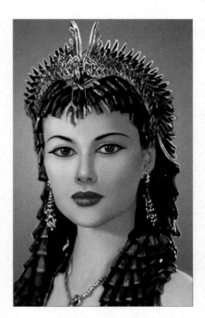

Figure 1–1a The Egyptians were the first to cultivate beauty in an extravagant fashion.

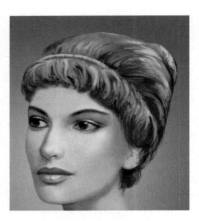

Figure 1–1b The Greeks were prominent in advancing grooming and skin care.

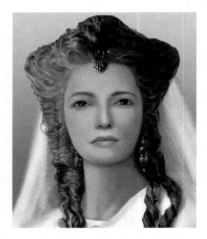

Figure 1–1c The Romans applied various preparations to the skin to maintain attractivness.

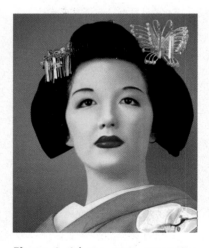

Figure 1–1d The geisha personifies the Japanese ideal of beauty.

The Romans

The ancient Romans are famous for their baths, which were magnificent public buildings with separate sections for men and women. Ruins of these baths survive to this day. Steam therapy, body scrubs, massage, and other physical therapies were all available at bathhouses. After bathing, Romans applied rich oils and other preparations to their skin to keep it healthy and attractive (Figure 1–1c). Fragrances made from flowers, saffron, almonds, and other ingredients were also part of bathing and grooming rituals.

The Asians

The Asians, like the Egyptians, blended nature, animal, and self into a sophisticated and elaborate culture that adhered to a high standard of grooming and appearance. Both the Chinese and Japanese cultures blended the edges of their natural scenery into their looks.

History also shows that during the Shang dynasty (1600 B.C.), Chinese aristocrats rubbed a tinted mixture of gum arabic, gelatin, beeswax, and egg whites onto their nails to turn them crimson or ebony.

The ancient geisha not only exemplified the ideal of beauty, she was also able to incorporate it into intricate rituals (Figure 1–1d). Geishas removed their body hair by a technique similar to what we call "threading" today—they wrapped a thread around each hair and plucked it out. From the tenth to the nineteenth centuries, blackened teeth were considered beautiful and appealing. It was common for both the married woman and the courtesan to black out their teeth with a paste made from sake, tea, and iron scraps.

The Africans

Traditional African medicine features diverse healing systems estimated to be about 4,000 years old. Since ancient times, Africans have created remedies and grooming aids from the materials found in their natural environment (Figure 1–1e). Even today in parts of North Africa, people use twigs from the mignonette tree as toothpicks. The twigs have an antiseptic quality and help prevent oral and tooth disease.

STYLE, SKIN CARE, AND GROOMING THROUGHOUT THE AGES

Style and personal grooming took many turns throughout history and reflected the mores of specific time periods. Beautification and adornment slowly moved away from the spiritual and the medicinal and began to reflect the popular culture of the day.

The Middle Ages

The Middle Ages is the period in European history between classical antiquity and the Renaissance. It began with the downfall of Rome in A.D. 476 and lasted until about 1450. During that time, religion played a prominent role in people's lives. Healing, particularly with herbs, was largely in the hands of the church. Beauty culture was also practiced. Tapestries, sculptures, and other artifacts from this period show towering headdresses,

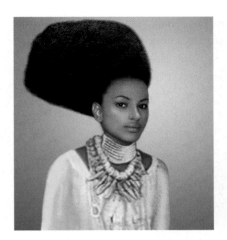

Figure 1–1e Africans created remedies and grooming aids from the materials found in their natural environment.

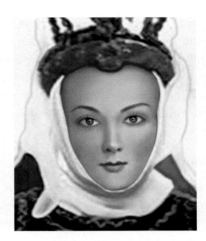

Figure 1–1f Tapestries, sculptures, and other artifacts from the Middle Ages show towering headdresses, intricate hairstyles, and the use of cosmetics on skin and hair.

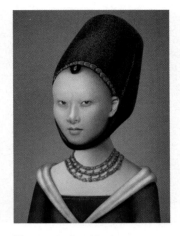

Figure 1–1g Shaving or tweezing the eyebrows and hairline to show a greater expanse of forehead was thought to make women appear more intelligent.

intricate hairstyles, and the use of cosmetics on skin and hair (Figure 1–1f). Women wore colored makeup on their cheeks and lips, but not on their eyes. Bathing was not a daily ritual, but those who could afford them used fragrant oils.

The Renaissance

During the Renaissance period, Western civilization made the transition from medieval to modern history. One of the most unusual practices was the shaving or tweezing of the eyebrows and the hairline to show a greater expanse of forehead—a bare brow was thought to give women a look of greater intelligence (Figure 1–1g). Fragrances and cosmetics were used, although highly colored preparations for lips, cheeks, and eyes were discouraged. The hair was carefully dressed and adorned with ornaments or headdresses. Many women used bleach to make their hair blond, which was a sign of beauty.

The Age of Extravagance

Marie Antoinette was queen of France from 1755 to 1793. This era was called the Age of Extravagance. Women of status bathed in strawberries and milk and used various extravagant cosmetic preparations, such as scented face powder made from pulverized starch (Figure 1–1h). Lips and cheeks were often brightly colored in pink and orange shades. Small silk patches were used to decorate the face and conceal blemishes. Some hairstyles extended high into the air, using elaborate wire cages with springs to adjust the height. The hairstyles might even contain gardens and menageries with live animals, which could attract lice and other parasites.

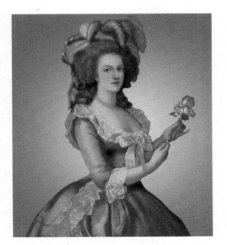

Figure 1–1h Women of status used various extravagant cosmetic preparations, such as scented face powder made from pulverized starch.

The Victorian Age

The Victorian Age spans the reign of Queen Victoria of England (1837–1901). Modesty was greatly valued, and makeup and showy clothing were discouraged

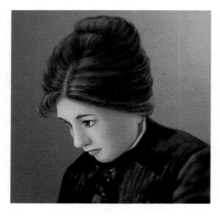

Figure 1–1i During the Victorian period, makeup and showy clothing were discouraged, except in the theater.

except in the theater (Figure 1–1i). Hairstyles were sleek and demure, often knotted in the back with hairpins. Men kept their hair short and grew sideburns, a mustache, and/or a beard. To preserve skin health and beauty, women used beauty masks and packs made from honey, eggs, milk, oatmeal, fruits, vegetables, and other natural ingredients. Victorian women are said to have pinched their cheeks and bitten their lips to induce natural color rather than use cosmetics such as lipstick and rouge.

Twentieth Century

The twentieth century brought about many changes in style, skin care, and innovation of the beauty culture. Each decade seemed to have an inherently different look, whereas in earlier history it may have taken a century to bring about a change (Figure 1–2). These changes were primarily due to greater

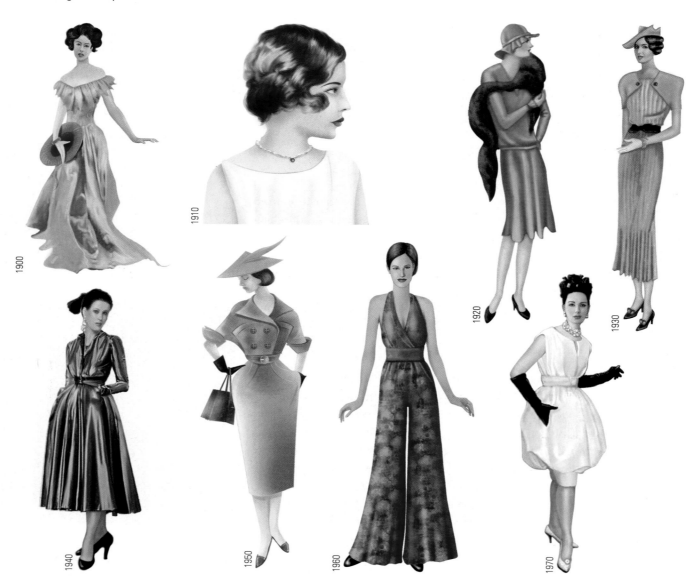

Figure 1–2 Beauty and fashion images through the decades.

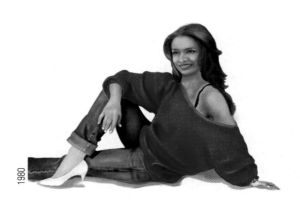

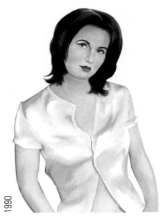

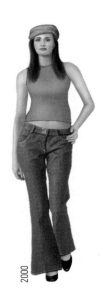

Figure 1–2 *(Continued.)*

exposure to other cultures, because more people were traveling, and to the industrialization of civilizations. Newspapers, magazines, radio, and motion pictures were important sources of information on fashions in the United States as well as in other countries. The twentieth century brought about Retin-A®, Botox®, alpha hydroxy acid, and a myriad of sought-after cosmetic surgery procedures.

Twenty-First Century

The beginning of the twenty-first century ushered in **nanotechnology,** the art of manipulating materials on an atomic or molecular scale—or the "micronization" of ingredients. By changing their chemistry and breaking them into smaller units, this technique has rejuvenated the older tried-and-true ingredients and created new ones. The future of skin health appears promising as researchers continually develop new products that will decrease adverse reactions to skin.

Today and Beyond

The birth of the medical spa has changed the skin care industry and has taken center stage to facilitate and support the cosmetic surgery phenomenon. Cosmetic surgery continues to be popular and has become a multibillion-dollar industry. According to the American Society for Aesthetic Plastic Surgery, in 2007, cosmetic procedures increased by 500 percent over those performed in the 1990s.

Customization is becoming even more important for the future. Professionals and consumers are looking for products made specifically for them. We will see more instruments being developed to create this customization, such as devices that will determine what the skin needs in the way of antioxidants, hydration, and protection.

Private Labeling and Branding

Private-label product lines have become important to many spas and medical spas (medi-spas). An esthetician can create a line as simple or as complex as desired, depending on the type of branding he or she chooses to promote sales.

Compounding Pharmacies

For estheticians working with and for physicians, skin care has a pharmaceutical component. Many compounding pharmacies have taken a market share of the cosmetic industry by offering more advanced preparations. These compounds may contain hormones such as estriol, for topical use, that are proven to demonstrate more substantial results than over-the-counter products do. These products, however, must be recommended and prescribed by a physician. A client or patient may have routine follow-up appointments to determine their tolerance levels for the product and be monitored for adverse effects.

New ingredients and therapies for wrinkles, skin cancer, and general skin health will continue to be developed. As the technology improves, these methods also will be less invasive, and will allow the client to spend less time away from her regular daily activities. Baby boomers will continue to retire and younger clients will take a lead in driving the market. The esthetician is well positioned to benefit from all of the future endeavors related to skin care development, technology, health, and fashion.

CAREER PATHS FOR AN ESTHETICIAN

Esthetics, from the Greek word *aesthetikos* (meaning "perceptible to the senses"), is a branch of anatomical science that deals with the overall health and well-being of the skin, the largest organ of the human body. An **esthetician** (or aesthetician) is a person devoted to, or professionally occupied with, skin health and beauty.

Estheticians provide preventive care for the skin and offer treatments to keep the skin healthy and attractive. They may also manufacture, sell, or apply cosmetics. They are trained to detect skin problems that may require medical attention. However, unless an esthetician is also a licensed dermatologist, physician, or physician's assistant, he or she cannot prescribe medication, make a diagnosis, or give medical treatments.

Esthetics is an exciting, ever-expanding field. Over the past few decades, it has evolved from a minor part of the beauty industry into an array of specialized services offered in elegant, full-service salons, day spas, and wellness centers. As a licensed esthetician, you can choose from a wide range of career options.

Salon or Day Spa Esthetician

Estheticians in a salon or day spa are skin care specialists and consultants. They perform facials and facial massage, waxing, and body treatments, applied both manually and with the aid of machines. They may also offer makeup. To be successful and build their clientele, estheticians must keep

---

? Did You Know

You will see the spelling of *esthetician* vary slightly depending on where you are working. In the medical realm, you will more often see the word spelled as *aesthetician* in reference to the original Greek word *aesthetikos*. Many cosmetic surgeons, nurses, and clinical estheticians prefer the original spelling. In recent history the initial letter *a* has been dropped in Western Europe and in the United States because the word *esthetician* relates more to the newer spa culture and has become a more modern term.

records of the services they provide and the products they use. They must always behave pleasantly toward clients, and they must become skillful at selling products.

Estheticians are employed in full-service salons, skin care salons, or day spas. These may be independent businesses or national chains, and they may operate within hotels or department stores.

As an esthetician, you can work your way up to management and supervisory positions. With the experience you gain in these positions, you may decide to open your own salon or buy an established business or franchise. Most private salon or franchise owners have multiple responsibilities. Besides running the business, you may perform any or all of the services your business offers; or, you may choose to limit your services to the areas of skin care and makeup.

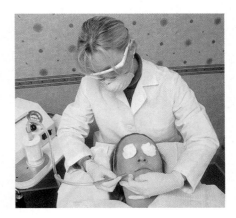

Figure 1–3 Microdermabrasion is a common treatment offered in a medical setting.

Medical Aesthetician

Medical aesthetics involves the integration of surgical procedures and esthetic treatments. In this setting, the physician concentrates on surgical work while the esthetician assists in esthetic treatments. Career opportunities are available in many different medical settings, where estheticians perform services ranging from working with pre- and postoperative patients to managing a skin care department in a medical spa. These tasks may involve patient education, marketing, buying and selling products, camouflage makeup, and—with a physician's supervision—performing advanced treatments including laser and light therapies (depending on state licensing rules). In addition, an experienced esthetician may manage the cosmetic surgery office or act as a patient care coordinator (Figures 1–3, 1–4, and 1–5). Some estheticians are also licensed practical nurses (LPNs) and registered nurses (RNs) or medical assistants. The settings for such work may include outpatient clinics, dermatology clinics, medical spas, laser clinics, and research and teaching hospitals.

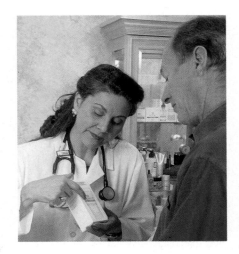

Figure 1–4 As an important part of treatment, dermatologists instruct patients on home care.

If you are interested in pursuing a career in medical aesthetics, you will want to learn not only basic skin care skills but also cosmetic chemistry, makeup and camouflage techniques, and business skills. A thorough understanding of skin anatomy, medical terminology, and skin disorders is also a must, as is the ability to communicate effectively and compassionately with clients. This type of work is very demanding, and it is important to be adaptable. Many rules and regulations must be observed and followed in a medical setting, and there is much at stake. You must be a good leader, but also be able to follow instructions explicitly. Teamwork is the number one priority in a medical organization.

Makeup Artist

A good makeup artist is skillful at highlighting a client's most attractive features and downplaying those that are less attractive. As a makeup artist, you must develop a keen eye for color and color coordination in order to select the most flattering cosmetics for each client. You may offer facials and facial massage as part of your services, or concentrate only on applying makeup.

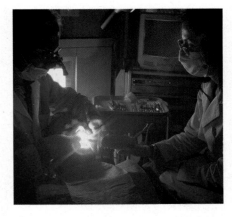

Figure 1–5 Depending on state licensing regulations, some estheticians may be trained as laser technicians.

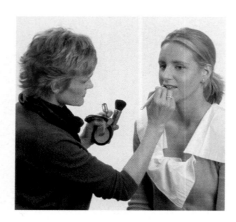

Figure 1–6 Makeup artists often work with models.

Makeup artists in salons, spas, and department stores work for an hourly wage, commission, or salary, or various combinations of all three.

- Commercial photographers often employ full- or part-time makeup artists. In fashion photography, a makeup artist works with models (Figure 1–6). Magazine and advertising layouts often require ultrafashionable hairstyles and makeup to call attention to products or clothing. The makeup artist may also be a photographer's assistant, helping with set designs or assisting with bridal photographs.

- Another exciting avenue for makeup artistry can be found in television, theater, movies, and fashion shows. In this highly competitive field, you may need a lengthy apprenticeship and acceptance into a union. Most major television and motion picture productions are shot on the East or West Coast, which may limit the number of jobs available. The same holds true for theatrical productions and large fashion shows. However, many cities and towns support community theater, and most large department stores produce fashion shows. In many cases, when full-time work as a makeup artist is not available, the position may be combined with other duties.

- A particularly rewarding field related to makeup artistry is camouflage therapy. Clients require this service for varying reasons: as a temporary measure while recovering from surgery, such as a face lift; to disguise a congenital defect; or to hide scars and other effects of an accident. The principles of standard makeup application also apply to camouflage makeup, particularly in terms of shading and blending. But working with clients desiring camouflage makeup also requires patience, compassion, a reassuring manner, and the ability to teach new techniques to an often traumatized individual.

- Another option for makeup artists is a career in mortuary science. Many people believe that viewing the deceased has a comforting psychological effect on the bereaved family and friends, and the custom is widely practiced. Training includes the study of restorative art, which is the preparation of the deceased. Restoration work requires a high degree of skill and must be performed under the direction of a mortician. In this career, the esthetician or cosmetologist works only on preparing and applying cosmetics.

Manufacturer's Representative

Manufacturers employ men and women to demonstrate to potential customers how to use the company's products. Representatives call on salons, drugstores, department stores, and specialty businesses to help build clientele and increase product sales. For this position, you must have a professional appearance, an outgoing personality, and sales ability. You can expect to travel a great deal, and you will often exhibit products at trade shows and conventions.

Salesperson or Sales Manager

Salons, spas, department stores, boutiques, and specialty businesses employ estheticians as salespersons and sales managers, who often work their way up to top management positions and ownership. As a salesperson, your duties would include keeping records of sales and stock on hand, demonstrating products, selling to clients, and cashiering (Figure 1–7). You must thoroughly know the products you sell and be able to help clients select cosmetics that suit their skin types and colors. Salespeople do not have to be licensed estheticians, but smart companies hire them because they are well trained to present cosmetics to the public, are polished in appearance, and are specialists in the art and science of skin care.

Cosmetics Buyer

A cosmetics buyer in department stores, salons, or specialty businesses must keep up with the latest products and trends in skin care. Buyers travel frequently, visiting markets, trade shows, and manufacturers' showrooms. As a buyer, you must estimate the amount of stock your operation will need over a particular period, and you must keep records of purchases and sales.

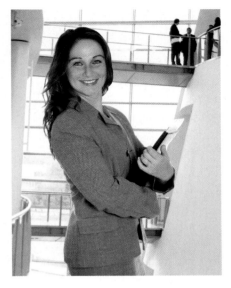

Figure 1–7 An esthetician can pursue a successful career in sales.

Esthetics Writer or Editor

If you have talent and training in journalism, you may wish to pursue a career as an esthetics writer or editor for a magazine or newspaper (Figure 1–8). Journalists in this field write feature articles, daily or weekly columns, and "question and answer" columns. Some also review new products, medical breakthroughs, and salon techniques. Writers produce educational books and brochures for the esthetics and cosmetology market, do fashion coordination and commentary, and make media appearances.

Cosmetics and skin care products are heavily advertised on television and radio and in magazines and newspapers. Copywriters design ads and commercials and write the information enclosed in packages and printed on labels. They often work with photographers and television producers to create commercial messages. Some are involved in producing the audiovisual programs used in classrooms to educate the consumer.

Travel Industry

Many cruise ships, airlines, and airport organizations are employing estheticians to work and manage esthetic departments. Airports today have licensed massage therapists as well as estheticians and manicurists to serve the traveling public. In addition, some private airline companies may employ estheticians to travel along to meet the needs of special clients with esthetics services. Cruise ship companies have mirrored the practices of land-based spa owners to keep up with demand for esthetic services onboard.

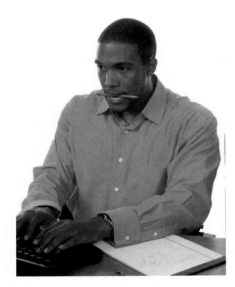

Figure 1–8 A writer with a background in esthetics can write for magazines, newspapers, television, or book publishers.

Educator

If you want to teach esthetics in a public, vocational, industrial, or technical high school, you must meet the same requirements as other teachers of career preparation courses. You must be trained in curriculum and lesson planning, classroom management, and presentation techniques. If you are

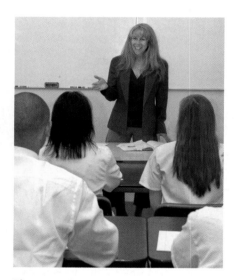

Figure 1–9 Some estheticians become instructors.

interested in heading a department of esthetics or cosmetology in a public or private school, you will need supervisory skills as well as the necessary certification.

Many private cosmetology or esthetics schools have teacher training programs for promising graduates (Figure 1–9). Some states require a teacher to train in teaching all subjects. Others require teachers to specialize in one area, such as skin care, makeup styling, theatrical makeup, or hair removal. Some basic teacher training courses are also generally required. As an instructor, you must keep up with developments in the education field as well as in beauty products and skin care techniques. Many teachers attend workshops and conferences to stay abreast of industry changes and trends.

Many private school owners and directors begin their careers as general practitioners. The director of a school or a department within a school has many duties, including preparing the curriculum and ensuring that the school's physical layout and equipment meet state standards. The director works closely with teachers, counsels students about licensing and placement, and maintains relationships with trade organizations and industry experts.

To be a successful teacher, supervisor, director, or school owner requires a good sense of commercial operations, a thorough knowledge of the business, and the ability to direct people and get along with them. Professionals in education dedicate themselves to improving the beauty industry by working together in associations at the national, state, and local level. They help establish, amend, and repeal state laws and regulations, improve and standardize curriculums, and ensure the professionalism of the entire industry.

Manufacturers of cosmetics and other products frequently employ licensed cosmetologists and estheticians as education directors. These professionals educate the public about the manufacturer's products and conduct seminars for teachers of consumer education. As part of the manufacturer's consumer education program, education directors appear at conventions to display products, talk with teachers about the merits of the products, and distribute educational materials for classroom use. Education directors may also be workshop or seminar leaders, lecturers, and/or writers.

State Licensing Inspector or Examiner

Most states have laws governing cosmetology and other personal services and give examinations for cosmetology and related licenses. As a licensed, experienced cosmetologist and/or esthetician, you may become a state inspector or examiner. Inspectors conduct regular salon and spa inspections to ensure that managers and employees are following state rules and regulations and meeting ethical standards. State examiners prepare and conduct examinations, enforce rules and regulations, investigate complaints, and conduct hearings.

State Board Member

Members of state licensing organizations must be highly qualified and experienced in their professions. They conduct examinations, grant licenses, and inspect schools to see that certain physical standards, such as those for space and equipment, are maintained. In addition, they make sure that educational materials meet certain specifications. The chairperson of the state board is usually a full-time employee, but other members may be school owners or people in related professions.

Researcher

Manufacturers are constantly competing with one another to produce safer and more effective consumer products. Research directors or assistants run laboratory tests (often on animals) to determine product safety before the company distributes them (Figure 1–10). Sometimes products are tested on volunteers to check for allergic reactions. Researchers may also conduct consumer surveys. For an esthetician with a science background, opportunities in this field are usually plentiful. Some positions require advanced scientific training in chemistry, physics, biology, and other subjects, but others offer on-the-job training.

A BRIGHT FUTURE

The future for esthetics is promising; experts predict that the skin care and medical industries will continue to work closely together to create products and treatments that promote dramatically younger-looking skin. Skin care products will be more potent, will contain both medical and natural ingredients, and will be available in more efficient delivery systems that penetrate deeper into the skin. More skin treatments will be targeted at menopausal women, and skin care in general will involve more preventive than corrective measures. Gene therapies—even skin transplants for wrinkled skin—are on the horizon as well.

All these trends bode well for the esthetician. The average life span of people in the United States has almost doubled since 1900. Life has become more fast-paced and stressful for most Americans, and environmental assaults on the skin have increased. These factors enhance the value of an esthetician's services, particularly to consumers who are more knowledgeable and more affluent than in previous generations. As skin care becomes more scientific and results more dramatic, consumers will consider spa and salon services a necessity rather than a luxury. The U.S. Department of Labor predicts the rapid growth of full-service day spas and a growing demand for practitioners licensed to provide a broad range of services.

There will be plenty of opportunities for estheticians in newer settings such as lifestyle and retirement centers. Whole communities are being designed for the baby boomers, who have grown accustomed to having these esthetic services. We are also seeing a multidisciplinary approach to medicine and a further blending of subspecialties such as esthetics, massage, wellness, and women's fitness centers that may be partnered with an OB-GYN facility, for example. Cosmetic dentists are partnering with cosmetic surgeons. Teaching hospitals that run clinical studies in human potential will also have medical spas and fitness centers to enhance the benefits of these studies. We will see more estheticians as independent practitioners

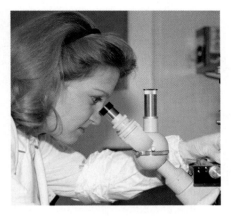

Figure 1–10 Research leads to scientific breakthroughs in skin care.

?   **Did You Know**

Look Good . . . Feel Better (LGFB) is a free public service program that teaches beauty techniques to women with cancer, helping them boost their self-image and camouflage their hair loss. The program is open to all women cancer patients actively undergoing treatment for cancer. Each year, approximately 30,000 women participate in LGFB group sessions, and more than 200,000 women have been served by the organization since it was founded in 1989.

Look Good . . . Feel Better

800-395-LOOK, 800-395-5665

http://www.lookgoodfeelbetter.org

WEB RESOURCES

For more information about the esthetics profession, visit these Web sites:

http://www.lookgoodfeelbetter.org

http://www.ncea.tv

http://www.dol.gov

http://www.cosmeticplasticsurgerystatistics.com

http://www.themakeupgallery.info

http://beauty.about.com

who make home, office, and hotel visits. Clinical esthetics will quite possibly become a subspecialty of dermatology, requiring a separate licensure altogether.

This is a time of revolutionary changes in what we know about the skin and the ways we care for it. Keeping the skin healthy and youthful looking for decades is no longer just a fantasy. As an esthetician, you are part of an exciting, rewarding, and well-respected profession that will only grow in importance and earning power in the years ahead. If you can dream of your ideal career, it is there waiting for you.

REVIEW QUESTIONS

1. Name some of the materials that ancient people used as color pigments in cosmetics.

2. What did the ancient Hebrews use to keep their skin healthy and moist?

3. The word *cosmetics* comes from what Greek word? What does it mean?

4. In ancient Rome, what body rituals were provided by bathhouses for patrons?

5. Describe the facial masks women used during the Victorian Age.

6. Which important cosmetic products were introduced in the late twentieth century?

7. What career options are available to estheticians in salons and day spas?

8. What is medical aesthetics? In what ways can estheticians practice their skills in a medical setting?

9. Describe the different environments in which makeup artists can be employed.

10. What are the duties of a manufacturer's representative? Of a cosmetics buyer?

11. Discuss the employment options open to an esthetics educator.

12. Describe the growth of esthetics from its beginnings as a component of cosmetology to its current status as a distinct, specialized profession.

CHAPTER GLOSSARY

esthetician (or aesthetician): person devoted to, or professionally occupied with, skin health and beauty.

esthetics (or aesthetics): branch of anatomical science that deals with the overall health and well-being of the skin, the largest organ of the human body; from the Greek word *aesthetikos,* meaning "perceptible to the senses."

henna: dye obtained from the powdered leaves and shoots of the mignonette tree; used as a reddish hair dye and in tattooing.

medical aesthetics: integration of surgical procedures and esthetic treatments.

nanotechnology: manipulation of materials on an atomic or molecular scale, or the "micronization" of ingredients.

YOUR PROFESSIONAL IMAGE

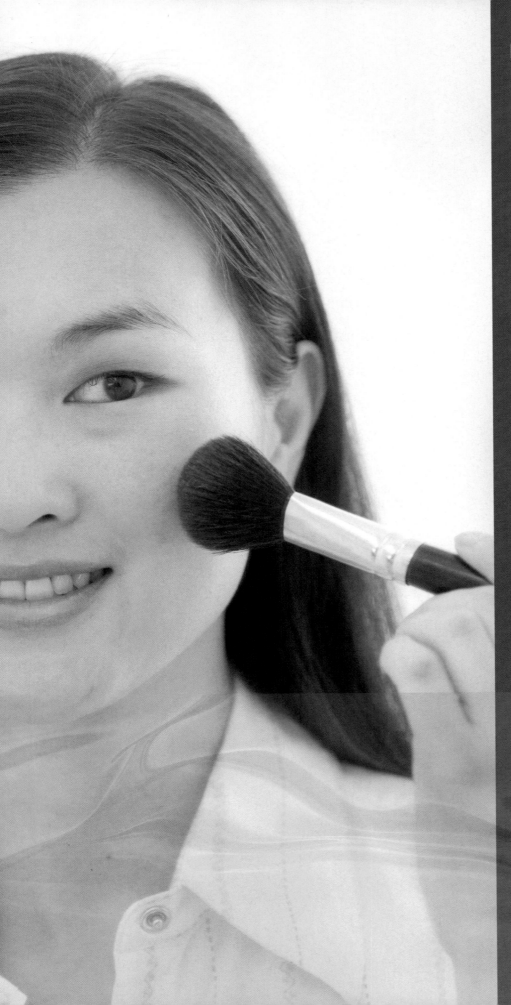

LEARNING OBJECTIVES

After completing this chapter, you will be able to:

- List the basic habits of daily personal hygiene.

- Demonstrate proper standing and sitting posture.

- List the characteristics of a healthy, positive attitude.

- Explain the attributes of a strong work ethic.

- Define ethics.

- List the most effective time management techniques.

Because you are in the image business, how you look and present yourself has a big influence on whether you will be successful working in your chosen career path within the field of esthetics. If you are talking style, then you need to look stylish; if you are advising your clients about makeup, then your makeup must be current and beautifully applied. If you are recommending skin care services, it is critical that your own skin be well cared for. When your appearance and the way that you conduct yourself are in harmony with the beauty business, your chances of being successful in any area of cosmetology increase by as much as 100 percent! After all, when you look great, your clients will assume that you can make them look great, too.

BEAUTY AND WELLNESS

Your **professional image** is the impression you project as a person engaged in the profession of esthetics (Figure 2–1). It consists of your outward appearance and the conduct you exhibit in the workplace. This image is extremely important. Your appearance, attitude, abilities, and energy create a mental picture in the minds of your clients and associates. You want that image to earn their respect, trust, and eagerness for your knowledge.

Your professional image is also tied to your role as a model for your clients. You not only help your clients look their best but also alert them to lifestyle decisions that can affect their beauty and health. That means you will need to look your best and make lifestyle choices that express your commitment to your own well-being. If you do not look good, your clients may assume that you cannot make *them* look good.

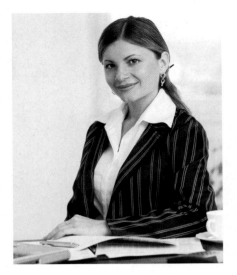

Figure 2–1 Project a professional image at all times.

Personal Hygiene

Personal hygiene is the daily maintenance of cleanliness and healthfulness through certain sanitary practices. The basics of personal hygiene include

- daily bathing or showering, shaving for men, and freshening up throughout the day as necessary.
- shampooing and conditioning your hair as required to keep it fresh and clean.
- following a regular skin care regimen.
- brushing and flossing your teeth, as well as using a mouthwash or breath mints throughout the day as needed.
- using underarm deodorant or antiperspirant.
- washing your hands throughout the day as required, such as when beginning and ending a service or after visiting the bathroom.
- be selective about wearing fragrances at work, because many people are allergic to them.

Nail care is particularly important for estheticians. Keep both fingernails and toenails clean, trimmed, and filed (Figure 2–2). Nails that are too long or pointed can scratch your client's skin or interfere with your work. Be meticulous about your manicure and pedicure. Take care of hangnails immediately. Keep your hands and feet well moisturized.

LOOKING GOOD

As a skin care specialist, your poised and attractive appearance will ensure that your clients think of you as a professional. Many salon and spa managers consider appearance and poise to be just as important for success as technical knowledge and skills. So it is a good idea to establish habits of good health and grooming from the start.

Creating Balance

Real beauty begins with health and stays grounded in health. Good health greatly affects your energy level, your attitude, and, ultimately, your appearance. One of the most important factors in promoting and maintaining health is balance.

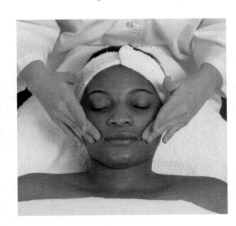

Figure 2–2 An esthetician's nails must be trimmed and filed smooth.

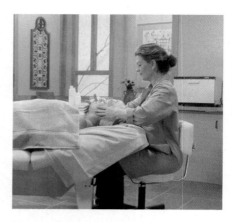

Figure 2–3 Clothing should be clean, functional and comfortable.

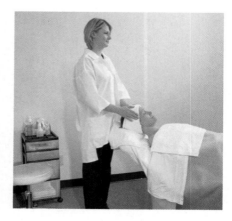

Figure 2–4 Good standing posture can help prevent back strain and other problems.

Balance can be hard to achieve in the fast pace of modern life. For many of us, it can be a challenge to manage stress. Being in balance enables us to make the right choices for ourselves. If you consistently undermine your well-being with poor choices, you may be putting yourself at risk for disease. Achieving balance is crucial to leading a healthy, productive life. You can help create balance by eating a nutritious diet, exercising regularly, getting adequate rest and recreation, and avoiding such habits as smoking, drinking excessively, and taking drugs.

Dress for Success

At the salon, strive to have your hair, makeup, and clothing express a professional image that is consistent with the image of the salon. You should always comply with the dress code, but the following guidelines are generally appropriate:

- Clothing should be clean and fresh. Uniforms should be comfortable and provide good mobility, especially in the shoulder and elbow areas, but should not be too loose fitting (Figure 2–3).
- Wear clean undergarments every day, and keep them out of view. Underwear elastic peeking out of your pants or exposed bra straps as well as cleavage exposure and a bare midriff are inconsistent with a professional image.
- Hair should be up and off the shoulders.
- Socks or hosiery should be free of runs and harmonize with your attire.
- Keep shoes clean and comfortable, with good support.
- A clean, natural approach is generally best when applying makeup.
- Dangling jewelry is inappropriate, and it is hazardous to your clients.

YOUR PHYSICAL PRESENTATION

Another important aspect of your professional image is **physical presentation.** To a large degree, your physical presentation is made up of your posture, walk, and movements. It can enhance or detract from your attractiveness and is an important part of your well-being. Unhealthy or defective body postures can cause a number of physical problems, particularly when these postures become a habit.

Posture

Good posture conveys an image of confidence and can prevent fatigue and other physical problems. As an esthetician, you will spend a lot of time on your feet, and good posture will be essential to getting you through the day.

Standing Posture

Here are some guidelines for achieving and maintaining good standing posture (follow Figure 2–4).

- Keep the neck elongated and balanced directly above the shoulders.
- Lift your upper body so that your chest is out and up (do not slouch).
- Hold your shoulders level and relaxed, not scrunched up.

- Keep your back straight.
- Pull your abdomen in so that it is flat.
- Flex your knees slightly and position them over your feet.

Sitting Posture

Guidelines for a proper sitting position (Figure 2–5) include

- keeping your back straight.
- keeping the soles of your feet entirely on the floor.
- not crossing your legs or your feet at the ankles.
- not bending forward from the waist or stooping forward from the shoulders. (Bend from the hips, or sit on a chair or wedge-shaped cushion that tilts forward.)

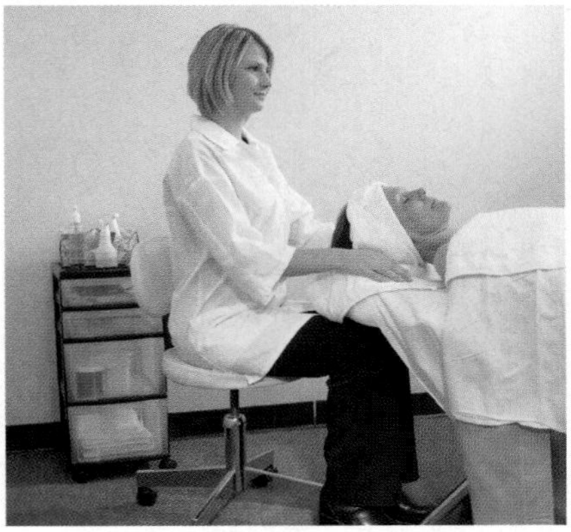

Figure 2–5 Proper body alignment while sitting is important for an esthetician.

PROFESSIONAL CONDUCT

In addition to your appearance, your professional image consists of your conduct in the workplace—how you get along with your clients, coworkers, and your employer. Your conduct, in turn, is affected by a number of related factors.

Attitude

Attitude can be defined as your outlook, and it underlies the way you live your life. Attitude stems from what you believe and can be influenced by your parents, teachers, friends, and even books and movies. You may not be able to change a characteristic that you were born with, but you can change your attitude.

In business and in your personal life, a pleasing attitude will gain you more associates, clients, and friends. Here are some ingredients of a healthy, well-developed attitude.

- *Diplomacy.* Be tactful in your dealings with others. This means being straightforward, but not critical.
- *Emotional stability.* It is essential to have feelings and express them appropriately. Self-control—learning how to handle a confrontation as well as letting people know how you feel without going overboard—is an important indicator of maturity.
- *Receptivity.* To be receptive means being interested in other people and being responsive to their opinions, feelings, and ideas. Receptivity involves taking the time to really listen instead of pretending to do so.
- *Sensitivity.* Your personality shines when you show concern for the feelings of others. Sensitivity is a combination of understanding, empathy, and acceptance. A sensitive person is aware of how damaging criticism can be and always offers criticisms constructively. Being sensitive does not mean you have to let people take advantage of you; it means being compassionate and responsive. It is strength, not weakness.
- *Values and goals.* Neither values nor goals are inborn characteristics. You acquire these as you move through life. It is important that you do acquire them, however, because they guide you on your journey through the world.

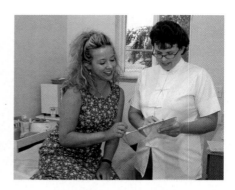

Figure 2–6 Communicating during a client consultation should be a two-way street.

- *Communication skills.* Communication is your way of ensuring that you understand the needs and desires of the people around you. And because communication is a two-way street, it ensures that your clients will understand your ideas and suggestions as well (Figure 2–6). Clients can go virtually anywhere and get good service, but they stay with estheticians who create the best atmosphere, treat them with respect, and have good interpersonal skills.
- *Discretion and confidentiality.* Do not share your personal problems with your clients or tell other people the concerns they may have shared with you.
- *Maintain boundaries.* Have a one-minute rule on sharing information about yourself. Remember the appointment is about the client and her skin, and you are an esthetician, not a counselor.

Work Ethic

We all want to be valued for the contributions we make. In today's competitive market, most employers are looking for people who are loyal and committed to doing a good job. But it takes more than getting up in the morning and showing up at work to earn that respect. Establishing a good work ethic requires that you be thoughtful about how you approach each day, how you treat others, and how you support your employer's needs. A willingness to give the best of yourself, accept constructive criticism, grow and learn from your mistakes, and adapt to changes in the workplace demonstrates a positive attitude that will get you off to a good start. A good work ethic includes being trustworthy, reliable, hardworking, respectful, and supportive of others.

Teamwork

Today's spa environment can be hectic and fast-paced. To maintain a stress-free and productive environment, every staff member must be focused on working cooperatively. Teamwork is essential to developing a positive work ethic in a salon environment. Staff members need to know they can rely on each other for help and support. When each person pulls their own weight and is dedicated to sharing responsibility, stress is alleviated and common goals are achieved.

Team members who are equally invested in providing quality service in a relaxing, supportive, and nurturing environment are also better able to encourage one another to do the best job possible. The result is a caring and respectful work environment where everyone can be successful.

Resolving Conflict

As long as we are working with people, there will always be those who appear more difficult. While they do present a challenge, you need to remember that you are in a professional setting, and your standards for dealing with others must be high. Difficult clients are still a source of income, and difficult coworkers may not go away. Learn to view them as an opportunity to practice positive communication skills.

FOCUS ON . . .

THE WHOLE PERSON

Some say that attitude is everything and that, with a winning attitude, you cannot miss being a success. So ask yourself: "Am I a winner?" "Do I have faith in my success?" "Do I get along with others?" If you can answer yes, then you may be able to create the life you want. If the answer is no, then you have more work to do on the attitude front. This is a process that continues throughout your life.

To be successful, you will need to develop coping mechanisms that encourage cooperation when conflicts arise. Consider the following techniques:

* Count to 10 and think before you speak.
* Distance yourself from a situation to regain your composure.
* Avoid engaging in a no-win situation or argument.
* Get another opinion before making a judgment.
* Be assertive and stand your ground.
* Direct a situation to a higher authority if necessary.
* Take the high road and refrain from criticizing.
* Help others meet their goals by assuming more responsibility (Figure 2–7).

Whatever circumstances you are forced to deal with, trust that you have the power to make positive choices. Ultimately, if you are invested in working cooperatively with others and practice good communication techniques, the potential for conflict is decreased.

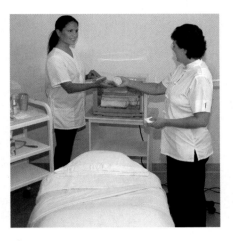

Figure 2–7 Pitching in wherever help is needed is part of being a team player.

PROFESSIONAL ETHICS

Ethics are the principles of good character, proper conduct, and moral judgment expressed through personality, human relations skills, and professional image. In other words, ethics are the moral principles by which we live and work. In different professions, codes of ethics are classified by boards or commissions. In cosmetology, for example, each state board sets the ethical standards that must be followed by all estheticians who work in that state.

Estheticians are expected to be knowledgeable about skin care. They are trained to perform specialized services and to advise and educate clients on products and techniques. To do this well, they must maintain competency, act responsibly, protect client confidentiality, avoid exploitation, and demonstrate exemplary conduct.

Obtaining the appropriate state license or certificate to practice esthetics is the first step in establishing credibility (Figure 2–8). Adhere to the regulations and guidelines of your license. Each state may vary in what an esthetician may or may not do in that state. But estheticians should also be aware of the Food and Drug Administration (FDA) and other government agencies whose

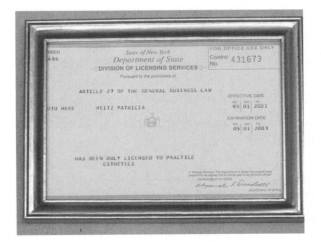

Figure 2–8 A license establishes that the esthetician is a qualified practitioner.

? Did You Know

When you smile, a number of physiological changes take place. Laughter can rev up your immune system, lower your blood pressure, and help you sleep better. Laughing is good for the soul, whether at work or at play.

? Did You Know

The National Coalition of Estheticians, Manufacturers/Distributors & Associations (NCEA) is an organization that was developed to support estheticians and the public in which they serve. Here is their mission statement:

> The mission of the NCEA is to represent the esthetic profession by defining and conveying standards of practice, while educating the industry and the public.

The code of ethics as printed by the NCEA is as follows:

CLIENT RELATIONSHIPS

- Estheticians* will serve the best interests of their clients at all times and will provide the highest quality service possible.

- Estheticians will provide clients with clear and realistic goals and outcomes and will not make false claims regarding the potential benefits of the techniques rendered or products recommended.

- Estheticians will adhere to the scope of practice of their profession and refer clients to the appropriate qualified health practitioner when indicated.

SCOPE OF PRACTICE

- Estheticians will offer services only within the scope of practice as defined by the state within which they operate, if required, and in adherence with appropriate federal laws and regulations.

- Estheticians will not utilize any technique/procedure for which they have not had adequate training and shall represent their education, training, qualifications and abilities honestly.

- Estheticians will strictly adhere to all usage instructions and guidelines provided by product and equipment manufacturers provided those guidelines and instructions are within the scope of practice as defined by the state, if required.

PROFESSIONALISM

- Estheticians will commit themselves to ongoing education and to provide clients and the public with the most accurate information possible.

- Estheticians will dress in attire consistent with professional practice and adhere to the Code of Conduct of their governing board.

*For the purpose of the NCEA Code of Ethics, the use of the term Esthetician applies to all licensed skin care professionals as defined by their state law.

All information printed with permission of NCEA.

function is to protect the consumer. Many regulations are in place to prevent the public from being duped by false claims and advertising.

As skin care professionals, we can all appreciate the consumer who is wary of purchasing "snake oil" or the ever-present "miracle in a jar." So how can we gain the public's trust? Here are some general guidelines that will help you maintain credibility and build confidence.

- Obtain the necessary credentials to practice in your state.
- Join and participate in professional organizations that take an unbiased approach to esthetics.
- Maintain your integrity by making sure your behavior and actions match your values. For example, if you believe it is unethical to sell products just to turn a profit, then do not do so. However, if you believe a client needs products and additional services for healthy skin maintenance, it would be unethical not to give the client that information. A sense of integrity also involves not making derogatory comments about other practitioners, not "stealing" clients, and not borrowing someone else's supplies. It does include endorsing your employer's price structure and other policies.
- Know your boundaries. Do only what you are trained to do. Do not offer advice or make recommendations outside of your area of expertise. This means understanding when to decline a service or opinion and refer the client to the appropriate professional.
- Keep client relationships professionally friendly. Clients often confide very personal information. Practice respectful listening, maintain professional boundaries, and do not gossip. Do not give advice or share personal information.

? Did You Know

In a medical setting, including skin care clinics and medical spas, federal privacy standards to protect clients and patients' medical records and health information has been enacted in the United States. The Department of Health and Human Services (HHS) developed the Health Insurance Portability Accountability Act (HIPAA) to protect individuals with regard to obtaining information about their health in a medical setting. But the act also states that all communication that takes place in a medical setting must be kept confidential. This means that clients or patients visiting a medical spa or clinical skin care setting can file formal complaints about practitioners engaging in a breach of confidentiality. Estheticians can be held liable for sharing information with others about clients or patients. The bottom line is, information shared about a client in the office is on a need-to-know basis as it pertains to properly treating a client. Do not gossip about clients with other estheticians or with other clients. For more information, visit http://www.hhs.gov/ocr/hipaa.

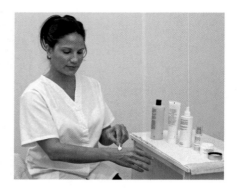

Figure 2–9 Always try products yourself before recommending them to others.

- Be honest and truthful. Do not make false claims about products and techniques. When you do not have the answer, simply say, "I don't know, but I'll find out for you."
- Do not rely on promotional literature by manufacturers to ensure a product's efficacy. Conduct your own research, particularly on controversial methods or ingredients, by having the staff try the products before you make claims about them (Figure 2–9). Also, it is fine to tell a client that a product is new in the office, and that you are trying it out. Make sure you can stand behind the products you use or recommend.
- Be open to seeking consultation from more experienced colleagues or other professionals.
- Keep informed. Attend as many continuing education seminars as you can (but recognize that one workshop does not make you an expert). Subscribe to professional trade publications, and read as much as possible.

LIFE SKILLS

All the technical skills you are now acquiring in school are vastly important. But the way you handle yourself and behave toward others will ultimately determine whether you can attain—and sustain—success. Even the best technical skills must rest on a solid foundation of life skills, which are tools and guidelines that prepare you for living as a mature adult in a complicated world. Acquiring life skills empowers you. Keeping an open mind and learning as much as you can about who you are will help you soar beyond your original dreams. Becoming a lifelong learner will keep you fresh, motivated, and engaged in your life and in the lives of those around you.

Be prepared to reinvent yourself from time to time. It is important to develop from the inside out. Take classes on interpersonal skills and communication. Seek out new friends who are on a path of personal growth, and meet regularly to share new and exciting information about what you are learning. Let people see you in new and different ways.

Guidelines for Success

Defining *success* is a very personal matter. Some basic principles, however, form the foundation of personal and professional success. You can begin your journey to success right now by examining and putting into practice these principles.

- *Build self-esteem.* Self-esteem is based on inner strength and begins with trusting your ability to reach your goals.
- *Visualize your success.* Imagine a movie screen. Picture yourself on this screen as a person of confidence, competence, and maturity. See yourself as well dressed and professional. The more you visualize, the more easily you can turn the possibilities in your life into realities.

- *Build on your strengths.* Practice doing whatever helps you maintain a positive self-image—playing the piano or cooking, for example (Figure 2–10). The things you are good at do not have to be things you can see. You could be good at helping someone less fortunate than yourself, or being a caring friend.
- *Be kind to yourself.* Put a stop to self-critical and negative thoughts that can work against you. If you make a mistake, tell yourself that it is okay and you will do your best next time.
- *Define success for yourself.* Do not depend on other people's definitions. What is right for your father, your sister, or your best friend may not be right for you.
- *Practice new behaviors.* Because creating success is a skill, you can help to develop it by practicing new behaviors such as speaking with confidence, standing tall, and using good grammar when you speak.
- *Keep your personal life separate from your work.* People who talk about themselves or others at work lower morale and make the whole team suffer.
- *Keep your energy up.* Get enough rest. Pace yourself. Success means having a clear head, a fit body, and the ability to refuel and recharge.
- *Respect others.* Use good manners. Avoid interrupting. Do not discuss your personal life with a neighboring coworker, even if you think clients cannot hear you. (They can and do.) As your awareness grows, this kind of respect will become a way of life. When you treat people well, they will respect you, and their respect helps build your self-esteem.
- *Stay productive.* Work on eliminating any bad habits that can keep you from maintaining peak performance: procrastination, perfectionism, and the lack of a career plan.

Setting Goals

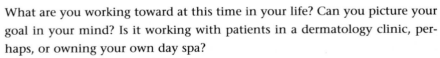

What are you working toward at this time in your life? Can you picture your goal in your mind? Is it working with patients in a dermatology clinic, perhaps, or owning your own day spa?

There are two types of goals: short term and long term. Examples of short-term goals are to get through a midterm exam successfully, or to finish your esthetics course. Short-term goals are usually those you wish to accomplish within a year at the most. Long-term goals, however, are measured in larger sections of time, such as 2 years, 5 years, 10 years, or even longer. Examples of long-term goals are owning your own salon, or doing the research to write a book on skin care.

The important thing is to have a plan and reexamine it often to make sure you are staying on track. The most successful professionals continue to set goals for themselves even after they have accumulated fame, fortune, and respect. They adjust their goals and action plans as they go along, but never forget that their goals are what keep them going (Figure 2–11).

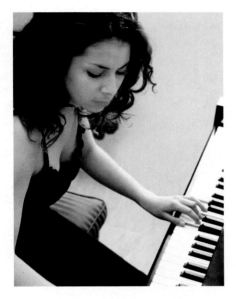

Figure 2–10 Spending time on the things you do well builds self-esteem.

FOCUS ON . . .

THE WHOLE PERSON

Invest in yourself by coming up with a game plan, the conscious act of planning your life instead of just letting things happen. You may think it is easier to just coast along from day to day, but the road to success is best reached with a clear plan that will lead you where you want to go. Begin by asking where you want to be in 10 years, or 10 months, or 10 days. What kind of resources and training will you need to get there? It may seem harder at first to approach life in this way, but you will find it brings greater rewards. Winners are people who decide what they want to do, set a goal, and stick to it. *Remember you are a winner.*

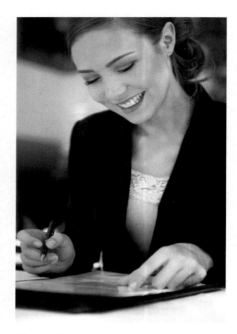

Figure 2–11 Write out a plan to help you reach your goals.

Time Management

Time management is essential to living a healthy life. We need time for rest, time to exercise, time to eat, time to play, time to work, and time to spend with friends and family. If we are able to manage our time carefully, we can live more fulfilling lives and actually contribute more to the lives of others. Some ideas for managing your time as efficiently as you can are as follows:

* Learn to prioritize. Make a list of tasks that need to be done in the order of most to least important. To-do lists for the day or week are very helpful (Figure 2–12).
* Never take on more than you can handle. Learn to say no firmly but kindly, and mean it. You will find it easier to complete your tasks if you limit your activities and do not spread yourself too thin.
* Learn problem-solving techniques, and use them.
* Give yourself a time-out whenever you are frustrated, overwhelmed, irritated, worried, or feeling guilty about something. Brooding loses you valuable time and energy.
* Plan to make dates with friends and family members; doing so makes us more well rounded and provides a solid support structure.
* Reward yourself with a special treat for work well done and time managed efficiently.
* Exercise to stimulate clear thinking and planning.
* Make time management a habit.
* Develop your own personal mission statement. This can help you stay on track, and it is useful to determine whether a project or job is good for you.

Time Management in Esthetics

Being on time is a large part of being professional. We would not stay in practice very long if we were unable to be on time, and balance that time with each client wisely. On the job, punctuality is a professional responsibility. Time is money. If you cannot perform a certain number of services or allow enough time to maximize your results, you will quickly fall behind in your monetary goals. To achieve long-term financial success and client satisfaction, you must carefully plan each day.

You must have a solid understanding of how long each treatment will take as well as a method for maintaining an organized approach. If you are just starting out, this means practicing each treatment until timing becomes second nature. Most facials require at least one hour to perform. When combined with additional consultation and retail responsibilities, the average treatment time generally totals about 1 hour and 15 minutes.

Getting used to working within these parameters requires training and discipline. Probably the most helpful advice you will receive as an esthetician is "Be prepared." The following guidelines will help you do that.

1. At the end of the day, begin organizing for the next day. Clean and organize your treatment room, and replenish supplies as needed.
2. Pull each scheduled client's record and review the last treatment. Decide on *possible* treatment procedures based on previous notations. Make sure all necessary equipment is sanitized and ready for use.

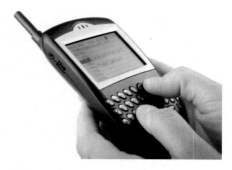

Figure 2–12 Organize your to-do-list for the day, weekly, as well as monthly.

3. Note any special considerations. Depending upon your employer's policy, ask a new client to arrive 10 minutes early to fill out a client intake form. While the client is changing, review the history.

4. For clients with special needs, know that you may need to spend more time with them, so ensure adequate scheduling.

5. Look at the retail products the client is using, and have them available. Leave enough time to review progress on home care or to recommend a program if the client is new.

6. Build time into your schedule for making important follow-up or sales calls.

7. Make time for lunch and a few minutes to visit with a friend or coworker to enjoy your day.

We live in a fast-paced world. An important part of your work that should not be overlooked is the added benefit of relaxation that most clients expect. If you are rushed, your clients will not be able to relax and fully enjoy the treatment. By taking time to prepare in advance, you can give your clients your undivided attention. Develop a method to appear relaxed and calm, and it will help you to be so. This is probably the best way to demonstrate your professionalism.

FOCUS ON . . .

THE GOAL

Make this commitment to yourself: I have taken my first steps on my journey to success. I have given myself the courage to enroll in school. By taking this step, I have made the conscious decision that I want more from my life for myself and for those for whom I am responsible. This decision will allow me to accomplish my dreams.

REVIEW QUESTIONS

1. Define the term *professional image*.

2. How does balance relate to good health?

3. List the basic habits of personal hygiene.

4. What is the role of posture in good health?

5. List the characteristics of a healthy, positive attitude.

6. How can you develop a strong work ethic?

7. Why is it important to be a team player?

8. Explain the best way to deal with an unhappy client.

9. Why is it so important to learn how to manage your time?

10. Name at least six ways you can practice ethical behavior.

11. List 10 life skills that can lead to success and a more productive life.

12. Why is setting goals important to success?

13. Discuss at least five ways to manage your time most efficiently.

CHAPTER GLOSSARY

ethics: principles of good character, proper conduct, and moral judgment, expressed through personality, human relations skills, and professional image.

personal hygiene: daily maintenance of cleanliness

and healthfulness through certain sanitary practices.

physical presentation: a person's physical posture, walk, and movements.

professional image: the impression projected by a person engaged in any profession, consisting of outward appearance and conduct exhibited in the workplace.

CHAPTER OUTLINE

COMMUNICATING FOR SUCCESS

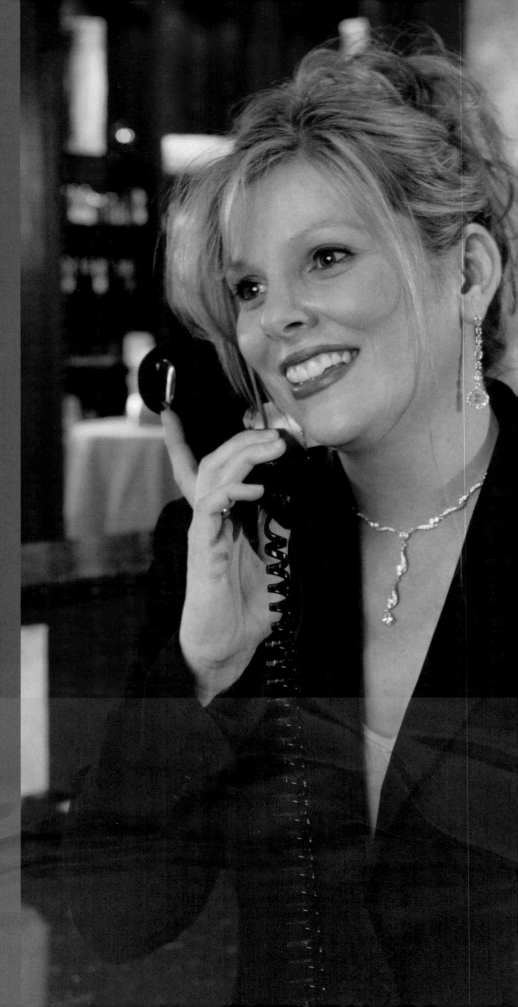

LEARNING OBJECTIVES

After completing this chapter, you will be able to:

- List the golden rules of human relations.

- Explain the importance of effective communication.

- Conduct a successful client consultation.

- Handle delicate communications with your clients.

- Build open lines of communication with coworkers and salon managers.

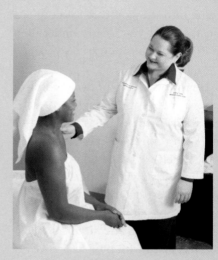

Figure 3–1 Good communication is essential to building positive client relations.

Do you have outstanding technical skills? Gifted hands? A flair for makeup artistry? If you do, you are definitely on your way to becoming successful in your chosen career path within the field of esthetics. It is important to realize, though, that technical and artistic skills can only take you so far. To thrive in the field of esthetics, you must also master the art of communication. Effective human relations and communication skills build lasting client relationships, aid in your growth as a practitioner, and help prevent misunderstandings and unnecessary tension in the workplace (Figure 3–1).

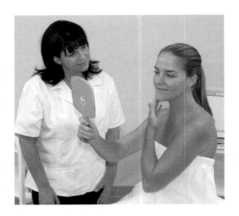

Figure 3–2 Be attentive to your client's needs.

HUMAN RELATIONS

No matter where you work, you will not always get along with everyone. It is not possible to always understand what people need, even when you know them well. Even if you do think you understand what people want, you cannot always be sure that you will satisfy them. This can lead to tension and misunderstanding.

The ability to understand people is the key to operating effectively in many professions. It is especially important in esthetics, where customer service is central to success. Most of your interactions will depend on your ability to communicate successfully with a wide range of people: your boss, coworkers, clients, and the different vendors who come into the skin care salon or spa to sell and educate you about their products. When you clearly understand the motives and needs of others, you are in a better position to do your job professionally and easily (Figure 3–2).

The best way to understand others is to begin with a firm understanding of yourself. When you are conscious of your own needs and desires, it is easier to appreciate others and to help them get what they need. Basically, we all have the same needs. When we are treated with respect and people listen to us, we feel good about them and ourselves. When we create an atmosphere where customers and staff have confidence in us, we will get the respect we deserve. Good relationships are built on mutual respect and understanding. Here is a brief look at the basics of human relations, along with some practical tips for dealing with situations that you are likely to encounter.

* A fundamental factor in human relations has to do with how secure we are feeling. When we feel secure, we are happy, calm, and confident, and we act in a cooperative and trusting manner. When we feel insecure, we become worried, anxious, overwhelmed, perhaps angry and suspicious, and usually we do not behave very well. We might be uncooperative, hostile, or withdrawn.

* Human beings are social animals. When we feel secure, we like to interact with other people. We enjoy giving our opinions, we take pleasure from having people help us, and we take pride in our ability to help others. When people feel secure with us, they are a joy to be with. You can help people feel secure around you by being respectful, trustworthy, and honest.

* No matter how secure you are, there will be times when you will be faced with people and situations that are difficult to handle. You may already have had such experiences. There are always some people who create conflict wherever they go. They can be rude, insensitive, or so self-centered that being considerate just does not enter their minds. Even though you may wonder how anyone could be so insensitive, just try to remember that this person at this particular time feels insecure, or he or she would not be acting this way.

To become skilled in human relations, learn to make the best of situations that could otherwise drain both your time and your energy. Here are some good ways to handle the ups and downs of human relations.

* *Respond instead of reacting.* A fellow was asked why he did not get angry when a driver cut him off. "Why should I let someone else dictate my emotions?" he replied. A wise fellow, don't you think? The ability to

think thoughtfully rather than react impulsively will help you to maintain control of your emotions. In situations like this, not reacting with "an eye for an eye" mentality might even have saved a life.

- *Believe in yourself.* When you do, you trust your judgment, uphold your own values, and stick to what you believe is right. It is easy to believe in yourself when you have a strong sense of self-worth. It comes with the knowledge that you are a good person and you deserve to be successful. Believing in yourself makes you feel strong enough to handle almost any situation in a calm, helpful manner.
- *Talk less, listen more.* There is an old saying that we were given two ears and one mouth for a reason. You get a gold star in human relations when you listen more than you talk. When you are a good listener, you are fully attentive to what the other person is saying. If there is something you do not understand, ask a question to gain understanding.
- *Be attentive.* Each client is different. Some are clear about what they want; others are aggressively demanding, while others may be hesitant. If you have an aggressive client who is not responding to your best efforts to communicate effectively, instead of trying to handle it by yourself, ask your manager for advice. You will likely be told that what usually calms difficult clients down is agreeing with them and then asking what you can do to make the service more to their liking. This approach works nine out of ten times.
- *Take your own temperature.* If you are tired or upset about a personal problem, or have had an argument with a fellow student, you may be feeling down about yourself and wish you were anywhere but in school. If this feeling lasts a short time, you will be able to get back on track easily enough and there is no cause for alarm. If, however, you begin to notice certain chronic behaviors about yourself once you are in a job, pay careful attention to what is happening. An important part of being in a service profession is taking care of yourself first and resolving whatever conflicts are going on so that you can take care of your clients. Trust can be lost in a second without even knowing it—and, once lost, trust is almost impossible to regain.

To conclude, human relations can be rewarding or frustrating. It all depends on how willing you are to give.

The Golden Rules of Human Relations

Keep the following guidelines in mind for a crash course in human relations that will always keep you in line and where you should be:

- Communicate from your heart; solve problems from your head.
- A smile is worth a million times more than a sneer.
- Be kind to others. Treat people in a way that allows them to maintain their dignity.
- Every action brings about a reaction.
- Learn to ask for help when you are overwhelmed.
- Show people you care by listening to them and trying to understand their point of view.
- Give compliments freely. An encouraging word at the right moment brings out the best in people.

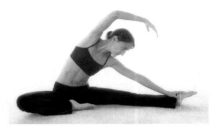

Figure 3–3 Learn to balance your professional life with personal time.

- Being right is different from acting righteous.
- Balance your service to others with personal time to renew your own mind, body, and spirit (Figure 3–3).
- Laugh often.
- Show patience with other people's flaws.
- Take time to evaluate your own attitude and actions.
- Make amends when you are wrong.
- Learn to forgive yourself and others.
- Be compassionate toward others, demonstrating your support in difficult times.
- Build shared goals; be a team player and a partner to your clients.
- A simple thank-you goes a long way in showing your appreciation to clients and colleagues.
- Remember that listening is the best relationship builder.

COMMUNICATION BASICS

Communication is the act of successfully sharing information between two people, or groups of people, so that it is effectively understood. There are many facets to communication. You can communicate through words, voice inflections, facial expressions, body language, and visual tools (e.g., before and after photos).

As you develop effective communication skills, consider that many times it is not *what* we say, but rather *how* we say it. Paying attention to the nonverbal cues we use can help us to improve the quality of our relations with both clients and colleagues. The following list of positive and negative nonverbal cues will help you to become more aware of how you are coming across to others (Table 3–1).

Table 3–1

| POSITIVE AND NEGATIVE NONVERBAL CUES ||
POSITIVE NONVERBAL CUES	NEGATIVE NONVERBAL CUES
A pleasant tone of voice	Rapid and jumbled speech
An even rate of speech	A loud and overpowering voice
A moderate tone of voice	A soft and unassertive voice
Good eye contact	Looking away from a person
A simple nod to demonstrate you are listening	Yawning or other distracting gesture
Warm and enthusiastic facial gestures	Pursing the lips or folding arms in an off-putting manner
A smile	A frown
Appropriate body distance	Standing uncomfortably close to a person
The gentle touch of a hand	Using hand gestures to scold or embarrass

When you and your client are both communicating clearly about an upcoming service, your chances of pleasing that person soar.

Meeting and Greeting New Clients

One of the most important communications you will have with a client is the first time you meet that person. Be polite, genuinely friendly, and inviting—and remember that your clients are coming to you for services they are paying for. This means it is your job to provide them with excellent customer service every time they come to see you; otherwise, you may lose them to another esthetician or salon (Figure 3–4).

To earn clients' trust and loyalty, you need to:

* Always approach a new client with a smile on your face. If you are having a difficult day or have a problem of some sort, keep it to yourself. The time you spend with your client is for her needs, not yours.
* Always introduce yourself. Names are powerful, and they are meant to be used. Many clients have had the experience of being greeted by the receptionist, ushered back to the service area, and when the service has been performed and the appointment is over, they have not learned the name of a single person.
* Set aside a few minutes to take new clients on a quick tour of the salon.
* Introduce clients to the people they may have interactions with while in the salon, including potential service providers for other services such as nail care or makeup.
* Be yourself. Do not try to trick your clients into thinking you are someone or something that you are not. Just be who you are. You will be surprised at how well this will work for you.

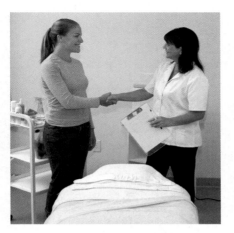

Figure 3–4 First impressions are often lasting impressions. When meeting a client for the first time, maintain good eye contact, smile, and extend a warm handshake.

Intake Form

An intake form—also called a *client questionnaire* or *consultation card*—should be filled out by every new client before receiving services. Whether in the salon or in school, this form can prove to be extremely useful (Figure 3–5).

Some salon intake forms ask for a lot of detailed information, and some do not. In esthetics school, the intake form may be accompanied by a release statement in which the client acknowledges that the service is being provided by a student who is still learning. This helps protect the school and the student from any legal action by a client who may be unhappy with the service.

How to Use the Client Intake Form

The client intake form should be mentioned the moment a new client calls the skin care salon or spa to make an appointment. When scheduling the appointment, let the client know that you and the salon will require some information before you can begin the service. Some salons ask clients to arrive 15 minutes before their appointment time for this purpose. You will also have to allow time in your schedule to conduct a 5 to 15-minute **client consultation,** depending on the type of service you will be performing and the client's needs (Figure 3–6).

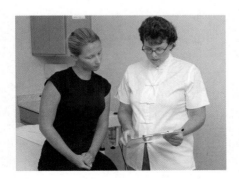

Figure 3–6 The client intake form gives you an opportunity to build an excellent relationship with your client.

Confidential Skin Health Survey

PLEASE PRINT

Today's Date _____

First Name _____ Last Name _____ Date of Birth __/__/____

Street _____ Apt. # _____ City _____ State _____ Zip _____

Phone: Home ( ) _____Work ( ) _____ Mobile ( ) _____

Dermatologist/Physician _____ Phone ( ) _____

Emergency Contact _____ Phone ( ) _____

Your Occupation _____

Referred By ❑ Friend ❑ Mailer ❑ Walk-by ❑ Yellow Pages ❑ Gift Certificate ❑ Other _____

Eesthetician Name _____

1. Is this your first facial? ❑ Yes ❑ No
2. What is the reason for your visit today?
   _____
3. What special areas of concern do you have?
   _____
   _____
4. Are you presently under a physician's care for any current skin condition or other problem? ❑ Yes ❑ No
   What?_____
5. Are you pregnant? ❑ Yes ❑ No
6. Are you taking birth control pills? ❑ Yes ❑ No
   If so, what type?_____
7. Hormone replacement? ❑ Yes ❑ No
   If so, what?_____
8. Do you wear contact lenses? ❑ Yes ❑ No
9. Do you smoke? ❑ Yes ❑ No
10. Do you often experience stress? ❑ Yes ❑ No
11. Have you had skin cancer? ❑ Yes ❑ No

12. Are you now using (or used in the past): ❑ Azelex
    ❑ Differin ❑ Renova ❑ Retin-A ❑ Tazarac
    ❑ Glycolic or alpha hydroxy acids
    If so, when and for how long? _____
13. Are you now using or have you ever used Accutane?
    ❑ Yes ❑ No
    If so, when and for how long? _____
14. Do you have acne? ❑ Yes ❑ No
    Experience frequent blemishes? ❑ Yes ❑ No
    If so, how frequently? _____
15. Do you have any allergies to cosmetics, foods, or drugs?
    ❑ Yes ❑ No
    Please list _____
16. Are you presently taking medications—oral or topical?
    ❑ Yes ❑ No If so, please list.
    _____
    _____
17. What products do you use presently? ❑ Soap
    ❑ Cleansing milk ❑ Toner ❑ Scrub ❑ Mask
    ❑ Creams ❑ Sunscreen ❑ Other

Please circle if you are affected by or have any of the following:

Asthma	Fever blisters	Hysterectomy	Sinus problems
Cardiac problems	Headaches—chronic	Immune disorders	Skin diseases—other
Depression or Anxiety	Hepatitis	Lupus	Urinary or kidney problems
Eczema	Herpes	Metal bone, pins, or plates	
Epilepsy	High blood pressure	Pacemaker	

Please explain above problems or list any other significant issues. _____

I understand that the services offered are not a substitute for medical care and any information provided by the therapist is for educational purposes only and not diagnostically prescriptive in nature. I understand that the information herein is to aid the therapist in giving better service and is completely confidential.

SPA POLICIES

1. Professional consultation is required before initial dispensing of products.
2. Our active discount rate is only effective for clients visiting every 4 weeks.
3. We do not give cash refunds.
4. We require a 24-hour cancellation notice.

I fully understand and agree to the above spa policies.

_____   _____

Client's Signature   Date

Figure 3–5 An intake form.

Consent Form

Having a client sign a *consent form* is standard practice for more aggressive treatments. However, it is important not to create an atmosphere of apprehension when introducing this form to clients. What you do want to accomplish is a thorough understanding of the benefits and features of the service or product in question. You also want the client to have a complete understanding of any contraindications to its use. Making these things clear at the outset can help reduce any fears or anxiety the client may have and allow the client to feel more comfortable with the treatment process.

How to Use the Consent Form

When introducing the consent form to clients, take time to review all the steps involved in the treatment process. Also carefully explain any home care directions that may be necessary. Provide the client with a copy of the consent form, and keep the original for your files. It is also wise to maintain a treatment log and have the client initial and date all subsequent treatment procedures. These extra precautionary measures go a long way in safeguarding both you and the client.

THE CLIENT CONSULTATION

The client consultation is the verbal communication that determines the desired results. It is the single most important part of any service and should always be done *before* beginning any part of the service. Some professionals skip the client consultation altogether, or they make time for it only on a client's first visit to the salon. These professionals are making a serious mistake. A consultation should be performed, to some degree, as part of every single service and salon visit. It keeps good communication

FOCUS ON . . .

UNDERSTANDING THE CLIENT'S GOALS

The initial consultation is the most important interaction you will have with a client. Information gathered at this point will help you to define the client's goals and objectives and create a positive working relationship. Remember that each client is an individual with a personal agenda. Some clients may be interested in age management, while others will be looking to remedy or control a certain skin condition. Many clients will simply want to experience the relaxation benefit associated with skin care services.

To determine the best outcome, you will want to gather as much information as possible without invading the client's privacy or making them feel uncomfortable. This generally includes information about any health problems, allergies, and medications as well as the use of any prescription skin care products, cosmeceuticals, or other skin care treatments the client has recently received that could adversely affect treatment. When conducting a consultation, remember that the information a client provides is considered privileged and should be held strictly confidential.

CONFIDENTIALITY

Estheticians can be held liable for a breach of confidentiality. This can result in lawsuits for both the salon and individuals. As a reminder, the intake information supplied by clients is strictly confidential and should be handled with the utmost discretion at all times and in all situations. Never discuss client information in public places or open salon areas.

going, and it allows you to keep your clients feeling satisfied with your services. More important, it helps to reduce the risk of doing harm to a client.

Once you are clear about what a client is looking for, and whether or not there are any contradictions to the desired treatments, you can work together to develop a strategy for meeting these needs.

Preparing for the Client Consultation

So that your time is well spent during the client consultation, it is important to be prepared. To facilitate the consultation process, you should have certain important items on hand. These may include vendor-supplied or salon-manufactured pamphlets, photos, articles, or clinical research papers that will help you to present the services or explain the benefits of certain ingredients that will be used to perform a treatment.

As skin care treatments become more sophisticated, many clients will have very specific questions about the outcome. Before and after photos are often a good way to demonstrate the results of a product or treatment. Step-by-step photos of the actual treatment process can also be helpful in letting clients know what to expect. Photos of satisfied customers are ideal for demonstrating the efficacy of a product or service, but they are not always suitable. Although many skin care clinics and medical spas will use before and after photos to document a client's progress, it is important to remember that such client information is confidential. If you have a client whose progress is significant, it is extremely important to gain her permission to use such photos for promotional purposes.

Vendor pamphlets that contain before and after photos are often a better resource for demonstrating the details of more aggressive treatments (Figure 3–7). When presenting such photos, be sure to explain how the procedure is conducted in your salon and to point out any differences. A discussion of who the best candidates are for specific treatments can help clients to decide if the treatment is suitable for them. Helping new clients understand why certain things can or cannot be achieved will also reassure them that you are knowledgeable and serious about their needs.

On occassion, you will find yourself consulting with a client who insists on a specific treatment or service that is not appropriate for them. In some cases a client may even misrepresent the truth about a situation to get you to perform a treatment that could have serious consequences. If you decide to perform a treatment that goes against your best judgment and causes harm to a client, guess who will catch the blame? In this situation, it is important to consult with a qualified superior. Refusing to perform a treatment can be difficult, but it is always better to be safe than sorry.

The Consultation Area

Presentation counts for a lot in a business that is concerned with appearances. Once you have brought the client to the consultation or treatment room to begin the consultation process, make sure she is comfortable. You and she are

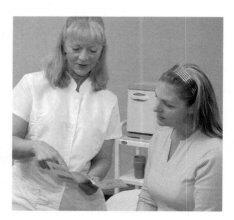

Figure 3–7 Before and after photos are an excellent way to demonstrate the results of a product or treatment.

about to begin an important conversation that will clue you in to her needs and preferences. Your work area needs to be freshly cleaned and uncluttered. Have any pamphlets, photos, and literature that you will use to describe the benefits, features, or any contraindications to a service available. All other appropriate tools to perform the desired service should be ready for use. Review the intake form carefully with the client, and refer to it often during the consultation process. Throughout the consultation, and especially once a course of action is decided on, make notes on the intake form. Record any formulations or products that you use, and include any specific techniques you follow, or goals you are working toward, so that you can remember them for future visits.

The 10-Step Consultation Method

Every complete consultation needs to be structured in such a way that you cover all the key points that consistently lead to a successful conclusion. While this may seem like a lot of information to memorize, it will become second nature as you become more experienced and conduct many consultations. Depending on the service requested, the consultation will vary to some degree. For example, a chemical peel will require a more detailed consultation than a makeup application. To ensure that you are always thorough, keep a list of the following 10 key points at your station for referral, and modify it as needed for the actual service.

1. **Review** the intake form that your client has filled out, and take a few minutes to develop rapport with the client and get the consultation going.
2. **Assess** your client's current goals and objectives. Is she looking to remedy a skin condition? Rejuvenate her appearance? Relax and unwind?
3. **Preference.** Ask your client what skin care products she is currently using. Does she love the fact that she only has to spend 10 minutes a day taking care of her skin? What professional treatments has she had in the past? Was she happy with the results? What is the reason for today's visit?
4. **Analyze.** Use a magnifying loupe and/or Wood's lamp to assess the client's skin. Note the skin type, texture, and any skin conditions on the consultation analysis form. Determine the client's Fitzpatrick type (more detailed information on the Fitzpatrick scale will be discussed in Chapter 11). Are there any contraindications, allergies, or sensitivities that will affect treatment (Figure 3–8)?
5. **Lifestyle.** Ask your client about her career and personal lifestyle.
   - Does she spend a great deal of time outdoors? Does she swim every day?
   - Is she a businesswoman? An artist? A stay-at-home mom?
   - Does she have a strong personal style that she wishes to project?
   - What are her skin care habits? How often does she have facials? How much time does she want to spend taking care of her skin each day?
   - Note all of the intrinsic and extrinsic factors.

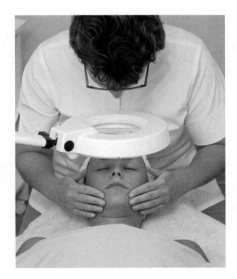

Figure 3–8 Analyze your client's skin for type, texture, and skin conditions.

6. **Show and tell.** Review the various treatment options. This is a good time to get a real grasp on whether the client's goals are realistic. What does the client hope to achieve? If she says she wants to look like a certain celebrity, does this mean she likes the shape of her eyebrows or is interested in having dermatological or plastic surgery? Reinforcing your words with literature and before and after photos is critical to having a clear understanding of what both of you are really saying.

   Listening to the client and then repeating, in your own words, what you think the client is telling you is known as **reflective listening.** Mastering this listening skill will help you to always be on target with your services, and to build a deep trust with your clients.

7. **Suggest.** Once you have enough information to make valid suggestions, narrow the treatment options based on the following factors:
   - *Lifestyle.* The products and services you recommend must fit the client's needs in terms of (time and effort), stress level, medical conditions, and other intrinsic and extrinsic factors such as hormonal issues, poor nutrition, smoking or alcohol habits, and personal appearance goals.
   - *Skin type.* You must base your recommendations on whether your client has dry, normal, oily, combination, or sensitive skin.
   - *Skin conditions.* Point out any contraindications to treatment or special considerations related to conditions, such as acne, hyper-, or hypopigmentation.
   - *Fitzpatrick typing.* Determine the client's Fitzpatrick type, and explain how this will affect any of the treatments or services you recommend. Advise the client on the appropriate sun protection products.

     When making suggestions, qualify them by referencing the preceding factors. For example: "I think this treatment will help to improve the overall tone and texture of your skin." Tactfully discuss any unreasonable expectations the client may have shared with you by pointing out any contraindications or limitations to the product or service that are unrealistic based on her personal goals. If the client's skin is damaged, you may need to address the need for a series of treatments, better home-care products, or lifestyle changes, or refer the client to a medical professional who is better able to meet her needs.

     Never hesitate to suggest additional services that will provide added value to the treatment or enhance the service. For example, adding an enzyme to a basic facial will help to improve skin tone and texture, while an eyebrow wax and new makeup palette can give the client a completely new look that will better suit her lifestyle, fulfill her desire to improve her appearance, and so on.

8. **Sun exposure.** Instructions regarding proper sun protection should be part of every consultation service. Use the Fitzpatrick scale to recommend the appropriate level of sun protection products, and caution all clients against the harmful effects of overexposure to the sun. Estheticians should stress to clients that overexposure to the sun may

not only lead to skin cancer but can also contribute to aging, hyperpigmentation, capillary damage, free-radical damage, and collagen and elastin deterioration (these will be discussed in detail in upcoming chapters). It is especially important to advise clients who have exfoliating treatments to keep out of the sun to avoid serious side effects.

9. **Maintenance.** Counsel every client on proper skin care, a regular schedule of salon treatments, the benefit of a series of treatments, lifestyle limitations, and home maintenance that she will need to commit to in order to look her best.

10. **Repeat.** Reiterate everything that you have agreed upon. Make sure to speak in measured, precise terms, and use visual tools to demonstrate the end result. This is the most critical step of the consultation process because it ultimately determines the service(s) you will perform. Take your time, and be thorough.

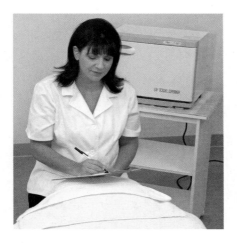

Figure 3–9 Take time to record your results on the client consultation form after each and every service.

Concluding the Service

Once the service is finished and the client has let you know whether she is satisfied, take a few more minutes to record the results on the consultation form. Ask for her reactions, and record them. Note anything you did that you might want to do again, as well as anything that does not bear repeating. Also make note of the final results and any retail products that you recommended. This is the perfect time to review the client's goals and objectives. Always supply the client with a written recommendation of the products and treatments you have suggested, with specific directions for product use and recommended time frames for in-salon treatments. This will help clients stay on track and increase the benefit of salon services. Be sure to date your notes and file them in the proper place (Figure 3–9).

SPECIAL ISSUES IN COMMUNICATION

Although you may do everything in your power to communicate effectively, you will sometimes encounter situations that are beyond your control. The solution is not to try to control the circumstances, but to communicate past the issue. Your reactions to situations, and your ability to communicate in the face of problems, are critical to being successful in a "people" profession such as the esthetics industry.

Handling Tardy Clients

Tardy clients are a fact of life in every service industry. Because skin care professionals are so dependent on appointments and scheduling to maximize working hours, a client who is very late for an appointment, or one who is habitually late, can cause problems. One tardy client can make you late for every other client you service that day, and the pressure involved in making up for lost time can take its toll. You also risk inconveniencing the rest of your clients who are prompt for their appointments.

Here are a few guidelines for handling late clients.

• Know and abide by the salon's tardy or late policy. Many salons set a limited amount of time they allow a client to be late before they require them to reschedule. Generally, if clients are more than 15 minutes late, they should be asked to reschedule. Most will accept responsibility and be understanding about the rule, but you may come across a few clients who insist on being seen immediately. In many cases, the front desk manager or receptionist handles this type of problem, but sometimes a client will insist on speaking to the service provider. If you are called upon, explain that you have other appointments and are responsible to those clients as well. Also explain that rushing through the service is unacceptable to both of you.

- If your tardy client arrives and you have the time to take her without jeopardizing other clients' appointments, let your client know why you are taking her even though she is late. You can deliver this information and still remain pleasant and upbeat. Say, "Oh, Ms. Lee, we're in luck! Even though you're a bit late, I can still take you because my next appointment isn't scheduled for another hour. Isn't it great that it worked out?" This lets her know that being late is not acceptable under normal circumstances, but that if you can accommodate her, you will.

- As you get to know your clients, you will learn who is habitually late. You may want to schedule such clients for the last appointment of the day, or ask them to arrive earlier than their actual appointments. In other words, if a client is always 30 minutes late, schedule her for 2:30 but tell her to arrive at 2:00!

- Imagine this scenario. Despite your best efforts, you are running late. You realize that no matter what has happened in the salon that day, your clients want and deserve your promptness. Have the receptionist look up your client's records and call them to advise them of the situation. Give them the opportunity to reschedule, or to come a little later than their scheduled appointments. If you cannot reach them beforehand, be sure to approach them when they come into the salon and let them know that you are delayed. Tell them how long you think the wait will be, and give them the option of changing their appointment. Apologize for the inconvenience and show a little extra attention by personally offering them a beverage. Even if these clients are not happy about the delay, or they need to change their appointment, at least they will feel informed and respected.

Handling Scheduling Mix-Ups

We are all human, and we all make mistakes. Chances are you have gone to an appointment on a certain day, at a certain time, only to discover that you are in the wrong place, at the wrong time. The way you are treated at that moment will determine if you ever patronize that business again. The number one thing to remember when you, as a professional, get involved with a scheduling mix-up is to be polite and never argue about who is correct. Being right may sound good, but this kind of situation is not about being right; it is about preserving your relationship with your client. If you handle the matter poorly, you run the risk of never seeing that client again.

Even if you know for sure that she is mistaken, tell yourself that the client is always right. Assume the blame if it helps keep her happy. *Do not, under any circumstances, argue the point with the client.*

Once you have the chance to consult your appointment book, you can say, "Oh, Mrs. Montez, I have you in my appointment book for 10:00, and unfortunately I already have a fully scheduled day. I'm so sorry about the mix-up. Can I reschedule you for tomorrow at 10:00?" Even though the client may be fuming, you need to stay disengaged. Your focus is to move the conversation away from who is at fault, and squarely in the direction of resolving the confusion. Make another appointment for the client, and be sure to get her telephone number so that you can call and confirm the details of the appointment in advance.

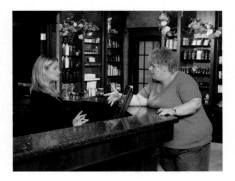

Figure 3–10 Accommodate an unhappy client promptly and calmly.

Handling Unhappy Clients

No matter how hard you try to provide excellent service to your clients, once in a while you will encounter a client who is dissatisfied with the service. The way you and the salon handle this difficult situation will have lasting effects on you, the client, and the salon, so you need to know how best to proceed (Figure 3–10).

Once again, it is important to remember the ultimate goal: make the client happy enough to pay for the service and return for more of the same.

Many salons and spas will have set guidelines for handling difficult situations. When in doubt, here are some guidelines to follow.

- Try to find out why the client is unhappy. Ask for specifics. If she has a difficult time expressing herself, break down the service for her piece by piece until you determine exactly what has caused the dissatisfaction.
- If it is possible to change what she dislikes, do so immediately. If that is not possible, look at your schedule to see how soon you can do it. You may need to enlist the help of the receptionist or front desk manager in rescheduling your other appointments or arranging for another practitioner to step in. If the client seems open to the suggestion of rescheduling, ask her to return to the salon at a time when you are free. If this is not possible, and you will be relying on help from another practitioner, explain who will be working with her and what the other practitioner will be doing. The bottom line is, do whatever you have to do to make her happy.
- If you cannot change what the client does not like, or it is simply impossible to change, you must honestly and tactfully explain the reason why you cannot make any changes. The client will not be happy, but you can offer any options that may be available.
- Again, never argue with the client or try to force your opinion. Unless you can change what has caused the dissatisfaction, arguing will just fuel the fire.
- Do not hesitate to call on the spa director, front desk manager, or a senior staff member for help. They have encountered a similar situation at some point in their careers and have insights that can help you.
- If, after you have tried everything, you are unable to satisfy the client, defer to your manager's advice on how to proceed. The client may be too upset to handle the situation maturely, and it may be easier for her

to deal with someone else. This does not mean that you have failed; it simply means that another approach is needed.

- Confer with your salon manager or spa director after the experience. A good manager will not hold the event against you, but view it instead as an inevitable fact of life that you can learn from. Follow your manager's advice and move on to your next client. Use whatever you may have learned from the experience to perform future client consultations and services better.

Handling Difficult People

The first thing you must realize when dealing with difficult clients, coworkers, and bosses is that the issues involved are not always about you. Do not take offensive words or actions personally. You must be prepared to deal with all kinds of personality types; not everyone who comes into your salon will be easygoing and trust your judgment. In fact, you may have clients who will take advantage of the fact that you are a novice.

Following some basic rules or coping strategies will help you maintain control.

- Respect boundaries.
- Keep conversation on a professional level. Steer inappropriate commentary back to the task at hand.
- Do not give personal or health advice.
- Post rules in a visible place. Make sure clients are aware of the salon's policies.
- Be assertive but respectful.
- Learn to censor your dialogue, and think before you speak. Avoid engaging in gossip.
- Practice positive communication skills such as active listening.
- Use language that evokes a positive response. Whenever possible, find a middle ground.
- Be clear. State the facts simply, courteously, and succinctly, in a manner that does not provoke controversy or argument.
- Acknowledge concerns, and state how you can address them. Assure clients as necessary.
- Compliment coworkers, managers, or bosses for a job well done. Everyone benefits from a well-deserved compliment.

Getting Too Personal

Sometimes when a client forms a bond of trust with her esthetician, she may have a hard time differentiating between a professional and a personal relationship. That will be *her* problem, but you must not make it *your* problem. Your job is to handle your client relationships tactfully and sensitively. You cannot become your clients' counselor, career guide, parental sounding board, or motivational coach. Your job and your relationship with your clients are very specific: the goal is to advise and service clients with their skin care needs, and nothing more.

FOCUS ON . . .

PROFESSIONALISM

A long-time client reveals to you one day that she and her husband are going through a messy divorce. You care for her and try to be understanding as she reveals increasingly personal details. You want to be helpful and supportive, but realize you need to establish boundaries. What can you do?

Try this: Tell her you understand the situation is very difficult, but while she is in the salon or spa, you want to do everything in your power to give her a break from it. Let her know that while she is in your care, you should both concentrate on her enjoyment of the services and not on the things that are stressing her.

She will appreciate the suggestion, and you will have put her back on the track of her real reason for coming to see you.

IN-SALON COMMUNICATION

Behaving in a professional manner is the first step in making meaningful in-salon communication possible. Unfortunately, some skin care professionals act immaturely and get overly involved in the salon rumor mill.

The salon community is usually a close-knit one in which people spend long hours working together. For this reason, it is important to maintain boundaries around what you will and will not do or say at the salon. Remember, the salon is your place of business and, as such, must be treated respectfully and carefully.

Communicating with Coworkers

As with all communication, there are basic principles that must guide your interactions. In a work environment, you will not have the opportunity to handpick your colleagues. There will always be people you like or relate to better than others, and people whose behaviors or opinions you find yourself in conflict with. These people can try your patience and your nerves, but they are your colleagues and are deserving of your respect.

Here are some guidelines to keep in mind as you interact and communicate with fellow staffers.

Treat everyone with respect. Regardless of whether you like someone, your colleagues are professionals who, just like you, provide services to clients who bring revenue into the salon. And, as practicing professionals, they have information they can offer you. Look at these people as having something to teach you, and hone in on their talents and their techniques.

Remain objective. Different types of personalities working in the same treatment rooms over long and intense hours are likely to breed some degree of dissension and disagreement. To learn and grow, you must make every effort to remain objective and resist being pulled into spats and cliques. When one or two people in the salon behave disrespectfully toward one another, the entire team suffers because the atmosphere changes. Not only will this be unpleasant for you, but it will also be felt by the clients who may decide to take their business elsewhere if they find the atmosphere in your salon too tense.

Be honest and be sensitive. Many people use the excuse of being honest as a license to say anything to anyone. While honesty is always the best policy, using unkind words or actions with regard to your colleagues is never a good idea. Be sensitive. Put yourself in the other person's place, and think through what you want to say before you say it. That way, any negative or hurtful words can be suppressed.

Remain neutral. Undoubtedly, there will come a time when you are called on to make a statement or to "pick a side." Do whatever you can to avoid getting drawn into the conflict. If you have a problem with a colleague, the best way to resolve it is to speak with her or him directly and privately.

Speaking to, or gossiping with, others about someone never resolves a problem. It only makes it worse and is often as damaging to you as it is to the object of your gossip.

Seek help from someone you respect. If you find yourself in a position where you are at odds with a coworker, you may want to seek out a third party—someone who is not involved and who can remain objective—such as the manager or a more experienced practitioner. Ask for advice about how to proceed, and really listen to what this mentor has to say. Since this person is not involved, he or she is more likely to see the situation as it truly is and can offer you valuable insights.

Do not take things personally. This is often easier said than done. How many times have you had a bad day, or been thinking about something totally unrelated, when a person asks you what is wrong, or wonders if you are mad at them? Just because someone is behaving in a certain manner and you happen to be there, do not interpret the words or behaviors as being meant for you. If you are confused or concerned by someone's actions, find a quiet and private place to ask the person about it. The person may not even realize he or she was giving off any signals.

Keep your private life private. There is a time and a place for everything, but the salon is never the place to discuss your personal life and relationships. It may be tempting to engage in that kind of conversation, especially if others in the salon are doing so, and to solicit advice and opinions, but that is why you have friends. Coworkers can become friends, but those whom you selectively turn into friends are different from the ones whose facial or massage room happens to be next to yours.

Communicating with Managers

Another important relationship for you within the salon is the one you will build with your manager. The salon manager is generally the person who has the most responsibility for how the salon is run in terms of daily maintenance, operations and client service. The manager's job is a demanding one. In some cases, in addition to running a hectic salon, the manager may also be a service provider.

Your manager is likely to be the one who hired you and is responsible for your training and for how well you move into the salon culture. Therefore, your manager has a vested interest in your success. As a salon employee, you will see the manager as a powerful and influential person, but it is also important to remember that she is a human being. She is not perfect, and she will not be able to do everything you think should be done in every instance. Whether she personally likes you or not, her job is to look beyond her personal feelings and make decisions that are best for the salon as a whole. The best thing you can do is to try to understand the decisions and rules that she makes whether you agree with them or not.

Many salon professionals utilize their salon managers in inappropriate ways by asking them to solve personal issues between staff members.

Inexperienced managers, hoping to keep everything flowing smoothly, may make the mistake of getting involved in petty issues. You and your manager must both understand that her job is to make sure the business is running smoothly, not to babysit temperamental practitioners.

Here are some guidelines for interacting and communicating with your salon manager.

Be a problem solver. When you need to speak with your manager about some issue or problem, think of some possible solutions beforehand. This will indicate that you are working in the salon's best interest and are trying to help, not make things worse.

Get your facts straight. Make sure that all your facts and information are accurate before you speak to your salon manager. This way you will avoid wasting time solving a "problem" that really does not exist.

Be open and honest. When you find yourself in a situation you do not understand or do not have the experience to deal with, tell your salon manager immediately and be willing to learn.

Do not gossip or complain about colleagues. Going to your manager with gossip or to "tattle" on a coworker tells your manager that you are a troublemaker. If you are having a legitimate problem with someone and have tried everything in your power to handle the problem yourself, then it is appropriate to go to your manager. But you must approach her with a true desire to solve the problem, not just to vent.

Check your attitude. The salon environment, although fun and friendly, can also be stressful, so it is important to take a moment between clients to "take your temperature." Ask yourself how you are feeling. Do you need an attitude adjustment? Be honest with yourself.

Be open to constructive criticism. It is never easy to hear that you need improvement in any area, but keep in mind that part of your manager's job is to help you achieve your professional goals. She is supposed to evaluate your skills and offer suggestions on how to increase them. Keep an open mind, and do not take her criticism personally (Figure 3–11).

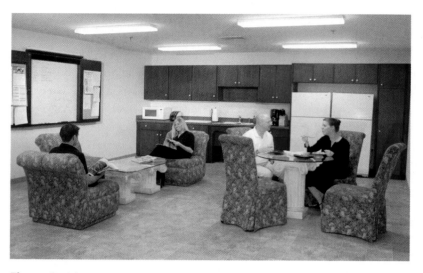

Figure 3–11 Getting along with coworkers is in everyone's best interest.

Communicating during an Employee Evaluation

Salons that are well run will make it a priority to conduct frequent and thorough employee evaluations. Sometime in the course of your first few days of work, your salon manager will tell you when you can expect your first evaluation. If she does not mention it, you might ask her about it and request a copy of the form she will use or the criteria on which you will be evaluated.

Take some time to look over this document. Be mindful that the behaviors and/or activities you will be evaluated on are most likely to be the ones listed on your job description. This is useful information. You can begin to watch and rate yourself in the weeks and months ahead so you can assess how you are doing. Remember, everything you are being evaluated on is there for the purpose of helping you improve. Make the decision to approach these communications positively. As the time draws near for the evaluation, try filling out the form yourself. In other words, give yourself an evaluation, even if the salon has not asked you to do so. Be objective, and carefully think about your comments. Then, when you meet with the manager, show her your evaluation and tell her you are serious about your improvement and growth. She will appreciate your input and your desire. And, if you are being honest with yourself, there should be no surprises (Figure 3–12).

Many salons are now drafting performance standards that clearly identify their human resource policies on wage increases and the protocol for advancement. If the salon you work at does not, be prepared to raise these important issues yourself. Before your evaluation meeting, write down any thoughts or questions you may have so you can share them with your manager. Do not be shy. If you want to know when you can take on more services, when your pay scale will be increased, or when you might be considered for promotion, this meeting is the appropriate time and place to ask. Many beauty professionals never take advantage of this crucial communication opportunity to discuss their future because they are too nervous, intimidated, or unprepared.

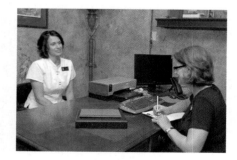

Figure 3–12 The employee evaluation provides an excellent opportunity to solicit your manager's advice on the best way to improve your skills.

Do not let that happen to you. Participate proactively in your career and in your success by communicating your desires and interests.

At the end of the meeting, thank your manager for taking the time to do an evaluation and for the feedback and guidance she has given you.

REVIEW QUESTIONS

1. List the golden rules of human relations.

2. Define communication.

3. How should you prepare for a client consultation?

4. List and describe the 10 elements of a successful client consultation.

5. Name some types of information that should go on a client consultation card.

6. How should you handle tardy clients?

7. How should you handle a scheduling mix-up?

8. How should you handle an unhappy client?

9. List at least five things to remember when communicating with your coworkers.

10. List at least four guidelines for communicating with salon managers.

CHAPTER GLOSSARY

client consultation: verbal communication with a client to determine desired results.

communication: the act of accurately sharing information between two people, or groups of people.

reflective listening: listening to the client and then repeating, in your own words, what you think the client is telling you.

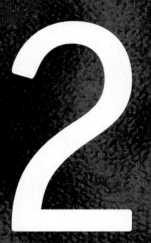

GENERAL SCIENCES

PART

2

INFECTION CONTROL: PRINCIPLES AND PRACTICE

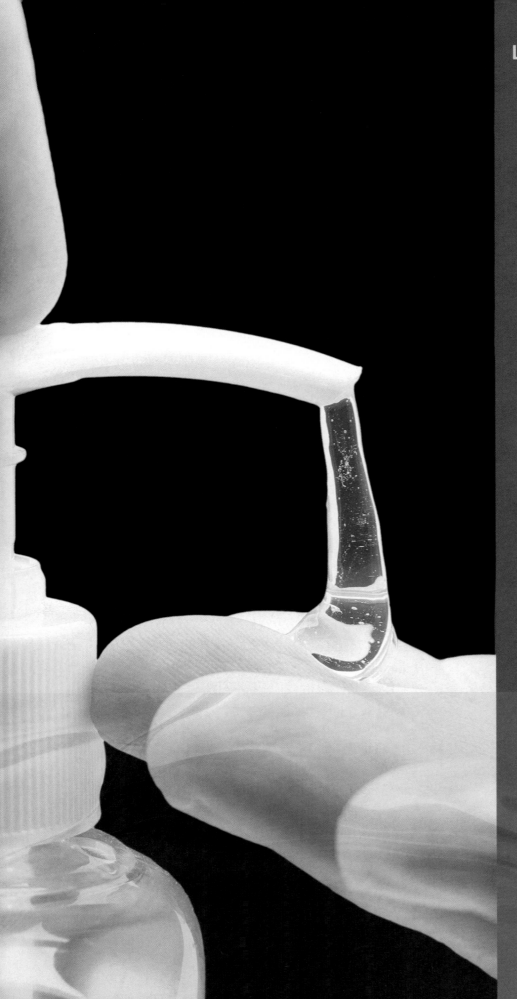

LEARNING OBJECTIVES

After completing this chapter,
you will be able to:

- List the types and
  classifications of bacteria.

- Define hepatitis and AIDS
  and explain how they are
  transmitted.

- Discuss the different types
  of disinfectants and how
  they are used.

- Describe how to safely
  sanitize and disinfect
  various salon tools and
  surfaces.

- Explain the differences
  between sterilization,
  disinfection, and
  sanitation.

- Understand the importance
  of sanitation for the health
  and safety of your clients,
  and for yourself.

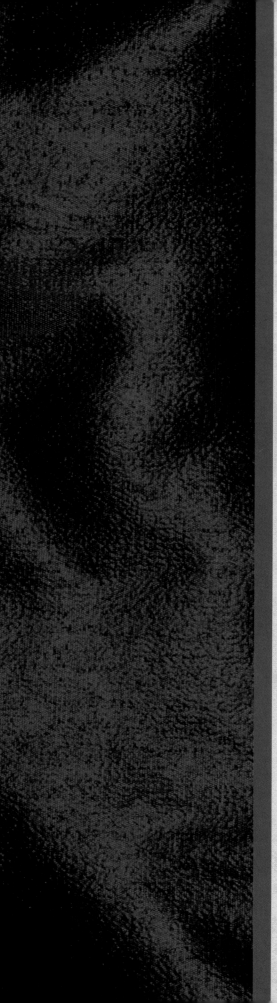

KEY TERMS

Page numbers indicate where in the chapter each term is used.

acquired immunity 70

AIDS (acquired immune deficiency syndrome) 67

antiseptics 71

aseptic procedure 80

asymptomatic 84

autoclave 73

bacilli (singular: bacillus) 63

bacteria 61

bactericidal 62

bloodborne pathogens 69

cilia 65

cocci 63

communicable 66

contagious 66

contaminants 73

contaminated 73

cross-contamination 78

decontamination 70

dermatophytes 70

diplococci 63

disinfectants 61, 73

disinfection 72

efficacy 74

exposure incident 84

flagella (singular: flagellum) 65

fungi (singular: fungus) 70

fungicidal 62

general infection 66

hepatitis 67

HIV (human immunodeficiency virus) 67

immunity 70

infection 65

local infection 66

Material Safety Data Sheet (MSDS) 59

Methicillin-resistant Staphylococcus aureus (MRSA) 66

microorganisms 62

motility 65

nitrile gloves 83

natural immunity 70

nonpathogenic 63

parasite 69

pathogenic 63

pediculosis 69

phenol 75

protozoa 69

pseudomonacidal 74

pus 65

quaternary ammonium compounds (quats) 74

sanitation 71

scabies 69

spirilla 65

staphylococci 63

sterilization 73

streptococci 63

tuberculocidal 61

tuberculosis 61

Universal Precautions 84

virucidal 62

virus 67

When reading this chapter, you may wonder if you are required to be part scientist or chemist to be a professional in the field of esthetics. Understanding the basics of cleaning and disinfecting and following state rules will ensure that you will protect yourself, clients, and your coworkers. This chapter will prepare you for a long and successful career in the field of esthetics.

REGULATION

Many different state and federal agencies regulate and set the guidelines for the practice of esthetics. Federal agencies set guidelines for manufacturing, sale, and use of equipment and chemical ingredients, and for safety in the workplace. State agencies regulate licensing, enforcement, and conduct when working in a salon, spa, or medical facility.

Federal Agencies

OSHA

The Occupational Safety and Health Administration (OSHA) was created as part of the U.S. Department of Labor to regulate and enforce safety and health standards to protect employees in the workplace. Regulating employee exposure to potentially toxic substances and informing employees about possible hazards of materials used in the workplace are key points of the Occupational Safety and Health Act of 1970. This regulation created the Hazard Communication Act, which requires that chemical manufacturers and importers assess the hazards associated with their products. Material Safety Data Sheets (MSDSs) are a result of this law.

The standards set by OSHA are important to the cosmetology industry because of the products used in salons, spas, and medical spas. These standards address issues relating to handling, mixing, storing, and disposing of products as well as general safety in the workplace. Most importantly, they address your right to know the hazardous ingredients in the products you use.

Material Safety Data Sheet

Federal laws require manufacturers to supply a **Material Safety Data Sheet (MSDS)** for all products sold (Figure 4–1). The MSDS includes information

Material Safety Data Sheet (MSDS)

Section I

Product Name or Number	Emergency Telephone No.
Manufacturer's Name	Manufacturer's D-U-N-5 No.
Address (Number, Street, City, State, Zip)	
Hazardous Materials Description and Proper Shipping Name (49.CFR 172.101)	Hazardous Class (49.CFR 172.101)
Chemical Family	Formula

Section II — Ingredients (list all ingredients)   CASE REGISTRY NO.   %

Section III — Physical Data

Boiling Point (F) (C)		Specific Gravity (H20 = 1)		
Vapor Pressure (mm Hg) ————		Percent Volatile by Volume (%)		
(psl) ————				
Vapor Density (Air = 1)		Evaporation Rate (= 1)		
Solubility in Water		pH =		
Appearance and Odor		Is material: Liquid Solid Gas Paste Powder		

Section IV — Fire & Explosion Hazard Data

Flash Point (method used)	Flammable Limits	LEL	UEL
( )			
( )			
Extinguishing Media			
Special Fire Fighting Procedures			
Unusual Fire and Explosion Hazards			

Figure 4–1 A sample of an MSDS.

about hazardous ingredients, safe use and handling procedures, precautions to reduce the risk of harm and overexposure, flammability and data in case of a fire, proper disposal guidelines, and medical information should anyone have a reaction to the product. When necessary, the MSDS can be sent to a doctor, so that any reaction can be properly treated. OSHA and state regulatory agencies require that MSDSs be kept available in the spa, salon, or skin care centers for all products that can cause harm. State inspectors can issue fines for any facility not having these sheets available.

You can get MSDSs from the product's manufacturer by downloading them from the product manufacturer or distributor's Web site. Not having an MSDS poses a health risk to anyone in a salon, spa, or skin care center who is exposed to hazardous materials and is a violation of federal regulations. Take the time to read all of this information to be certain that you are protecting yourself and your clients to the best of your ability.

Environmental Protection Agency (EPA)

The EPA registers different types of **disinfectants.** The two types that are used in salons and spas are chemical disinfectants and hospital-grade disinfectants, also known as **tuberculocidal.** Hospital-grade disinfectants are safe for cleaning blood and body fluids in hospitals.

Tuberculocidal disinfectants are proven to kill the **bacteria** that cause **tuberculosis,** which are more difficult to kill. This does not mean that you should use a tuberculocide; in fact, these products can be harmful to salon and spa tools and equipment, and they require special methods of disposal. Check the rules in your state to be sure that the product that you choose complies with requirements.

It is against federal law to use any disinfecting product contrary to its labeling. This means that if you do not follow the instructions for mixing, contact time, and the type of surface the disinfecting product can be used on, you have broken federal law.

State Regulatory Agencies

State regulatory agencies exist to protect the consumers' health, safety, and welfare while receiving services in a salon, spa, or medical spa. Regulatory agencies include licensing agencies, state boards of cosmetology, commissions, and health departments. They protect consumers by requiring everyone working in the facility to follow specific procedures. Enforcement of the rules through inspections and investigations of consumer complaints is also part of the agency's responsibility. The agency can issue penalties, against both the salon owner and the operator's license, ranging from warnings to fines, probation, and suspension or revocation of licenses. It is vital that you understand and follow the laws and rules in your state at all times—your license and your client's safety depend upon strict adherence.

? Did You Know

The term *hospital grade* is a myth. The EPA verifies the efficacy of infection control disinfectants. Once the effectiveness of a product has been approved, the product is then given a registration number and label that lists whether a product is approved for use in a hospital or it is not.

 WEB RESOURCES

OSHA Web site:
http://www.osha.com

Laws and Rules—What Is the Difference?

Laws are written by legislature. Laws determine the scope of practice (what each license allows the holder to do) and establish guidelines for regulatory agencies to make rules. Laws are also called *statutes*. Rules (also called *regulations*) are more specific than laws. Rules are written by the regulatory agency or board and determine how the law will be applied. Rules establish specific standards of conduct, and they can be changed and updated.

PRINCIPLES OF INFECTION

Being an esthetician is fun and rewarding, but it is also a great responsibility. One careless action could cause injury or infection, and you can lose your license to practice. Fortunately, preventing the spread of infection is easy if you know what to do and you practice what you have learned at all times. Safety begins and ends with *you*.

Infection Control

There are four classifications of potentially infectious microorganisms: bacteria, fungi, viruses, and parasites. Remember, when practicing infection control we are not seeking to treat any disease or condition; instead, we are taking steps so that the tools and equipment we use are safe to use on clients. These steps are designed to prevent infection or disease.

Disinfectants used in salons must be **bactericidal** (back-teer-uh-SYD-ul), **fungicidal** (fun-jih-SYD-ul), and **virucidal** (vy-rah-SYD-ul), meaning that when these solutions are mixed and used according to the instructions on the label, these will kill potentially infectious bacteria, fungi, and viruses. Dirty tools and equipment may spread infections from client to client. You have an obligation to provide safe services and prevent consumers from harm by practicing safely. If your clients are infected or harmed because you did not correctly follow sanitary guidelines, you may be found legally responsible for their condition, injury, or infection.

Bacteria

Microorganisms (my-kroh-OR-gah-niz-ums) are microscopic plants or animals. Also known as microbes, bacteria can exist almost everywhere: in and on our bodies, on our clothing, in water, on the surfaces of objects, and even in the air. They cannot be seen with the naked eye. One must use a microscope, and in some cases an electron microscope, to see them. The study of these organisms is known as microbiology. A microbiologist studies pathogenic organisms to prevent the spread of disease. The study of bacteria is known as bacteriology.

Types of Bacteria

There are thousands of different kinds of bacteria, but they are grouped into just two primary types—pathogenic and nonpathogenic. Most bacteria

Table 4–1

DEFINITIONS RELATING TO CAUSES OF DISEASE	
TERM	**DEFINITION**
Bacteria (singular: bacterium)	One-celled microorganisms with both plant and animal characteristics. Some are harmful, some are harmless. Also known as microbes or germs.
Infectious	Communicable by infection from one person to another person or from one infected body part to another.
Microbes/germs	Nonscientific synonyms for disease-producing bacteria.
Microorganism	Any organism of microscopic to submicroscopic size.
-ology	Suffix meaning "study of" (e.g., microbiology).
Parasite	An organism that grows, feeds, and shelters on or in another organism, while contributing nothing to the survival of that organism.
Toxin	Any of various poisonous substances produced by some microorganisms.
Virus (plural: viruses)	A parasitic submicroscopic particle that infects cells of biological organisms. A virus is capable of replication only through taking over the host cell's reproduction machinery.

are **nonpathogenic** (completely harmless; do not cause disease). They can perform many useful functions. In the human body, nonpathogenic bacteria help the body breakdown food, protect against infection, and stimulate the immune system. **Pathogenic** (path-uh-JEN-ik) bacteria are considered harmful because they may cause disease or infection when they invade the body. Preventing the spread of pathogenic microorganisms is vital in salons and schools, and it is why they must maintain sanitary standards. Tables 4–1 and 4–2 present terms and definitions related to pathogens.

Classifications of Pathogenic Bacteria

Bacteria have distinct shapes that help to identify them. Pathogenic bacteria are classified as follows:

1. **Cocci** (KOK-sy) are round-shaped bacteria that appear either singly (alone) or in the following groups (Figure 4–2).
   - **Staphylococci** (staf-uh-loh-KOK-sy)—Pus-forming bacteria that grow in clusters like a bunch of grapes. They cause abscesses, pustules, and boils (Figure 4–3).
   - **Streptococci** (strep-toh-KOK-sy)—Pus-forming bacteria arranged in curved lines resembling a string of beads. They cause infections such as strep throat and blood poisoning (Figure 4–4).
   - **Diplococci** (dip-lo-KOK-sy)—Spherical bacteria that grow in pairs and cause diseases such as pneumonia (Figure 4–5).
2. **Bacilli** (bah-SIL-ee; **singular: bacillus**) are short, rod-shaped bacteria. They are the most common bacteria and produce diseases such as tetanus (lockjaw), typhoid fever, tuberculosis, and diphtheria (Figure 4–6).

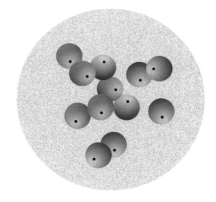

Figure 4–2 Cocci.

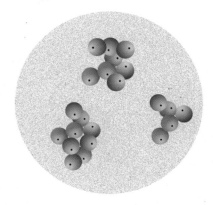

Figure 4–3 Staphylococci.

Table 4–2

GENERAL TERMS RELATING TO DISEASE	
TERM	**DEFINITION**
Allergy	Reaction due to extreme sensitivity to certain foods, chemicals, or other normally harmless substances.
Contagious Disease	Disease that is communicable or transmittable by contact.
Contamination	The presence, or the reasonably anticipated presence, of blood or other potentially infectious materials on an item's surface or visible debris/residues such as dust, hair, skin, etc.
Diagnosis	Determination of the nature of a disease from its symptoms.
Disease	Abnormal condition of all or part of the body, organ, or mind that makes it incapable of carrying on normal function.
Exposure Incident	Contact with non-intact skin, blood, body fluid or other potentially infectious materials that results from performance of an employees duties (previously called Blood Spill).
Infectious Disease	Disease caused by pathogenic microorganisms that are easily spread.
Inflammation	Condition in which a part of the body reacts to protect itself from injury, irritation, or infection, characterized by redness, heat, pain, and swelling.
Occupational Disease	Illnesses resulting from conditions associated with employment, such as prolonged and repeated overexposure to certain products or ingredients.
Parasitic Disease	Disease is caused by parasites, such as lice and ringworm.
Pathogenic Disease	Disease produced by disease-causing organisms, including bacteria, virus, and fungi.
Systemic Disease	Disease that affects the body generally, often due to under- or overfunctioning of internal glands/organs.

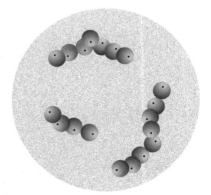

Figure 4–4 Streptococci.

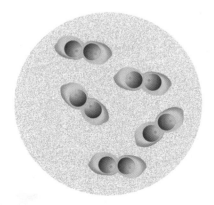

Figure 4–5 Diplococci.

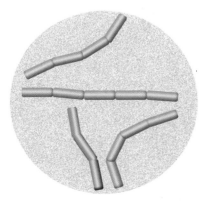

Figure 4–6 Bacilli.

3. **Spirilla** (spy-RIL-ah) are spiral or corkscrew-shaped bacteria. They are subdivided into subgroups, such as *Treponema pallida,* which causes syphilis, a sexually transmitted disease (STD), or *Borrelia burgdorferi,* which causes Lyme disease (Figure 4–7).

Movement of Bacteria

Different bacteria move in different ways. Cocci rarely show active **motility** (self-movement). They are transmitted in the air, in dust, or within the substance in which they settle. Bacilli and spirilla are both motile and use slender, hairlike extensions, known as **flagella** (flu-JEL-uh; **singular: flagellum**) or **cilia** (SIL-ee-uh), for locomotion (moving about). A whiplike motion of these hairlike extensions moves the bacteria in liquid.

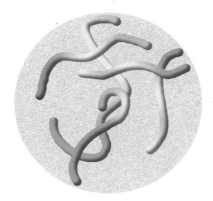

Figure 4–7 Spirilla.

Bacterial Growth and Reproduction

Bacteria generally consist of liquid, called protoplasm, enclosed by an outer cell wall. Cells absorb food from the surrounding environment. They give off waste products, grow, and reproduce. The life cycle of bacteria consists of two distinct phases: the active stage and the inactive or spore-forming stage.

Active Stage During the active stage, bacteria grow and reproduce. Bacteria multiply best in warm, dark, damp, or dirty places where food is available. When conditions are favorable, bacteria grow and reproduce. When they mature, bacteria divide into two new cells. This division is called *mitosis* (my-TOH-sis). The cells that are formed are called daughter cells. When conditions become unfavorable and difficult for them to thrive, the bacteria either die or become inactive.

Inactive or Spore-Forming Stage Certain bacteria, such as the anthrax and tetanus bacilli, coat themselves with waxy outer shells that are able to withstand long periods of famine, dryness, and unsuitable temperatures. In this stage, spores can be blown about and are not harmed by disinfectants, heat, or cold. When favorable conditions are restored, the spores change into the active form and begin to grow and reproduce. Spores are dangerous if they enter the body during a surgical procedure and become active.

Bacterial Infections

An **infection** occurs when body tissues are invaded by disease-causing or pathogenic microorganisms. These microorganisms are called *infectious agents.* There can be no bacterial infection without the presence of pathogenic bacteria. The presence of pus is one sign of bacterial infection. **Pus** is a fluid, created by tissue inflammation, that contains white blood cells, the debris of dead cells, tissue elements, and bacteria.

Staphylococci ("staph") are among the most common human bacteria. They are normally carried by about a third of the population. Although staph can be picked up on doorknobs, countertops, and other surfaces, it is more frequently spread through skin-to-skin contact, such as by shaking hands or using unclean implements.

?   Did You Know

Some states and provinces prohibit the use of invasive procedures in the salon, including those requiring needles, lancets, and probes. Check with your state regulatory agency for the rules in your state.

CAUTION!

Discard any unused makeup every six months and purchase a new supply. Makeup is a breeding ground for bacteria, so it is best to keep your makeup as fresh as possible. Do not share it with anyone else. Conjunctivitis, sties, and herpes are just a few of the diseases you may contract—or spread—if you share makeup.

A single practitioner can put many of her clients at risk if she does not practice stringent cleaning and disinfection guidelines. A case in point was the spread of a bacterium called *Mycobacterium fortuitum furunculosis* (MY-koh-bak-TIR-ee-um for-TOO-i-tum fur-UNK-yoo-LOH-sis), a microorganism that normally exists in tap water and in small numbers is completely harmless. In 2000, over 100 clients of a California salon developed serious skin infections on their legs after receiving pedicures. The infection was resistant to conventional antibiotics; it caused stubborn, ugly sores that lingered for months; and, in some cases, it caused scarring. The source of the infection was traced to the salon's whirlpool foot spas. Salon staff did not clean the foot spas properly, resulting in a buildup of hair and debris in the spas; in turn, this buildup created the perfect breeding ground for bacteria.

The outbreak was a catalyst for change in the industry. For instance, the California state government issued specific requirements for pedicure equipment aimed at preventing future outbreaks. Despite these efforts in California and elsewhere, other outbreaks affecting hundreds of women have occurred since 2000. In 2006 alone, several lengthy hospital stays resulting from pedicures were documented. Such developments have led to increased measures by state agencies (and salon owners) as well as more stringent cleaning instructions and warnings by pedicure equipment manufacturers.

Staph is responsible for food poisoning and a wide range of diseases including toxic shock syndrome. Some staph bacteria are resistant to certain antibiotics—for example, the staph infection called **Methicillin-resistant Staphylococcus aureus,** (meth-uh-SILL-in resistant staf-uh-loh-KOK-is OR-ee-us) also called **MRSA.** Historically, MRSA occurred most frequently among persons with weakened immune systems, or in people who have undergone medical procedures. Today, it has become more common in otherwise healthy people—and ironically, the increased incidence of MRSA could be due to the overuse of antibiotics. The symptoms usually appear as skin infections, such as pimples and boils that can be difficult to cure and have resulted in death. Because of these highly resistant strains, it is important to clean and disinfect all tools and equipment used in the salon or spa. You owe it to yourself and your clients!

A **local infection,** such as a pimple or abscess, is one that is confined to a particular part of the body and is indicated by a lesion containing pus. A **general infection** results when the bloodstream carries the bacteria or virus and their toxins (poisons) to all parts of the body. AIDS is an example. When a disease spreads from one person to another by contact, it is said to be **contagious** (kon-TAY-jus) or **communicable** (kuh-MYOO-nih-kuh-bul). Some of the more common contagious diseases that will prevent an esthetician from servicing a client are the common cold, ringworm, conjunctivitis (pinkeye), and viral infections. The chief sources of spreading these infections are dirty hands and implements; open sores, pus, mouth and nose discharges; and shared drinking cups, telephone receivers, and towels. Uncovered coughing or sneezing and spitting in public also spread germs. The need for constant and consistent hand washing cannot be taken lightly.

Viruses

A **virus** (VY-rus) is a microscopic organism, capable of infesting almost all plants and animals, including bacteria. In humans, viruses cause the common cold, influenza, herpes, measles, chicken pox, smallpox, hepatitis, polio, and AIDS.

One difference between viruses and bacteria is that viruses live only by penetrating cells and becoming part of them, while bacteria can live on their own. Viral infections cannot be successfully treated with antibiotics, and they are hard to kill without harming the body in the process.

HIV

HIV (human immunodeficiency virus) is the virus that causes **AIDS (acquired immune deficiency syndrome).** AIDS, the disease, breaks down the body's immune system. HIV is passed from person to person through blood and other body fluids such as semen and vaginal secretions. A person can be infected with HIV for many years without having symptoms; but according to the Centers for Disease Control and Prevention, testing can determine if a person is infected within six months after exposure to the virus.

Sometimes people who are HIV-positive have never been tested and do not know they are infecting other people. HIV is transmitted through unprotected sexual contact, the sharing of needles by intravenous (IV) drug users, and accidents with needles in health-care settings. It can enter the bloodstream through cuts and sores and can be transmitted in the salon by a contaminated sharp implement. It is *not* transmitted by holding hands, hugging, kissing, sharing food or household items like the telephone, or sitting on toilet seats.

Hepatitis

Hepatitis (hep-uh-TY-tus) is a bloodborne pathogen that causes a disease marked by inflammation of the liver. This disease is caused by a virus similar to HIV in transmission. It is more easily contracted than HIV, however, because it is present in all body fluids. Unlike HIV, hepatitis can live on a surface outside the body for long periods of time. In the salon or spa facility, it is vital for all surfaces that contact a client to be thoroughly cleaned, especially if someone sneezes or coughs on them. Be sure to clean your hands after coughing or sneezing.

Three types of hepatitis are of concern for practicing estheticians and other personal service workers. They are hepatitis A, B, and C. Hepatitis B is the most difficult to kill on a surface, so check the label of the disinfectant you use to be sure that the product is effective against it. Those who work closely with the public can be vaccinated against hepatitis B. It is imperative for those working in a medical environment to receive the vaccine. In fact, if you decline to have the vaccine, you must sign a waiver relieving the clinic

THE BLOODBORNE PATHOGENS STANDARD

The likelihood of exposure to blood and body fluids increases for estheticians when performing extractions during facials, using microdermabrasion equipment, or working with postoperative patients in a medical office or spa. The OSHA Bloodborne Pathogens Standard was created to minimize the transmission of HIV and hepatitis B infections among health-care workers. Here are a few key points of the guideline:

1. *Use Universal Precautions.* This means to treat all body fluids as if they are infectious, and assume all tissue (even dead skin) is hazardous. Frequent hand washing and wearing nitrile gloves and appropriate body protection devices during treatments and cleanup are essential.

2. *Apply all work practice controls and guidelines.* This means the employer must provide protection devices such as antiseptic soaps and cleaning supplies, masks, lab coats/uniforms, eye flush stations, sharps containers (for lancets if your state allows the use), gloves, and appropriate labels for hazardous materials.

3. *Cleanliness of work areas.* The employer is to ensure a work environment that is clean and sanitary; gloves must be worn anytime during a potential exposure to blood or other potentially infected material (OPIM). All linens are to be appropriately cleaned and laundered after each client use. Eating or drinking is not allowed in work areas.

5. *Hepatitis B vaccine.* As estheticians we are considered a Group One Classification, which means that we do come in contact with body fluids while performing our jobs. It is imperative that we have the hepatitis B vaccine.

6. *Follow up after exposure.* The *employer* must make a documented confidential evaluation, called an Incident Report, detailing

   * the circumstances surrounding the event of exposure (i.e., blood or body fluid of a client or esthetician on the broken skin or an open sore of another person).

   * the route of the exposure. (Where did it come from? Where did it go?)

   * identification of the person. (Who was the source of exposure?)

   * immediate washing of the exposed area with soap and water, or flush in the case of eye exposure.

   * screening of employee and client by qualified medical personnel (Emergency Medical Occupational Medicine facility).

In addition, OSHA requires the following measures:

* The exposed employee must be tested for hepatitis A, hepatitis C, and HIV (providing consent is given).

* The source of the individual's blood must be tested for hepatitis A, hepatitis C, and HIV (providing consent is given).

* The employee must be offered medication prophylaxis, gamma globulin, or hepatitis B vaccine.

* The employee must be counseled regarding precautions to take to avoid transmission.

* OSHA 200 form must be filled out.

* The medical record of employee exposure is to be kept for 30 years, and confidentiality must be guaranteed.

of all responsibility should you contract hepatitis. All estheticians should be vaccinated for hepatitis B and remain current on any other infection control measures that become available. Under the OSHA Bloodborne Pathogens Standard, it is necessary to use personal protection devices such as gloves and eye protection during treatments because you will undoubtedly come into contact with blood or body fluids.

Bloodborne Pathogens

Disease-causing bacteria or viruses that are carried through the body in the blood or body fluids, such as hepatitis and HIV, are called **bloodborne pathogens.** If you perform extractions on a client who is HIV-positive or is infected with hepatitis and you continue to use that implement without disinfecting it, you risk puncturing your skin or cutting another client with a contaminated tool. Similar risks are present during waxing and tweezing.

How Pathogens Enter the Body

Pathogens enter the body through

* a break in the skin, such as a cut, pimple, or scratch.
* the mouth (contaminated water or food).
* the nose (air).
* the eyes.
* the ears.
* unprotected sex.

The body fights infection by means of

* unbroken skin, which is the body's first line of defense.
* body secretions, such as perspiration and digestive juices.
* white cells within the blood that destroy bacteria.
* antitoxins that counteract the toxins produced by bacteria and viruses.

Parasites

There are two types of **parasites**—those living inside (endoparasites) a host and those living outside (ectoparasites). Parasites that affect humans internally may have been acquired by ingesting raw fish or meat. The external parasites, such as ticks, fleas, or mites, have burrowed in from the skin. All parasites require a host to survive; they cannot live on their own.

Protozoa (pro-toe-ZOH-ah) are single-celled parasites with the ability to move. This type of parasitic infection is spread by eating or drinking contaminated food or water, and it causes infections such as malaria and gastroenteritis.

Parasites such as head lice can also cause contagious diseases and conditions such as **pediculosis** (puh-dik-yuh-LOH-sis) (Figure 4–8). **Scabies** (SKAY-beez), a contagious skin disease, is caused by the itch mite, which burrows under the skin (Figure 4–9).

Other types of parasites are worms such as tapeworms, hookworms, and roundworms. These parasites are typically found in areas of the world where unsanitary conditions support their growth. They can enter the body through ingestion (internal) or can burrow in from the skin (external). When traveling in tropical locations, wearing covered footwear is highly recommended to avoid a risk of a parasitic infection; also be sure that all foods ingested are fully cooked.

Contagious diseases and conditions caused by parasites should never be treated in a esthetics school or salon. Clients should be referred to a physician. Contaminated countertops should be cleaned with a pesticide or insecticide according to manufacturer's directions.

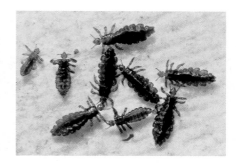

Figure 4–8 Head lice.

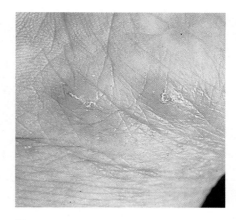

Figure 4–9 Scabies.

Fungi

Commonly known types of **fungi** (FUN-jy; **singular: fungus**) are yeast, molds, and mildew. Depending upon the type, they grow in single cells or in colonies. Fungi, also called vegetable parasites, obtain nourishment from dead organic matter, or from living organisms. Most fungi are nonpathogenic and make up many of the body's normal flora. Fungal infections usually affect the skin as they live off of *keratin*, a protein that makes up the skin. The most basic cause of fungal infections are **dermatophytes** (DUR-mah-toh-fytes), the fungi that cause skin, nail, and hair infections.

Common types of fungal infections are *Tinea pedis,* or athlete's foot; *Tinea corporis,* or ringworm; and *Onychomycosis,* a nail infection.

Other types of fungal infections are those brought about by yeast—such as *Tinea versicolor,* also called "sun spots," which is characterized by white or varicolored patches on the skin and is often found on arms and legs. *Intertrigo* is found in the body folds of the skin, such as underarms and in the groin; and *thrush* is found in the mouth and vaginal areas; both are caused by *Candida albicans,* a yeast that thrives in dark, moisture-rich environments.

Immunity

Immunity is the ability of the body to resist disease and prevent infection. Immunity against disease can be natural or acquired, and it is a sign of good health.

Natural immunity is a naturally inherited resistance to disease. A healthy individual produces white blood cells and antibodies to fight disease-causing invaders. Unbroken skin protects the body from pathogens that can invade through openings such as cuts and scratches. So we can say that our unbroken skin protects our body from invaders.

Acquired immunity is developed after the body overcomes a disease, or through inoculation (such as vaccination). Vaccinations stimulate the body's immune system so that invaders are fought off before they can cause disease. The immune system is the body's army of pathogen fighters that continue to work around the clock to keep us healthy. This is why it is so important to have a strong immune system—it has a big job to do.

PRINCIPLES OF PREVENTION

The principles of prevention are used in developing a practical plan toward infection control and decontamination in an environment. There are three levels of **decontamination.** These are sanitation, disinfection, and sterilization. Due to the low risk of infection in salons as compared to medical facilities, salons are concerned primarily with the first two. The three levels of decontamination and infection control are summarized here and described in more detail in the following sections.

1. Sanitation is the lowest level of decontamination and infection control. *Sanitation* means "to significantly reduce the number of pathogens or disease-producing organisms found on a surface." Examples of sanitation devices are ultraviolet (UV) sanitizers, antiseptics, soaps, and detergents.

2. Disinfection, the second level of decontamination and infection control, kills most microorganisms (bacteria, except bacterial spores, and some viruses) on hard, nonporous surfaces. Disinfectants are chemical agents and hospital-grade products that must be used carefully.

3. Sterilization, the highest level of decontamination and infection control, kills all microorganisms including bacteria and bacterial spores, viruses, and fungi. The primary method of sterilization is an autoclave.

Sanitation

The third, or lowest, level of decontamination is **sanitation.** To *sanitize* means "to significantly reduce the number of pathogens or disease-producing organisms found on a surface." Cleaning with soaps or detergents sanitizes salon tools and other surfaces. Putting antiseptics designed for hands or feet on your skin or washing your hands are other examples of sanitation. (Keep in mind, however, that although your hands may appear very clean when you are finished, they still harbor pathogens found in the tap water and on the towel.)

UV sanitizers, sometimes referred to as sterilizers, are metal cabinets that utilize ultraviolet rays to sanitize and store disinfected implements. UV rays are invisible, have short wavelengths, and are the least penetrating. These rays, also known as cold rays or actinic rays, produce chemical effects and kill some germs. UV sanitizers will *not* sterilize or disinfect but can be useful as clean storage containers.

Antiseptics (ant-ih-SEP-tiks) can kill, retard, or prevent the growth of bacteria, but they are not classified as disinfectants. Antiseptics are weaker than disinfectants and are safe for application to skin. They are considered sanitizers and are not adequate for use on instruments and surfaces.

All areas of the salon or spa require regular sanitizing (see the guidelines in Table 4–3). In addition, pay attention to the following:

- *Trash cans.* All receptacles should be made of a nonporous material that can be cleaned and sanitized (Figure 4–10). The most appropriate receptacle for treatment rooms is one made of metal with a lid and operated by a foot pedal. It can be lined with a disposable plastic bag.

- *Treatment rooms.* Treatment rooms normally have dim lighting and are often damp from steam or showers (Figure 4–11). If sink trim and drains are not sealed properly during initial installation, or are old, contaminated water can seep under these areas, causing mold and mildew to breed. Periodically inspect all wet rooms. Watch for rusting, mold, and other signs of deterioration.

- *Air systems.* Inadequately engineered air systems can be a means to transport allergens and pathogens through the salon or spa. Placing both an air supply and a cold air return in closed treatment rooms will result in a healthier, more comfortable environment. Other closed areas, such as showers and wet rooms, should include ventilation systems that remove steam. Ceiling grates should be cleaned monthly—or more frequently if they collect dust. Areas where caustic substances are used, such as manicuring or hairstyling areas, should have their own ventilation systems

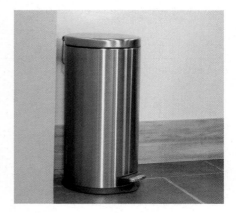

Figure 4–10 A covered, nonporous trash can with a lid should be in every treatment room, along with a trash can that has a red biohazard bag and is used for gloves and blood- or body-fluid-soaked disposable materials.

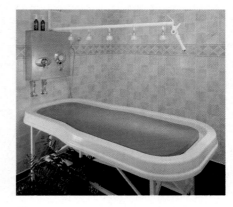

Figure 4–11 Monitor treatment rooms for mold and mildew.

Table 4–3

GUIDELINES FOR PREVENTING INFECTION		
	LEVEL OF DECONTAMINATION	**PROCEDURE**
Lancets or other facial tools and implements used to puncture or break the skin, or anything that comes in contact with pus or blood	Sterilization	Steam autoclave and dry heat. Dispose of all sharps and other disposables in a puncture-proof container.
Nonporous tools and implements such as tweezers, scissors, plastic spatulas, and so on, that have *not* come in contact with body fluids or blood	Disinfection	Complete immersion in EPA-registered, hospital-grade, bactericidal, pseudomonacidal, fungicidal, and virucidal disinfectant for amount of time specified by the manufacturer.
Nonporous tools and implements that have accidentally come in contact with blood or body fluids	Disinfection	Complete immersion in an EPA-registered disinfectant with demonstrated efficacy against HIV-1/HBV or tuberculosis for the amount of time specified by the manufacturer.
Electrotherapy tools	Disinfection	Spraying or wiping with an EPA-registered, hospital-grade disinfectant specifically made for electrical equipment.
Countertops, sinks, floors, toilets, doorknobs, mirrors, magnifying lamps, dispensary, facial beds	Sanitation	Use an EPA-registered cleaning product designed for surfaces. The efficacy label states what is appropriate for such surfaces as floors, countertops, toilets, towels, sinks, and the like.
Towels, linens, headbands	Sanitation	Laundering in hot water and detergent, with bleach or Lysol added to rinse water.
Your hands prior to each service	Sanitation	Washing with liquid antibacterial soap and warm water.

because hair care products and chemicals from nail services can cause allergic reactions in sensitive individuals. Babies and young children should never be allowed in these areas.

Disinfection

Disinfection is the process of killing most microorganisms on hard, nonporous surfaces. It is a level of decontamination second only to sterilization. Disinfection provides the level of protection required in the salon to kill most microorganisms, with one exception: it does not kill bacterial spores.

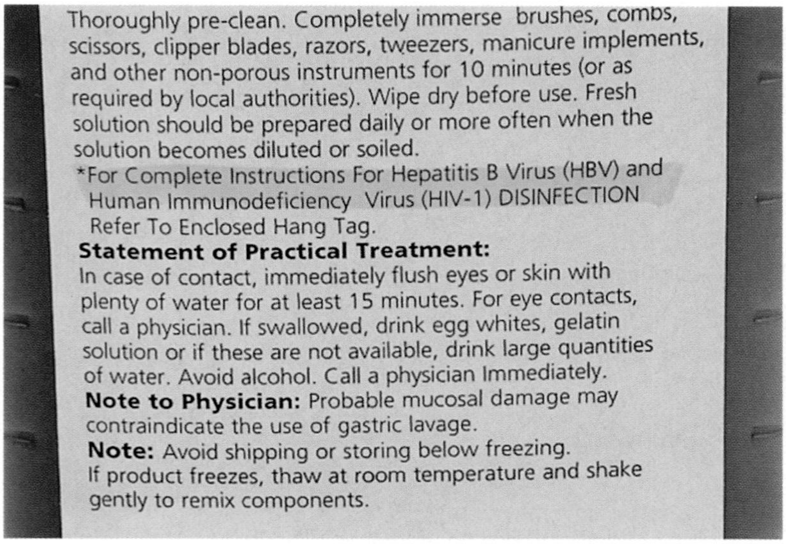

Thoroughly pre-clean. Completely immerse brushes, combs, scissors, clipper blades, razors, tweezers, manicure implements, and other non-porous instruments for 10 minutes (or as required by local authorities). Wipe dry before use. Fresh solution should be prepared daily or more often when the solution becomes diluted or soiled.

*For Complete Instructions For Hepatitis B Virus (HBV) and Human Immunodeficiency Virus (HIV-1) DISINFECTION Refer To Enclosed Hang Tag.

Statement of Practical Treatment:
In case of contact, immediately flush eyes or skin with plenty of water for at least 15 minutes. For eye contacts, call a physician. If swallowed, drink egg whites, gelatin solution or if these are not available, drink large quantities of water. Avoid alcohol. Call a physician Immediately.

Note to Physician: Probable mucosal damage may contraindicate the use of gastric lavage.

Note: Avoid shipping or storing below freezing. If product freezes, thaw at room temperature and shake gently to remix components.

Figure 4–12 A product label.

No matter how clean an object or surface may appear to the naked eye, chances are it is **contaminated**—that is, microorganisms are in or on it. Dirt, oils, and microbes are **contaminants,** which are any substances that can cause disease. Many things can be contaminants, such as makeup on a brush or cleansing cream on a cotton pad. Even tools that appear to be clean are usually covered with contaminants. It is necessary to assume that all materials are contaminated.

Of course, a salon, skin care center, spa, or even a medical spa can never be completely free from all contamination, and it would not make sense to attempt such a goal. However, it is your responsibility as a skin care professional to be on constant alert for disease-causing contaminants.

Disinfectants are chemical agents used to destroy most bacteria and some viruses and to disinfect implements and surfaces. Disinfectants are not for use on human skin, hair, or nails. Never use disinfectants as hand cleaners. Any substance powerful enough to quickly and efficiently destroy pathogens can also damage skin. Always look for the EPA registration number on the product label when choosing a disinfectant. The label will also tell you exactly which organisms the disinfectant is effective against. (Figure 4–12).

Sterilization

Sterilization is the highest level of decontamination. Sterilization kills all microorganisms, including bacteria, viruses, fungi, and bacterial spores. Comedo extractors and other tools that come into contact with blood or bodily fluids require sterilization. Methods of sterilization include the steam autoclave and dry heat.

An **autoclave** is an apparatus for sterilization by steam under pressure (Figure 4–13). Autoclaves are used in hospitals and medical offices as well as in some spas and salons. Objects such as comedone extractors, tweezers, and

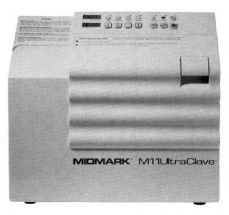

Figure 4–13 Example of an autoclave.

> ## CAUTION!
>
> In the past, formalin (a solution of formaldehyde in water) was recommended as a disinfectant and fumigant in dry cabinet sanitizers. However, formalin is not safe for salon use. Formaldehyde, a pungent gas, is a suspected cancer-causing agent. It is poisonous when inhaled and is extremely irritating to the eyes, nose, throat, and lungs. It can also cause skin allergies, irritation, dryness, and rash. After long-term use, formaldehyde vapors can cause symptoms similar to chronic bronchitis or asthma. These symptoms usually worsen over time with continued exposure.

REGULATORY AGENCY ALERT

Each state board of cosmetology has its own set of rules and regulations for sanitation. Check with your state board for your state sanitation regulations.

electrolysis needles can be autoclaved. Some items, such as glass electrodes, cannot be autoclaved because they will break. If there is an autoclave in your salon or facility, read the manufacturer's instructions to find out exactly what objects can and cannot be autoclaved.

Choosing a Disinfectant

Disinfectants are chemicals. To use a disinfectant properly, you must read and follow the manufacturer's instructions. Such variables as mixing precautions and exposure times demand particular attention. The product label will explain what the disinfectant has been tested for. To meet facility requirements, a disinfectant must have the correct **efficacy** (effectiveness) to be used against bacteria, fungi, and viruses. For a disinfectant to be considered a broad-spectrum disinfectant, and suitable for use in hospitals and health-care facilities, it must be **pseudomonacidal** (SOO-dum-ohn-uh-SIDE-ul; effective against *Pseudomonas* bacteria, "swimmers ear" and "hot tub rash" which cause itching, swelling and redness, which can be spread in spas), *bactericidal* (back-teer-uh-SYD-ul), *fungicidal* (fun-jih-SYD-ul), and *virucidal* (vy-ruh-SYD-ul). In addition, the label must state that the disinfectant is effective against specific organisms. If a disinfectant has been tested for additional organisms such as HIV-1, that information will be stated on the label.

To comply with the OSHA Bloodborne Pathogens Standard, salon and spa implements that accidentally come into contact with blood or body fluids should be cleaned and completely immersed in an EPA-registered tuberculocidal (tuh-bur-kyoo-loh-SYD-ul) disinfectant and/or a disinfectant that kills HIV-1 and hepatitis B virus.

Types of Disinfectants

A variety of disinfectants are used in the salon and spa (Figure 4–14). **Quaternary ammonium compounds** (KWAT-ur-nayr-ree uh-MOH-nee-um), commonly called **quats,** are a type of disinfectant considered non-toxic, odorless, and fast acting. Most quat solutions disinfect implements

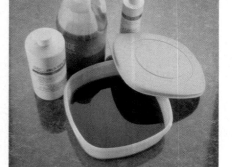

Figure 4–14 A variety of disinfectants are available for salon and spa use.

in 10 to 15 minutes. Quats are also very effective for cleaning tables and countertops.

Like quats, **phenol** (FEE-nohl; carbolic acid) has been used reliably over the years to disinfect implements. Phenol is a caustic poison, but it can be safe and extremely effective if used according to instructions. One disadvantage is that most rubber and plastic materials may be softened or discolored by phenols. Phenols in 5 percent solution are used mostly for metal implements.

In the salon, *ethyl* and *isopropyl alcohol* are sometimes used to disinfect implements. To be effective, the strength of ethyl alcohol must be no less than 70 percent, and the strength of isopropyl alcohol must be 99 percent. Because alcohol is not an EPA-registered disinfectant, it is not permitted for use with implements in states requiring hospital disinfection. This means it is not legal to use alcohol as a disinfectant in most states.

Household bleach (*sodium hypochlorite*) is an effective disinfectant, but it shares some of the same drawbacks as alcohols. Neither bleach nor alcohols are professionally designed and tested for disinfection of salon implements. Bleach is, however, an effective laundering additive.

An EPA-registered cleaning product should be used on floors, and an appropriate disinfectant specifically made for sanitizing implements should be used on all tools.

Disinfectant Safety

Disinfectants may cause serious skin and eye damage. They can be poisonous if ingested and can cause serious skin and eye damage, especially in concentrated form. A good rule is: Use caution! In addition, you should observe the following guidelines.

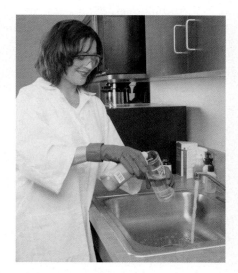

Figure 4–15 Wear gloves and safety goggles when handling disinfectants.

- Always follow manufacturer's recommendations for mixing and using, and check the efficacy to make sure you are using the right disinfectant.
- Always wear gloves and safety glasses when mixing chemicals with water (Figure 4–15).
- Always add disinfectant to water, not water to disinfectant.
- Use tongs, gloves, or a draining basket to remove implements from disinfectants.
- Never pour quats, phenol, alcohol, or any other disinfectant over your hands.
- Carefully weigh and/or measure all products to ensure that they perform at peak efficiency.
- Never place any disinfectant or other product in an unmarked container (Figure 4–16).

Jars or containers used to disinfect implements are often incorrectly called *wet sanitizers*. Of course, the purpose of these containers is not to sanitize but to disinfect. The disinfecting soak solution must be changed daily and kept free from debris, always follow the manufacturer's instructions. Containers must be large enough to completely immerse tools, materials, and implements.

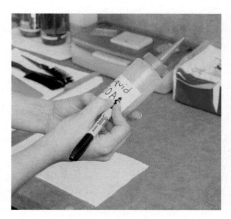

Figure 4–16 Make sure all containers are labeled.

PROCEDURE 4–1

IMPLEMENTS AND MATERIALS

Most tools and implements can be disinfected. These include scissors, tweezers, plastic spatulas, and other nonporous implements.

SUPPLIES
- gloves
- disinfectant
- disinfectant container
- water
- soap
- paper towels
- safety goggles
- implements

PROPER USE OF DISINFECTANTS

Any item that is used on a client must be disinfected or discarded after each use. Items that cannot be disinfected, such as sponges or cotton swabs, must be discarded. Electrodes, tweezers, and other nonporous tools must be sterilized or disinfected.

All implements should be thoroughly cleaned before soaking to avoid contaminating the disinfecting solution. Creams, oils, and makeup lessen the effectiveness of the solution. Always disinfect your tools or other implements according to the guidelines listed for EPA wet disinfectants. This means complete immersion for the required amount of time. The following are guidelines for specific salon materials.

Preparation

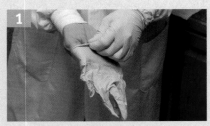

Put on gloves, goggles, or safety glasses. *(Figure P4-1-1)*

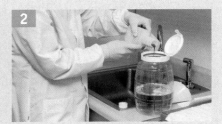

Always add disinfectant to water. *(Figure P4-1-2)*

1 Put on gloves, goggles, or safety glasses (Figure P4-1-1).

2 Mix disinfectant according to manufacturer's directions, always adding disinfectant to the water in the disinfectant container so no disinfectant can splash up or out of the container. (Figure P4-1-2).

Procedure

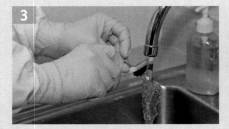

Preclean to remove all visible debris and reside from tools and implements. *(Figure P4–1-3)*

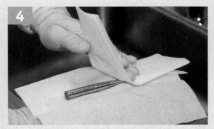

Rinse items thoroughly and pat dry with a clean towel. *(Figure P4-1-4)*

3 Pre-clean to remove hair, filings and debris, and other such loose matter by scrubbing implements with soap and water (Figure P4-1-3).

4 Rinse items thoroughly and pat dry with a clean towel (Figure P4-1-4).

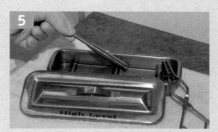

Completely immerse implements or tools for the required amount of time. *(Figure P4–1-5)*

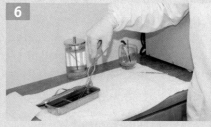

Remove implements with tongs, basket, or gloves. *(Figure P4–1-6)*

5 Using gloves or tongs, completely immerse implements or tools and leave for the required amount of time, per manufacturer's instructions (Figure P4–1-5).

6 Remove implements with clean tongs, basket, or gloves so as not to contaminate the disinfectant. Rinse thoroughly and dry (Figure P4–1-6).

Clean-up

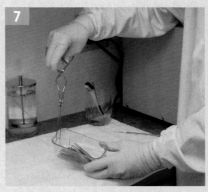

Place disinfected implements in a clean, closed, dry, disinfected container. *(Figure P4–1-7)*

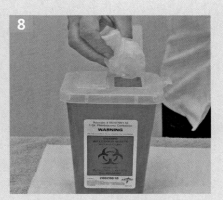

Clean up the work station, including glove disposal and other sanitation measures. *(Figure P4–1-8)*

7 Place disinfected implements in a clean, closed, dry, disinfected container (such as a plastic container with a lid) (Figure P4–1-7).

8 Clean up the workstation, including glove disposal and other sanitation measures (Figure P4–1-8).

Linens

All linens should be used once and then sanitized by laundering with bleach. Soiled laundry should be handled with gloves and placed in a closed, lined receptacle until it is washed. Add chlorine bleach along with the soap powder. Keep clean towels in a closed closet or cabinet until needed.

Laundry hampers or bins should be cleaned daily with disinfectant. Laundry should be done regularly rather than left for the next day. If damp linens are left in a laundry cart, fungus and mold may grow not only on the linens, but on the cart as well if it is made of canvas.

Electrical Equipment

The contact points of equipment (parts that come in contact with a client's skin) that cannot be immersed in liquid, such as electrotherapy tools, should be wiped or sprayed with an EPA-registered, hospital-grade disinfectant created especially for electrical equipment. Electrical equipment must be kept in good repair.

Workstation

Before and after performing services on each client, an EPA-registered, hospital-grade disinfectant should be used on the workstation, facial chair, stainless steel bowls, and other supplies. Leave the disinfectant on the surface for the full amount of time prescribed by the manufacturer's directions. Remember to disinfect *all* surfaces, including doorknobs, handles, and so on.

Cross-Contamination

Any disinfected item that has been touched or exposed to air is contaminated. **Cross-contamination** occurs when you, the esthetician, touch an object such as the skin without sanitizing your hands, and then touch an object or product with the same hand or utensil. You must use properly disinfected tools, and you must never touch clean items with hands that have been exposed to the client's skin (Figure 4–17).

Spatulas are flexible implements with blunt blades used to remove a product from its jar without contaminating the product by touching it with your hands. A product can be safely used after it is removed from the container, as long as it is used only on one client. Once a product has been removed from a jar or container, it should never be put back into the container and spatulas should never be put back into the container to avoid contaminating the product. Spatulas must be properly disinfected or disposed of after each use. Some estheticians use children's tongue depressors as spatulas. These are disposable and are used only once. Plastic spatulas can be disinfected and reused.

Any nondisposable object that touches a client's skin must be properly disinfected before it is reused. Nondisposable items include plastic spatulas; mask brushes; towels, sheets, and linens; machine attachments; electrodes;

CAUTION!

Mixing chemicals in higher concentrations than recommended by the manufacturer counteracts their effectiveness and may create noxious fumes or harm instruments.

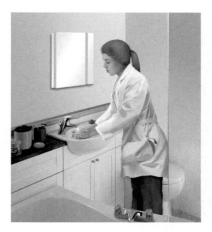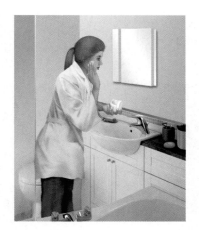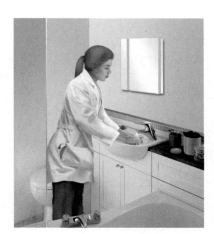

Figure 4–17 Preventing cross-contamination.

headbands; and client gowns. Any object that is exposed to blood or bodily fluids must be discarded, autoclaved, or sterilized.

All disposable supplies should be thrown away after use. These include esthetician's gloves, sponges, cotton, cotton swabs, tongue depressors, paper towels, tissues, and disposable makeup utensils such as mascara wands and disposable lip brushes (Figure 4–18).

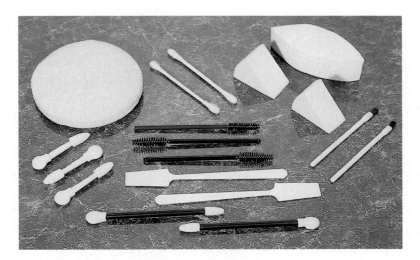

Figure 4–18 Use disposable makeup applicators.

PROCEDURE 4–2

ASEPTIC PROCEDURE

SUPPLIES
- cotton
- swabs
- sponges
- gauze
- brushes
- spatulas
- tweezers
- comedo extractors
- electrodes
- wax strips
- gloves

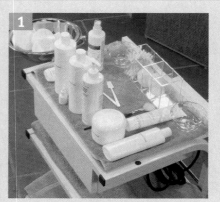

Lay out implements and materials before beginning a service. *(Figure P4–2-1)*

An **aseptic procedure** is the process of properly handling sterilized and disinfected equipment and supplies so that they do not become contaminated by microorganisms before they are used on a client. The following is a good example of an aseptic procedure.

1 Set up for the service. Before beginning any treatment, wash your hands using proper sanitizing methods. Lay out on a clean towel all implements that you will use during the treatment (Figure P4–2-1), such as cotton, swabs, sponges, and so forth. To prevent airborne contact, cover with another clean towel until you are ready to start the treatment. By prearranging these utensils, you will be less likely to need to open a container to get more supplies. This not only prevents cross-contamination but is also more efficient. Once you have begun a treatment, never open any package or container or touch a product without a spatula or tongs. Touching any object with gloved hands that have touched the client will contaminate that object. Any object touched during treatment must be discarded, disinfected, or autoclaved.

Procedure

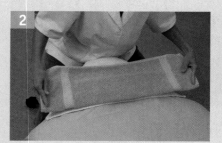

Use clean, towels, sheets, headband or plastic cap, and gown for each client. *(Figure P4–2-2)*

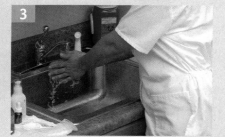

Wash and sanitize your hands after touching a client's hair. *(Figure P4–2-3)*

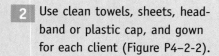

2 Use clean towels, sheets, headband or plastic cap, and gown for each client (Figure P4–2-2).

3 Wash and sanitize your hands after touching a client's hair (Figure P4–2-3).

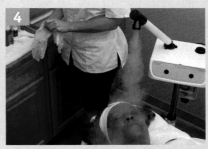

Gloves should be worn for safety and hygiene. *(Figure P4–2-4)*

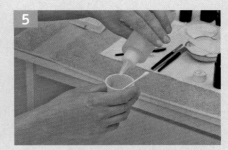

Remove products before the treatment and place them in small disposable cups. *(Figure P4–2-5)*

4 Put on gloves at the beginning of every treatment, and wear them throughout the treatment (Figure P4-2-4). This is especially important during and after extraction, waxing, or electrolysis.

5 Remove creams and products from containers using pumps, squeeze bottles with dispenser caps, or disinfected spatulas. It is best to remove products before the treatment and place them in small disposable cups

(Figure P4–2-5). This way you will not have to touch bottles or jars with soiled gloved hands. Spatulas should be disinfected or discarded after each use.

Clean-Up

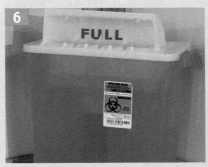

Dispose of lancets and other sharp implements in a sharps box. *(Figure P4-2-6)*

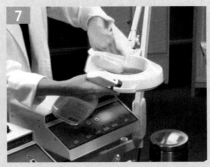

Wipe down all surfaces touched during treatment with a disinfectant before your next client. *(Figure P4–2-7)*

6 After completing the treatment, place linens in a covered laundry receptacle. Throw away disposable items in a closed trash container. Place sharps in a sharps box (Figure P4–2-6). Disinfect or sterilize all items to be reused. Discard any unused product that has been removed from its container.

7 Wipe down all surfaces touched during treatment with a disinfectant before the next client is seated. (Figure P4–2-7).

PROCEDURE 4-3

HAND WASHING

SUPPLIES
- paper towels
- soap
- nail brush
- warm water

Procedure

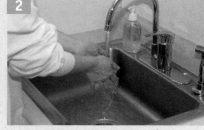

Turn on faucet with a clean, dry paper towel. *(Figure P4–3-1)*

1 Use a paper towel to turn faucet on, if it is not automatic (Figure P4-3-1).

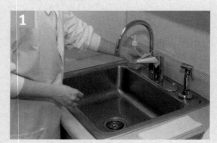

Dampen hands with warm water. *(Figure P4-3-2)*

2 Dampen hands with warm water (Figure P4-3-2).

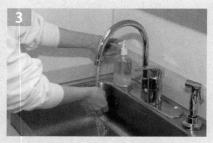

Apply soap and massage hands thoroughly, including nails and fingers. *(Figure P4–3-3)*

3 Apply soap and massage hands thoroughly, including nails and fingers (Figure P4-3-3).

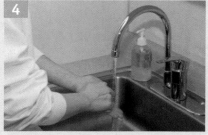

Lather with soap and scrub hands for 20–30 seconds. *(Figure P4-3-4)*

4 Lather with soap and scrub hands thoroughly for 20 to 30 seconds (Figure P4-3-4).

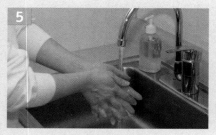

Rinse hands with warm water. *(Figure P4–3-5)*

5 Rinse hands with warm water (Figure P4-3-5).

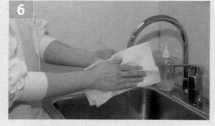

Dry with paper towel. *(Figure P4-3-6)*

6 Dry hands with paper towel (Figure P4-3-6).

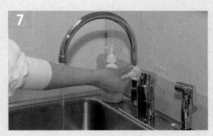

Turn faucet off with additional clean paper towel. *(Figure P4–3-7)*

7   Turn faucet off using an additional clean paper towel (Figure P4–3-7).

Clean-up

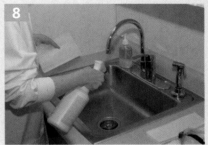

Disinfect sink after each service. *(Figure P4–3-8)*

8   Disinfect sink after each service (Figure P4-3-8).

CAUTION!

All gloves are to be removed by turning them inside out and pulling them off. Think dirty to dirty, and clean to clean. After removing gloves, dispose of them in the appropriately marked (biohazard) trash can. This prevents the transfer of microorganisms and accidental contamination.

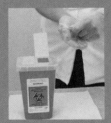

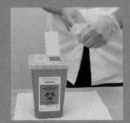

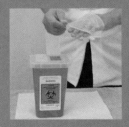

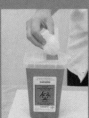

Figure 4–19 Pull top of glove inside out from the outside with opposite gloved hand.

Figure 4–20 Pull glove completely off inside out with opposite gloved hand.

Figure 4–21 With free hand, pull off remaining glove, touching only the inside.

Figure 4–22 Dispose off gloves in an appropriate biohazard container.

UNIVERSAL PRECAUTIONS

The **Universal Precautions** are a set of guidelines published by OSHA that require the employer and the employee to assume that all human blood and body fluids are infectious for bloodborne pathogens. Because it is impossible to identify clients with infectious diseases, the same infection control practices should be used with all clients. In most instances, clients who are infected with hepatitis B virus or other bloodborne pathogens are **asymptomatic**, which means that they show no symptoms or signs of infection. Bloodborne pathogens are more difficult to kill than germs that live outside the body.

OSHA sets safety standards and precautions that protect employees when they are potentially exposed to bloodborne pathogens. Precautions include hand washing, wearing gloves, and proper handling and disposal of sharp instruments and items that have been contaminated by blood or other body fluids. It is important that specific procedures are followed if blood or body fluid is present.

Contact with Blood or Body Fluid

Accidents happen. If a client's skin is cut during a salon service, blood or body fluid can be present—this is called an **exposure incident.** If this should occur, follow these steps for the client's safety as well as yours:

1. If a cut occurs during service, stop the service.
2. Wear gloves to protect yourself against contact with the client's blood.
3. Clean the injured area with an antiseptic—each salon must have a first aid kit.
4. Bandage the cut with an adhesive bandage.
5. Clean your workstation as necessary.
6. Discard contaminated objects. Discard all disposable contaminated objects such as wipes or cotton balls by double-bagging (place the waste in a plastic bag and then in a trash bag). Use a biohazard sticker (red or orange) or a container for contaminated waste. Deposit sharp disposables in a sharps box (Figure 4–23).
7. Disinfect tools and implements. Remember, before removing your gloves, that all tools and implements that have come into contact with blood or other body fluids must be thoroughly cleaned and completely immersed in an EPA-registered, hospital-grade disinfectant solution. Because blood can carry pathogens, you should never touch an open sore or wound.
8. Remove your gloves. Wash your hands with soap and warm water before returning to the service.

FIRST AID

Because emergencies arise in every line of business, knowledge of basic first aid is invaluable. Every esthetician should know CPR (cardiopulmonary resuscitation) and should have some first aid training. You

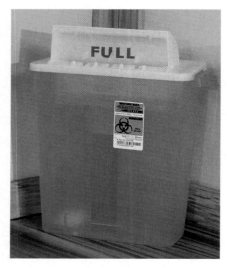

Figure 4–23 Dispose off lancets and other sharp implements in a sharps box.

CAUTION!

Because blood can carry many pathogens, you should never touch a client's open sore or wound without wearing gloves.

CAUTION!

Avoid using bar soap in the salon. Bar soap can actually encourage bacterial growth. It is a better practice to provide pump-type liquid soaps.

can obtain this training through your local trade or technical college. Emergency medical technicians (EMTs) or an ambulance should be called as soon as possible after any accident has occurred. Do *not* recommend treatment for specific emergencies—always call a medical professional or 911.

In Case of Emergency

Every salon, spa, and medical facility should have current emergency contact information posted clearly by each telephone. The emergency contact list should include the following information: fire department, police (local and state), ambulance, nearest hospital emergency room, poison control center.

Each employee should know where exits are located and how to evacuate the building efficiently in case of fire or other emergency. Yearly fire drills or evacuation procedures should be performed just to keep everyone informed on how to clear safely out of a building. Fire extinguishers should be placed where they can be reached easily, and employees should know how to use them. Employees should have regular training on how to operate these devices, and they should know exactly where they are located. A well-stocked first aid kit should be kept within easy reach.

Basic First Aid Knowledge

Estheticians are not medical personnel. However, anyone who works with the public should have a working knowledge of first aid as it pertains to the work environment. People who can administer first aid are also good citizens in their community. It makes good sense to know how to apply pressure to a bleeding wound, or how to dress a burn, or what to do if someone chokes, and it will certainly come in handy should you come across a situation that requires such knowledge (Figure 4–24).

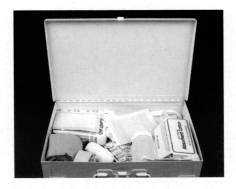

Figure 4–24 Having a well-stocked first aid kit is necessary.

Burns

There are four levels of burns (Figure 4–25, a–d). They are identified as follows:

1. *First degree.* A minor burn affecting the upper layers of the skin, primarily the epidermis, with some redness and irritation, but no blisters or open skin.
2. *Second degree.* This level of burn affects the top two layers of the skin, the epidermis and the dermis. It is more painful than the first-degree burn and will show redness and blisters.
3. *Third degree.* This burn affects all layers of the skin and will blister, swell, and scar. The pain associated with a third-degree burn depends on the amount of nerve damage that has taken place.
4. *Fourth degree.* These are burns that have injured the muscle, ligaments, tendons, nerves, blood vessels, and bones. These burns always require medical attention.

> **? Did You Know**
>
> A first aid kit at a minimum should include these items: small bandages, gauze, antiseptic, and a blood spill kit that contains disposable bags, gloves, and hazardous waste stickers.

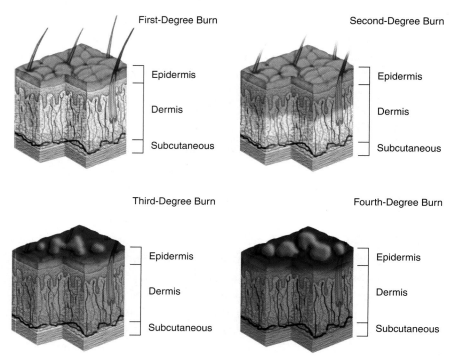

Figure 4–25a–d The four degrees of burns.

Eye Flush

Eye-flushing stations are important to an esthetician working in any type of setting. As always, prevention is the best answer to warding off problems with product getting into a client's eye. Have them wear eye protection during treatments. However, accidents do happen; and when they do, you must be proactive. Take the client to the nearest available sink or eye-flushing station. Gently flush the eye with water for 15 minutes, and have the client seek medical attention immediately.

THE PROFESSIONAL SALON AND SPA IMAGE

Cleanliness should be a part of your normal routine as well as of those who work with you. This way, you and your coworkers can project a steadfast professional image. Here are some simple guidelines that will keep the salon/spa looking its best.

- Keep floors clean. Mop floors and vacuum carpets every day.
- Keep trash in a waste receptacle; covered containers may be necessary by mandate of your state regulatory agency and to reduce odors and to look more professional.
- Control dust, hair, and other debris.
- Clean fans, ventilation systems, and humidifiers at least once each week.
- Keep all work areas well lit.
- Keep restrooms clean, including door handles.
- Provide toilet tissue, paper towels, liquid soap, and clean, soft-bristle nail brushes in the restroom.

WEB RESOURCES

Check out these Web sites for more information on the topics discussed in this chapter:

http://www.hipaacompliance.biz

http://www.osharegulations101.com

http://www.ncea.com

http://www.medicinenet.com

http://www.cellsalive.com

http://www.niehs.nih.gov

- Do not allow the salon/spa to be used for cooking or living quarters.
- Never place food in the refrigerators used to store products.
- Prohibit eating, drinking, and smoking in areas where services are performed or where clients may be.
- Empty waste receptacles regularly throughout the day. A waste receptacle with a self-closing lid works best.
- Make sure all containers are properly marked and properly stored.
- Never place any tools or implements in your mouth or pockets.
- Properly clean and disinfect all tools after each use.
- Store clean and disinfected tools in a clean container, or use another sanitary method. Clean drawers may be used for storage if only clean items are stored in them.
- Avoid touching your face, mouth, or eye areas during services.
- Clean all work surfaces after every client service. This includes manicure and facial chairs and tables, workstations, and bowls.
- Always use clean linens on clients, and use disposable towels and linens. Keep soiled linens separate from clean linens.
- Use exhaust systems in the salon. Replacing the air in the salon with fresh air at least four times every hour is recommended to ensure proper air quality.

YOUR PROFESSIONAL RESPONSIBILITY

You have many responsibilities as a salon professional. Nothing is more important than your responsibility to protect your clients' health and safety as well as your own. Never take shortcuts when it comes to sanitation and disinfection. Understand and comply with all government regulations. Remember, this is a hands-on profession. If you are to be an effective practitioner you must learn the rules, and you must always follow them to the letter of the law. This is how you, your colleagues, and your clients can maintain a sense of mutual trust and respect.

REVIEW QUESTIONS

1. What is an MSDS?

2. What are bacteria?

3. Name and describe the two main classifications of bacteria.

4. Name and describe the three forms of pathogenic bacteria.

5. How are viruses different from bacteria?

REVIEW QUESTIONS

6. How does AIDS affect the body? How is it transmitted? How is it not transmitted?

7. What is a contagious or communicable disease?

8. What is the difference between a local and a general infection?

9. Define immunity, and name the two types.

10. What is decontamination? Explain the three levels of decontamination.

11. List and describe three types of disinfectants.

12. Explain how to disinfect the following: nonporous implements, linens, electrical tools that cannot be immersed, and work surfaces.

13. List at least six precautions to follow when using disinfectants.

14. Describe the procedure for taking care of an exposure incident.

15. What are Universal Precautions?

CHAPTER GLOSSARY

acquired immunity: immunity developed after the body overcomes a disease, or through inoculation.

AIDS: acquired immune deficiency syndrome; a disease caused by the HIV virus that breaks down the body's immune system.

antiseptics: agents that may kill, retard, or prevent the growth of bacteria.

aseptic procedure: process of properly handling sterilized and disinfected equipment and supplies so that they do not become contaminated by microorganisms until they are used on a client.

asymptomatic: showing no symptoms or signs of infection.

autoclave: apparatus for sterilization by steam under pressure.

bacilli (singular: bacillus): short, rod-shaped bacteria; the most common bacteria; produce diseases such as tetanus (lockjaw), typhoid fever, tuberculosis, and diphtheria.

bacteria: one-celled microorganisms with both plant and animal characteristics; also known as microbes.

bactericidal: capable of destroying bacteria.

bloodborne pathogens: disease-causing bacteria or viruses that are carried through the body in the blood or body fluids.

cilia: hairlike extensions that protrude from cells and help to sweep away fluids and particles.

cocci: round bacteria that appear alone or in groups.

communicable: when a disease spreads from one person to another by contact.

contagious: communicable or transmittable by contact.

contaminants: substances that can cause contamination.

contaminated: when an object or product has microorganisms in or on it.

cross-contamination: contamination that occurs when you touch an object, such as the skin, and then touch an object or product with the same hand or utensil.

decontamination: removal of pathogens and other substances from tools and surfaces.

dermatophytes: a type of fungi that cause skin, hair, and nail infections.

diplococci: spherical bacteria that grow in pairs and cause diseases such as pneumonia.

disinfectants: chemical agents used to destroy most bacteria, fungi, and viruses and to disinfect implements and surfaces.

disinfection: second-highest level of decontamination, nearly as effective as sterilization but does not kill bacterial spores; used on hard, nonporous surfaces.

efficacy: effectiveness.

exposure incident: a specific contact of a client's blood or other potentially infectious materials (OPIM) with the esthetician's eyes, mouth, or other mucous membranes as a result of performing services and duties.

flagella (singular: flagellum): long threads attached to the cell to help it move.

fungi (singular: fungus): vegetable (plant) parasites, including molds, mildews, and yeasts.

fungicidal: capable of destroying fungi.

general infection: infection that results when the bloodstream carries pathogens and their toxins (poisons) to all parts of the body.

hepatitis: disease marked by inflammation of the liver and caused by a bloodborne virus.

HIV: human immunodeficiency virus; virus that causes AIDS.

immunity: ability of the body to resist infection and destroy pathogens that have infected the body.

infection: the invasion of body tissues by disease-causing pathogenic bacteria.

local infection: infection that is confined to a particular part of the body and is indicated by a lesion containing pus.

Material Safety Data Sheet (MSDS): material Safety Data Sheet; information compiled by a manufacturer about its product, ranging from ingredient content and associated hazards to combustion levels and storage requirements.

Methicillin-resistant Staphylococcus aureus (MRSA): a highly resistant form of staph infection that can be caused by the overuse of antibiotics.

microorganism: any organism of microscopic to submicroscopic size.

motility: cell motility refers to single-celled organisms and their ability to move in their environment.

natural immunity: an inherent resistance to disease.

nitrile gloves: gloves made from synthetic rubbers known as acrylonitrile and butadiene; these gloves are resistant to tears, punctures, chemicals, and solvents.

nonpathogenic: not harmful; not disease producing.

parasite: organism that lives in or on another organism and draws its nourishment from that organism.

pathogenic: causing disease; harmful.

pediculosis: skin disease caused by infestation with head lice.

phenol: carbolic acid; a caustic poison; used for peels and to sanitize metallic implements.

protozoa: single-celled parasites with the ability to move; they can divide and grow only when inside a host.

pseudomonacidal: capable of destroying *Pseudomonas* bacteria.

pus: fluid product of inflammation that contains white blood cells and the debris of dead cells, tissue elements, and bacteria.

quaternary ammonium compounds (quats): disinfectants that are considered nontoxic, odorless, and fast acting.

sanitation: third level of decontamination; significantly reduces the number of pathogens or disease-producing organisms found on a surface.

scabies: contagious skin disease caused by an itch mite burrowing under the skin.

spirilla: spiral or corkscrew-shaped bacteria that cause syphilis, Lyme disease, and other diseases.

CHAPTER GLOSSARY

staphylococci: pus-forming bacteria that grow in clusters like a bunch of grapes; cause abscesses, pustules, and boils.

sterilization: highest level of decontamination; completely kills every organism on a nonporous surface.

streptococci: pus-forming bacteria arranged in curved lines resembling a string of beads; cause infections such as strep throat and blood poisoning.

tuberculocidal: capable of destroying the bacteria that cause tuberculosis.

tuberculosis: a bacterial disease that usually affects the lungs.

Universal Precautions: set of guidelines and controls, published by OSHA, that require the employer and the employee to assume that all human blood and specified human body fluids are infectious for HIV, hepatitis B virus, and other bloodborne pathogens.

virucidal: capable of destroying viruses.

virus: microorganism that can invade plants and animals, including bacteria.

CHAPTER OUTLINE

GENERAL ANATOMY AND PHYSIOLOGY

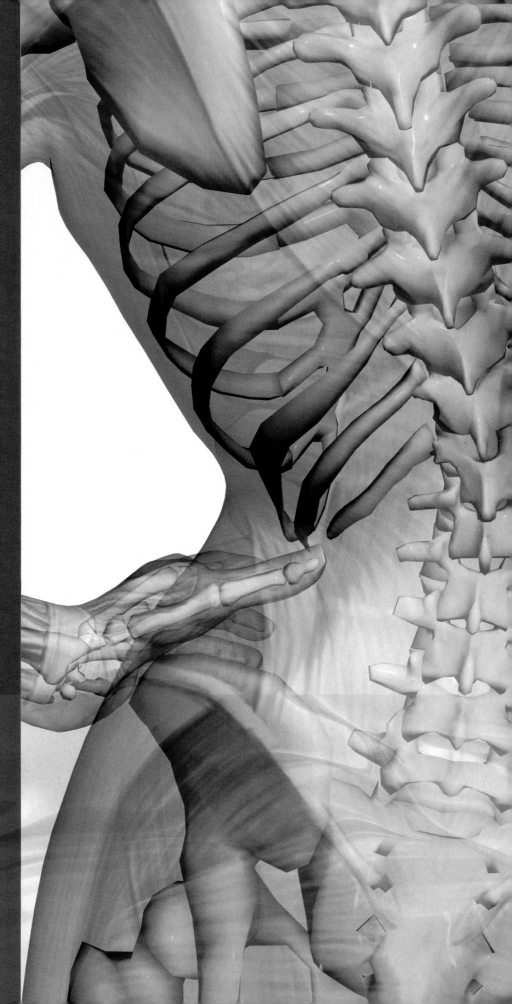

LEARNING OBJECTIVES

After completing this chapter, you will be able to:

- Explain why the study of anatomy, physiology, and histology is important to the esthetician.

- Describe cells, their structure, and their reproduction.

- Define tissue and identify the types of tissues found in the body.

- Name the 11 main body systems and explain their basic functions.

KEY TERMS

Page numbers indicate where in the chapter each term is used.

absorption 119

anabolism 97

anatomy 95

angular artery 116

anterior auricular
   artery 116

aponeurosis 103

arteries 114

atrium 114

auricularis anterior 103

auricularis posterior 103

auricularis superior 103

auriculotemporal
   nerve 110

autonomic nervous
   system 108

axon 110

belly (muscle) 103

biceps 106

blood 114

brain 109

brain stem 109

buccal nerve 112

buccinator 105

capillaries 114

cardiac muscle 103

carpus 102

catabolism 97

cell membrane 96

cells 95

central nervous
   (cerebrospinal)
   system 107

cerebellum 109

cerebrum 109

cervical cutaneous
   nerve 112

cervical nerves 112

cervical vertebrae 101

circulatory system 113

clavicle 102

common carotid
   arteries 115

connective tissue 97

corrugator muscle 104

cranium 100

cytoplasm 96

defecation 119

deltoid 106

dendrites 110

deoxyribonucleic acid
   (DNA) 96

depressor labii
   inferioris 105

diaphragm 119

diencephalon 109

digestion 119

digestive enzymes 118

digestive system 118

digital nerve 113

eleventh cranial
   nerve (accessory) 112

endocrine (ductless)
   glands 117

endocrine system 117

epicranius 103

epithelial tissue 97

ethmoid bone 101

excretory system 119

exocrine (duct)
   glands 117

extensors 106

external carotid
   artery 115

external jugular
   vein 116

facial artery 116

fifth cranial nerve 110

flexors 106

frontal artery 116

frontal bone 101

frontalis 103

glands 117

greater auricular
   nerve 112

greater occipital
   nerve 112

heart 113

hemoglobin 115

histology 95

hormones 117

humerus 102

hyoid bone 101

immune or lymphatic
   system 117

inferior labial artery 116

infraorbital artery 116

infraorbital nerve 110

infratrochlear nerve 111

ingestion 119

insertion 103

integumentary
   system 120

internal carotid artery 115

internal jugular vein 116

interstitial 117

joint 100

lacrimal bones 101

latissimus dorsi 106

levator anguli oris 105

levator labii superioris 105

lungs 119

lymph 117

lymph capillaries 117

lymph nodes 117

lymphatic or immune
   system 117

mandible 101

mandibular nerve 110, 112

masseter 104

maxillary bones 101

maxillary nerve 110

median nerve 113

W hether applying product, giving a treatment or doing a skin care analysis, as licensed estheticians, we are permitted to touch people as part of our profession. This is true of very few other occupations, and it is an honor to be able to aid others in a greater sense of well-being.

WHY STUDY ANATOMY?

As an esthetic professional, an overview of human anatomy and physiology will enable you to

- understand how the human body functions as an integrated whole.
- recognize changes from the norm.
- determine a scientific basis for the proper application of services and products such as facials and hand and arm massages.

Anatomy (ah-NAT-oh-me) is the study of the structures of the human body that can be seen with the naked eye, and what they are made up of. It is the science of the structure of organisms, or of their parts.

Physiology (fiz-ih-OL-oh-jee) is the study of the functions and activities performed by the body structures.

Histology (his-TAHL-uh-jee) is the study of the tiny structures found in living tissue, that is, microscopic anatomy.

Estheticians focus primarily on the muscles, bones, nerves, and circulation of the head, neck, arms, and hands. Understanding this anatomy and physiology will help you develop your skills and perform your work safely.

CELLS

Any discussion of anatomy and physiology must begin with **cells,** the basic unit of all living things, from bacteria to plants to animals to human beings. Without cells, life does not exist. As a basic functional unit, the cell is responsible for carrying on all life processes. There are trillions of cells in the human body, and they vary widely in size, shape, and purpose.

Basic Construction of the Cell

The cells of all living things are composed of a substance called **protoplasm** (PROH-toh-plaz-um). Protoplasm is a colorless, jellylike substance in which food elements such as proteins, fats, carbohydrates, mineral salts, and water are present. You can visualize the protoplasm of a cell as being similar to the white of a raw egg.

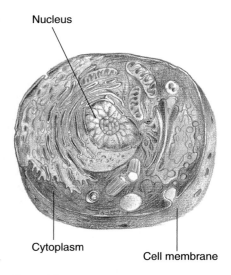

Figure 5–1 Anatomy of the cell.

In addition to protoplasm, most cells also include the following (Figure 5–1).

* The **nucleus** (NOO-klee-us) is the dense, active protoplasm found in the center of the cell. It plays an important part in cell reproduction and metabolism. You can visualize the nucleus as the yolk of a raw egg. Within the nucleus of the cell is the **nucleoplasm,** which is a fluid that contains proteins, and a very important acid known as **deoxyribonucleic acid** (DEE-ok-see-RYE-boh-noo-KLEE-ik ASS-id) or **DNA.** DNA is what determines our genetic makeup including the color of our eyes, skin, and hair.
* The **cytoplasm** (sy-toh-PLAZ-um) is all the protoplasm of a cell except that found in the nucleus. This watery fluid contains the food material necessary for cell growth, reproduction, and self-repair.
* The **cell membrane** encloses the protoplasm and permits soluble substances to enter and leave the cell.

Cell Reproduction and Division

Cells have the ability to reproduce, thus providing new cells for the growth and replacement of worn or injured ones. Most cells reproduce by dividing into two identical cells called daughter cells (Figure 5–2). This process is known as **mitosis** (my-TOH-sis). As long as conditions are favorable, the cell will grow and reproduce. Favorable conditions include an adequate supply of food, oxygen, and water; suitable temperatures; and the ability to

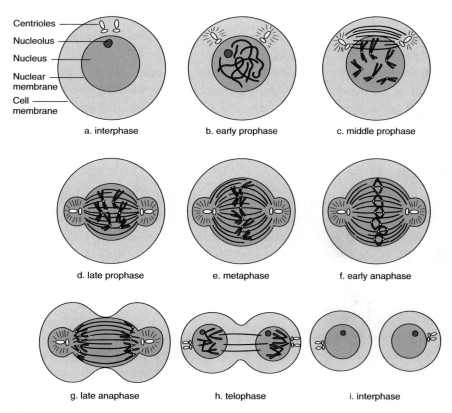

Figure 5–2 Phases of mitosis.

eliminate waste products. If conditions become unfavorable, the cell will become impaired or may be destroyed. Unfavorable conditions include toxins (poison), environmental damage, and disease.

Cell Metabolism

Metabolism (muh-TAB-uh-liz-um) is a chemical process that takes place in living organisms. Through metabolism, the cells are nourished and carry out their activities. Metabolism has two phases, anabolism and catabolism, that are carried out simultaneously and continually within the cells.

1. **Anabolism** (uh-NAB-uh-liz-um) is constructive metabolism, the process of *building up* larger molecules from smaller ones. During this process, the body stores water, food, and oxygen for the time when these substances will be needed for cell growth and repair.

2. **Catabolism** (kuh-TAB-uh-liz-um) is the phase of metabolism in which complex compounds within the cells are *broken down* into smaller ones. This process releases energy that is stored by special molecules to be used in muscle contractions, body secretions, or heat production.

TISSUES

A **tissue** (TISH-oo) is a collection of similar cells that perform a particular function. Each tissue has a specific function and can be recognized by its characteristic appearance. Body tissues are composed of large amounts of water, along with various other substances. There are four types of tissue in the body.

1. **Connective tissue** supports, protects, and binds together other tissues of the body. Examples of connective tissue are bone, cartilage, ligaments, tendons, fascia (which separates muscles), and fat or adipose tissue. Collagen and elastin are protein fibers also located in the connective tissue.

2. **Epithelial tissue** (ep-ih-THEE-lee-ul) is a protective covering on body surfaces. Examples are skin, mucous membranes, and the lining of the heart, digestive and respiratory organs, and glands.

3. **Muscular tissue** contracts and moves the various parts of the body.

4. **Nerve tissue** carries messages to and from the brain and controls and coordinates all bodily functions. Nerve tissue is composed of special cells known as neurons, which make up the nerves, brain, and spinal cord.

ORGANS AND BODY SYSTEMS

Organs are groups of tissues designed to perform a specific function. Table 5–1 lists some of the most important organs of the body.

Body systems are groups of bodily organs acting together to perform one or more functions. The human body is composed of 11 major systems (Table 5–2).

?   Did You Know

Have you ever wondered why someone has green eyes instead of brown, or red hair instead of blond? It is because of the genetic information enclosed within the DNA (deoxyribonucleic acid) located in the nucleus of the cell. The DNA determines all of the cell's functions and characteristics, and the information is transferred at conception. As an esthetician working with all sorts of people, you will become aware of how a person's genetic code will largely determine his or her appearance.

?   Did You Know

An average adult body is 50 to 65 percent water—which equals roughly 45 quarts. Men's bodies contain more water than women's bodies do. A man's body is 60 to 65 percent water, compared to 50 to 60 percent for a woman. In infants, the figure is a whopping 70 percent. Water content differs throughout various tissues in the body; for instance, blood is made up of 83 percent water, and muscle is 75 percent water.

Table 5–1

SOME MAJOR BODY ORGANS AND THEIR FUNCTIONS	
ORGAN	**FUNCTION**
brain	Controls the body.
eyes	Control vision.
heart	Circulates the blood.
kidneys	Excrete water and waste products.
lungs	Supply oxygen to the blood.
liver	Removes toxic products of digestion.
skin	Forms external protective covering of the body.
stomach and intestines	Digest food.

Table 5–2

BODY SYSTEMS AND THEIR FUNCTIONS	
SYSTEM	**FUNCTION**
circulatory	Controls the steady circulation of the blood through the body by means of the heart and blood vessels.
digestive	Changes food into nutrients and wastes; consists of mouth, stomach, intestines, salivary and gastric glands, and other organs.
endocrine	Affects the growth, development, sexual activities, and health of the entire body; consists of specialized glands.
excretory	Purifies the body by the elimination of waste matter; consists of kidneys, liver, skin, intestines, and lungs.
integumentary	Serves as a protective covering and helps in regulating the body's temperature; consists of skin, accessory organs such as oil and sweat glands, sensory receptors, hair, and nails.
muscular	Covers, shapes, and supports the skeleton tissue; also contracts and moves various parts of the body; consists of muscles.
nervous	Controls and coordinates all other systems and makes them work harmoniously and efficiently; consists of brain, spinal cord, and nerves.
reproductive	Responsible for processes by which plants and animals produce offspring.
respiratory	Enables breathing, supplying the body with oxygen, and eliminating carbon dioxide as a waste product; consists of lungs and air passages.
skeletal	Physical foundation of the body; consists of the bones and movable and immovable joints.
lymphatic or immune	Protects the body from disease by developing immunities and destroying disease-causing microorganisms.

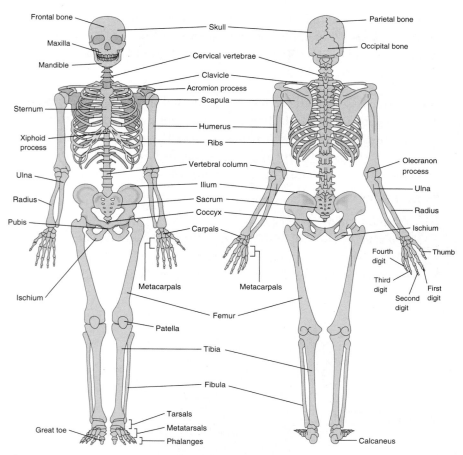

Figure 5–3 The skeletal system.

THE SKELETAL SYSTEM

The **skeletal system** is the physical foundation of the body (Figure 5–3). The skeletal system serves many important functions; it provides the shape and form for our bodies in addition to supporting, protecting, allowing bodily movement, producing blood for the body, and storing minerals.

The skeleton has 206 bones that form a rigid framework to which the softer tissues and organs of the body are attached. Muscles are connected to bones by tendons. Bones are connected to each other by ligaments. The place where bones meet one another is typically called a joint.

The bone tissue is composed of several types of bone cells embedded in a web of inorganic salts (mostly calcium and phosphorus) to give the bone strength, and collagenous fibers and ground substance to give the bone flexibility.

The primary functions of the skeletal system are to

- give shape and support to the body.
- protect various internal structures and organs.
- serve as attachments for muscles and act as levers to produce body movement.
- help produce both white and red blood cells (one of the functions of bone marrow).
- store most of the body's calcium supply as well as phosphorus, magnesium, and sodium.

A **joint** is the connection between two or more bones of the skeleton. There are two types of joints: movable, such as elbows, knees, and hips; and immovable, such as the pelvis or skull, which allow little or no movement.

Bones of the Skull

The human head contains 22 bones divided into two groups: the **cranium** (KRAY-nee-um) and the facial bones. The cranium is formed by 8 bones; and the face consists of 14 bones including the maxilla (upper jaw) and mandible (lower jaw). The skull has many little holes in its base that allow the cranial nerves to travel to their destinations (Figure 5–4).

Bones of the Cranium

The cranium is made up of eight bones:

* The **occipital** (ahk-SIP-ih-tul) **bone** is the hindmost bone of the skull; it forms the back of the skull above the nape.
* The two **parietal** (puh-RY-uh-tul) **bones** form the sides and crown (top) of the cranium.

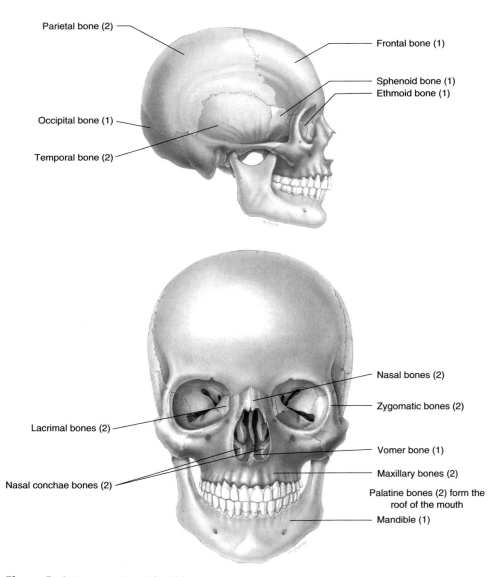

Figure 5–4 The cranial and facial bones.

- The **frontal** (FRUNT-ul) **bone** forms the forehead.
- The two **temporal** (TEM-puh-rul) **bones** form the sides of the head in the ear region.
- The **ethmoid** (ETH-moyd) **bone** is the light, spongy bone between the eye sockets that forms part of the nasal cavities.
- The **sphenoid** (SFEEN-oyd) **bone** joins all the bones of the cranium together.

Bones of the Face

The 14 bones of the face include the following

1–2. Two **nasal** (NAY-zul) **bones** form the bridge of the nose.

3–4. Two **lacrimal** (LAK-ruh-mul) **bones,** the smallest and most fragile bones of the face, are situated at the front inside part of the eye socket.

5–6. Two **zygomatic** (zy-goh-MAT-ik) or **malar bones** form the prominence of the cheeks, or cheekbones.

7–8. Two **maxillary** (mak-SIL-AIR-EE: maxillary) **bones** form the upper jaw.

9. The **mandible** (MAN-duh-bul) forms the lower jawbone, the largest and strongest bone of the face.

10–11. Two **turbinal** (TUR-bih-nahl) **bones** (also referred to as turbinate bones); these are thin layers of spongy bone on either of the outer walls of the nasal depression.

12. The **vomer** (VOH-mer), is a flat, thin bone that forms part of the nasal septum.

13–14. Two **palatine bones** form the hard palate of the mouth.

Bones of the Neck

The main bones of the neck are the **hyoid** (HY-oyd) **bone,** a U-shaped bone at the base of the tongue that supports the tongue and its muscles; and the **cervical vertebrae** (SUR-vih-kul VURT-uh-bray), the seven bones of the top part of the vertebral column located in the neck region (Figure 5–5).

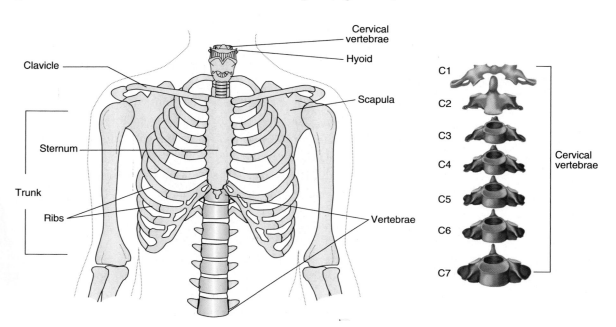

Figure 5–5 Bones of the neck, shoulder, and back.

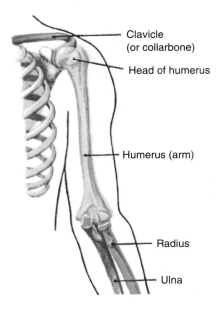

Figure 5-6 Bones of the arm.

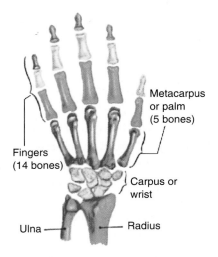

Figure 5-7 Bones of the hand.

Bones of the Chest

The **thorax** (THOR-aks), or chest, is an elastic, bony cage made up of the **sternum** (breastbone), spine, 12 pairs of ribs, and connective cartilage. It serves as a protective framework for the heart, lungs, and other internal organs.

Bones of the Shoulder, Arm, and Hand

Each shoulder consists of one **clavicle**, or collarbone, and one **scapula**, or shoulder blade. The arm and hand consist of the following bones (Figures 5–6 and 5–7).

* The **humerus** (HYOO-muh-rus) is the uppermost and largest bone of the arm, extending from the elbow to the shoulder.
* The **ulna** (UL-nuh) is the inner and larger bone of the forearm (lower arm), attached to the wrist and located on the side of the little finger.
* The **radius** (RAY-dee-us) is the smaller bone in the forearm on the same side as the thumb.
* The **carpus** (KAR-pus) is the wrist, a flexible joint composed of eight small, irregular bones (carpals) held together by ligaments.
* The **metacarpus** (met-uh-KAR-pus) is the palm, consisting of five long, slender bones called metacarpal bones.
* The **phalanges** (fuh-LAN-jeez) are the bones in the fingers, three in each finger and two in each thumb, totaling 14 bones.

THE MUSCULAR SYSTEM

The **muscular system** covers, shapes, and supports the skeletal tissue. It contracts and moves various parts of the body. The human body has over 600 muscles, which are responsible for approximately 40 percent of the body's weight. Out of the more than 600 muscles, 30 of them are facial muscles.

Muscles are fibrous tissues with the ability to stretch and contract according to the demands of the body's movements.

There are three types of muscular tissue. **Striated** (STRY-ayt-ed) **muscles,** also called skeletal or voluntary muscles, are attached to the bones and make up a large percentage of body mass (Figure 5–8). Nerve impulses trigger a reaction from the muscle which contracts, moving its associated bone or joint. **Nonstriated muscles,** also called involuntary, visceral, or smooth muscles, function automatically, without conscious will (Figure 5–9). These muscles are found in the digestive and circulatory systems as well as some internal organs of the body. **Cardiac muscle** is the involuntary muscle that makes up the heart (Figure 5–10). This type of muscle is unique and not found in any other part of the body. It is striated and has a crossing, banding pattern that allows contraction and thus the beating of the heart. It is under the control of the autonomic nervous system.

A muscle has three parts. The **origin** is the part that does not move; it is attached to the skeleton and serves as a basis for action. The movable attachment, where the effects of contraction are seen, is called the **insertion.** The **belly** is the middle part of the muscle. Pressure in massage is usually directed from the insertion to the origin.

Muscular tissue can be stimulated by

* massage (hand or electric vibrator).
* electrical current (high-frequency or faradic current).
* light rays (infrared rays or ultraviolet rays).
* heat rays (heating lamps or heating caps).
* moist heat (steamers or moderately warm steam towels).
* nerve impulses (through the nervous system).
* chemicals (certain acids and salts).

Muscles of the Scalp

The following muscles are attached to the scalp.

* The **epicranius** (ep-ih-KRAY-nee-us) or occipito-frontalis (ahk-SIP-ihtoh-frun-TAY-lus) is a broad muscle that covers the top of the skull. It consists of two parts, occipitalis and frontalis (Figure 5–11).
* The **occipitalis** (ahk-SIP-i-tahl-is), the back of the epicranius, is the muscle that draws the scalp backward.
* The **frontalis** (frun-TAY-lus) is the anterior (front) portion of the epicranius. It is the scalp muscle that raises the eyebrows, draws the scalp forward, and causes wrinkles across the forehead.
* The **aponeurosis** (ap-uh-noo-ROH-sus) is a tendon connecting the occipitalis and the frontalis.

Muscles of the Ear

These muscles are attached to the ear.

* The **auricularis** (aw-rik-yuh-LAIR-is) **superior** is the muscle above the ear that draws the ear upward.
* The **auricularis anterior** is the muscle in front of the ear that draws the ear forward.
* The **auricularis posterior** is the muscle behind the ear that draws the ear backward.

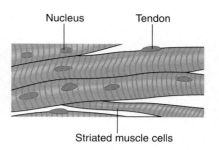

Figure 5–8 Striated muscle cells.

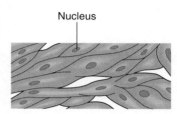

Figure 5–9 Nonstriated muscle cells.

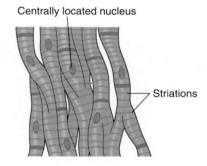

Figure 5–10 Cardiac muscle cells.

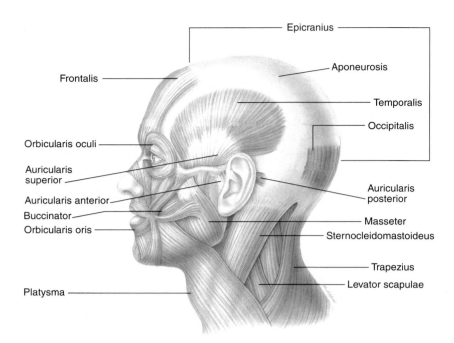

Figure 5–11 Muscles of the head, face, and neck.

Muscles of Mastication (Chewing)

The **masseter** (muh-SEE-tur) and the **temporalis** (tem-poh-RAY-lis) muscles coordinate in opening and closing the mouth and are sometimes referred to as chewing muscles.

Muscles of the Neck

Muscles of the neck include the following.
- The **platysma** (plah-TIZ-muh) is a broad muscle extending from the chest and shoulder muscles to the side of the chin. It is responsible for lowering the lower jaw and lip.
- The **sternocleidomastoideus** (STUR-noh-KLEE-ih-doh-mas-TOY-dee-us) is the muscle extending along side of the neck from the ear to the collarbone. It acts to rotate the head from side to side and up and down.

Muscles of the Eyebrow

Muscles of the eyebrow include the following.
- The **corrugator** (KOR-oo-gay-tohr) **muscle** is the muscle located beneath the frontalis and orbicularis oculi. It draws the eyebrow down and wrinkles the forehead vertically (Figure 5–12).
- The **orbicularis oculi** (or-bik-yuh-LAIR-is AHK-yuh-lye) is the ring muscle of the eye socket; it closes the eyes.

Muscle of the Nose

Only one muscle is attached to the nose. The **procerus** (proh-SEE-rus) muscle covers the bridge of the nose, lowers the eyebrows, and causes wrinkles across the bridge of the nose.

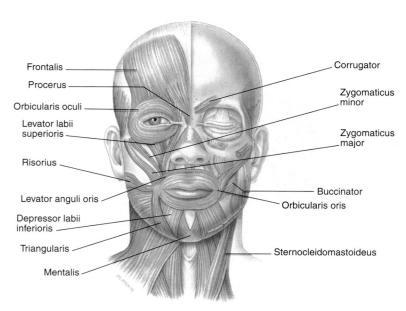

Figure 5–12 Muscles of the face.

Muscles of the Mouth

The following are important muscles of the mouth.

- The **buccinator** (BUK-sih-nay-tur) is the thin, flat muscle of the cheek between the upper and lower jaw that compresses the cheeks and expels air between the lips, as in when blowing a whistle.
- The **depressor labii inferioris** (dee-PRES-ur LAY-bee-eye in-FEER-eeor-us), also known as quadratus labii inferioris, is a muscle surrounding the lower lip that depresses the lower lip and draws it to one side.
- The **levator anguli oris** (lih-VAYT-ur ANG-yoo-ly OH-ris), also known as caninus (kay-NY-nus), is a muscle that raises the angle of the mouth and draws it inward.
- The **levator labii superioris** (lih-VAYT-ur LAY-bee-eye soo-peer-ee-OR-is), also known as quadratus (kwah-DRA-tus) labii superioris, is a muscle surrounding the upper lip that elevates the upper lip and dilates the nostrils, as in expressing distaste.
- The **mentalis** (men-TAY-lis) is the muscle that elevates the lower lip and raises and wrinkles the skin of the chin.
- The **orbicularis oris** (or-bik-yuh-LAIR-is OH-ris) is the flat band around the upper and lower lips that compresses, contracts, puckers, and wrinkles the lips.
- The **risorius** (rih-ZOR-ee-us) is the muscle that draws the corner of the mouth out and back, as in grinning.
- The **triangularis** (try-ang-gyuh-LAY-rus) is the muscle extending alongside the chin that pulls down the corners of the mouth.
- The **zygomaticus** (zy-goh-MAT-ih-kus) **major** and **minor** are muscles extending from the zygomatic bone to the angle of the mouth that elevate the lip, as in laughing.

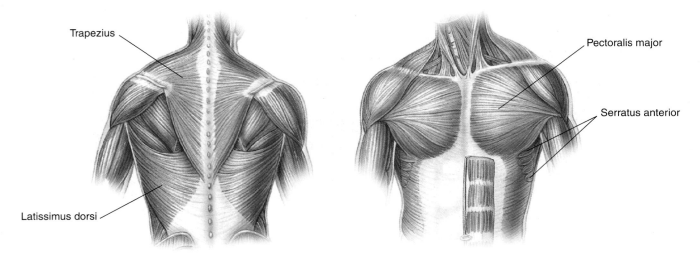

Figure 5–13 Muscles of the back and neck.

Figure 5–14 Muscles of the chest.

Muscles That Attach the Arms to the Body

Muscles attaching the arms to the body include the following.

- The **latissimus dorsi** (lah-TIS-ih-mus DOR-see) is a large, flat, triangular muscle that covers the lower back. It comes up from the lower half of the vertebral column and iliac crest (hip bone) and narrows to a rounded tendon attached to the front of the upper part of the humerus (Figure 5–13).
- The **pectoralis major** (pek-tor-AL-is) and **minor** are muscles of the chest that assist the swinging movements of the arm.
- The **serratus anterior** (ser-RAT-us an-TEER-ee-or) is a muscle of the chest that assists in breathing and in raising the arm (Figure 5–14).
- The **trapezius** (trah-PEE-zee-us) muscle covers the back of the neck and upper and middle region of the back; shrugs shoulders and stabilizes the scapula.

Muscles of the Shoulder and Arm

Here are the principal muscles of the shoulders and upper arms (Figure 5–15).

- The **biceps** (BY-seps) muscles produce the contour of the front and inner side of the upper arm; they lift the forearm, flex the elbow, and turn the palms outward.
- The **deltoid** (DEL-toyd) is a large, triangular muscle covering the shoulder joint that allows the arm to extend outward and to the side of the body.
- The **triceps** (TRY-seps) is a large muscle that covers the entire back of the upper arm and extends the forearm.

The forearm is made up of a series of muscles and strong tendons. As an esthetician, you will be concerned with the following muscles.

- The **extensors** (ik-STEN-surs) are muscles that straighten the wrist, hand, and fingers to form a straight line.
- The **flexors** (FLEK-surs), extensor muscles of the wrist, are involved in bending the wrist.

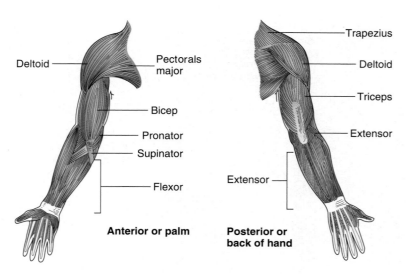

Figure 5–15 Muscles of the shoulder and arm.

- The **pronators** (proh-NAY-tohrs) are muscles that turn the hand inward so that the palm faces downward.
- The **supinator** (SOO-puh-nayt-ur) muscle rotates the radius outward and the palm upward.

Muscles of the Hand

The hand has many small muscles that overlap from joint to joint, giving it strength and flexibility. During the aging process, these muscles lose mobility, causing stiffness in the joints. Massage can help relax and maintain the pliability of these muscles.

THE NERVOUS SYSTEM

The **nervous system** is an exceptionally well-organized system that is responsible for coordinating all the many activities that are performed by the body. Every square inch of the human body is supplied with fine fibers known as *nerves;* there are over 100 billion nerve cells, known as *neurons,* in the body. An understanding of how nerves work will help you perform massage more proficiently and understand the effects of these treatments on the body as a whole.

Divisions of the Nervous System

The principal components of the nervous system are the brain, spinal cord, and the nerves themselves (Figure 5–16). The nervous system can be divided into two major categories: the *central nervous system* (CNS), which is the primary control center for the whole system; and the *peripheral nervous system* (PNS), which is divided into many smaller units.

The **central nervous** or **cerebrospinal** (ser-ree-bro-SPY-nahl) **system** consists of the brain and the spinal cord. It controls consciousness and all mental activities, voluntary functions of the five senses (seeing, hearing, feeling, smelling, and tasting), and voluntary muscle actions, including all body movements and facial expressions.

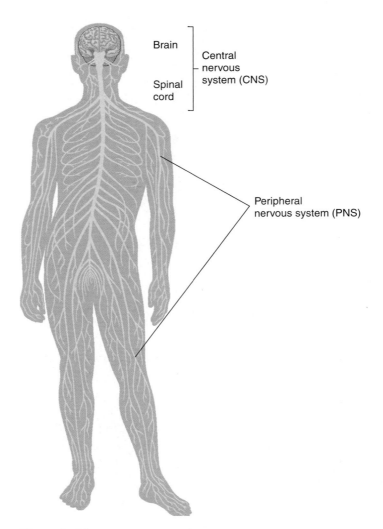

Labels in figure:
Brain
Spinal cord
Central nervous system (CNS)
Peripheral nervous system (PNS)

Figure 5–16 Principal parts of the nervous system.

The **peripheral** (puh-RIF-uh-rul) **nervous system** connects the peripheral (outer) parts of the body, such as the muscles and glands, to the central nervous system. It has both sensory and motor nerves. Its function is to carry impulses, or messages, to and from the central nervous system.

The peripheral nervous system (PNS) is further divided into two sections, the *afferent peripheral system* and the *efferent peripheral system*. From the efferent peripheral system, there are two subcategories, the *somatic nervous system*, which causes us to react to our external environment; and the **autonomic nervous system** (ANS), which causes the internal regulation of impulses from the central nervous system to smooth muscles such as the heart, blood vessels, and glands. The autonomic nervous system is considered involuntary. The organs affected by the autonomic system receive nerve cells or fibers from its two divisions, the *sympathetic* and the *parasympathetic*. The **sympathetic division** stimulates or speeds up activity and prepares the body for stressful situations, whereas the **parasympathetic division** operates under normal nonstressful conditions and helps restore and slow down activity, thus keeping the balance in the body.

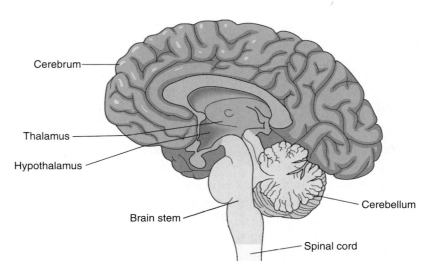

Cerebrum

Thalamus

Hypothalamus

Brain stem

Cerebellum

Spinal cord

Figure 5–17 Principal parts of the brain.

The Brain and Spinal Cord

The **brain** is the largest and most complex mass of nerve tissue in the body. The brain is contained in the cranium, weighs an average of 44 to 48 ounces, and has four main parts. They are the **cerebrum,** the **cerebellum,** the **diencephalon,** and the **brain stem.** The brain controls sensation, muscles, glandular activity, and the power to think and feel. It sends and receives tele-graphic messages through 12 pairs of cranial nerves that originate in the brain and reach various parts of the head, face, and neck (Figure 5–17).

The brain can be divided into four parts.

1. The **cerebrum** makes up the bulk of the brain. It is located in the front, upper part of the cranium. It has an inner core of white matter, com-posed of bundles of axons each coated with a sheath of myelin; and an outer core of gray matter, composed masses of cell bodies and dendrites. Within the cerebrum is the *cerebral cortex*, in the part of the cerebrum from which most messages from the brain are sent—such as those con-veying thought, hearing, and sight.

2. The term **cerebellum** is Latin for "little brain." It lies at the base of the cere-brum and is attached to the brain stem. It acts to control movement, coordi-nate voluntary muscular activity, and maintain balance and equilibrium.

3. The **diencephalon** (Dy-en-sef-ah-lon) is located in the uppermost part of the midbrain and has two main parts, known as the *thalamus* and the *hypothalamus*. The thalamus, located in the upper part of the diencepha-lon, acts as a relay station for sensory impulses and plays a role in the recognition of pain and temperature in the body. The hypothalamus, located in the lower part of the diencephalon, controls many bodily functions such as body temperature; it also controls the pituitary gland.

4. The **brain stem** connects the spinal cord to the brain. It consists of three parts—the *midbrain, pons,* and *medulla oblongata*—all of which connect parts of the brain with the spinal cord. The brain stem is involved in regu-lating such vital functions as breathing, heartbeat, and blood pressure.

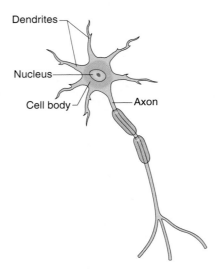

Figure 5–18 Parts of a neuron.

The **spinal cord** is the portion of the central nervous system that originates in the brain, extends down to the lower extremity of the trunk, and is protected by the spinal column. Thirty-one pairs of spinal nerves extending from the spinal cord are distributed to the muscles and skin of the trunk and limbs.

Nerve Cell Structure and Function

A **neuron** (NOO-rahn), or nerve cell, is the primary structural unit of the nervous system (Figure 5–18). It is composed of a cell body and nucleus; **dendrites** (DEN-dryts), nerve fibers extending from the nerve cell that receive impulses from other neurons; and an **axon** (AK-sahn), which sends impulses away from the cell body to other neurons, glands, or muscles.

Nerves are whitish cords, made up of bundles of nerve fibers held together by connective tissue, through which impulses are transmitted. Nerves have their origin in the brain and spinal cord and send their branches to all parts of the body.

Types of Nerves

Sensory or **afferent** (AF-uh-rent) **nerves** carry impulses or messages from the sense organs to the brain, where sensations of touch, cold, heat, sight, hearing, taste, smell, pain, and pressure are experienced. **Motor** or **efferent** (EF-uh-rent) **nerves** carry impulses from the brain to the muscles. The transmitted impulses produce movement. **Mixed** nerves contain both sensory and motor fibers and have the ability to send and receive messages.

A **reflex** (REE-fleks) is an automatic nerve reaction to a stimulus that involves the movement of an impulse from a sensory receptor along the afferent nerve to the spinal cord, and a responsive impulse along an efferent neuron to a muscle, causing a reaction (for example, the quick removal of the hand from a hot object). Reflexes do not have to be learned.

Nerves of the Head, Face, and Neck

There are 12 cranial nerves arising at the base of the brain and the brain stem. The cranial nerves activate the muscles and sensory structure of the head and neck, including skin, membranes, eyes, and ears (Figure 5–19).

Estheticians are primarily concerned with nerves V, VII, and XI, and each one has several branches.

The largest of the cranial nerves is the **fifth cranial nerve,** also known as the trifacial (try-FAY-shul) or trigeminal (try-JEM-un-ul) nerve. It is the chief sensory nerve of the face, and it serves as the motor nerve of the muscles that control chewing. It consists of three branches: **ophthalmic** (ahf-THAL-mik), **mandibular** (man-DIB-yuh-lur), and **maxillary** (MAK-suh-lair-ee) (Figure 5–20).

The following branches of the fifth cranial nerve are affected by facial or lymphatic massage.

- The **auriculotemporal** (aw-RIK-yuh-loh-TEM-puh-rul) **nerve** affects the external ear and skin above the temple, up to the top of the skull.
- The **infraorbital** (in-fruh-OR-bih-tul) **nerve** affects the skin of the lower eyelid, side of the nose, upper lip, and mouth.

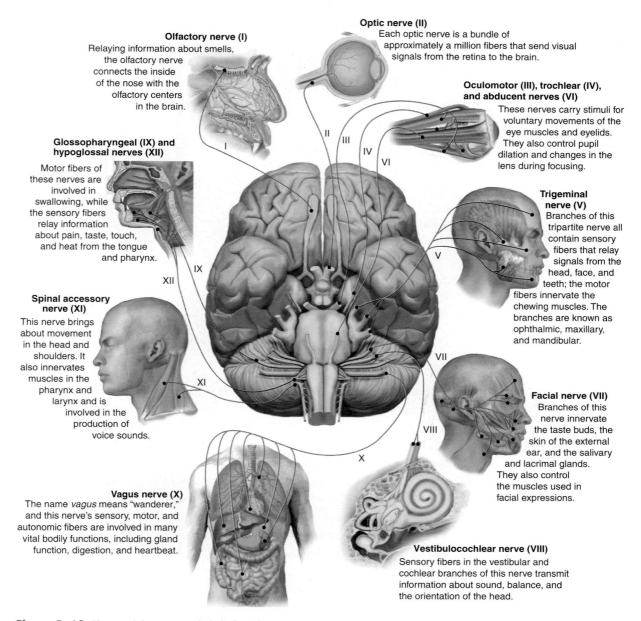

Olfactory nerve (I)
Relaying information about smells, the olfactory nerve connects the inside of the nose with the olfactory centers in the brain.

Optic nerve (II)
Each optic nerve is a bundle of approximately a million fibers that send visual signals from the retina to the brain.

Oculomotor (III), trochlear (IV), and abducent nerves (VI)
These nerves carry stimuli for voluntary movements of the eye muscles and eyelids. They also control pupil dilation and changes in the lens during focusing.

Glossopharyngeal (IX) and hypoglossal nerves (XII)
Motor fibers of these nerves are involved in swallowing, while the sensory fibers relay information about pain, taste, touch, and heat from the tongue and pharynx.

Trigeminal nerve (V)
Branches of this tripartite nerve all contain sensory fibers that relay signals from the head, face, and teeth; the motor fibers innervate the chewing muscles. The branches are known as ophthalmic, maxillary, and mandibular.

Spinal accessory nerve (XI)
This nerve brings about movement in the head and shoulders. It also innervates muscles in the pharynx and larynx and is involved in the production of voice sounds.

Facial nerve (VII)
Branches of this nerve innervate the taste buds, the skin of the external ear, and the salivary and lacrimal glands. They also control the muscles used in facial expressions.

Vagus nerve (X)
The name *vagus* means "wanderer," and this nerve's sensory, motor, and autonomic fibers are involved in many vital bodily functions, including gland function, digestion, and heartbeat.

Vestibulocochlear nerve (VIII)
Sensory fibers in the vestibular and cochlear branches of this nerve transmit information about sound, balance, and the orientation of the head.

Figure 5–19 The cranial nerves and their functions.

- The **infratrochlear** (in-frah-TRAHK-lee-ur) **nerve** affects the membrane and skin of the nose.
- The **mental nerve** affects the skin of the lower lip and chin.
- The **nasal nerve** affects the point and lower side of the nose.
- The **supraorbital** (soo-pruh-OR-bih-tul) **nerve** affects the skin of the forehead, scalp, eyebrow, and upper eyelid.
- The **supratrochlear** (soo-pruh-TRAHK-lee-ur) **nerve** affects the skin between the eyes and upper side of the nose.
- The **zygomatic** (zy-goh-MAT-ik) **nerve** affects the muscles of the upper part of the cheek.

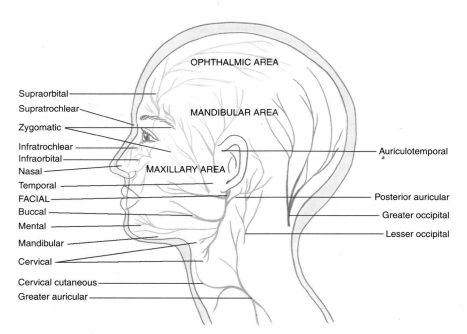

Figure 5–20 Nerves and nerve branches of the head, face, and neck.

The **seventh (facial) cranial nerve** is the chief motor nerve of the face. It emerges near the lower part of the ear and extends to the muscles of the neck. Its divisions and their branches supply and control all the muscles of facial expression and secretions of saliva. The following are the most important branches of the facial nerve.

- The **buccal** (BUK-ul) **nerve** affects the muscles of the mouth.
- The **cervical** (SUR-vih-kul) **nerves** (branches of the facial nerve) affect the side of the neck and the platysma muscle.
- The **mandibular nerve** affects the muscles of the chin and lower lip.
- The **posterior auricular nerve** affects the muscles behind the ear at the base of the skull.
- The **temporal nerve** affects the muscles of the temple, side of the forehead, eyebrow, eyelid, and upper part of the cheek.
- The **zygomatic nerve (upper and lower)** affects the muscles of the upper part of the cheek.

The **eleventh cranial nerve (accessory)** is a type of motor nerve that controls the motion of the neck muscles. This nerve is important to estheticians because it is affected during facials, primarily with massage.

Cervical nerves originate at the spinal cord, and their branches supply the muscles and scalp at the back of the head and neck as follows.

- The **cervical cutaneous** (kyoo-TAY-nee-us) **nerve,** located at the side of the neck, affects the front and sides of the neck as far down as the breastbone.
- The **greater auricular nerve,** located at the side of the neck, affects the face, ears, neck, and parotid gland.
- The **greater occipital nerve,** located in the back of the head, affects the scalp as far up as the top of the head.

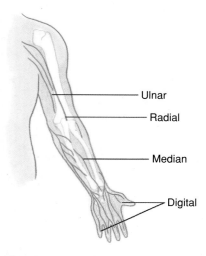

Figure 5–21 Nerves of the arm and hand.

- The **smaller (lesser) occipital nerve,** located at the base of the skull, affects the scalp and muscles behind the ear.

Nerves of the Arm and Hand

The principal nerves supplying the superficial parts of the arm and hand are as follows (Figure 5–21).

- The **digital nerve** (DIJ-ut-tul) is a sensory-motor nerve that, with its branches, supplies the fingers.
- The **radial** (RAY-dee-ul) **nerve** is a sensory-motor nerve that, with its branches, supplies the thumb side of the arm and back of the hand.
- The **median** (MEE-dee-un) **nerve** is a smaller sensory-motor nerve than the ulnar and radial nerves; with its branches, it supplies the arm and hand.
- The **ulnar** (UL-nur) **nerve** is a sensory-motor nerve that, with its branches, affects the little-finger side of the arm and palm of the hand.

THE CIRCULATORY SYSTEM

The **circulatory system,** also referred to as the *cardiovascular* or *vascular system,* controls the steady circulation of the blood through the body by means of the heart and blood vessels (veins and arteries). The **vascular system** consists of the heart, arteries, veins, and capillaries for the distribution of blood throughout the body.

The Heart

The **heart** is often referred to as the body's pump (Figure 5–22). It is a muscular, cone-shaped organ that keeps the blood moving within the circulatory system. It is enclosed by a membrane known as the **pericardium**

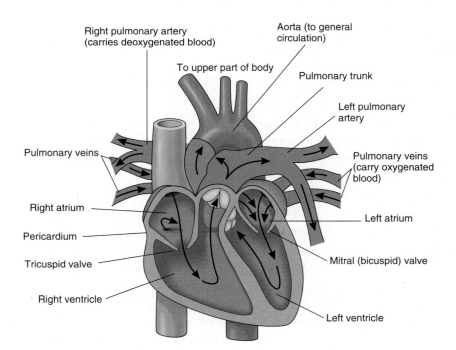

Figure 5–22 Anatomy of the heart.

(payr-ih-KAR-dee-um). The heart is about the size of a closed fist, weighs approximately 9 ounces, and is located in the chest cavity. The heartbeat is regulated by the vagus (tenth cranial) nerve and other nerves in the autonomic nervous system. In a normal resting state, the heart beats 72 to 80 times per minute.

The interior of the heart contains four chambers and four valves. The upper, thin-walled chambers are the right **atrium** (AY-tree-um) and left atrium. The lower, thick-walled chambers are the right **ventricle** (VEN-truh- kul) and left ventricle. **Valves** between the chambers allow the blood to flow in only one direction. With each contraction and relaxation of the heart, the blood flows in, travels from the atria (plural of *atrium*) to the ventricles, and is then driven out, to be distributed throughout the body.

The blood is in constant and continuous circulation from the time it leaves the heart until it returns to the heart. Two systems attend to this circulation. **Pulmonary circulation** sends the blood from the heart to the lungs to be oxygenated. **Systemic** or **general circulation** carries the oxygenated blood from the heart throughout the body and back to the heart again.

Blood Vessels

The blood vessels are tubelike structures that transport blood to and from the heart, and then on to various tissues of the body. **Arteries** are thick-walled, muscular, flexible tubes that carry oxygenated blood away from the heart to the capillaries. The largest artery in the body is the aorta. **Capillaries** are minute, thin-walled blood vessels that connect the smaller arteries to the veins. They bring nutrients to the cells and carry away waste materials. **Veins** are thin-walled blood vessels that are less elastic than arteries. They carry blood containing waste products from the various capillaries back to the heart. Veins contain valves that prevent backflow (Figure 5–23).

The Blood

Blood is a nutritive fluid flowing through the circulatory system. There are 8 to 10 pints of blood in the human body, accounting for about one-twentieth of the body's weight. Blood is approximately 80 percent water. It is sticky and salty, with a normal temperature of 98.6° Fahrenheit (36° Celsius). It is bright red in the arteries (except for the pulmonary artery) and dark red in the veins. The color change occurs during the exchange of carbon dioxide for oxygen as the blood passes through the lungs, and the exchange of oxygen for carbon dioxide as the blood circulates throughout the body.

Blood performs the following critical functions.

* It carries water, oxygen, food, and secretions to all cells of the body.
* It carries away carbon dioxide and waste products to be eliminated through the lungs, skin, kidneys, and large intestines.
* It helps to equalize the body's temperature, thus protecting the body from extreme heat and cold.
* It aids in protecting the body from harmful bacteria and infections through the action of the white blood cells.
* It closes injured minute blood vessels by forming clots, thus preventing blood loss.

Blood flow toward the heart

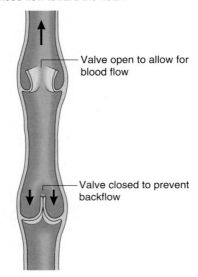

— Valve open to allow for blood flow

— Valve closed to prevent backflow

Figure 5–23 Valves in the veins.

Composition of the Blood

Blood is composed of red blood cells, white blood cells, plasma, and platelets.

Red blood cells, also called red corpuscles (KOR-pus-uls) or *erythrocytes* (ih-RITH-ruh-syts), are produced in the red bone marrow. They contain **hemoglobin** (HEE-muh-gloh-bun), a complex iron protein that gives the blood its bright red color. The function of red blood cells is to carry oxygen to the body cells. **White blood cells,** also called *white corpuscles* or *leukocytes* (LOO-koh-syts), perform the function of destroying disease causing germs. **Platelets,** or *thrombocytes* (THRAHM-buh-syts), are much smaller than red blood cells. They contribute to the blood-clotting process, which stops bleeding.

Plasma (PLAZ-muh) is the fluid part of the blood in which the red and white blood cells and platelets flow. It is about 90 percent water and contains proteins, sugars, and oxygen. The main function of plasma is to carry food and secretions to the cells and to take carbon dioxide away from the cells.

Arteries of the Head, Face, and Neck

The **common carotid** (kuh-RAHT-ud) **arteries** are the main source of blood supply to the head, face, and neck. They are located on either side of the neck, and each one is divided into an internal and external branch.

The **internal carotid artery** supplies blood to the brain, eyes, eyelids, forehead, nose, and internal ear. The **external carotid artery** supplies blood to the anterior (front) parts of the scalp, ear, face, neck, and side of the head (Figure 5–24). The external carotid artery subdivides into several branches. Of particular interest to the esthetician are the following arteries:

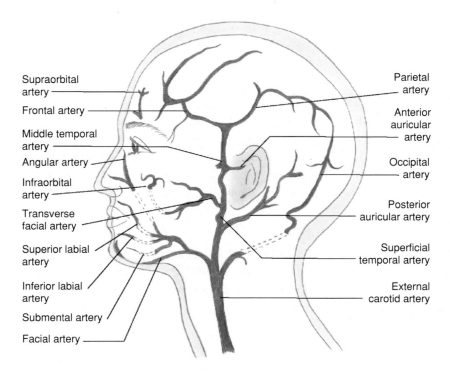

Figure 5–24 Arteries of the head, face, and neck.

The **facial artery** or external maxillary artery supplies blood to the lower region of the face, mouth, and nose. Here are some of its branches.

- The **submental** (sub-MEN-tul) **artery** supplies blood to the chin and lower lip.
- The **inferior labial** (LAY-bee-ul) **artery** supplies blood to the lower lip.
- The **angular artery** supplies blood to the side of the nose.
- The **superior labial artery** supplies blood to the upper lip and region of the nose.

The **superficial temporal artery** is a continuation of the external carotid artery and supplies blood to the muscles of the front, side, and top of the head. Some of its important branches are as follows.

- The **frontal artery** supplies blood to the forehead and upper eyelids.
- The **parietal artery** supplies blood to the side and crown of the head.
- The **transverse facial** (tranz-VURS) **artery** supplies blood to the skin and masseter.
- The **middle temporal artery** supplies blood to the temples.
- The **anterior auricular artery** supplies blood to the front part of the ear.

Two other arteries that branch from the external carotid artery are as follows.

- The **occipital artery** supplies blood to the skin and muscles of the scalp and back of the head up to the crown.
- The **posterior auricular artery** supplies the scalp, the area behind and above the ear, and the skin behind the ear.

Here are two branches of the internal carotid artery that are important to know.

- The **supraorbital** (soo-pruh-OR-bih-tul) **artery** supplies blood to the upper eyelids and forehead.
- The **infraorbital** (in-frah-OR-bih-tul) **artery** supplies blood to the muscles of the eye.

Veins of the Head, Face, and Neck

The blood returning to the heart from the head, face, and neck flows on each side of the neck in two principal veins: the **internal jugular** (JUG-yuh-lur) and **external jugular.** The most important veins of the face and neck are parallel to the arteries and take the same names as the arteries. However, there are no jugular arteries; rather, they are known as the carotid arteries.

Blood Supply of the Arm and Hand

The ulnar and radial arteries are the main blood supply of the arms and hands and are branches of the brachial artery (Figure 5–25). The **ulnar artery** and its numerous branches supply the little-finger side of the arm and palm of the hand. The **radial artery** and its branches supply the thumb side of the arm and the back of the hand.

The important veins are located almost parallel with the arteries and take the same names as the arteries. While the arteries are found deep in the tissues, the veins lie nearer to the surface of the arms and hands.

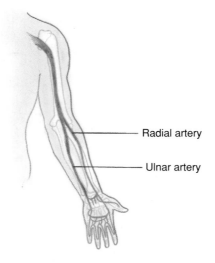

Radial artery

Ulnar artery

Figure 5–25 Arteries of the arm and hand.

THE LYMPHATIC/IMMUNE SYSTEM

The **lymphatic, or immune system,** is made up of **lymph,** lymph nodes, the thymus gland, the spleen, and lymph vessels. Its function is to protect the body from disease by developing immunities and destroying disease-causing microorganisms as well as to drain the tissue spaces of excess **interstitial** fluids to the blood. It carries waste and impurities away from the cells.

The lymphatic system is closely connected to the blood and the cardiovascular system. They both transport fluids, like rivers throughout the body. The difference is that the lymphatic system transports lymph, which eventually returns to the blood where it originated.

The lymphatic vessels start as tubes that are closed at one end. They can occur individually or in clusters that are called **lymph capillaries.** The lymph capillaries are distributed throughout most of the body (except the nervous system).

The lymphatic vessels are filtered by the **lymph nodes,** which are glandlike bodies in the lymphatic vessels. This filtering process helps to fight infection.

The primary functions of the lymphatic system are
* to carry nourishment from the blood to the body cells.
* to act as a defense against invading bacteria and toxins.
* to remove waste material from the body cells to the blood.
* to provide a suitable fluid environment for the cells.

THE ENDOCRINE SYSTEM

The **endocrine** (EN-duh-krin) **system** is a group of specialized glands that affect the growth, development, sexual activities, and health of the entire body. **Glands** are specialized organs that remove certain elements from the blood to convert them into new compounds. There are two main types of glands.

1. **Exocrine** (EK-suh-krin) **glands** or **duct** glands produce a substance that travels through small, tubelike ducts. Sweat and oil glands of the skin belong to this group.

2. **Endocrine glands** or **ductless** glands release secretions called **hormones** directly into the bloodstream, which in turn influence the welfare of the entire body (Figure 5–26). Hormones, such as insulin, adrenaline, and estrogen, stimulate functional activity or secretion in other parts of the body.

Here is a list of the endocrine glands and their functions.
* The pineal gland plays a major role in sexual development, sleep, and metabolism.
* The pituitary gland is the most complex organ of the endocrine system. It affects almost every physiologic process of the body: growth, blood pressure, contractions during childbirth, breast-milk production, sex organ functions in both women and men, thyroid gland function, the conversion of food into energy (metabolism), and osmolarity regulation in the body.

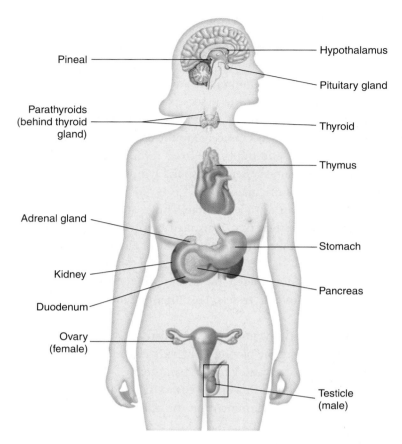

Figure 5–26 The endocrine glands.

- The thyroid gland controls how quickly the body burns energy (metabolism), makes proteins, and how sensitive the body should be to other hormones.
- The parathyroid glands regulate blood calcium and phosphorus levels so that the nervous and muscular systems can function properly.
- The pancreas secretes enzyme-producing cells that are responsible for digesting carbohydrates, proteins, and fats. The islet of Langerhans cells within the pancreas control insulin and glucagons production.
- The adrenal glands secrete about 30 steroid hormones and control metabolic processes of the body, including the fight-or-flight response.
- The ovaries and testes function in sexual reproduction as well as determining male and female sexual characteristics.

THE DIGESTIVE SYSTEM

The **digestive system,** also called the *gastrointestinal* (gas-troh-in-TES-tun-ul) *system*, is responsible for changing food into nutrients and waste. **Digestive enzymes** (EN-zymz) are chemicals that change certain kinds of food into a form that can be used by the body. The food, now in soluble form, is transported by the bloodstream and used by the body's cells and tissues.

The digestive system prepares food for use by the cells through five basic activities.

1. Eating or **ingestion**—taking food into the body
2. Moving food along the digestive tract—known as **peristalsis**
3. Breakdown of food by mechanical and chemical means—known as **digestion**
4. **Absorption** of the digested food into the circulatory systems for transportation to the tissues and cells
5. Elimination from the body—known as **defecation**

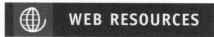
WEB RESOURCES

http://www.innerbody.com

http://www.getbodysmart.com

THE EXCRETORY SYSTEM

The **excretory** (EK-skre-tor-ee) **system** is responsible for purifying the body by eliminating waste matter. The metabolism of body cells forms various toxic substances that, if retained, could poison the body. Each of the following organs plays a crucial role in the excretory system.

- The kidneys excrete urine.
- The liver discharges bile.
- The skin eliminates perspiration.
- The large intestine eliminates decomposed and undigested food.
- The lungs exhale carbon dioxide.

THE RESPIRATORY SYSTEM

The **respiratory system** enables breathing (respiration) and consists of the lungs and air passages. The **lungs** are spongy tissues composed of microscopic cells in which inhaled air is exchanged for carbon dioxide during one breathing cycle. The respiratory system is located within the chest cavity and is protected on both sides by the ribs. The **diaphragm** is a muscular wall that separates the thorax from the abdominal region and helps control breathing (Figure 5–27).

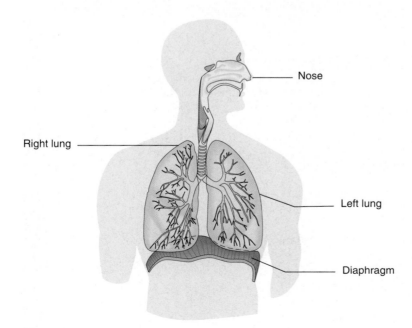

Figure 5–27 The respiratory system.

With each breathing cycle, an exchange of gases takes place. During inhalation (in-huh-LAY-shun), or breathing in, oxygen is absorbed into the blood. During exhalation (eks-huh-LAY-shun), or breathing outward, carbon dioxide is expelled from the lungs.

THE INTEGUMENTARY SYSTEM

The **integumentary system** is made up of the skin and its various accessory organs, such as the oil and sweat glands, sensory receptors, hair, and nails. (Skin anatomy and physiology are discussed in detail in Chapter 9.)

THE REPRODUCTIVE SYSTEM

The **reproductive system** performs the function of reproducing and perpetuating the human race. Although important to the perpetuation of the species, it is not of major importance to the esthetician, except as the sex hormones, testosterone in males and estrogen in females, affect skin functions.

As an esthetician you will see how the hormones affect the skin in many ways. They include acne, facial hair color and growth, and a condition known as **melasma** that causes darker pigmentation of the skin such as on the upper lip and around the eyes and cheeks.

Luckily, estheticians today have many resources—including products, treatments, and lifestyle modifications—for helping clients with skin changes due to fluctuating hormones.

REVIEW QUESTIONS

1. Define *anatomy, physiology,* and *histology.*

2. Why is the study of anatomy, physiology, and histology important to the esthetician?

3. Name and describe the basic structures of a cell.

4. Explain cell metabolism and its purpose.

5. List and describe the functions of the five types of tissue found in the human body.

6. What are organs?

7. List and describe the functions of the most important organs found in the body.

8. Name the 11 body systems and their main functions.

9. List the primary functions of the bones.

10. Name and describe the three types of muscular tissue found in the body.

11. Name and describe the three types of nerves found in the body.

12. Name and briefly describe the three types of blood vessels found in the body.

13. List and describe the components of blood.

14. What two types of glands make up the endocrine system?

15. List the organs of the excretory system and their function.

CHAPTER GLOSSARY

absorption: the transport of fully digested food into the circulatory system to feed the tissues and cells.

anabolism: constructive metabolism; the process of building up larger molecules from smaller ones.

anatomy: the study of the structure of the body that can be seen with the naked eye and what it is made up of; the science of the structure of organisms or of their parts.

angular artery: artery that supplies blood to the side of the nose.

anterior auricular artery: artery that supplies blood to the front part of the ear.

aponeurosis: tendon that connects the occipitalis and the frontalis.

arteries: thick-walled muscular and flexible tubes that carry oxygenated blood from the heart to the capillaries throughout the body.

atrium: one of the two upper chambers of the heart through which blood is pumped to the ventricles (plural: atria).

auricularis anterior: muscle in front of the ear that draws the ear forward.

auricularis posterior: muscle behind the ear that draws the ear backward.

auricularis superior: muscle above the ear that draws the ear upward.

auriculotemporal nerve: nerve that affects the external ear and skin above the temple, up to the top of the skull.

autonomic nervous system: the part of the nervous system that controls the involuntary muscles; regulates the action of the smooth muscles, glands, blood vessels, and heart.

axon: the process, or extension, of a neuron by which impulses are sent away from the body of the cell.

belly (muscle): middle part of a muscle.

biceps: muscle producing the contour of the front and inner side of the upper arm.

blood: nutritive fluid circulating through the circulatory system (heart, veins, arteries, and capillaries).

brain: part of the central nervous system contained in the cranium; largest and most complex nerve tissue; controls sensation, muscles, glandular activity, and the power to think and feel.

brain stem: structure that connects the spinal cord to the brain.

buccal nerve: nerve that affects the muscles of the mouth.

buccinator: thin, flat muscle of the cheek between the upper and lower jaw that compresses the cheeks and expels air between the lips.

CHAPTER GLOSSARY

capillaries: thin-walled blood vessels that connect the smaller arteries to the veins.

cardiac muscle: the involuntary muscle that makes up the heart.

carpus: the wrist; flexible joint composed of a group of eight small, irregular bones held together by ligaments.

catabolism: the phase of metabolism that involves the breaking down of complex compounds within the cells into smaller ones, often resulting in the release of energy to perform functions such as muscular efforts, secretions, or digestion.

cell membrane: part of the cell that encloses the protoplasm and permits soluble substances to enter and leave the cell.

cells: basic unit of all living things; minute mass of protoplasm capable of performing all the fundamental functions of life.

central nervous (cerebrospinal) system: cerebrospinal nervous system; consists of the brain, spinal cord, spinal nerves, and cranial nerves.

cerebellum: lies at the base of the cerebrum and is attached to the brain stem; this term is Latin for "little brain."

cerebrum: makes up the bulk of the brain and is located in the front, upper part of the cranium.

cervical cutaneous nerve: nerve located at the side of the neck that affects the front and sides of the neck as far down as the breastbone.

cervical nerves: nerves that originate at the spinal cord, whose branches supply the muscles and scalp at the back of the head and neck.

cervical vertebrae: the seven bones of the top part of the vertebral column, located in the neck region.

circulatory system: system that controls the steady circulation of the blood through the body by means of the heart and blood vessels.

clavicle: collarbone; bone joining the sternum and scapula.

common carotid arteries: arteries that supply blood to the face, head, and neck.

connective tissue: fibrous tissue that binds together, protects, and supports the various parts of the body such as bone, cartilage, and tendons.

corrugator muscle: facial muscle that draws eyebrows down and wrinkles the forehead vertically.

cranium: oval, bony case that protects the brain.

cytoplasm: all the protoplasm of a cell except that which is in the nucleus; the watery fluid containing food material necessary for cell growth, reproduction, and self-repair.

defecation: elimination of foods from the body.

deltoid: large, triangular muscle covering the shoulder joint that allows the arm to extend outward and to the side of the body.

dendrites: tree-like branching of nerve fibers extending from a nerve cell; short nerve fibers that carry impulses toward the cell.

deoxyribonucleic acid (DNA): the blueprint material of genetic information; contains all the information that controls the function of every living cell.

depressor labii inferioris: muscle surrounding the lower lip; depresses the lower lip and draws it to one side; also known as quadratus labii inferioris.

diaphragm: muscular wall that separates the thorax from the abdominal region and helps control breathing.

diencephalon: located in the uppermost part of the midbrain; consists of two main parts, the thalamus and the hypothalamus.

digestion: breakdown of food by mechanical and chemical means.

digestive enzymes: chemicals that change certain kinds of food into a form that can be used by the body.

digestive system: the mouth, stomach, intestines, and salivary and gastric glands that change food into nutrients and wastes.

digital nerve: nerve that, with its branches, supplies the fingers and toes.

eleventh cranial nerve (accessory): a type of motor nerve that controls the motion of the neck muscles.

endocrine (ductless) glands: ductless glands that release hormonal secretions directly into the bloodstream.

endocrine system: group of specialized glands that affect the growth, development, sexual activities, and health of the entire body.

epicranius: broad muscle that covers the top of the skull; also called occipito-frontalis.

epithelial tissue: protective covering on body surfaces, such as the skin, mucous membranes, and lining of the heart; digestive and respiratory organs; and glands.

ethmoid bone: light, spongy bone between the eye sockets that forms part of the nasal cavities.

excretory system: group of organs—including the kidneys, liver, skin, large intestine, and lungs—that purify the body by elimination of waste matter.

exocrine (duct) glands: duct glands that produce a substance that travels through small tubelike ducts, such as the sudoriferous (sweat) glands and the sebaceous (oil) glands.

extensors: muscles that straighten the wrist, hand, and fingers to form a straight line.

external carotid artery: artery that supplies blood to the anterior parts of the scalp, ear, face, neck, and side of the head.

external jugular vein: vein located on the side of the neck that carries blood returning to the heart from the head, face, and neck.

facial artery: artery that supplies blood to the lower region of the face, mouth, and nose; also called external maxillary artery.

fifth cranial nerve: chief sensory nerve of the face; controls chewing; also known as trifacial or trigeminal nerve.

flexors: extensor muscles of the wrist, involved in flexing the wrist.

frontal artery: artery that supplies blood to the forehead and upper eyelids.

frontal bone: bone forming the forehead.

frontalis: anterior or front portion of the epicranium; muscle of the scalp.

glands: a cell or group of cells that produce and release substances used nearby or in another part of the body.

greater auricular nerve: nerve at the sides of the neck affecting the face, ears, neck, and parotid gland.

greater occipital nerve: nerve located in the back of the head, affecting the scalp.

heart: muscular cone-shaped organ that keeps the blood moving within the circulatory system.

hemoglobin: iron-containing protein in red blood cells that binds to oxygen.

histology: study of the structure and composition of tissue.

hormones: secretions produced by one of the endocrine glands and carried by the bloodstream or body fluid to another part of the body, or a body organ, to stimulate functional activity or secretion.

humerus: uppermost and largest bone in the arm, extending from the elbow to the shoulder.

hyoid bone: u-shaped bone at the base of the tongue that supports the tongue and its muscle.

immune or lymphatic system: body system made up of lymph, lymph nodes, the thymus gland, the spleen, and lymph vessels. Functions protect the body from disease by developing immunities and destroying disease-causing microorganisms as well as draining the tissue spaces of excess interstitial fluids to the blood. It carries waste and impurities away from the cells.

inferior labial artery: supplies blood to the lower lip.

infraorbital artery: artery that originates from the internal maxillary artery and supplies blood to the eye muscles.

infraorbital nerve: nerve that affects the skin of the lower eyelid, side of the nose, upper lip, and mouth.

infratrochlear nerve: nerve that affects the membrane and skin of the nose.

ingestion: eating or taking food into the body.

insertion: the point where the skeletal muscle is attached to a bone or other more movable body part.

integumentary system: the skin and its accessory organs, such as the oil and sweat glands, sensory receptors, hair, and nails.

internal carotid artery: artery that supplies blood to the brain, eyes, eyelids, forehead, nose, and internal ear.

internal jugular vein: vein located at the side of the neck to collect blood from the brain and parts of the face and neck.

interstitial: the fluid in spaces between the tissue cells.

joint: connection between two or more bones of the skeleton.

lacrimal bones: small, thin bones located in the anterior medial wall of the orbits (eye sockets).

latissimus dorsi: broad, flat, superficial muscle covering the back of the neck and upper and middle region of the back; controls the shoulder blade and the swinging movements of the arm.

levator anguli oris: muscle that raises the angle of the mouth and draws it inward.

levator labii superioris: muscle surrounding the upper lip; elevates the upper lip and dilates the nostrils, as in expressing distaste.

CHAPTER GLOSSARY

lungs: spongy tissues composed of microscopic cells in which inhaled air is exchanged for carbon dioxide during one respiratory cycle.

lymph: clear, yellowish fluid that circulates in the lymph spaces (lymphatic) of the body; carries waste and impurities away from the cells.

lymph capillaries: lymphatic vessels that occur in clusters and are distributed throughout most of the body.

lymph nodes: glandlike bodies in the lymphatic vessels that filter lymph products.

mandible: lower jawbone; largest and strongest bone of the face.

mandibular nerve: branch of the fifth cranial nerve that supplies the muscles and skin of the lower part of the face; also, nerve that affects the muscles of the chin and lower lip.

masseter: one of the muscles of the jaw used in mastication (chewing).

maxillary bones: form the upper jaw.

maxillary nerve: branch of the fifth cranial nerve that supplies the upper part of the face.

median nerve: nerve, smaller than the ulnar and radial nerves, that supplies the arm and hand.

melasma: a condition of the skin that is triggered by hormones; causes darker pigmentation in areas such as on the upper lip and around the eyes and cheeks.

mental nerve: nerve that affects the skin of the lower lip and chin.

mentalis: muscle that elevates the lower lip and raises and wrinkles the skin of the chin.

metabolism: chemical process taking place in living organisms whereby the cells are nourished and carry out their activities.

metacarpus: bones of the palm of the hand; parts of the hand containing five bones between the carpus and phalanges.

middle temporal artery: artery that supplies blood to the temples.

mitosis: cells dividing into two new cells (daughter cells); the usual process of cell reproduction of human tissues.

motor (efferent) nerves: nerves that carry impulses from the brain to the muscles.

muscular system: body system that covers, shapes, and supports the skeleton tissue; contracts and moves various parts of the body.

muscular tissue: tissue that contracts and moves various parts of the body.

nasal bones: bones that form the bridge of the nose.

nasal nerve: nerve that affects the point and lower sides of the nose.

nerve tissue: tissue that controls and coordinates all body functions.

nerves: whitish cords made up of bundles of nerve fibers held together by connective tissue, through which impulses are transmitted.

nervous system: body system composed of the brain, spinal cord, and nerves; controls and coordinates all other systems and makes them work harmoniously and efficiently.

neuron: nerve cell; basic unit of the nervous system, consisting of a cell body, nucleus, dendrites, and axon.

nonstriated muscles: also called involuntary, visceral, or smooth muscles; muscles that function automatically, without conscious will.

nucleoplasm: a fluid within the nucleus of the cell that contains proteins and DNA; determines our genetic makeup.

nucleus: dense, active protoplasm found in the center of the cell; plays an important part in cell reproduction and metabolism.

occipital artery: artery that supplies blood to the skin and muscles of the scalp and back of the head up to the crown.

occipital bone: hindmost bone of the skull, located below the parietal bones.

occipitalis: back of the epicranius; muscle that draws the scalp backward.

ophthalmic nerve: branch of the fifth cranial nerve that supplies the skin of the forehead, upper eyelids, and interior portion of the scalp, orbit, eyeball, and nasal passage.

orbicularis oculi: the ring muscle of the eye socket; closes the eyelid.

orbicularis oris: flat band around the upper and lower lips that compresses, contracts, puckers, and wrinkles the lips.

organs: structures composed of specialized tissues and performing specific functions.

origin: part of the muscle that does not move; it is attached to the skeleton and is usually part of a skeletal muscle.

palatine bones: the two bones that form the hard palate of the mouth.

parasympathetic division: as part of the autonomic nervous system, it operates under normal nonstressful situations, such as resting. It also helps to restore calm and balance to the body after a stressful event.

parietal artery: artery that supplies blood to the side and crown of the head.

parietal bones: bones that form the sides and top of the cranium.

pectoralis major and minor: muscles of the chest that assist the swinging movements of the arm.

pericardium: double-layered membranous sac enclosing the heart.

peripheral nervous system: system of nerves and ganglia that connects the peripheral parts of the body to the central nervous system; has both sensory and motor nerves.

peristalsis: moving food along the digestive tract.

phalanges: bones of the fingers or toes (singular: phalanx).

physiology: study of the functions or activities performed by the body's structures.

plasma: fluid part of the blood and lymph that carries food and secretions to the cells and carbon dioxide from the cells.

platelets: blood cells that aid in the forming of clots.

platysma: broad muscle extending from the chest and shoulder muscles to the side of the chin; responsible for depressing the lower jaw and lip.

posterior auricular artery: artery that supplies blood to the scalp, behind and above the ear.

posterior auricular nerve: nerve that affects the muscles behind the ear at the base of the skull.

procerus: muscle that covers the bridge of the nose, depresses the eyebrows, and causes wrinkles across the bridge of the nose.

pronators: muscles that turn the hand inward so that the palm faces downward.

protoplasm: colorless, jellylike substance in cells; contains food elements such as protein, fats, carbohydrates, mineral salts, and water.

pulmonary circulation: process of blood circulation from heart to lungs to be purified.

radial artery: artery that supplies blood to the thumb side of the arm and the back of the hand.

radial nerve: nerve that, with its branches, supplies the thumb side of the arm and back of the hand.

radius: smaller bone in the forearm on the same side as the thumb.

red blood cells: also called red corpuscles; blood cells that carry oxygen from the lungs to the body cells.

reflex: automatic nerve reaction to a stimulus; involves the movement of an impulse from a sensory receptor along the afferent nerve to the spinal cord, and a responsive impulse along an efferent neuron to a muscle, causing a reaction.

reproductive system: body system responsible for processes by which plants and animals produce offspring.

respiratory system: body system consisting of the lungs and air passages; enables breathing, which supplies the body with oxygen and eliminates carbon dioxide as a waste product.

risorius: muscle of the mouth that draws the corner of the mouth out and back, as in grinning.

scapula: one of a pair of shoulder blades; large, flat triangular bone of the shoulder.

sensory (afferent) nerves: nerves that carry impulses or messages from the sense organs to the brain, where sensations of touch, cold, heat, sight, hearing, taste, smell, pain, and pressure are experienced.

serratus anterior: muscle of the chest that assists in breathing and in raising the arm.

seventh (facial) cranial nerve: chief motor nerve of the face, emerging near the lower part of the ear.

skeletal system: physical foundation of the body, composed of the bones and movable and immovable joints.

smaller (lesser) occipital nerve: nerve located at the base of the skull, affecting the scalp and muscles behind the ear.

sphenoid bone: bone that joins all the bones of the cranium together.

spinal cord: portion of the central nervous system that originates in the brain, extends down to the lower extremity of the trunk, and is protected by the spinal column.

sternocleidomastoideus: muscle of the neck that depresses and rotates the head.

sternum: the flat bone, or breastbone, that forms the ventral support of the ribs.

striated muscles: also called voluntary or skeletal muscles; muscles that are controlled by the will.

submental artery: artery that supplies blood to the chin and lower lip.

CHAPTER GLOSSARY

superficial temporal artery: artery that supplies blood to the muscles of the front, side, and top of the head.

superior labial artery: artery that supplies blood to the upper lip and region of the nose.

supinator: muscle of the forearm that rotates the radius outward and the palm upward.

supraorbital artery: artery that supplies blood to the upper eyelid and forehead.

supraorbital nerve: nerve that affects the skin of the forehead, scalp, eyebrow, and upper eyelid.

supratrochlear nerve: nerve that affects the skin between the eyes and upper side of the nose.

sympathetic division: part of the autonomic nervous system that stimulates or speeds up activity and prepares the body for stressful situations, such as in running from a dangerous situation, or competing in a sports event.

systemic (general) circulation: circulation of blood from the heart throughout the body and back again to the heart; also called *general circulation*.

temporal bones: bones forming the sides of the head in the ear region.

temporal nerve: nerve affecting the muscles of the temple, side of the forehead, eyebrow, eyelid, and upper part of the cheek.

temporalis: temporal muscle; one of the muscles involved in mastication (chewing).

thorax: the chest; elastic, bony cage that serves as a protective framework for the heart, lungs, and other internal organs.

tissue: collection of similar cells that perform a particular function.

transverse facial artery: artery that supplies blood to the skin and the masseter.

trapezius: muscle that covers the back of the neck and upper and middle region of the back; stabilizes the scapula and shrugs the shoulders.

triangularis: muscle extending alongside the chin that pulls down the corner of the mouth.

triceps: large muscle that covers the entire back of the upper arm and extends the forearm.

turbinal bones: thin layers of spongy bone on either of the outer walls of the nasal depression.

ulna: inner and larger bone of the forearm, attached to the wrist on the side of the little finger.

ulnar artery: artery that supplies blood to the muscle of the little-finger side of the arm and palm of the hand.

ulnar nerve: nerve that affects the little-finger side of the arm and palm of the hand.

valves: structures that temporarily close a passage or permit flow in one direction only.

vascular system: body system consisting of the heart, arteries, veins, and capillaries for the distribution of blood throughout the body.

veins: thin-walled blood vessels that are less elastic than arteries; they contain cuplike valves to prevent backflow and carry impure blood from the various capillaries back to the heart and lungs.

ventricle: the lower thick-walled chamber of the heart.

vomer: a flat, thin bone that forms part of the nasal septum.

white blood cells: blood cells that perform the function of destroying disease-causing germs; also called white corpuscles or leukocytes.

zygomatic or malar bones: bones that form the prominence of the cheeks; the cheekbones.

zygomatic nerve: nerve that affects the skin of the temple, side of the forehead, and upper part of the cheek.

zygomaticus major and minor: muscles extending from the zygomatic bone to the angle of the mouth; they elevate the lip, as in laughing.

CHAPTER OUTLINE

CHAPTER 6

BASICS OF CHEMISTRY

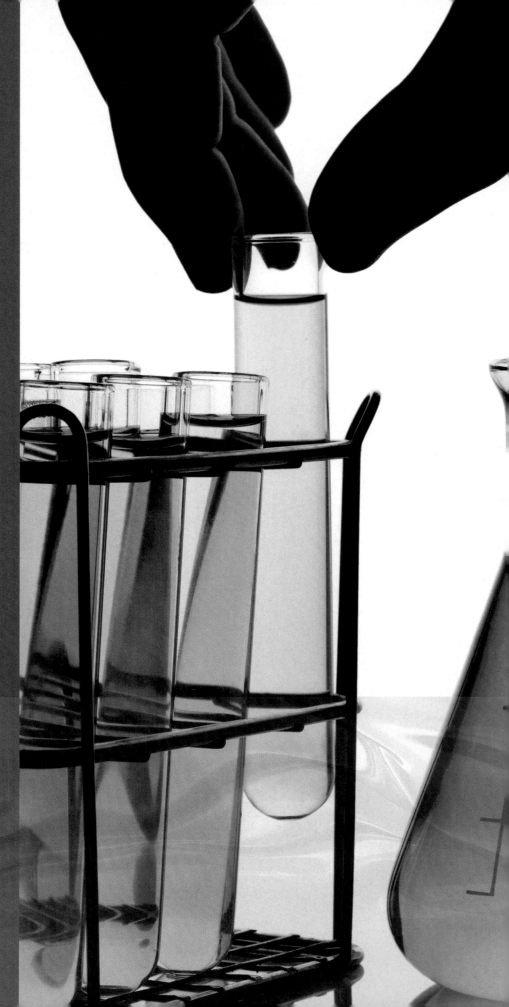

After completing this chapter, you will be able to:

- Define chemistry and its branches.

- Explain matter and its structure.

- Discuss the properties of matter and how matter changes.

- Explain the differences between solutions, suspensions, and emulsions.

- Understand how acid, alkaline, and pH affects the skin.

KEY TERMS

Page numbers indicate where in the chapter each term is used.

acid-alkali neutralization
   reactions 135

acid mantle 135

acids 134

air 134

alkalies 134

antioxidants 136

atoms 131

chemical change 133

chemical compounds 133

chemical properties 133

chemistry 130

combustion 136

compound molecules 132

element 131

elemental molecules 131

emulsions 138

free radicals 136

hydrogen 133

hydrogen peroxide 134

hydrophilic 138

immiscible 137

inorganic chemistry 130

lipophilic 138

logarithmic scale 135

matter 130

miscible 137

molecule 131

nitrogen 134

oil-in-water (O/W)
   emulsion 138

organic chemistry 130

oxidation 135

oxidation-reduction
   (redox) reactions 135

oxidize 136

oxygen 134

pH 134

physical change 132, 133

physical mixture 133

physical properties 133

redox 135

redox reactions 135

reduction 135

solute 137

solutions 137

solvent 137

surfactants 138

suspensions 137

water 134

water-in-oil (W/O)
   emulsion 139

A s an esthetician, you will be working with chemistry every day. As you will see, chemistry (one of the physical sciences), along with chemicals and chemical changes, make life on earth possible. The daily functioning of our bodies is based on chemical reactions. The skin is made of chemicals. So are all creams, lotions, masks, and makeup—whether they come from natural sources such as plant extracts or from ingredients manufactured in a laboratory (Figure 6–1).

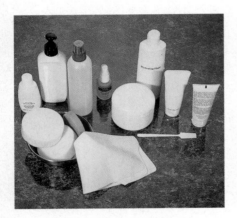

Figure 6–1 All skin care products are made of chemicals.

The effects of cosmetics and skin care products are based on chemical reactions. To understand how different chemicals affect the skin, and to choose the correct products and cosmetics for each client's skin type, estheticians must have a basic knowledge of chemistry.

CHEMISTRY

Chemistry is the science that deals with the composition, structure, and properties of matter and with how matter changes under different conditions. There are two branches of chemistry—organic and inorganic.

Organic chemistry is the study of substances that contain carbon. All living things, whether they are plants or animals, contain carbon. Although the term *organic* is often used to mean "natural" because of its association with living things, the term also applies to anything that has ever been alive. Gasoline, plastics, synthetic fabrics, pesticides, and fertilizers are all organic substances. These products are manufactured from natural gas and oil, which are the remains of plants and animals that died millions of years ago. Organic compounds will burn.

Inorganic chemistry is the branch of chemistry dealing with compounds that do not contain carbon. Inorganic substances are not, and never were, alive. Metals, minerals, pure water, and clean air are examples of inorganic substances. Inorganic substances will not burn.

MATTER

Matter is any substance that occupies space and has mass (weight). Although matter has physical properties that we can touch, taste, smell, or see, not everything that we can see is matter. For instance, we can see visible light and electric sparks, but these are forms of energy, and energy is not matter. Energy does not occupy space or have physical properties, such as mass (weight). Energy is discussed in Chapter 7.

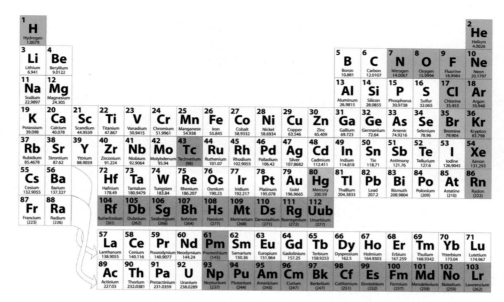

Figure 6–2 The periodic table of elements.

Elements

An **element** is the simplest form of matter and cannot be broken down into a simpler substance without loss of identity. There are about 90 naturally occurring elements, each with its own distinctive physical and chemical properties. All matter in the universe is made up of one or more of these 90 different elements.

Each element is identified by a letter symbol, such as O for oxygen, C for carbon, and H for hydrogen (Figure 6–2).

Atoms

Atoms are the structural units that make up elements. Atoms are the particles from which all matter is composed. An atom is the smallest particle of an element that still retains the properties of that element.

The atoms of each element are different in structure from the atoms of all other elements. The structural differences of the 90 different atoms accounts for the 90 different elements and their distinct properties. All the atoms of the same element are identical. Atoms cannot be divided into simpler substances by ordinary chemical means. Atoms consist of smaller particles; protons, which have a positive electrical charge; neutrons, with a neutral charge; and electrons, with a negative charge (Figure 6–3). The number of protons in an atom equals the number of electrons.

Molecules

A **molecule** is formed by joining two or more atoms chemically. There are two types of molecules.

1. **Elemental** (el-uh-MEN-tuhl) **molecules** that contain two or more atoms of the same element that are united chemically. (Figure 6–4). When all the atoms that form a molecule are the same, the molecule is made of the same element, and the molecule is called an elemental molecule. Atmospheric

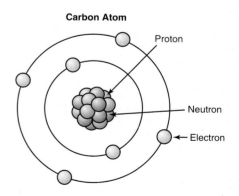

Figure 6–3 An atom consists of negatively charged electrons, positively charged protons, neutral neutrons, and electrons orbiting the unit.

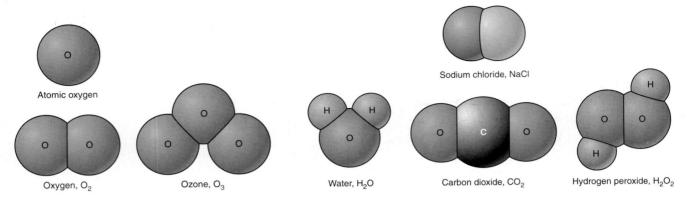

Figure 6–4 Elemental molecules.

Figure 6–5 Compound molecules.

oxygen, in the air we breathe, is the elemental molecule O_2. In the atmosphere, the ozone that protects us from ultraviolet radiation is the elemental molecule O_3.

2. **Compound** (KAHM-pownd) **molecules,** also called *compounds,* are chemical combinations of two or more atoms of different elements that are united chemically. (Figure 6–5).

States of Matter

All matter exists in one of three different physical forms: solid, liquid or gas. These three different physical forms are called the *states of matter.* The difference in these physical forms depends on temperature (Figure 6–6).

Like most other substances, water (H_2O) can exist in all three states of matter, depending on its temperature. Ice turns to water as it melts, and water turns to steam as it boils. The form of water is different due to a change of state, but it is still water (H_2O). It is not a different chemical. It is the same chemical in a different physical form. This is called a **physical change.**

The three different states of matter have the following distinct characteristics:

Solids have a definite size (volume) and a definite shape. Ice is an example of a solid. Ice has a definite size and shape. Ice is solid water (H_2O) at a temperature of less than 32°F/0°C.

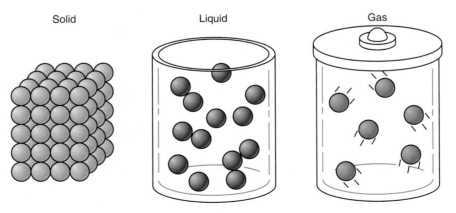

Figure 6–6 The states of matter: solid, liquid, and gas.

Liquids have a definite size (volume) but not a definite shape. Liquids take on the shape of the container they are in. Water is an example of a liquid. Water has a definite size, but it does not have a definite shape. Water is liquid water (H_2O) at a temperature between 32°F/0°C and 211°F/100°C.

Gases do not have a definite size (volume) or a definite shape. Steam is an example of a gas. Steam does not have a definite size or a definite shape. Steam is gaseous water (H_2O) at a temperature above 212°F/100°C.

Physical and Chemical Properties

Every substance has unique physical and chemical properties that allow us to identify it.

Physical properties are those characteristics that can be determined without a chemical reaction and that do not cause a chemical change in the identity of the substance. Physical properties include color, odor, weight, density, specific gravity, melting point, boiling point, and hardness.

Chemical properties are those characteristics that can be determined only with a chemical reaction and that cause a chemical change in the identity of the substance. Rusting iron and burning wood are examples of a change in chemical properties. In both these examples, the chemical reaction known as oxidation creates a chemical change in the identity of the substance. The iron is chemically changed to rust, and the wood is chemically changed to ash.

Physical and Chemical Changes

Matter can be changed in two different ways: physically and chemically.

1. A **physical change** is a change in the form or physical properties of a substance without the formation of a new substance. There is no chemical reaction involved, and no new chemicals are formed. A change in the state of matter is an example of a physical change. Solid ice undergoes a physical change when it melts into liquid water (Figure 6–7).

2. A **chemical change** is a change in the chemical composition of a substance, in which a new substance or substances are formed having properties different from the original. It is the result of a chemical reaction (Figure 6–8). As previously described (iron into rust, wood into ash), oxidation is an example of a chemical reaction that causes a chemical change.

Properties of Common Elements, Chemical Compounds, and Physical Mixtures

A familiarity with the properties of some of the most common elements, chemical compounds, and **physical mixtures** can help you understand why certain cosmetic products act the way they do. **Chemical compounds** are a combination of two or more atoms of different elements united chemically with a fixed chemical composition, definite proportions, and distinct properties.

Hydrogen (H) is a colorless, odorless, tasteless gas and is the lightest element known. It is found in chemical combination with oxygen in water, and with other elements in most organic substances. Elemental hydrogen is flammable and explosive when mixed with air.

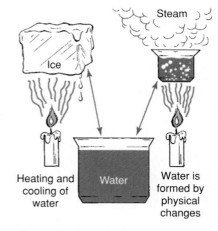

Figure 6–7 Physical changes.

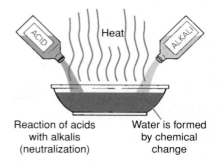

Figure 6–8 Chemical changes.

Oxygen (O), the most abundant element found on earth, is a colorless, odorless, tasteless gas. It comprises about half of the earth's crust, half of the rock, one-fifth of the air, and 90 percent of the water. It combines with most other elements to form an infinite variety of compounds, called oxides. One of the chief chemical characteristics of this element is its ability to support combustion.

Nitrogen (N) is a colorless, gaseous element. It makes up about four-fifths of the air in our atmosphere and is found chiefly in the form of ammonia and nitrates.

Air is the gaseous mixture that makes up the earth's atmosphere. It is odorless, colorless, and generally consists of about 1 part oxygen and 4 parts nitrogen by volume. It also contains a small amount of carbon dioxide, ammonia, and organic matter, which are all essential to plant and animal life.

Water (H_2O) is the most abundant of all substances, comprising about 75 percent of the earth's surface and about 65 percent of the human body. Water is seldom pure. Natural spring water contains dissolved minerals, bacteria, and other substances.

Water makes up a large part of the skin. All cells require water to live, and even dying cells in the upper layer of the skin contain water. Water is also the most commonly used cosmetic ingredient. It replenishes moisture on the surface of the skin, helps keep other ingredients in solution, and helps spread products across the skin.

Hydrogen peroxide (H_2O_2), a chemical compound of hydrogen and oxygen, is a colorless liquid with a characteristic odor and a slightly acid taste. The substance known as 20 volume peroxide is a solution of 6 percent hydrogen peroxide that is used as the developer in haircoloring; 10 volume peroxide is a solution of 3 percent hydrogen peroxide that is used as an antiseptic.

POTENTIAL HYDROGEN (pH)

The **pH** (potential hydrogen) of a substance is its relative degree of acidity or alkalinity and is measured on a scale of 0 to 14. **Acids** are substances that have a pH below 7.0, taste sour, and turn litmus paper from blue to red. The lower the pH number, the greater the degree of acidity. **Alkalies,** or bases, have a pH above 7.0, taste bitter, and turn litmus paper from red to blue. The higher the pH number, the greater the degree of alkalinity (Figure 6–9).

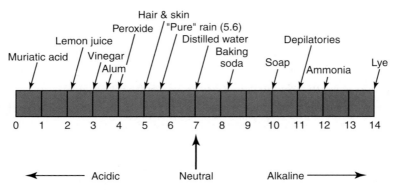

Figure 6–9 The pH scale.

The natural pH of the skin is 5.5; so although a pH of 7 is neutral for water, a pH of 5.5 is considered neutral for the skin.

The skin produces both sebum and sweat, which on the surface of the skin create a barrier known as the **acid mantle.** The acid mantle is a protective barrier against certain forms of bacteria and microorganisms, and it may be a factor in the natural skin-shedding and renewal process. Although the pH of the acid mantle varies with different individuals, the average pH is 5.5. When the skin is exposed to low or high pH, inflammation can occur. Strong acids, such as sulfuric acid, can produce chemical burns that destroy the epidermis. Likewise, highly alkaline substances, such as lye, can also produce inflammation and, in some cases, chemical burns. These acids and alkaline substances are, of course, never used in esthetic services.

Even at levels that are not nearly as severe, extreme variations in pH can damage the skin's barrier function and cause irritation. Buffering agents are frequently added to skin care products to maintain the pH at the correct level to produce the desired effect while keeping the product safe and nonirritating to the skin. This is why it is important for estheticians to understand the chemistry of products and to make selections based on the skin type and condition being treated.

CHEMICAL REACTIONS

Two types of chemical reactions are of importance to estheticians because they explain how skin care products work. They are **acid-alkali neutralization reactions** and **oxidation-reduction (redox) reactions.**

Acid-Alkali Neutralization Reactions

Acid-alkali neutralization reactions occur when an acid is mixed with an alkali, also called a base, in equal proportions to neutralize each other and form water (H_2O) and a salt. For example, hydrochloric acid (HCl) reacts with sodium hydroxide (NaOH) to form sodium chloride (NaC1), common table salt, and water (H_2O).

Oxidation-Reduction (Redox) Reactions

Oxidation-reduction (redox) reactions are one of the most common types of chemical reactions and are prevalent in all areas of chemistry. When oxygen is added to a substance, the substance is oxidized; for example, rust forms when oxygen is added to iron. **Oxidation** chemically changes the iron into iron oxide.

When oxygen is removed from a substance, the substance is *reduced*. An oxidation reaction is a transfer of oxygen from the oxidizer to the substance that is oxidized. In an oxidation reaction, the substance that gains oxygen is oxidized and, at the same time, the oxidizer that lost oxygen is reduced.

Oxidation cannot happen without **reduction.** Because oxidation and reduction always happen at the same time, they are also called **redox reactions.** The same oxidation reaction that causes iron to rust also causes the oxidizer (atmospheric oxygen) to be reduced.

> **? Did You Know**
>
> The pH scale is a **logarithmic scale.** This means that in a pH scale, a change of one whole number represents a tenfold change in pH. A pH of 8 is 10 times more alkaline than a pH of 7. A change of two whole numbers indicates a change of 10 times 10, or a hundredfold change. A pH of 9 is 100 times more alkaline than a pH of 7.

Combustion is the rapid oxidation of a substance, accompanied by the production of heat and light. Lighting a match is an example of rapid oxidation. You cannot have a fire without oxygen.

As estheticians we learn about the process of oxidation by using **antioxidants** in skin care products. Antioxidants are used to stabilize skin care products by preventing or retarding the oxidation that would otherwise cause a product to turn rancid and spoil. They are vitamins such as vitamin A, C, and E, which can be applied topically in products and taken internally to increase healthy body functions.

Antioxidants prevent oxidation by neutralizing **free radicals.** Free radicals are "super" oxidizers that cause an oxidation reaction and produce a new free radical in the process. Because they are created by highly reactive atoms or molecules (often oxygen) that have an unpaired number of electrons, free radicals are unstable. They are looking to partner, so by stealing electrons from other molecules they begin to damage the chemical processes in the body and further the oxidation process. If left alone they will create inflammation, damage DNA, and eventually cause disease and death. One free radical can **oxidize** millions of other substances. Antioxidants are free radical scavengers that stop the oxidation reaction from continuing.

CHEMISTRY AS APPLIED TO COSMETICS

To better serve their clients, estheticians should have an understanding of the chemical composition, preparation, and uses of cosmetics that are intended to cleanse and beautify the skin. Most of the products an esthetician uses are solutions, suspensions, and emulsions.

Solutions, Suspensions, and Emulsions

Solutions, suspensions, and emulsions are all physical mixtures of two or more different substances (Table 6–1). The distinction between solutions, suspensions, and emulsions depends on the size of the particles and the solubility of the components.

Table 6–1

SOLUTIONS, SUSPENSIONS, AND EMULSIONS		
SOLUTIONS	**SUSPENSIONS**	**EMULSIONS**
Miscible	Slightly miscible	Immiscible
No surfactant	No surfactant	Surfactant
Small particles	Larger particles	Largest particles
Usually clear	Usually cloudy	Usually a solid color
Stable mixture	Unstable mixture	Limited stability
Solution of hydrogen peroxide	Calamine lotion	Shampoos and conditioners

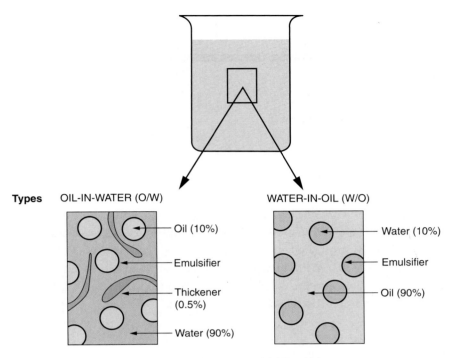

Figure 6–10 Oil-in-water (left side). Water-in-oil (right side).

Solutions

Solutions (soh-LOO-shuns) are uniform mixtures of two or more mutually mixable substances. A **solute** (SOL-yoot) is any substance that is dissolved by a solvent to form a solution. A **solvent** (SOL-vent) is any substance that dissolves the solute to form a solution.

Miscible (MIS-eh-bel) liquids are mutually soluble. Water and alcohol are examples of miscible (mixable) liquids. **Immiscible** liquids are not mutually soluble (Figure 6–10). Water and oil are examples of immiscible (nonmixable) liquids. You have probably heard the saying, "oil and water don't mix."

Solutions contain particles the size of a small molecule that are invisible to the naked eye. Solutions are usually transparent, although they may be colored. Solutions do not separate on standing. Salt water is a solution of a solid dissolved in a liquid. Water is the solvent that dissolves the salt and holds it in solution. Air, salt water, and hydrogen peroxide are examples of solutions.

Suspensions

Suspensions are uniform mixtures of two or more substances. Suspensions differ from solutions due to the size of the particles. Suspensions contain larger particles than solutions do. The particles in a suspension are large enough to be visible to the naked eye. Suspensions are not usually transparent and may be colored. Suspensions have a tendency to separate over time.

Oil and vinegar salad dressing is an example of a suspension with oil suspended in vinegar. Salad dressing will separate on standing and should be shaken well before use. Salad dressing, paint, and aerosol hair spray are examples of suspensions.

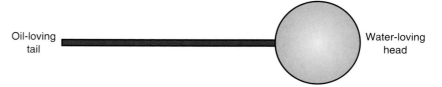

Figure 6–11 A surfactant molecule.

Emulsions

Emulsions (ee-MUL-shuns) are suspensions (mixtures) of an unstable mixture of two or more immiscible substances united with the aid of an emulsifier. The term *emulsify* means "to form an emulsion," which is a suspension of one liquid dispersed in another. Although emulsions tend to separate over time, a properly formulated emulsion, when stored correctly, should be stable for at least 3 years. Without adequate dispersion, emulsions can become unstable over time and break (separate) into two insoluble layers. Once this occurs, the emulsion should usually be discarded.

Surfactants

Surfactants are used to emulsify oil and water to create an emulsion. The word *surfactant* (sur-FAK-tant) is an acronym for surface active agent (*surf*ace *act*ive age*nt*). Surfactants are able to wet the skin and disperse oil in water. A surfactant molecule has two distinct parts that make the emulsification of oil and water possible (Figure 6–11). One end of the surfactant molecule is **hydrophilic** (water loving), and the other end is **lipophilic** (oil loving). Since "like dissolves like," the hydrophilic end dissolves in water and the lipophilic end dissolves in oil. So, a surfactant molecule dissolves in both oil and water and joins them together to form an emulsion.

Most skin care products are emulsions of oil and water. Two types of emulsions are used in cosmetic preparations: oil-in-water (O/W) and water-in-oil (W/O). As a skin moisturizer, the purpose of an emulsion is to apply a uniform layer of the emulsion's oil phase evenly on the skin. Once contact is made with the skin, the finely dispersed oil phase is deposited on the surface. The oil phase acts as an external lubricant to smooth and protect the surface of the epidermis. The water phase restores the natural moisture content of the epidermis, making the skin soft and smooth. Thus, the water in the emulsion acts as an internal lubricant. One advantage of O/W emulsions is that they are easily rinsed away with water. An O/W cleansing lotion, for example, can be removed easily with wet cotton pads or sponges.

O/W emulsions are often milky, free-flowing liquids, although thickeners may be added to form gels or thick creams. O/W emulsions include moisturizing lotions, cleansing lotions, and suntan lotions.

Oil-in-Water (O/W) Emulsions

In an **oil-in-water emulsion,** droplets of oil are dispersed in water. The droplets of oil (micelles) are surrounded by surfactants with their "tails" (lipophilic ends) pointing in and their "heads" (hydrophilic ends) pointing out,

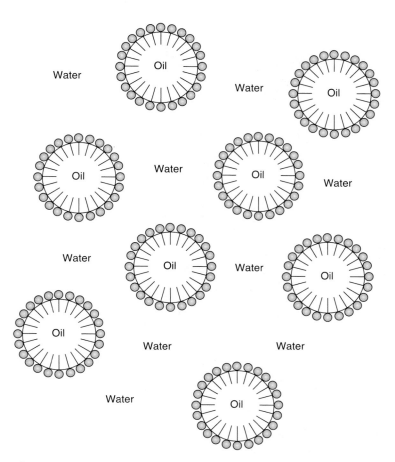

Figure 6–12 Oil-in-water emulsion.

which keeps the oil dispersed in water. In O/W emulsions, the water is the continuous or external phase and the oil is the discontinuous or internal phase (Figure 6–12). O/W emulsions usually contain a small amount of oil and a greater amount of water. Salons primarily use O/W emulsions.

Mayonnaise is an O/W emulsion of two immiscible liquids. Although oil and water are immiscible, the egg yolk in mayonnaise emulsifies the oil and disperses it uniformly in the water. Without the egg yolk as an emulsifying agent, the oil and water would separate into two insoluble layers. Mayonnaise should not separate on standing. Most of the lotions and creams used by estheticians are O/W emulsions. Mayonnaise, skin cleansers, moisturizers, and body washes are examples of O/W emulsions.

Water-in-Oil (W/O) Emulsions

In a **water-in-oil emulsion,** droplets of water are dispersed in oil. The droplets of water (inverse micelles) are surrounded by surfactants with their "heads" (hydrophilic ends) pointing in and their "tails" (lipophilic ends) pointing out. In W/O emulsions, the oil is the continuous or external phase and the water is the discontinuous, or internal phase (Figure 6–13).

W/O emulsions usually contain a smaller amount of water and a greater amount of oil. W/O emulsions are heavier, greasier, and more water resistant

ACTIVITY

Have you ever heard the saying, "Oil and water don't mix?" Pour some water into a glass, and then add a little cooking oil (or other oil). What happens? Stir the water briskly with a spoon, and then observe for a minute or two. What does the oil do?

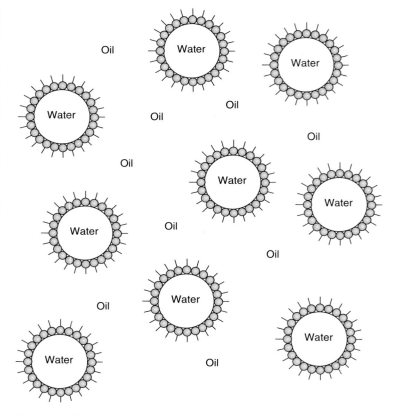

Figure 6–13 Water-in-oil emulsion.

than O/W emulsions because the oil is in the external phase. These emulsions remove grime and help prevent moisture loss from the skin. Examples include cleansing creams, cold creams, night creams, massage creams, baby creams, and hair-grooming creams.

REVIEW QUESTIONS

1. Define *chemistry*.
2. What is the difference between organic and inorganic chemistry?
3. Define *matter*.
4. What are the differences between solids, liquids, and gases?
5. Define *element*.
6. What are atoms?
7. Define *molecule*.

8. What is the difference between a compound and a mixture?

9. What are physical properties? How are they different from chemical properties?

10. How can matter be changed? Give an example of each kind of change.

11. Describe hydrogen, oxygen, and nitrogen.

12. How is water important in skin care?

13. Define *pH*. Why do you need to know the pH of products you work with?

14. Define *oxidation* and *reduction*.

15. Explain the differences between solutions, suspensions, and emulsions.

16. Explain the structure of the two types of emulsion products used in skin care.

CHAPTER GLOSSARY

acid mantle: protective lipids and secretions on top of the skin.

acid-alkali neutralization reactions: when an acid is mixed with an alkali, also called a base, in equal proportions to neutralize each other and form water (H_2O) and a salt.

acids: substances that have a pH below 7.0, taste sour, and turn litmus paper from blue to red.

air: the gaseous mixture that makes up the earth's atmosphere. It is odorless, colorless, and generally consists of about 1 part oxygen and 4 parts nitrogen by volume.

alkalies: also called bases; have a pH above 7.0, taste bitter, and turn litmus paper from red to blue.

antioxidants: free radical scavengers, vitamins, and ingredients. Antioxidants also inhibit oxidation. They are used both to help the condition of the skin and to stop the oxidation that causes products to turn rancid and spoil.

atoms: the smallest particle of an element that still retains the properties of that element.

chemical change: change in the chemical composition of a substance, in which a new substance or substances are formed that have properties different from the original.

chemical compounds: combinations of two or more atoms of different elements united chemically with a fixed chemical composition, definite proportions, and distinct properties.

chemical properties: those characteristics that can be determined only with a chemical reaction and that cause a chemical change in the identity of the substance.

CHAPTER GLOSSARY

chemistry: science that deals with the composition, structures, and properties of matter and with how matter changes under different conditions.

combustion: rapid oxidation of any substance, accompanied by the production of heat and light.

compound molecules: chemical combinations of two or more atoms of different elements.

element: the simplest form of matter; cannot be broken down into a simpler substance without loss of identity.

elemental molecules: chemical combinations of two or more atoms of the same element.

emulsions: an unstable mixture of two or more immiscible substances united with the aid of an emulsifier.

free radicals: "super" oxidizers that cause an oxidation reaction and produce a new free radical in the process; are created by highly reactive atoms or molecules (often oxygen) having an unpaired number of electrons. Free radicals are unstable and can damage DNA, causing inflammation and disease in the body.

hydrogen: colorless, odorless, tasteless gas; the lightest element known.

hydrogen peroxide: chemical compound of hydrogen and oxygen; a colorless liquid with a characteristic odor and a slightly acid taste.

hydrophilic: capable of combining with or attracting water.

immiscible: not capable of being mixed.

inorganic chemistry: branch of chemistry dealing with elements that do not contain carbon.

lipophilic: having an affinity or attraction to fat and oils.

logarithmic scale: a method of displaying data in multiples of 10.

matter: any substance that occupies space and has mass (weight).

miscible: capable of being mixed with another liquid in any proportion without separating.

molecule: a chemical combination of two or more atoms.

nitrogen: colorless, gaseous element that makes up four-fifths of the air in the atmosphere.

oil-in-water (O/W) emulsion: oil droplets dispersed in a water with the aid of an emulsifying agent.

organic chemistry: study of substances that contain carbon.

oxidation: chemical reaction that combines a substance with oxygen to produce an oxide.

oxidation-reduction (redox) reactions: one of the most common types of chemical reactions; prevalent in all areas of chemistry. When oxygen is added to a substance, the substance is oxidized; for example, rust forms when oxygen is added to iron.

oxidize: to combine or cause a substance to combine with oxygen.

oxygen: the most abundant element on earth.

pH: relative degree of acidity and alkalinity of a substance.

physical change: change in the form or physical properties of a substance without a chemical reaction or the formation of a new substance.

physical mixture: combination of two or more substances united physically, not chemically, without a fixed composition and in any proportions.

physical properties: characteristics that can be determined without a chemical reaction and that do not cause a chemical change in the identity of the substance.

redox: acronym for *reduction-oxidation*; chemical reaction in which the oxidizing agent is reduced and the reducing agent is oxidized.

redox reactions: oxidation and reduction happening at the same time.

reduction: the loss of oxygen from a substance.

solute: a substance that is dissolved by a solvent to form a solution.

solutions: a uniform mixture of two or more mutually miscible substances.

solvent: a substance that dissolves another substance to form a solution.

surfactants: surface active agents that reduce surface tension between the skin and the product to increase product spreadability; also allow oil and water to mix; detergents and emulsifiers.

suspensions: state in which solid particles are distributed throughout a liquid medium.

water: most abundant of all substances, comprising about 75 percent of the earth's surface and about 65 percent of the human body.

water-in-oil (W/O) emulsion: droplets of water dispersed in an oil.

CHAPTER 7

BASICS OF ELECTRICITY

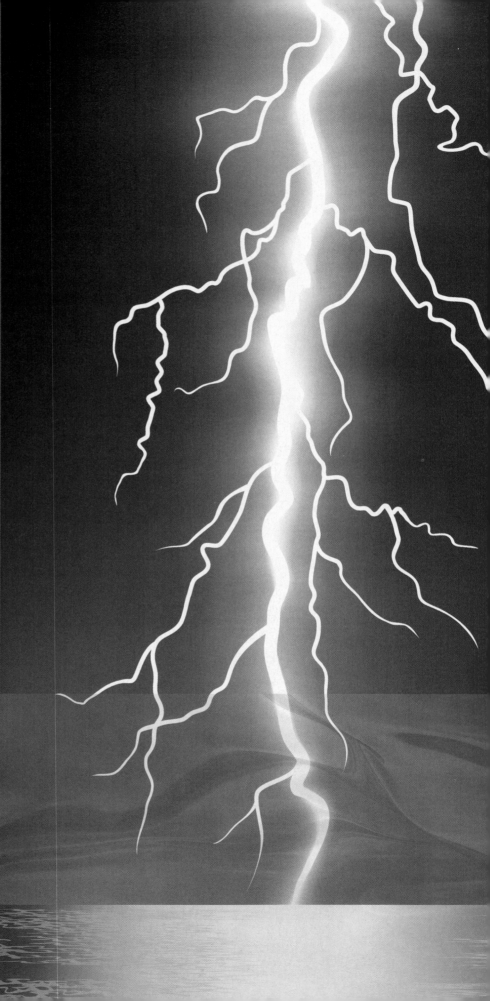

LEARNING OBJECTIVES

After completing this chapter, you will be able to:

- Define the nature of electricity and the two types of electric current.

- Describe the four types of electrotherapy and their uses.

- Explain electromagnetic radiation and the visible spectrum of light.

- Describe the rays used in light therapy and their benefits.

- Describe what the acronym *laser* stands for.

KEY TERMS

Page numbers indicate where in the chapter each term is used.

active electrode 151

alternating current (AC) 148

amp (A) 148

anaphoresis 152

anode 151

blue light 157

cataphoresis 152

cathode 151

circuit breaker 149

complete circuit 146

conductor 146

converter 148

desincrustation 152

direct current (DC) 148

electric current 146

electricity 146

electrode 151

electromagnetic radiation 155

electrotherapy 151

faradic current 152

fuse 149

galvanic current 151

inactive electrode 151

infrared rays 156

insulator (nonconductor) 146

iontophoresis (ionization) 152

kilowatt (K) 149

laser 158

light therapy 156

microcurrent 153

milliampere 149

modalities 151

ohm (O) 149

phototherapy 156

photothermolysis 158

plug 149

polarity 151

rectifier 148

red light 157

sinusoidal current 152

Tesla high-frequency current 153

ultraviolet (UV) rays 156

visible light 155

volt (V) 148

watt (W) 149

wavelength 155

white light 157

E stheticians use electricity to enhance their work with the skin. Electricity powers all of our machines, including galvanic current, high frequency, steamers, microdermabrasion, microcurrent, magnifying lamps, and many more to come.

Just getting to work requires a fair amount of electricity when we consider the hair dryer, curling iron, lights, heat, hot water, and even some cars. So what is really happening when we turn on the light and turn or flip a switch? In this chapter, we will explore the basics of electricity and gain an understanding of how to use electrical machines safely (Figure 7–1).

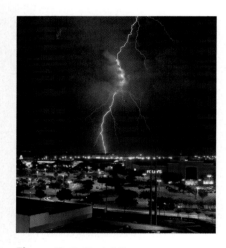

Figure 7–1 Electricity.

ELECTRICITY

We have already provided you with a general overview of chemistry, and we will do the same with electricity because it, too, plays an important role in your work. Lightning on a stormy night is an effect of electricity. If you plug a poorly wired appliance into a socket and sparks fly out, you are also seeing the effects of electricity. You are not really "seeing'" electricity, but its effects on the surrounding air. Electricity does not occupy space or have physical or chemical properties; therefore, it is not matter. If it is not matter, then what is it? **Electricity** is a form of energy that, when in motion, exhibits magnetic, chemical, or thermal effects. It is a flow of electrons, which are negatively charged particles that swirl around atoms like a swarm of bees.

An **electric current** is the flow of electricity along a conductor. All substances can be classified as conductors or insulators, depending on how easily an electric current can be transmitted through them.

A **conductor** is any substance that easily transmits electricity. Most metals are good conductors. Copper is a particularly good conductor and is used in electric wiring and electric motors. The ionic compounds in ordinary water make it a good conductor. This explains why you should not swim in a lake during an electrical storm.

An **insulator** (IN-suh-lay-tur) or **nonconductor** is a substance that does not easily transmit electricity. Rubber, silk, wood, glass, and cement are good insulators. Electric wires are composed of twisted metal threads (conductor) covered with rubber (insulator). A **complete circuit** (SUR-kit) is the path of an electric current from the generating source through conductors and back to its original source (Figure 7–2).

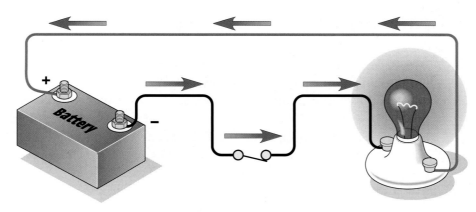

Figure 7–2 A complete electrical circuit.

Hydropower (water-powered) plants today make up our country's largest renewable energy source. Hydropower plants rely on a dam that holds back water and creates a large lake known as a reservoir. The water comes from melting snow from the mountains, traveling via groundwater, creeks, streams and rivers, and of course, rain.

When large doors on the dam open, water flows from the reservoir into a pipe. As the water flows into the pipe it builds up pressure, which turns a turbine (a big disc with blades) attached to a generator. As the turbine blades turn, so do a series of magnets inside the generator. Giant magnets rotate past copper coils, producing alternating current (more later on alternating current) by moving electrons. The alternating current (AC) is converted to a higher-voltage current by a transformer. Going out of the power plant are large wires that become power lines, and the electrical current that is passing through the lines supplies the community with electricity (Figure 7–3).

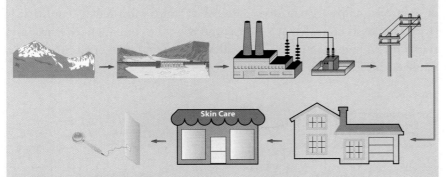

Figure 7–3 Electricity flow chart.

Types of Electric Current

There are two kinds of electric current.

Direct current (DC) is a constant, even-flowing current that travels in one direction only. Flashlights, cellular telephones, and cordless electric drills use the direct current produced by batteries. The battery in your car stores electrical energy. Without it, your car would not start in the morning. A **converter** is an apparatus that changes direct current to alternating current. Some cars have converters that allow you to use appliances that would normally be plugged into an electrical wall outlet.

Alternating current (AC) is a rapid and interrupted current, flowing first in one direction and then in the opposite direction. This change in direction happens 60 times per second. Hair dryers and curling irons that plug into a wall outlet use alternating current produced by mechanical generators.

A **rectifier** is an apparatus that changes alternating current to direct current. Battery chargers use a rectifier to convert the AC current from an electrical wall outlet to the DC current needed to recharge their DC batteries.

Electrical Measurements

The flow of an electric current can be compared to water flowing through a garden hose. Individual electrons flow through a wire in the same way that individual water molecules flow through a hose.

A **volt (V),** or voltage, is the unit that measures the pressure or force that pushes the flow of electrons forward through a conductor, much like the water pressure that pushes the water molecules through the hose (Figure 7–4). Without pressure, neither water nor electrons would flow. Car batteries are 12 volts, normal wall sockets that power your hair dryer and curling iron are 110 volts, and most air conditioners and clothes dryers run on 220 volts. A higher voltage indicates more pressure or force.

An **amp (A),** or ampere (AM-peer), is the unit that measures the strength of an electric current (the number of electrons flowing through a wire). Like a water hose, which must be able to expand as the amount of water flowing through it increases, a wire also must expand with an increase in the amount of electrons (amps). A hair dryer rated at 12 amps must have a cord that is twice as thick as one rated at 5 amps; otherwise, the cord might overheat and start a fire. A higher amp rating indicates a greater number of electrons and a stronger current (Figure 7–5).

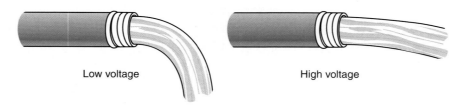

Low voltage   High voltage

Figure 7–4 Volts measure the pressure or force that pushes electrons forward.

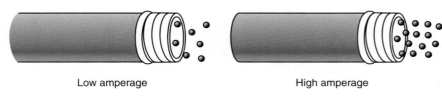

Figure 7–5 Amps measure the number of electrons flowing through the wire.

Low amperage   High amperage

A **milliampere** (mill-ee-AM-peer) is one-thousandth of an ampere. The current for facial and scalp treatments is measured in milliamperes; an ampere current would be much too strong and would damage the skin or body.

An **ohm (O)** is a unit that measures the resistance of an electric current. Current will not flow through a conductor unless the force (volts) is stronger than the resistance (ohms).

A **watt (W)** is a measurement of how much electric energy is being used in one second. A 40-watt light bulb uses 40 watts of energy per second.

A **kilowatt (K)** is 1,000 watts. The electricity in your house is measured in kilowatts per hour (kwh). A 1,000-watt (1-kilowatt) hair dryer uses 1,000 watts of energy per second.

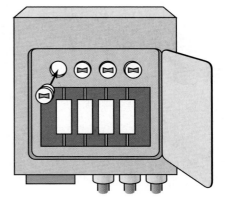

Figure 7–6 Fuse box.

ELECTRICAL EQUIPMENT SAFETY

When working with electricity, you must always be concerned with your own safety as well as that of your clients. All electrical equipment should be inspected regularly to determine whether it is in safe working order. Poor electrical connections and overloaded circuits can result in an electrical shock, a burn, or even a serious fire.

Safety Devices

A **fuse** (FYOOZ) is a special device that prevents excessive current from passing through a circuit. It is designed to blow out or melt when the wire becomes too hot from overloading the circuit with too much current (i.e., too many appliances or faulty equipment). To reestablish the circuit, disconnect the appliance, check all connections and insulation, and insert a new fuse (Figure 7–6).

A **circuit breaker** is a switch that automatically interrupts or shuts off an electric circuit at the first indication of overload. Circuit breakers have replaced fuses in modern electric circuits. They have all the safety features of fuses but do not require replacement, and they can simply be reset. Your hair dryer has a circuit breaker located in the electric **plug** designed to protect you and your client in case of an overload or short circuit. When a circuit breaker shuts off, you should disconnect the appliance and check all connections and insulation before resetting (Figure 7–7).

The principle of "grounding" is another important way of promoting electrical safety. All electrical appliances must have at least two electrical connections. The "live" connection supplies current to the circuit. The ground connection completes the circuit and carries the current safely away to the ground. If you look closely at electrical plugs with two rectangular prongs,

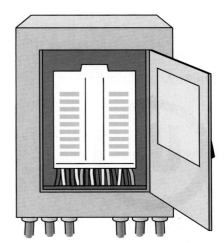

Figure 7–7 Circuit breaker.

CAUTION!

Underwriter's Laboratory (UL®) certifies the safety of electrical appliances. Electric mitts, masks, and other tools that are UL approved are certified to be safe when used according to the manufacturer's directions. Always look for the UL symbol on electrical appliances, and take the time to read and follow the manufacturer's directions.

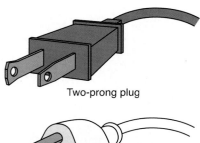

Two-prong plug

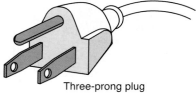

Three-prong plug

Figure 7–8 Two-prong and three-prong plugs.

Underwriter's Laboratory

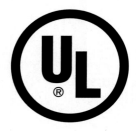

Figure 7–9 Always check for the UL symbol.

you will see that one is slightly larger than the other. This guarantees that the plug can be inserted only one way, and it protects you and your client from electrical shock in the event of a short circuit.

For added protection, some appliances have a third, circular, electrical connection that provides an additional ground. This extra ground is designed to guarantee a safe path for electricity if the first ground fails or is improperly connected. Appliances with a third circular ground offer the most protection for you and your client (Figure 7–8).

Guidelines for Safe Use of Electrical Equipment

Careful attention to electrical safety helps to eliminate accidents and to ensure greater client satisfaction. The following reminders will help ensure the safe use of electricity.

- All the electrical appliances you use should be UL certified (Figure 7–9).
- Read all instructions carefully before using any piece of electrical equipment.
- Disconnect all appliances when not in use.
- Inspect all electrical equipment regularly.
- Keep all wires, plugs, and electrical equipment in good repair.
- Use only one plug to each outlet; overloading may cause the circuit breaker to pop (Figure 7–10).
- You and your client should avoid contact with water and metal surfaces when using electricity; do not handle electrical equipment with wet hands.
- Do not leave your client unattended while he or she is connected to an electrical device.
- Keep electrical cords off the floor and away from people's feet; getting tangled in a cord could cause you or your client to trip.
- Do not attempt to clean around electric outlets while equipment is plugged in.
- Do not touch two metal objects at the same time if either is connected to an electric current.
- Do not step on or place objects on electrical cords.

Safe

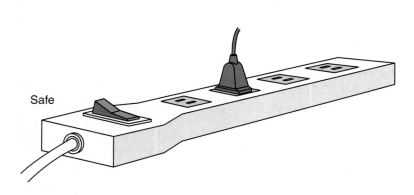

Unsafe

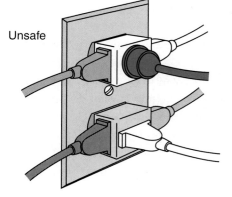

Figure 7–10 Safe and unsafe use of outlets.

- Do not allow an electrical cord to become twisted; this can cause a short circuit.
- Disconnect appliances by pulling on the plug, not the cord.
- Do not attempt to repair electrical appliances unless you are qualified.

ELECTROTHERAPY

Electrical facial treatments are commonly referred to as **electrotherapy.** These treatments are often called **modalities.** Each modality produces a different effect on the skin.

An **electrode** is an applicator for directing the electric current from the machine to the client's skin. It is usually made of carbon, glass, or metal. Each modality (except for Tesla high frequency) requires two electrodes—one negative and one positive—to conduct the flow of electricity through the body (Figure 7–11).

Polarity

Polarity indicates the negative or positive pole of an electric current. Electrotherapy devices always have one negatively charged pole and one positively charged pole. The positive electrode is called an **anode** (AN-ohd). The anode is usually red and is marked with a "P" or a plus (+) sign. The negative electrode is called a **cathode** (KATH-ohd). It is usually black and is marked with an "N" or a minus (−) sign (Figure 7–12). If the electrodes are not marked, the following polarity tests will tell you which is which.

Separate the two tips of the conducting cords from each other and immerse them in a glass of salt water. Turn the selector switch of the appliance to galvanic current, and then turn up the intensity. More active bubbles will accumulate at the negative pole than at the positive pole.

Another test involves placing the tips of the conducting cords on two separate pieces of moist blue litmus paper. The paper under the positive pole will turn red, while the paper under the negative pole will stay blue. If you use red litmus paper, the paper under the positive pole will remain red, and the paper under the negative pole will turn blue.

Modalities

The four main modalities used in esthetics are galvanic, faradic, sinusoidal, and Tesla high frequency.

Galvanic Current

The most commonly used modality is **galvanic current.** It is used for unblocking clogged pores and to drive solutions deeper into the epidermis. It is a constant and direct current (DC), having a positive and negative pole, and produces chemical changes when it passes through the tissues and fluids of the body.

Galvanic current works by creating two different chemical reactions, depending on the polarity (negative or positive) that is used (Table 7–1). The **active electrode** is the electrode used on the area to be treated. The **inactive electrode** is the opposite pole from the active electrode. Note that the effects produced by the positive pole are the exact opposite of those produced by the negative pole.

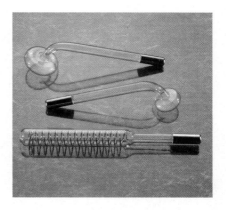

Figure 7–11 Electrodes come in a variety of shapes.

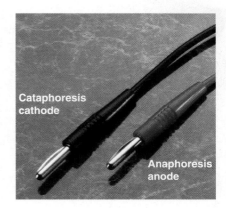

Cataphoresis cathode

Anaphoresis anode

Figure 7–12 Cathode and anode.

Table 7–1

EFFECTS OF GALVANIC CURRENT	
POSITIVE POLE (ANODE)	**NEGATIVE POLE (CATHODE)**
Produces acidic reactions	Produces alkaline reactions
Closes the pores	Opens the pores
Soothes nerves	Stimulates and irritates the nerves
Decreases blood supply	Increases blood supply
Contracts blood vessels	Expands blood vessels
Hardens and firms tissues	Soften tissues

Iontophoresis

Iontophoresis (eye-ahn-toh-foh-REE-sus) **(ionization)** is a term for the process of introducing water-soluble products into the skin with the use of electric current, such as that from the positive and negative poles of a galvanic machine.

Cataphoresis (kat-uh-fuh-REE-sus) forces acidic substances into deeper tissues by using galvanic current from the positive toward the negative pole.

Anaphoresis (an-uh-for-EES-sus) is the process of forcing alkaline liquids into the tissues from the negative toward the positive pole.

Desincrustation (des-in-krus-TAY-shun) is a process which uses the negative pole to soften and emulsify grease deposits (oil) and blackheads in the hair follicles. This process is frequently used to treat acne, milia (small, white cyst-like pimples), and comedones (blackheads and whiteheads).

Faradic Current

Faradic current is an alternating and interrupted current that produces a mechanical reaction without a chemical effect. It is used during scalp and facial manipulations to cause visible muscular contractions. Benefits derived from faradic current include

- improved muscle tone.
- removal of waste products.
- increased blood circulation.
- relief of blood congestion.
- increased glandular activity.
- stimulation of hair growth.
- increased metabolism.

Sinusoidal Current

Sinusoidal (sy-nuh-SOYD-ul) **current** is similar to faradic current and is also used during scalp and facial manipulations. It is an alternating current that produces mechanical contractions that tone the muscles. Sinusoidal current has the following advantages:

- supplies greater stimulation, deeper penetration, and is less irritating than faradic current
- soothes the nerves and penetrates into deeper muscle tissue
- is best suited for the nervous client

> **CAUTION!**
>
> Do not use negative galvanic current on skin with broken capillaries or pustular acne conditions, or on a client with high blood pressure or metal implants.

> **CAUTION!**
>
> Do not use faradic or sinusoidal current if it causes pain or discomfort, if the face is very ruddy (red in color), or if your client has gold-filled teeth, high blood pressure, broken capillaries, or pustular skin conditions. Never use faradic or sinusoidal currents longer than 15 to 20 minutes.

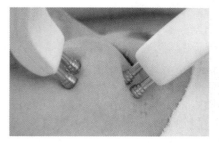 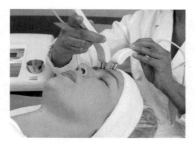

Figure 7–13 A, B A microcurrent treatment. (Courtesy David Suzuki, Bio Therapeutic, Inc.)

Microcurrent

Microcurrent is an extremely low level of electricity that mirror's the body's own natural electrical impulses. Through electrical stimulation, microcurrent works by mimicking the way that the brain relays messages to the muscles. It is reported to aid in the healing and repairing of tissue and to influence cellular activity. The goal is to speed up the body's natural regenerative processes, using the proper amount of low-level current, less than 400uA's. Microcurrent requires a manual manipulation to reeducate the muscles, but it does not cause a visible or physical contraction of the face via the electrical current. Microcurrent can be effective in the following ways:

- improves blood and lymph circulation
- increases muscle tone
- restores elasticity
- reduces redness and inflammation
- minimizes post-surgical healing time
- increases collagen and elastin production

When used in treatments for aging skin, the results may be a firmer appearance of the skin. Microcurrent treatments have also been shown to benefit stroke and paralysis patients (Figure 7–13 A, B).

As with all electrical equipment, microcurrent should not be used on people with pacemakers, epilepsy, pregnancy, phlebitis, or thrombosis; or on anyone currently "under a doctor's care."

Tesla High-Frequency Current

Tesla high-frequency current is a thermal or heat-producing current with a high rate of oscillation or vibration. It is commonly called the violet ray and is used for both scalp and facial treatments. Tesla current does not produce muscle contractions, and its effects can be either stimulating or soothing, depending on the method of application. The electrodes are made from either glass or metal, and only one electrode is used to perform a service. Here are some benefits of using Tesla high-frequency current.

- stimulates blood circulation
- improves glandular activity
- increases elimination and absorption
- increases metabolism
- improves germicidal action
- relieves congestion

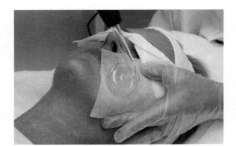

Figure 7–14 Direct high-frequency application.

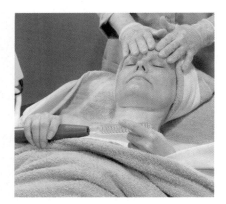

Figure 7–15 Indirect high-frequency application.

CAUTION!

As with all facial treatments, it is important to take a full history before performing electrotherapy. If your client has any of the following conditions, it is not advisable to treat them with electrotherapy:

- Pacemaker/Heart conditions/High blood pressure
- Epilepsy
- Open cuts, sores, pustular acne, or abrasions
- Diabetes
- Metal dental or facial implants including braces, pins, or plates
- Pregnancy
- Dilated capillaries (telangiectasias, or spider veins)
- Recent laser resurfacing or chemical peel
- Clients using Accutane® or retinoids

There are two methods for applying high-frequency current.

1. *Direct surface application.* The esthetician holds the handpiece, where the glass electrode is inserted, and applies it directly to the client's skin, moving it slowly over the entire face for stimulation (Figure 7–14). When applying and removing the electrode from the skin, you must hold your finger on the glass electrode to prevent sparking. Remove your finger once the electrode has been placed on the skin. Apply the electrode to areas for healing acne and disinfecting.

2. *Indirect application.* The client holds the tube electrode (with the metal coil inside) while the esthetician massages the face with her hands (Figure 7–15). At no time should the esthetician hold the electrode. To prevent shock, turn on the current only after the client has firmly grasped the electrode. Turn the current off before removing the electrode from the client's hand. The indirect application stimulates all cell functions without the irritation that could occur with direct application. This treatment is beneficial for sensitive, dehydrated skin.

LIGHT WAVES/LIGHT RAYS

Light or electrical waves travel at a tremendous speed—186,000 miles per second. There are many kinds of light rays, but in esthetics work we are concerned with only three—those producing heat, known as infrared rays; those producing chemical and germicidal reaction, known as ultraviolet rays; and visible light, all of which are contained within the spectrum of the sun.

If a ray of sunshine is passed through a glass prism, it will appear in seven different colors, known as the rainbow, arrayed in the following manner: red, orange, yellow, green, blue, indigo, and violet. These colors, which are visible to the eye, constitute the visible rays.

Scientists have discovered that at either end of the visible spectrum are rays of the sun that are invisible to us. The rays beyond the violet are the ultraviolet rays, also known as cold rays or actinic rays. These rays are the shortest and least penetrating rays of the spectrum. Beyond the red rays of the spectrum are the infrared rays. These are pure heat rays.

Visible light is electromagnetic radiation that we can see. **Electromagnetic radiation,** also called radiant energy, carries, or radiates, energy through space on waves. These waves are similar to the waves caused when a stone is dropped on the surface of the water. The distance between two successive peaks is called the **wavelength.** Long wavelengths have low frequency, meaning the number of waves is less frequent (fewer waves) within a given length. Short wavelengths have higher frequency because the number of waves is more frequent (more waves) within a given length (Figure 7–16).

The entire range of wavelengths of electromagnetic radiation (radiant energy) is called the electromagnetic spectrum. Visible light is the part of the electromagnetic spectrum that we can see. Visible light makes up 35 percent of natural sunlight (Figure 7–17).

Ultraviolet rays and infrared rays are also forms of electromagnetic radiation, but they are invisible because their wavelengths are beyond the visible spectrum of light. Invisible rays make up 65 percent of natural sunlight.

Within the visible spectrum of light, violet has the shortest wavelength and red has the longest. The wavelength of infrared is just below red, and the wavelength of ultraviolet is just above violet. Infrared and ultraviolet rays are not really light at all. Again, they are the wavelengths of electromagnetic radiation that are just beyond the visible spectrum.

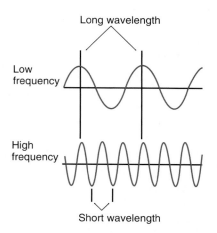

Figure 7–16 Long and short wavelengths.

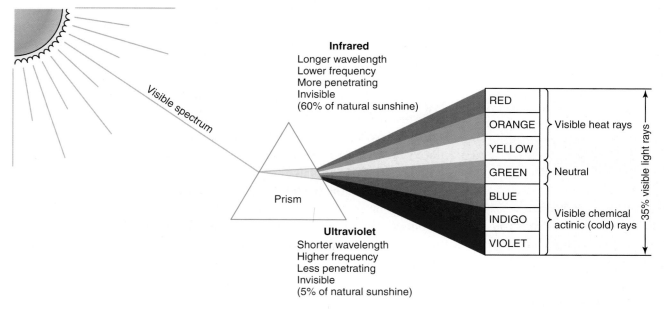

Figure 7–17 The visible spectrum.

Ultraviolet Rays

We need sunlight to survive on the planet. Through a process called photosynthesis, green plants use sunlight to form carbohydrates from carbon dioxide and water and then release oxygen as a by-product. Sunlight also controls our weather and is considered our ultimate energy source. **Ultraviolet (UV) rays** make up 5 percent of natural sunlight. UV rays have shorter wavelengths, penetrate less, and produce less heat than visible light does. UV rays also produce chemical effects and kill germs.

Small amounts of exposure to the sun can be beneficial in the production of vitamin D; however, recent studies have shown that overexposure to the sun causes skin damage, premature aging, and skin cancer. There are three types of ultraviolet rays.

1. *Ultraviolet A (UVA).* Ultraviolet A rays are the longest of the UV rays and penetrate directly into the dermis of the skin, damaging the collagen and elastin, UVA rays are often used in tanning beds.
2. *Ultraviolet B (UVB).* Ultraviolet B rays are often called the burning rays, because they are most associated with sunburns. UVB rays penetrate the epidermis to the basal layer, stimulate melanin, and are the cause of most skin cancers.
3. *Ultraviolet C (UVC).* Ultraviolet rays are short rays that are blocked by the ozone layer. They have germicidal properties, but in larger amounts will eliminate life as we know it. We do not want to deplete the ozone layer, because it protects us from UVC radiation.

We all need to strike a delicate balance with sunlight exposure. Keep in mind that tanned skin is damaged skin. Tanning will eventually cause photoaging (premature aging due to sun exposure) and irreversibly damage the skin's collagen-building properties.

Light Therapy

Light therapy, also called **phototherapy,** has evolved throughout time. Some of the original techniques are still valid today. From dermatologists using ultraviolet rays for treating psoriasis to estheticians using blue- and red-light therapy for acne to surgeons using the most high-tech lasers for advanced surgical procedures the power of light is here to stay.

Although the application of UV rays can be beneficial, it must be done with the utmost care in a carefully measured manner by a qualified professional. It has been used to kill bacteria on the skin and to help the body produce vitamin D. Dermatologists use UV therapy in addition to drugs such as psoralen for the treatment of psoriasis.

Depending on the type of therapy, UV application should begin with exposure times of 2 to 3 minutes, with a gradual increase in exposure time to 7 or 8 minutes. Overexposure to UV rays can produce painful burns and blistering, increase the risk of skin cancer, and cause premature aging of the skin. Clients are not left unattended during the exposure time.

Infrared Rays

Infrared rays make up 60 percent of natural sunlight. Infrared rays have longer wavelengths, penetrate deeper, and produce more heat than visible light does.

Infrared lamps are often used in salons for heating conditioners and chemicals in hair treatments. They are also used in spas and saunas for relaxation and for warming up muscles.

Visible Light Rays

Visible light rays are the primary light source used for facial and scalp treatments. The bulbs used for therapeutic visible light therapy are white, red, and blue.

White light is referred to as combination light because it is a combination of all the visible rays of the spectrum. White light has the benefits of all the rays of the visible spectrum. **Blue light** should be used only on oily skin that is bare. It contains few heat rays, is the least penetrating, and has some germicidal and chemical benefits. **Red light** is used on dry skin in combination with oils and creams. Red light penetrates the deepest and produces the most heat. Table 7–2 lists the effects of the different rays used in light therapy.

WEB RESOURCES

Several Web sites can provide additional information about electricity. Try these:

http://www.ezistim.com

http://www.eia.doe.gov

http://howto.altenergystore.com

http://www.loc.gov

http://www.bio-therapeutic.com

Table 7–2

EFFECTS OF DIFFERENT TYPES OF RAYS USED IN LIGHT THERAPY	
TYPES OF LIGHT	**BENEFICIAL EFFECTS**
Ultraviolet	Increases the elimination of waste products Improves the flow of blood and lymph Has a germicidal and antibacterial effect Produces vitamin D in the skin Can be used to treat rickets, psoriasis, and acne
Infrared	Heats and relaxes the skin Dilates blood vessels and increases circulation Produces chemical changes Increases metabolism Increases production of perspiration and oil Deep penetration relieves pain in sore muscles Soothes nerves
White light	Relieves pain in the back of the neck and shoulders Produces some chemical and germicidal effects Relaxes muscles
Blue light	Soothes nerves Improves acne Improves skin tone Provides some chemical and germicidal effects Used for mild cases of skin eruptions Produces little heat
Red light	Improves dry, scaly, wrinkled skin Increases rate of collagen building Relaxes muscles Penetrates the deepest Produces the most heat

Lasers and Light Therapy (Phototherapy) Devices

Lasers and light therapy devices have been in use for many decades. One of the many differences between light therapies and lasers is that lasers are made to have all of the light power going to a certain level, in all the same color, in one direction. In contrast, light therapies will have multiple depths, colors, and wavelengths, and the light may be more scattered. The equipment to be used is based on the condition you are treating.

Lasers

Laser is an acronym that stands for *light amplification stimulation emission of radiation*. Because lasers are used to treat a variety of conditions, there are many kinds of lasers to choose from. All lasers work by selective **photothermolysis**, a process that turns the light from the laser into heat. Depending on the intended use and type, lasers can remove blood vessels, disable hair follicles, remove tattoos, or eliminate some wrinkles without destroying surrounding tissue. Lasers work by means of a medium (solid, liquid or gas, or semiconductor) that emits light when excited by a power source. The medium is placed in a specifically designed chamber with mirrors located at both ends of the inside. The chamber is stimulated by an energy source such as electrical current, which in turn excites the particles. The reflective surfaces create light that becomes trapped and goes back and forth through the medium, gaining energy with each pass. The light becomes a laser light. The medium determines the wavelength of the laser and thus its use (Figure 7–18).

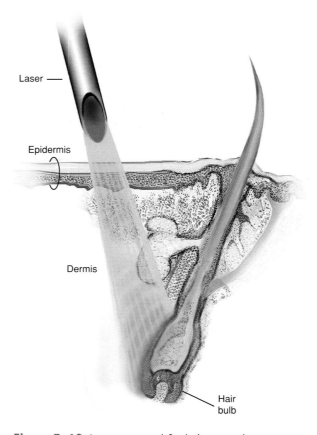

Figure 7–18 Lasers are used for hair removal.

LED or Light-Emitting Diode

Depending on the type of equipment, the LED can be blue, red, yellow, or green. LED in blue has been shown to reduce acne, and red is good for increasing circulation and improving the collagen content in the skin. Yellow light has been shown to reduce swelling and inflammation, and green light is good for hyperpigmented areas. The LED works by releasing flashing light onto the skin to stimulate specific responses such as, with the blue light, killing bacteria that causes acne or, with the red light, increasing circulation and stimulation of the skin (Figure 7–19).

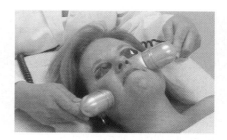

Figure 7–19 LED treatment shown to reduce redness and improve collagen content in the skin. (Courtesy of Revitalight.)

As with all light therapies, it is important to make certain that you have viewed the client consultation form for any contraindications. Light therapy should not be performed on anyone who has light sensitivities (photosensitivities), phototoxic reactions, is taking antibiotics, has cancer or epilepsy, is pregnant, or is under a physician's care.

Intense Pulse Light

Intense pulse light is a light device that uses *a broad spectrum* of focused light to treat spider veins and brown spots (hyperpigmentation). As with most devices, multiple treatments of this type are required.

REVIEW QUESTIONS

1. Why is it important for estheticians to have a basic understanding of electricity?

2. What is the difference between conductors and insulators?

3. Describe the two types of electric current, and give examples of each.

4. Define *volt, amp, ohm,* and *watt.*

5. Why should you look for the UL symbol on electrical devices?

6. What are the four modalities used in electrotherapy? What kind of current is each one?

7. List the effects of the positive pole and the negative pole of a galvanic current.

8. What is iontophoresis? What is desincrustation?

9. Name the benefits of Tesla high-frequency current.

10. What is electromagnetic radiation? What is visible light?

11. List and describe the five main types of light therapy.

12. Why must exposure to ultraviolet rays be carefully monitored?

13. What does the acronym *laser* stand for?

CHAPTER GLOSSARY

active electrode: electrode used on the area to be treated.

alternating current (AC): rapid and interrupted current, flowing first in one direction and then in the opposite direction.

amp (A): unit that measures the amount of an electric current (quantity of electrons flowing through a conductor).

anaphoresis: process of forcing liquids into the tissues from the negative toward the positive pole.

anode: positive electrode.

blue light: therapeutic light that should be used only on oily skin that is bare; contains few heat rays, is the least penetrating, and has some germicidal and chemical benefits.

cataphoresis: process of forcing acidic substances into deeper tissues using galvanic current from the positive toward the negative pole.

cathode: negative electrode.

circuit breaker: switch that automatically interrupts or shuts off an electric circuit at the first indication of overload.

complete circuit: the path of an electric current from the generating source through conductors and back to its original source.

conductor: any substance, material, or medium that easily transmits electricity.

converter: apparatus that changes direct current to alternating current.

desincrustation: galvanic current is used to create an alkaline chemical reaction that emulsifies or liquefies sebum and debris.

direct current (DC): constant, even-flowing current that travels in one direction only.

electric current: flow of electricity along a conductor.

electricity: form of energy that, when in motion, exhibits magnetic, chemical, or thermal effects; a flow of electrons.

electrode: applicator for directing the electric current from the machine to the client's skin.

electromagnetic radiation: energy in the form of electromagnetic waves; also called radiant energy because it carries, or radiates, energy through space on waves.

electrotherapy: the use of electrical devices for therapeutic benefits.

faradic current: alternating and interrupted current that produces a mechanical reaction without a chemical effect.

fuse: special device that prevents excessive current from passing through a circuit.

galvanic current: a constant and direct current (DC); uses a positive and negative pole to produce the chemical changes of desincrustation, an iontophoresis.

inactive electrode: opposite pole from the active electrode.

infrared rays: invisible rays that have longer wavelengths, penetrate deeper, and produce more heat than visible light does.

insulator (nonconductor): substance that does not easily transmit electricity.

iontophoresis (ionization): process of introducing water-soluble products into the skin by using electric current such as that from the positive and negative poles of a galvanic machine.

kilowatt (K): 1,000 watts.

laser: acronym for *light amplification stimulation emission of radiation;* a medical device used for hair removal and skin treatments.

light therapy: the application of light rays to the skin for the treatment of acne, wrinkles, capillaries, pigmentation, or hair removal.

microcurrent: a device that mimics the body's natural electrical energy to reeducate and tone facial muscles; improves circulation and increases collagen and elastin production.

milliampere: one-thousandth of an ampere.

modalities: currents used in electrical facial and scalp treatments.

ohm (O): unit that measures the resistance of an electric current.

phototherapy: Phototherapy (light therapy), is a form of treatment used for various skin conditions using artificial light wavelengths from the ultraviolet (blue light) part of the sun's spectrum.

photothermolysis: process by which light from a laser is turned into heat.

plug: two- or three-prong connector at the end of an electrical cord that connects an apparatus to an electrical outlet.

polarity: negative or positive pole of an electric current.

rectifier: apparatus that changes alternating current to direct current.

red light: therapeutic light used on dry skin in combination with oils and creams; penetrates the deepest and produces the most heat.

sinusoidal current: alternating current similar to faradic current; produces mechanical contractions and is used during scalp and facial manipulations.

Tesla high-frequency current: thermal or heat-producing current with a high rate of oscillation or vibration; also called violet ray.

ultraviolet (UV) rays: invisible rays that have short wavelengths, are the least penetrating rays, produce chemical effects, and kill germs; also called cold rays or actinic rays.

visible light: the primary source of light used in facial and scalp treatments.

volt (V): unit that measures the pressure or force that pushes the flow of electrons forward through a conductor.

watt (W): measurement of how much electric energy is being used in one second.

wavelength: distance between two successive peaks of electromagnetic waves.

white light: referred to as combination light because it is a combination of all the visible rays of the spectrum.

CHAPTER 8

BASICS OF NUTRITION

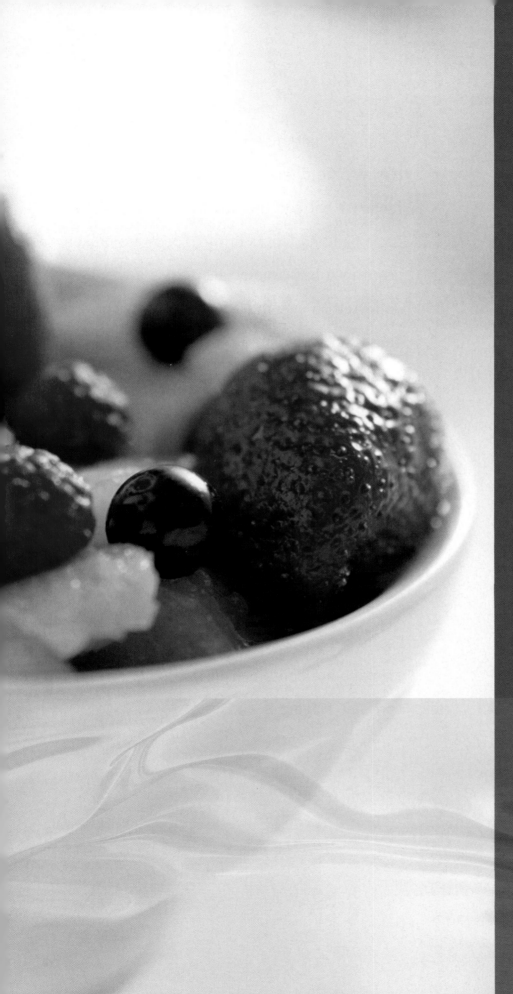

All bodily functions, including the building of tissues, are directly related to nutrition. The foods we eat and the water we drink are the basic building blocks of life. Foods are broken down into basic molecules that are then delivered to every cell in the human body. These molecules are used by the cells to repair damage, form new cells, and conduct all biochemical reactions that run the body's systems. They provide energy that enables our bodies to perform numerous functions. The skin is nourished by the blood and lymph through the arteries and capillaries in the circulatory system. Think of the body or the cell as a machine. All the necessary motors and parts to run the machine are contained in the foods we consume (Figure 8–1).

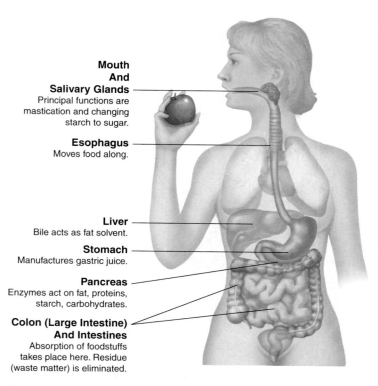

Mouth And Salivary Glands
Principal functions are mastication and changing starch to sugar.

Esophagus
Moves food along.

Liver
Bile acts as fat solvent.

Stomach
Manufactures gastric juice.

Pancreas
Enzymes act on fat, proteins, starch, carbohydrates.

Colon (Large Intestine) And Intestines
Absorption of foodstuffs takes place here. Residue (waste matter) is eliminated.

Figure 8–1 The digestive system and food consumption.

Estheticians are not dietitians. Dietitians have degrees in nutrition, and most are licensed practitioners. Estheticians are not adequately trained in nutrition to legally recommend dietary changes to their clients. Clients may have medical conditions such as diabetes or high blood pressure that can be negatively affected by misleading advice. However, it is beneficial for anyone practicing personal care services, such as esthetics, to have a good working knowledge of nutrition and how the body is affected by the foods we consume. Good nutrition is necessary for healthy skin.

NUTRITION RECOMMENDATIONS

Nutritional needs depend on various factors such as age, sex, weight, physical activity, and body type. The United States Department of Agriculture (USDA) is the governmental agency that regulates nutrition-related affairs. The USDA issues recommended dietary allowances (RDAs) for certain nutrients, including vitamins and minerals.

The USDA food pyramid is a recommended guideline for foods in food groups that individuals should consume daily. The pyramid is now personalized for individual needs and can be found at http://www.mypyramid.gov. Grains, vegetables, dairy, fruits, and meat and beans are the basic food categories in the pyramid (Figure 8–2). Three examples of food guidelines are the USDA Food Guide; the Dietary Approaches to Stop Hypertension (DASH) Eating Plan; and the Institute of Medicine's nutrient intake recommendations.

Many nutritional reports say that much of the population consumes more calories than needed. To safeguard against this, choose foods that are high in

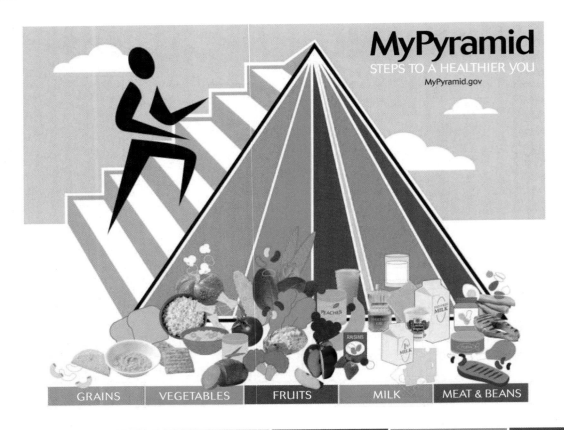

MyPyramid
STEPS TO A HEALTHIER YOU
MyPyramid.gov

| GRAINS | VEGETABLES | FRUITS | MILK | MEAT & BEANS |

GRAINS	VEGETABLES	FRUITS	MILK	MEAT & BEANS
Make half your grains whole	Vary your veggies	Focus on fruits	Get your calcium-rich foods	Go lean with protein
Eat at least 3 oz. of whole-grain cereals, breads, crackers, rice, or pasta every day

1 oz. is about 1 slice of bread, about 1 cup of breakfast cereal, or ½ cup of cooked rice, cereal, or pasta | Eat more dark-green veggies like broccoli, spinach, and other dark leafy greens

Eat more orange vegetables like carrots and sweetpotatoes

Eat more dry beans and peas like pinto beans, kidney beans, and lentils | Eat a variety of fruit

Choose fresh, frozen, canned, or dried fruit

Go easy on fruit juices | Go low-fat or fat-free when you choose milk, yogurt, and other milk products

If you don't or can't consume milk, choose lactose-free products or other calcium sources such as fortified foods and beverages | Choose low-fat or lean meats and poultry

Bake it, broil it, or grill it

Vary your protein routine — choose more fish, beans, peas, nuts, and seeds |

For a 2,000-calorie diet, you need the amounts below from each food group. To find the amounts that are right for you, go to MyPyramid.gov.

| Eat 6 oz. every day | Eat 2½ cups every day | Eat 2 cups every day | Get 3 cups every day; for kids aged 2 to 8, it's 2 | Eat 5½ oz. every day |

Find your balance between food and physical activity
- Be sure to stay within your daily calorie needs.
- Be physically active for at least 30 minutes most days of the week.
- About 60 minutes a day of physical activity may be needed to prevent weight gain.
- For sustaining weight loss, at least 60 to 90 minutes a day of physical activity may be required.
- Children and teenagers should be physically active for 60 minutes every day, or most days.

Know the limits on fats, sugars, and salt (sodium)
- Make most of your fat sources from fish, nuts, and vegetable oils.
- Limit solid fats like butter, margarine, shortening, and lard, as well as foods that contain these.
- Check the Nutrition Facts label to keep saturated fats, *trans* fats, and sodium low.
- Choose food and beverages low in added sugars. Added sugars contribute calories with few, if any, nutrients.

MyPyramid.gov
STEPS TO A HEALTHIER YOU

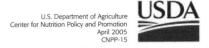

U.S. Department of Agriculture
Center for Nutrition Policy and Promotion
April 2005
CNPP-15

USDA is an equal opportunity provider and employer.

Figure 8–2 The USDA daily food pyramid.

nutrients but lower in calories. People of all ages are encouraged to eat foods with more calcium, potassium, fiber, magnesium, and vitamins A, C, and E. Other recommended dietary changes are to reduce calories, saturated and trans fats, cholesterol, sugars, and salt.

Individual needs such as pregnancy and lactation can affect women's nutritional needs. Diseases or medications that affect the ability to digest food interrupt the normal process of nutrients reaching the bloodstream and, consequently, the cells. See a dietitian or doctor for nutritional advice.

NUTRITION FOR THE SKIN

Understanding how to maintain skin and body health is beneficial to the esthetician personally, as well as to the client. Healthy skin begins with diet and water intake. The adage "You are what you eat" still holds true. Proper dietary choices help to regulate hydration (maintaining a healthy level of water in the body), oil production, and overall cell function. Skin disorders, fatigue, stress, depression, and some diseases are often the result of a poorly balanced diet. Vitamins and minerals are a necessary part of a balanced diet. The benefits and effects of nutrients and their food sources are discussed in this chapter (Figure 8–3).

MACRONUTRIENTS

Macronutrients are the basic building blocks necessary for bodily functions, including the functioning of the skin. The **macronutrients** are the three basic food groups: proteins, carbohydrates, and fats. They make up the largest part of the nutrition we take in. Eating foods found in all three of these basic food groups is necessary to support the health of the body. The recommended intake is protein, 20 percent (105 grams); carbohydrates, 54 percent (281 grams); and fat, 26 percent (60 grams). This is based on an intake of 2,000 calories per day according to the USDA's DASH Eating Plan.

Proteins

Proteins are chains of **amino acid** molecules that are used by every cell of the body to make other usable proteins. These building blocks carry out various functions required by the cells and the body. Proteins are used in the duplication of **deoxyribonucleic acid** (DNA; dee-ox-ee-RYE-bow-new-KLAY-ik AH-sid), the blueprint material containing all the information that controls the function of every living cell. Proteins are needed to make muscle tissue, blood, and enzymes as well as the keratin that is present in skin, nails, and hair. Proteins are used by the immune system in making antibodies. Collagen is also made from protein.

Proteins contain all essential amino acids. Although there are more than 100 naturally occurring amino acids, the proteins of all plants and animals are made from just 20 "common amino acids." Eleven of the 20 common amino acids are called the **nonessential amino acids** because they can be synthesized by the body and do not have to be in our diet. The remaining 9 are

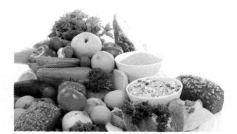

Figure 8–3 Find beneficial nutrients from an abundance of food sources.

the essential amino acids that must be in our daily diet because they cannot be synthesized by the human body.

Dietary Sources of Proteins

Although meat, fish, poultry, eggs, and dairy products are complete proteins that provide all of the essential amino acids, they should be limited in the diet because they are also high in fat. Many plant sources are low in fat and also a good source of fiber, but they are not complete proteins because they all lack at least one of the essential amino acids. **Complementary foods** are combinations of two incomplete proteins that provide all the essential amino acids and make a complete protein. Some complementary proteins are peanut butter and bread, rice and beans, beans and corn, and black-eyed peas and cornbread.

Vegetarians must be careful to obtain their daily protein requirements. Those who consume dairy products have an easier time obtaining a sufficient amount of protein. Vegans, people who eat strictly plant products with no dairy products, must be especially careful to consume enough protein in their diets through nuts, grains, legumes, and vegetables. Soy products are particularly beneficial in the vegetarian diet.

Dietary sources of protein come from animal meats as well as fish, eggs, dairy products, nuts, grains, and beans. Although most vegetables also contain protein, it is in smaller proportions. Protein deficiencies can cause anemia, low resistance to infection, and organ impairment.

Carbohydrates

Carbohydrates break down the basic chemical sugars that supply energy for the body. They are frequently called "carbs." The most important carbohydrate is glucose because it provides most of the body's energy. Glucose is stored in the muscles and liver as glycogen, or animal starch. When muscles are used, glycogen is broken down to provide the energy needed for muscular work. Nutrients are broken down into **adenosine triphosphate** (ATP; uh-DEE-nuh-zeen tri-FOS-fate), the substance that provides energy to cells. ATP also converts oxygen to carbon dioxide, a waste product we breathe out.

Carbohydrates can be combined with proteins to produce many important body chemicals. For example, **mucopolysaccharides** (mew-ko-poly-SACK-uh-rides) are carbohydrate–lipid complexes that are good water binders. These are important to the skin and are present in the dermis as **glycosaminoglycans** (gly-kose-ah-mee-no-GLY-cans), a water-binding substance between the fibers of the dermis.

Monosaccharides, Disaccharides, and Polysaccharides

There are three basic structural carbohydrate divisions: monosaccharides, disaccharides, and polysaccharides.

Monosaccharides. The most basic unit of a carbohydrate is glucose, the simplest of all carbohydrates. The glucose molecule is known as a **monosaccharide** (mah-no-SACK-uh-ride; *mono* means "one," and *saccharide* means "sugar"), a one-unit sugar molecule that all cells use for energy. Fruit sugar (fructose) is a naturally occurring monosaccharide.

Disaccharides (dye-SACK-uh-rides). These are made up of two molecular sugar units (*di* means "two"). Lactose (milk sugar) and sucrose (sugar) are both disaccharides.

Polysaccharides (poly-SACK-uh-rides). These complex compounds consist of a chain of sugar unit molecules (*poly* is from the Greek *polu*, meaning "many"). A digestible polysaccharide starch can be broken down by the digestive system into simpler, usable glucose molecules. Starch is the storage form of glucose for plants. Fiber is also a polysaccharide but is not digestible.

The Three Basic Types of Carbohydrates

The three basic types of carbohydrates are simple sugars, starches, and fiber.

Simple sugars. These are present in table sugar (also known as sucrose), fruit sugars (fructose), and milk sugars (lactose).

Starches. These also called complex carbohydrates, are present in many vegetables and grains. Starch is a white, odorless, complex carbohydrate that is an important food. In plants, carbohydrates are stored chiefly as starch.

Fiber. Fiber is made of a carbohydrate called cellulose, which is not digested by humans and is important in helping push wastes out of the colon. This is necessary for proper digestion. Lack of fiber is associated with constipation and, in the long term, with colon cancer.

Dietary Sources of Carbohydrates

The dietary sources of carbohydrates include:

*   simple carbohydrates such as sweets, syrups, honey, fruits, candy, and many vegetables.
*   starches, including grains, cereals, breads, and other flour products; potatoes; rice; legumes (beans); and pasta.
*   high-fiber foods, including grain, brans (such as oat bran or wheat bran), whole-grain breads, beans, apples, and vegetables such as carrots and corn.

Some foods are listed in two different categories because there is more than one type of saccharide group in many foods. For example, potatoes are a starch source and also contain fiber. Fruits and vegetables have both simple sugars and fiber.

Glucose

Blood glucose or blood sugar can drop too low without adequate carbohydrates. This condition is known as **hypoglycemia** (high-poh-gly-SEE-me-ah). Low blood sugar causes symptoms such as fatigue, anxiety, and food cravings. Fluctuating blood sugar levels and food cravings are triggered if the brain is energy starved. Simple carbs, such as table sugar, have no fiber and are quickly absorbed into the bloodstream. Refined carbohydrates such as white bread have their natural fiber and bran milled away, so they enter the bloodstream more quickly but do not provide long-term energy. Eating "good" or complex carbohydrates such as whole grains will help to slow absorption of glucose into the bloodstream and balance glucose levels.

The hormone insulin, produced in the pancreas, brings nutrients and glucose into cells and stores fat. Without insulin, the body cannot utilize glucose. Consequently, there is a high level of glucose in the blood and a low level of glucose absorption by the tissues. Diabetes results from this imbalance. Regulating hormone and glucose levels through proper nutrition is important to maintain good health.

Fats

Fats, or **lipids,** are the third group of macronutrients. Fats are used as energy, but not as readily as carbohydrates. Although many people associate fats with obesity, some fat is required in the diet, and it is an essential component of good health. The layer of fat in the body also helps retain heat. Fats are used to produce the materials in the sebaceous glands that lubricate the skin. Lipids are fats or fatlike substances used by the body to make hormones, create cell membranes, and assist in absorption of the fat-soluble vitamins A, D, E, and K.

Fatty Acids

Fats are organic compounds made up of a glycerol molecule and fatty acids. The chemical composition of the carbon and hydrogen molecules that combine with glycerol determine the types of fatty acid. Fatty acids make up triglycerides, the main fat in foods. Triglycerides are fats and oils representing 95 percent of fat intake. Phospholipids and sterols are the remaining 5 percent.

The three types of fatty acids are *saturated, monounsaturated,* and *polyunsaturated.*

- Saturated fats are more rigid molecules, and this can cause hardening of the arteries.
- Monounsaturated fats from olive oil and canola oil are more fluid molecules and are important for cell integrity and membrane phospholipids.
- Polyunsaturated fats are liquid at room temperature and are more easily oxidized. Polyunsaturated fats are found in fish, corn, safflower, and nut oils.

The body has the capacity to manufacture fats for use as needed. These fats can be made from carbohydrates and proteins. Essential fatty acids are acids that the body cannot manufacture on its own and therefore they need to be taken internally from food. Fatty acids from food protect against disease and help produce hormones.

Disease-preventing omega-3 and omega-6 fatty acids are polyunsaturated fatty acids necessary for brain and body development, metabolism, and hair and skin growth. However, too much omega-6 in the diet can lead to health problems; and the typical American diet has an excess of omega-6. The healthy Mediterranean diet has more omega-3. The dietary amount for omega-3 is recommended to be three times more than omega-6.

Linoleic acid (lyn-uh-LAY-ick AH-sid) is omega-6, an essential fatty acid used to make important hormones and the lipid barrier of the skin. Linoleic acid is found in oils made from safflower, sunflower, corn, soybean, borage, and flaxseed.

Omega-3 fatty acids (Alpha-linolenic) are a type of "good" polyunsaturated fat that may decrease the likelihood of cardiovascular diseases by reducing

arteriosclerosis (are-TEER-ee-oh-sklur-OH-sis), clogging and hardening of the arteries. Omega-3 fatty acids are largely present in cold-water fish. Salmon is highest in omega-3 acids, but mackerel, tuna, herring, trout, and cod are also high in omega-3. Nutritionists suggest that these fish should be a regular part of the diet and consumed two to three times a week. Alpha-linoleic acid, omega-3, is a popular nutrient for healthy skin and reducing inflammation. Sources of omega-3 include fish oil, walnuts, flax, pumpkin seeds, and algae.

Trans Fatty Acids

Trans fatty acids can increase the "bad" type of cholesterol in the blood, known as low-density lipoprotein (LDL; lie-po-PRO-teen). LDLs are composed largely of cholesterol. Conversely, high-density lipoproteins (HDLs) are "good" lipoproteins with high protein content. Lipoproteins contain protein and lipids that transport water-insoluble lipids through the blood.

The body makes cholesterol, so it does not need to be consumed in the diet. Cholesterol is a necessary component of cell membranes, nerve and brain cells, and bile synthesis. It is also a precursor of vitamin D and steroid hormones. Cholesterol and phospholipids, along with some triglycerides, are absorbed into the lymph system because they are insoluble in water (blood).

Saturated fats are unhealthy, highly processed fats that raise serum cholesterol. Hydrogenated fats are also detrimental to health because they elevate blood lipids and cholesterol. Saturated fats are found mostly in animal sources and coconut and palm oils.

Too much cholesterol or fat in the diet can result in clogged blood vessels, slowing and blocking blood flow. High levels of blood cholesterol can lead to high blood pressure, heart disease, and stroke. Yellow or white papules around the eyes may indicate an elevated cholesterol level. High cholesterol is also genetically determined.

Calories

Fats are very high in **calories,** the measure of heat units. Calories fuel the body by making energy available for work. A gram of fat has 9 calories, while a gram of carbohydrate or a gram of protein has 4 calories. When people take in too many calories, and do not use them in body functions, the body stores the excess calories as body fat. It takes about 3,500 extra calories for the body to store 1 pound of fat. These extra calories can come from the intake of fat, carbohydrates, or even protein.

The number of calories required to run the body varies with individual lifestyles. Obesity in the United States has doubled in the past two decades. Nearly one-third of adults are obese; that is, they have a body mass index (BMI) of 30 or greater. Changing our diets and lifestyle is necessary to slow down this prevalent trend. Conversely, some individuals are underweight and malnourished, which is not healthy either. An average weight and balanced diet are the optimum goals for good health.

Dietitians generally believe that 55 to 60 percent of all calories should be obtained from carbohydrates—mainly grains, breads, pasta, vegetables,

USDA Guidelines are recommended daily allowances (RDAs) for a balanced nutritional consumption. Recommended intake for calories is 2,300 to 3,000 for men and 1,900 to 2,200 for women. As a general range for food categories, 45 to 65 percent of the diet should be complex carbohydrates; 15 to 35 percent proteins; and 30 percent unsaturated fats.

 WEB RESOURCES

To calculate your BMI, check out http://www.healthatoz.com.

and fruit. Candy is also a carbohydrate, but sweets should be limited to no more than 240 calories per day for women and 310 calories per day for men.

Most nutritional authorities generally recommend limiting fats to no more than 30 percent of the diet. No more than 10 percent of this amount should come from saturated fats. Saturated fats come primarily from meats and dairy products. Polyunsaturated and monounsaturated oils come primarily from vegetable oils. Foods such as pastries, fast foods, fried foods, snack foods (junk foods), and products containing cream are high in fat and should be avoided or eaten in moderation.

Protein requirements make up the balance of the diet, around 15 to 20 percent. Remember that protein sources, such as meat, also contain fats and carbohydrates.

Enzymes

Enzymes are biological catalysts made of protein and vitamins. Enzymes break down complex food molecules into smaller molecules to utilize the energy extracted from food. Enzymes are also necessary to bring about reactions or speed up reactions in the body. Materials in the body are reduced by enzymes into carbon dioxide, water, and unnecessary end products that are excreted. Vitamins also assist in breaking down molecules.

MICRONUTRIENTS: VITAMINS

Vitamins, or **micronutrients,** are substances that have no calories and no real nutritional value, yet they are necessary for many nutrients to be properly processed by the body. They are also needed for many processes carried out by the cells and for the production of many biochemicals necessary for life. Most vitamins must be part of the diet because the body cannot synthesize all vitamins on its own. Vitamins are required for many chemical reactions that break down and reconstruct proteins, convert amino acids, and synthesize fatty acids. Many vitamins are also involved in energy release from carbohydrates. Without vitamins, the body cannot operate and will eventually die.

Vitamins play an important role in the skin's health by aiding in healing, softening, and fighting diseases of the skin. Antioxidant vitamins such as A, C, and E have all been shown to have positive effects on skin health. Although experts agree that taking vitamins internally is still the best way to support skin health, some external applications of vitamins also nourish the skin.

Ideally, the nutrients the body needs for proper functioning and survival should come primarily from the foods we eat (Table 8–1). If a person's daily food consumption is lacking in nutrients, vitamin and mineral supplements can help provide some additional nutrients (making sure not to exceed the RDA). Medications can interfere with the body's ability to absorb vitamins and minerals.

Vitamins fall into two categories: fat-soluble (vitamins A, D, E, and K), and water-soluble (vitamins B and C).

Table 8–1

A NUTRITION CHART: VITAMINS, MINERALS, AND FOOD SOURCES			
VITAMIN RDA	**NATURAL SOURCES**	**FUNCTIONS**	**DEFICIENCY SYMPTOMS**
A 5,000 IU	Yellow and green fruits and vegetables, carrots, dairy products, fish liver oil, yellow fruits	Growth and repair of body tissues, bone formation, vision	Night blindness, dry scaly skin, loss of smell and appetite, fatigue, bone deterioration
B-1 Thiamine 1.5 mg	Grains, nuts, wheat germ, fish, poultry, legumes, meat	Metabolism, appetite maintenance, nerve function, healthy mental state, and muscle tone	Nerve disorders, cramps, fatigue, loss of appetite, loss of memory, heart irregularity
B-2 Riboflavin 1.7 mg	Whole grains, green leafy vegetables, liver, fish, eggs	Metabolism, health in hair, skin, nails; cell respiration, formation of antibodies and red blood cells	Cracks and lesions in corners of mouth, digestive disturbances
B-6 Pyridoxine 2 mg	Whole grains, leafy green vegetables, yeast, bananas, organ meats	Metabolism, formation of antibodies sodium/ potassium balance	Dermatitis, blood disorders, nervousness, weakness, skin cracks, loss of memory
B-7 Biotin 300 mcg	Legumes, eggs, grains, yeast	Metabolism, formation of fatty acids	Dry, dull skin; depression, muscle pain, fatigue, loss of appetite
B-12 Cobalamine 6 mcg	Eggs, milk/milk products, fish, organ meats	Metabolism, healthy nervous system, blood cell formation	Nervousness, neuritis, fatigue
Choline (no RDA)	Lecithin, fish wheat germ, egg yolk, soybeans	Nerve metabolism, and transmission, regulates liver, kidneys, and gall-bladder	Hypertension, stomach ulcers, liver and kidney conditions
Folic acid Folacin 400 mcg	Green leafy vegetables, organ meats, yeast, milk products	Red blood cell formation, growth and cell division (RNA and DNA)	Gastrointestinal disorders, poor growth, loss of memory, anemia
Inositol (no RDA)	Whole grains, citrus fruits, yeast molasses, milk	Hair growth, metabolism, lecithin formation	Elevated cholesterol, hair loss, skin disorders, constipation, eye abnormalities
B complex (Niacin) 20 mg	Meat, poultry, fish milk products, peanuts	Metabolism, healthy skin, tongue, and digestive system, blood circulation, essential for synthesis of sex hormones	Fatigue, indigestion irritability, loss of appetite, skin conditions
B complex PABA (no RDA)	Yeast, wheat germ, molasses	Metabolism, red blood cell formation, intestines, hair-coloring, sunscreen	Digestive disorders, fatigue, depression, constipation

continues on next page

Table 8–1 *(continued)*

VITAMIN RDA	NATURAL SOURCES	FUNCTIONS	DEFICIENCY SYMPTOMS
B-15 Pantothenic acid 10 mg	Whole grains, pumpkin and sesame seeds	Metabolism, stimulates nerve and glandular systems, cell respiration	Heart disease, glandular and nerve disorders, poor circulation
C Ascorbic acid 60 mg	Citrus fruits, vegetables, tomatoes, potatoes	Aids in healing, collagen maintenance, resistance to disease	Gum bleeding, bruising, slow healing of wounds, nosebleeds, poor digestion
D 400 IU	Egg yolks, organ meats, fish, fortified milk	Health bone formation, healthy circulatory functions, nervous system	Rickets, osteoporosis, poor bone growth, nervous system irritability
E 30 IU	Green vegetables, wheat germ, organ meats, eggs, vegetable oils	Red blood cells, inhibits coagulation of blood, cellular respiration	Muscular atrophy, abnormal fat deposits in muscles, gastrointestinal conditions, heart disease, impotency
F (no RDA)	Wheat germ, seeds, vegetable oils	Respiration of body organs, lubrication of cells, blood coagulation, glandular activity	Brittle nails and hair, dry dandruff, diarrhea, varicose veins, underweight, acne, gallstones
K (no RDA)	Green leafy vegetables, milk, kelp, safflower oil	Blood clotting agent, important to proper liver function and longevity	Hemorrhage
P Bioflavonoids (no RDA)	Fruits	For healthy connective tissue, aids in utilization of vitamin C	Tendency to bleed easily, gum bleeding, bruising, similar to vitamin C's symptoms
Calcium 1000–1400 mg	Dairy products, bone meal	Resilient bones, teeth, muscle tissue, regulating heartbeat, blood clotting	Soft, brittle bones; osteoporosis, heart palpitations
Chromium (no RDA)	Corn oil, yeast, clams, whole grains	Body's use of glucose, energy, effective use of insulin	Atherosclerosis, diabetic sugar intolerance
Copper 2 mg	Whole grains, leafy green vegetables, seafood, almonds	Healthy red blood cells, bone growth and formation, joins with vitamin C to form elastin	Skin lesions, general weakness, labored respiration
Iodine .15 mg	Iodized table salt, shellfish	Part of the hormone thyroxine which controls metabolism	Dry skin and hair, obesity, nervousness, goiters
Iron 18 mg	Meats, fish, leafy green vegetables	Hemoglobin formation, blood quality, resistance to stress and disease	Anemia, constipation, breathing difficulties
Magnesium 400 mg	Nuts, green vegetables, whole grains	Metabolism	Nervousness, agitation, disorientation, blood clots

VITAMIN RDA	NATURAL SOURCES	FUNCTIONS	DEFICIENCY SYMPTOMS
Manganese 2 mg	Egg yolks, legumes, whole grains	Carbohydrate and fat production, sex hormone production, bone development	Dizziness, lacking muscle coordination
Phosphorus 800mg	Proteins, grains	Bone development, important in protein, fat and carbohydrate utilization	Soft bones, rickets, loss of appetite, irregular breathing
Potassium 2000 mg	Grains, vegetables, bananas, fruits, legumes	Fluid balance; controls activity of heart muscle, nervous system, and kidneys	Irregular heartbeat, muscle cramps (legs), dry skin, general weakness
Sodium 500 mg	Table salt, shellfish, meat and poultry	Maintains muscular, blood and lymph, and nervous systems, regulates body fluid	Muscle weakness and atrophy, nausea, dehydration
Sulphur (no RDA)	Fish, eggs, nuts, cabbage, meat	Collagen and body tissue formation, gives strength to keratin	N/A
Zinc 15 mg	Whole grains, wheat bran	Healthy digestion and metabolism, reproductive system, aids in healing	Stunted growth, delayed sexual maturity, prolonged wound healing
Selenium 055 mcg	Whole grains, liver, meat, fish	Part of important antioxidant, glutathione peroxidase	Heart damage, reduces body's resistance to chronic illnesses
Fluoride	Fluoridated water and toothpaste	Bone and tooth formation	Increased tooth decay

Fat-Soluble Vitamins

Fat-soluble vitamins A, D, E, and K are generally present in fats within foods. The body stores them in the liver and in adipose (fat) tissue. Because they can be stored in the body, it is possible to get too much of certain vitamins, namely vitamins A and D. Fat-soluble vitamins protect the outside membrane of cells.

Vitamin A

Vitamin A is formally known as **retinol,** which is an ingredient used in skin care products designed for aging skin. Vitamin A is also a group of compounds called retinoids. Retinol, **retinoic acid** (re-tuh-NO-ik AH-cid)**,** and **Retin-A®** are all examples of retinoids.

Vitamin A is necessary for proper eyesight, especially at night. A deficiency in vitamin A can result in a condition known as night blindness, or the impaired ability of the eyes to adapt to the dark. Vitamin A is also important for the proper maintenance of epithelial tissue, which makes up the surface of the lungs, intestines, mucous membranes, the bladder, and the skin. These surfaces produce mucus, which is important for protection and flexibility.

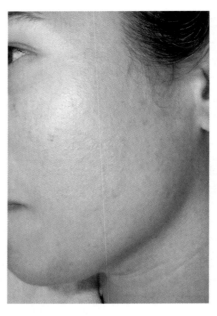
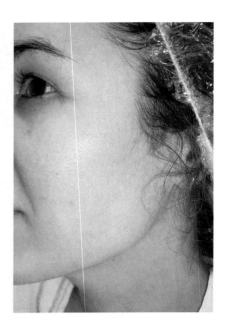

Figure 8–4 A, B Examples of using Retin-A on the skin.

Vitamin A supports the overall health of the skin. This vitamin aids in the functioning and repair of skin cells. Vitamin A is an antioxidant that can help prevent certain types of cancers, including skin cancer, and it has been shown to improve the skin's elasticity and thickness.

Topically, vitamin A can be used to treat many different types of acne and other skin conditions, primarily wrinkles. It is found in many over-the-counter (OTC) creams and lotions. Derivatives of vitamin A are used in many skin prescription creams called retinoic acid or Retin-A, known as retinoids. Tretinoin, better known as Retin-A or Renova™, is used to treat both acne and sun-damaged skin. Retinoids are also used in skin care formulations. Retinol helps improve the appearance of sun-damaged skin, and it may help other esthetic disorders (Figure 8–4 A, B). Retinyl palmitate polypeptide and beta-carotene are also used in skin care, primarily for their antioxidant properties.

Without vitamin A, a hard keratin protein forms in the body, impairing cellular function of epithelial tissues, replacing mucus, and sometimes resulting in bacterial infection. These surfaces are also a frequent site for cancer development. Research is ongoing to determine the role of vitamin A in preventing cancer.

Since the body stores vitamin A, consuming too much of it can result in vitamin A toxicity. This condition can be serious, resulting in hair loss, very dry lips, and damage to the liver, spleen, and other organs. People should avoid taking more than about 15,000 retinol equivalents (RE) per day. This condition is generally a problem only when people take too many vitamin A supplements.

Beta-carotene is a provitamin A. Provitamins, also called precursors, are vitamin-containing substances that are converted to the actual vitamin once they are in the body. Beta-carotene is responsible for the bright color of many fruits and vegetables. The carotenes consumed in the diet are important in controlling the free radicals formed during biochemical reactions in the body. Research also points to the possibility that carotenes may play an important role in the formation and function of immune system cells.

Beta-carotene is found in colorful vegetables such as carrots, dark green vegetables such as spinach, and in fruits that are orange in color.

Most people get about half their vitamin A from retinol, and half from beta-carotene. Milk that has been fortified contains vitamin A. *Fortified* means that a vitamin has been added to a food product. Carrots, pumpkin, yams, fish, and eggs all contain vitamin A.

Vitamin D

Vitamin D is sometimes called the "sunshine vitamin" because the skin synthesizes vitamin D from cholesterol when exposed to sunlight. This is not a recommendation for tanning, because the skin is also severely damaged by sun exposure. Minimal amounts of sunshine are all that is necessary for vitamin D synthesis.

The main function of vitamin D is to enable the body to properly absorb and use calcium, the element needed for proper bone development and maintenance. Vitamin D also promotes healthy, rapid healing of the skin. Because vitamin D helps to support the bone structure of the body, it is found in many fortified foods and dietary supplements. Dietary sources include fortified milk, fish oils, egg yolks, and butter. Foods from plants are not a good source of vitamin D.

Deficiencies of vitamin D result in a condition called rickets, which is seen in children. Children with rickets do not develop bones normally. In adults, vitamin D deficiency results in a condition called osteomalacia, or adult rickets, which is the gradual softening and bending of the bones. This disease is more common in women than men, and it often first develops during pregnancy.

Osteoporosis (ahs-tee-oh-puh-ROH-sis) is a reduction in the quality of bone or atrophy of the skeletal tissue. It is an age-related disorder affecting 20 million Americans, 80 percent of them women age 45 and older. Lack of vitamin D is a contributory cause of the disorder. Psoriasis also appears to be linked to deficiency of vitamin D.

Vitamin D is stored in the body, so it is possible—though rare—to have toxic symptoms from too much vitamin D. Most vitamin D toxicity is the result of taking too many vitamin D supplements.

Vitamin E

Vitamin E, or **tocopherol** (toe-KAH-fah-roll), is primarily an antioxidant. Antioxidants are important in protecting the body from damage caused by free radicals (the wild molecules that steal electrons from other molecules).

Tocopherol helps to stop free radicals so that cell membranes are not damaged. Continual damage from free radicals is associated with many diseases, tumor formation, and the aging process of the body as well as the skin. Vitamin E generally works to protect many tissues of the body from damage so that they can function normally.

Used in conjunction with vitamin A, vitamin E helps protect the skin from the harmful effects of the sun's rays. Vitamin E also helps heal damage

FOCUS ON . . .

YOUR SKIN

Although a healthy diet does not always guarantee healthy skin, you are what you eat. Your body cannot produce healthy skin without the proper nutrients. Antioxidants are your skin's best friend.

to tissues when used both internally and externally. When used externally in topical lotions or creams, vitamin E may help heal structural damage to the skin, including burns and stretch marks.

Good sources of vitamin E include vegetable oils and seed oils (safflower oil is very high in vitamin E); green, leafy vegetables; and avocados, wheat germ, egg yolks, and butter.

Vitamin K

Vitamin K is essential for the synthesis of proteins necessary for blood coagulation. Coagulation is the clotting factor that allows bleeding to stop. Vitamin K helps to diminish the presence of abnormal capillaries, or spider veins, by strengthening capillary walls.

Vitamin K is found in beans; dark, leafy vegetables such as spinach and broccoli; and egg yolks. Deficiencies of vitamin K, although rare, result in hard-to-control bleeding and can be related to certain disorders that prevent proper absorption of fats by the intestines.

Water-Soluble Vitamins

Water-soluble vitamins, B and C, benefit the inside of cells. Water-soluble vitamins do not stay in the body very long. The body must have regular supplies of the water-soluble vitamins because they are used in almost every metabolic reaction and are then excreted—not retained by the body. Most of these are easily obtained through many foods.

B Vitamins

There are eight **B vitamins:** *B complex (niacin), B_1 (thiamine), B_2 (riboflavin), B_6 (pyridoxine), B_7 (biotin), B_{12} (cobalamine), folic acid (folacin), and B_{15} (pantothenic acid).* These interact with other water-soluble vitamins and act as coenzymes (catalysts) to facilitate enzymatic reactions.

- *Niacin* is a necessary part of many metabolic reactions. Most of these complex reactions are important in the release of energy from carbohydrates. Niacin is required by the body for manufacturing steroids as well as red blood cells. Proteins are the best source of niacin: peanuts, beans, milk, eggs, and meats. Some niacin is found in whole-grain products and in enriched foods. Pellagra is a disease associated with niacin deficiency. Pellagra can affect the skin, mental functions, the intestinal tract, and can cause death.

- *Riboflavin* (vitamin B_2) is a water-soluble vitamin that works with enzymes to produce energy in cells. Cells use vitamin B_2 to manufacture various amino acids and fatty acids. Vitamin B_2 is found in milk; meats; liver; dark green, leafy vegetables; broccoli; eggs; and salmon and tuna. Grains and bread are often fortified with riboflavin. Deficiencies can result in retarded growth, nerve tissue damage, dryness of the skin, and cracks at the corners of the mouth, known as cheilosis.

- *Thiamine* (vitamin B_1) removes carbon dioxide from cells and converts carbohydrates stored as fat. Vitamin B_1 is found in pork, beef, fortified cereals, whole wheat products, and nuts. Beriberi is the disease caused by B_1 deficiency. Beriberi affects the nervous system, and it can slow the heart rate as well as cause mental dysfunction. In children it can stunt growth. Vitamin B_1 deficiency can also be caused by alcohol abuse.

- *Pyridoxine* (vitamin B_6) is important in the metabolism of proteins, both for breaking down and reconstructing amino acids as needed by the body. Several important chemicals, including histamine, are produced in conjunction with vitamin B_6. Research has shown vitamin B_6 can help improve the effects of premenstrual syndrome (PMS) and irritability. Vitamin B_6 is present in meats, soybeans, fish, and walnuts as well as in vegetables and fruits such as bananas, potatoes, prunes, and avocados. Vitamin B_6 deficiency results in many symptoms, including poor coordination and mental acuity problems, and it can affect the levels of white blood cells. Vitamin B_6 is strongly connected to protein synthesis. Many problems are associated with a deficiency and create a domino effect on many other reactions.

- *Folacin,* also known as folic acid, is an important B vitamin. It is involved in processing amino acids and in transporting certain molecules. This is important for cells that make chemicals conducive to mental health. Vitamin B_{12} and vitamin C must be present for folacin to work properly. Like many other important vitamins, folacin is found in dark green, leafy vegetables. Asparagus, cantaloupe, sweet potatoes, and green peas are all good sources of folacin. Deficiencies can cause various mental problems, including moodiness, hostility, and loss of memory. There is a connection between low intakes of folacin and birth defects, as well as colorectal cancer.

- *Biotin* (vitamin B_7) is involved in energy formation by cells, as well as in the synthesis of both proteins and fatty acids. It is produced in the intestinal tract by microbes ("good" bacteria) and is present in milk, liver, and other organ meats. Deficiencies are primarily caused by intestinal disorders or by poor absorption. Antibiotics can kill off good bacteria along with the bad, causing lower levels of biotin.

- *Cobalamine* (vitamin B_{12}) is important in the activation of folacin, fatty acid synthesis, and DNA synthesis in conjunction with proper red blood vessel formation by the bone marrow. Liver, salmon, clams, oysters, and egg yolks are some good food sources of vitamin B_{12}. A disorder known as pernicious anemia is caused by a lack of vitamin B_{12}, or from poor absorption of the vitamin caused by other diseases. Absorption of this vitamin decreases with age, making deficiency symptoms more likely to occur in older persons.

- *Pantothenic acid* (vitamin B_{15}) is important in various processes involved in synthesizing fatty acids and in metabolizing proteins and carbohydrates. Its role in fatty acid synthesis includes the synthesis of hormones, cholesterol, and phospholipids. The latter two are important in the barrier function of skin (the lipid matrix that protects the skin's surface). This vitamin also aids in the functioning of the adrenal glands. Pantothenic acid deficiency is practically nonexistent. Pantothenic acid is present in many foods, but not in fruits.

Vitamin C

Vitamin C, also known as **ascorbic acid** (uh-SKOR-bick AH-cid), is an antioxidant that helps protect the body from many forms of oxidation and from problems involving free radicals. Research indicates that an adequate intake of vitamin C may help prevent cancer because of its ability to scavenge free radicals that attack DNA. DNA damage can lead to the formation of cancerous cells. Vitamin C performs numerous functions in the body.

Vitamin C is an important vitamin needed for proper repair of the skin and tissues. Vitamin C is important in fighting the aging process and promotes collagen production in the dermal tissues, keeping the skin healthy and firm. It is required for collagen formation in skin as well as in cartilage and spinal discs. Vitamin C also renews vitamin E by allowing it to neutralize more free radicals.

Vitamin C also helps prevent damage to capillary walls that can cause easy bruising, bleeding gums, and capillary distension. Vitamin C acts to prevent cardiovascular disease by helping to maintain blood vessel walls and by preventing oxidation of bad cholesterol, which can lead to clogging in the blood vessels. Vitamin C assists the body in dealing with stress, and it is easily depleted during times of great stress. This vitamin supports the healing process of the body. Studies also show that vitamin C helps reduce the time and severity of colds.

Vitamin C is found in citrus fruits; dark green, leafy vegetables; tomatoes; and other fruits and vegetables. Vitamin C is easily depleted in smokers, which is important because smokers have more free radicals forming in their bodies. Researchers suggest that smokers need twice as much vitamin C as nonsmokers do. Symptoms of scurvy from vitamin C deficiency include easy bruising, bleeding gums, poor wound healing, and anemia. Scurvy is rare, but it can occur in people with very poor diets and is occasionally seen in senior citizens.

Bioflavonoids (by-oh-FLAH-vuh-noids), which are referred to as vitamin P, enhance absorption of vitamin C. Bioflavonoids relieve pain and bruises. They also protect capillary blood vessels. Bioflavonoids promote circulation, have an antibacterial effect, and can reduce the symptoms of oral herpes. Bioflavonoids are antioxidants found in citrus peel, peppers, grapes, garlic, berries, and green tea.

MINERALS

The body requires many **minerals.** These inorganic materials are essential in many cell reactions and bodily functions. Most are required in relatively small quantities, but they are nevertheless necessary for life.

Essential Minerals

Some of the important minerals and their functions are as follows:

- *Calcium* is important in forming and maintaining teeth and bones. It helps prevent osteoporosis, a degenerative disease that results in brittle bones.

- *Magnesium* is required for energy release and protein synthesis, preventing tooth decay, and nerve and muscle movement.
- *Phosphorus* is present in DNA and is involved in energy release. It is needed for bone formation and cell growth, and it assists vitamins and food energy processes.
- *Potassium* is required for energy use, water balance and muscular movement. It aids in maintaining blood pressure and regulates cell nutrient transfer and reactions. It is also important in heart and nervous system functions.
- *Sodium* moves carbon dioxide, regulates water levels, and transports materials through cell membranes. It also regulates blood pH and helps in stomach, nerve, and muscle function. To limit sodium intake, people should consume less than 2,300 mg (approximately 1 tsp of salt) of sodium per day. Choose and prepare foods with little salt. Sodium and potassium need to be balanced, so consume potassium-rich foods such as fruits and vegetables. On average, the higher an individual's salt (sodium chloride) intake is, the higher his or her blood pressure will be. Nearly all Americans consume substantially more salt than they need. Decreasing salt intake is advisable to reduce the risk of elevated blood pressure.

Trace Minerals

Other minerals needed in the body are trace minerals. These are required in very small quantities. All of these minerals are necessary for correct body functions, and many are present in cells and tissues. The following are brief descriptions of trace mineral functions, but they are by no means complete.

- Iron is used in the production of hemoglobin and oxygenation of red blood cells. It is also essential for enzymes and for the immune system.
- Iodine helps metabolize excess fat and is important in development and thyroid health.
- Zinc is important for protein synthesis and collagen formation. It also promotes wound healing and helps the immune system.
- Copper aids in formation of bone, hemoglobin, cells, and elastin. It is involved in healing, energy production, and is essential for collagen formation.
- Chromium helps with energy and the metabolism of glucose and aids in synthesizing fats and proteins. Chromium also stabilizes blood sugar levels.
- Fluoride is needed for healthy teeth and bone formation.
- Selenium is a vital antioxidant protecting the immune system. It works with vitamin E to produce antibodies and to maintain a healthy heart; it is also needed for tissue elasticity.
- Manganese assists protein and fat metabolism, promotes healthy nerves, and supports immune system function. Manganese also aids in energy production and bone growth.

? Did You Know

Vegetarians need more protein, iron, and vitamin B_{12} as well as calcium and vitamin D. One egg, ½ ounce of nuts, or ¼ cup of legumes is equivalent to 1 ounce of meat.

FYI

The term *moderately active* means an activity level equal to walking 1.5 to 3 miles at a pace of 3 to 4 mph and daily light physical activity. The term *active* includes activity equal to walking more than 3 miles per day.

Walking burns 280 calories per hour. Running burns 590 calories per hour.

ACTIVITY

Keep a log of your day's food intake by reading labels and recording calories and nutritional values. Compare these values to the RDAs. How close did you come to eating the recommended portions? A daily food log can help you be more aware of what you are eating and inspire healthy habits.

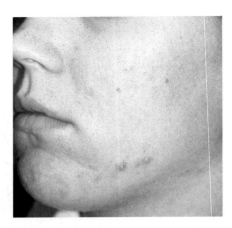

Figure 8–5 Excess iodine can trigger acne.

NUTRITION AND ESTHETICS

Proper nutrition is a primary factor in maintaining the skin's health. Some foods directly affect certain conditions of the skin, but there are also many myths about food and the skin. An example is the widely held belief that chocolate can cause or worsen acne. The truth is that junk foods and sweets are unhealthy and should not be consumed in large quantities, but they may not directly affect acne. However, excess iodine may trigger acne (Figure 8–5).

As scientific studies continue, the correlation between foods and acne will become clearer. It is well known that spicy foods and alcohol consumption can induce rosacea flare-ups. Diet will affect the skin, and skin is an indicator of the body's overall health. Some women have such low-fat diets that their body fat drops too low, resulting in hormonal imbalances that can cause skin problems, including hyperpigmentation and forms of acne. Chapter 12 discusses the effects of topical vitamins and antioxidants on the skin.

Client Health Concerns

Obesity and weight loss are concerns for many clients. Although clients may talk to you about their health-related issues, it is important to remember that unless you are formally educated in nutrition, you are not a source of counsel for persons with nutritional concerns. To do so might endanger your client's health and have legal consequences. All clients who have serious questions about nutritional issues should be referred to a registered dietitian. Fad diets are rampant. Every week there is some new, magical weight-loss gimmick or plan.

Here is the truth about weight loss:

- The only way to lose weight is to burn more calories than you consume.
- Certain diets can cause chemical imbalances that may damage the body.
- Vitamins and supplements are not substitutes for proper nutrition. You can get most of the vitamins and minerals you need from a balanced diet.
  - Vitamin and mineral supplements have little nutritional value because they do not provide the basics—the carbohydrates, proteins, and fats necessary for life processes.
  - You must eat a balanced diet for the vitamins and minerals to have any effect. If you look at nutrition as building and maintaining a house, the nails (vitamins and minerals) are no good without the wood and the bricks (macronutrients).
- No magical ingredient can cause weight loss without having other, sometimes harmful, effects on the body.
- The best way to lose weight, and to maintain proper weight, is to adopt a healthy diet along with proper exercise.

Food Choices

Healthier food choices are more readily available in today's health-conscious world. The abundance of choices makes it easier to eat nutritious, high-quality foods.

Education and scientific advances have increased our knowledge of nutrition and how foods affect our health. Organic foods are grown without pesticides and added chemicals and are becoming more popular as awareness increases. Farmer's markets and health-food sections of grocery stores have become more common. Fast-food restaurants are offering healthier alternatives. Selecting what we put in our bodies is a choice, and eating fresh foods without preservatives is one of them. Nutritional and herbal supplements are another topic altogether. A wealth of information is available on nutrition and health. As with anything else, doing research and checking facts for accuracy is recommended. As scientific research improves, what may be true today could change tomorrow.

WATER AND THE SKIN

There is one essential nutrient no person can live without, and that is water (Figure 8–6). To function properly, the body and skin both rely heavily on water. Water composes 50 to 70 percent of the body's weight. Drinking pure water is essential to keeping the skin and body healthy; it sustains cell health, aids in elimination of toxins and waste, helps regulate body temperature, and aids in proper digestion. When all of these functions perform properly, they help the skin stay healthy, vital, and attractive. Drinking 9 to 12 cups of water a day is an average recommendation.

Water Facts

An estimated 75 percent of Americans are chronically dehydrated. Research suggests that the benefits of water on human health and functioning are many:

- Even mild dehydration will slow metabolism by as much as 3 percent.
- Drinking lots of water can help stop hunger pangs for many dieters.
- Lack of water is the number one cause of daytime fatigue.
- A 2 percent drop in body water can trigger fuzzy short-term memory, trouble with basic math, and difficulty in focusing on a computer screen or printed page.

Water Intake Requirements

The amount of water needed by an individual varies, depending on body weight and level of daily physical activity. Here is an easy formula to help you determine how much water is needed every day for maximum physical health: Take your body weight and divide by 2. Divide this number by 8. The resulting number approximates how many 8-ounce glasses of water you should drink every day. For instance, if you weigh 160 pounds, you should drink 10 glasses of water a day. If you engage in intense physical activity each day, add two extra glasses of water to the final number. This will help replace extra fluids lost while exercising. Drinking excessive amounts of water is not recommended, so increase the amount only if you are thirsty or dehydrated. As with all healthy habits, moderation is usually the best choice for nutritional balance.

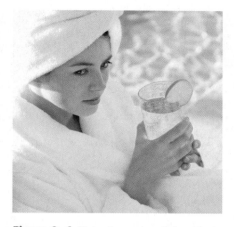

Figure 8–6 Water is an essential nutrient.

Here's a Tip

Keep a large bottle of water on hand daily to keep the body hydrated. Offer clients water during their services (Figure 8–7).

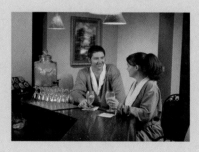

Figure 8–7 Encourage clients to drink water to maintain healthy skin.

ACTIVITY

We have presented a basic overview of nutrition in this chapter. If you are interested in learning more about this subject, check out nutrition courses or textbooks to give you a better knowledge base for both nutrition and health issues.

REVIEW QUESTIONS

1. What is a food pyramid?

2. What are calories?

3. What are the three macronutrients?

4. What are proteins?

5. What are carbohydrates?

6. Why is fat necessary in the diet?

7. What are the micronutrients?

8. What are the fat-soluble vitamins?

9. What are the water-soluble vitamins?

10. Which vitamins are antioxidants?

11. How is vitamin A beneficial for the skin?

12. Name the eight B vitamins.

13. List the minerals and trace minerals.

14. Why is water essential for the body?

15. How does vitamin C affect the skin?

CHAPTER GLOSSARY

adenosine triphosphate (ATP): the substance that provides energy to cells and converts oxygen to carbon dioxide, a waste product we breathe out.

amino acid: organic acids that form the building blocks of protein.

arteriosclerosis: clogging and hardening of the arteries.

bioflavonoids: biologically active flavonoids; also called vitamin P; considered an aid to healthy skin and found most abundantly in citrus fruits.

B vitamins: these water-soluble vitamins interact with other water-soluble vitamins and act as coenzymes (catalysts) by facilitating enzymatic reactions. B vitamins include niacin, riboflavin, thiamine, pyridoxine, folacin, biotin, cobalamine, and pantothenic acid.

calories: a measure of heat units; measures food energy for the body.

carbohydrates: compounds that break down the basic chemical sugars and supply energy for the body.

complementary foods: combinations of two incomplete foods; complementary proteins eaten together provide all the essential amino acids and make a complete protein.

deoxyribonucleic acid (DNA): the blueprint material of genetic information; contains all the information that controls the function of every living cell.

disaccharides: sugars made up of two simple sugars such as lactose and sucrose.

enzymes: catalysts that break down complex food molecules to utilize extracted energy.

fats (lipids): macronutrients used to produce energy in the body; the materials in the sebaceous glands that lubricate the skin.

glycosaminoglycans: a water-binding substance between the fibers of the dermis.

hypoglycemia: a condition in which blood glucose or blood sugar drops too low; caused by either too much insulin or low food intake.

linoleic acid: omega 6, an essential fatty acid used to make important hormones; also part of the skin's lipid barrier.

macronutrients: nutrients that make up the largest part of the nutrition we take in; the three

basic food groups: protein, carbohydrates, and fats.

micronutrients: vitamins and substances that have no calories or nutritional value, yet are essential for body functions.

minerals: inorganic materials required for many reactions of the cells and body.

monosaccharides: carbohydrates made up of one basic sugar unit.

mucopolysaccharides: carbohydrate–lipid complexes that are also good water binders.

nonessential amino acids: amino acids that can be synthesized by the body and do not have to be obtained from the diet.

omega-3 fatty acids: alpha-linolenic acid; a type of "good" polyunsaturated fat that may decrease cardiovascular diseases. It is also an anti-inflammatory and beneficial for skin.

osteoporosis: a thinning of bones, leaving them fragile and prone to fractures; caused by the reabsorption of calcium into the blood.

polysaccharides: carbohydrates that contain three or more simple carbohydrate molecules.

proteins: chains of amino acid molecules used in all cell functions and body growth.

retinoic acid (Retin-A): a vitamin A derivative. It has demonstrated an ability to alter collagen synthesis and is used to treat acne and visible signs of aging. Side effects are irritation, photosensitivity, skin dryness, redness, and peeling.

vitamin A (retinol): an antioxidant that aids in the functioning and repair of skin cells.

vitamin C (ascorbic acid): an antioxidant vitamin needed for proper repair of the skin and tissues.

vitamin D: fat-soluble vitamin sometimes called the "sunshine vitamin" because the skin synthesizes vitamin D from cholesterol when exposed to sunlight. Essential for growth and development.

vitamin E (tocopherol): primarily an antioxidant; helps protect the skin from the harmful effects of the sun's rays.

vitamin K: vitamin responsible for the synthesis of factors necessary for blood coagulation.

SKIN SCIENCES

PART

3

CHAPTER 9

PHYSIOLOGY AND HISTOLOGY OF THE SKIN

CHAPTER OUTLINE

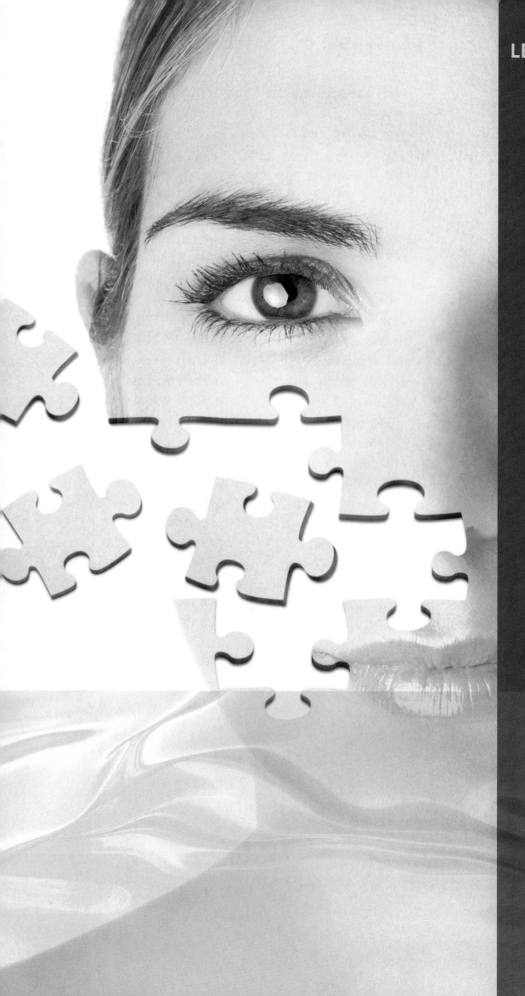

KEY TERMS

Page numbers indicate where in the chapter each term is used.

Estheticians have an opportunity to study a most fascinating science. The science of skin histology and physiology includes the functions, layers, and anatomy of the skin. Skin **histology** is the study of the structure and composition of the skin tissue. **Physiology** is the study of the functions of living organisms. These sciences are the foundations estheticians need to learn before caring for the skin.

There is much more to being an esthetician than simply performing facials and selling products. Estheticians who specialize in the health and beauty of the skin, waxing, and makeup and are sometimes referred to as *technicians, skin therapists,* or *specialists.* As scientific research in the industry changes constantly, estheticians must continue their education at all times. By educating clients, estheticians are sharing their knowledge and expertise. Clients appreciate an esthetician's understanding of their skin and treatment suggestions (Figure 9–1). An esthetician's primary focus is on preserving, protecting, and nourishing the skin.

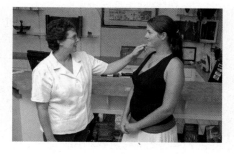

Figure 9–1 Consulting with a client.

The complexity of the integumentary system is amazing. The layers, components, and functions all work to protect and regulate the skin and the body. There is much to study about the body's largest organ and how to best maintain its optimum health. The aging process, sun exposure, hormones, and nutrition affect the skin's health and appearance. By understanding skin physiology, estheticians can be confident in treating this intricate system.

SKIN FACTS

Skin, the **integumentary system** (in-TEG-yuh-ment-uh-ree SIS-tum), is the largest organ in the body. It is a strong barrier designed to protect us from the outside elements. The body systems that make up our outermost layer are incredibly complex. Skin layers, nerves, cellular functions, hair follicles, and glands all work together harmoniously to regulate and protect the body. Healthy skin is slightly moist, soft, smooth, and somewhat acidic. Skin is thickest on the palms of the hands and soles of the feet. It is thinnest on the eyelids.

Our skin is a cell-making factory with miles of blood vessels, millions of sweat glands, and an array of nerves within a network of fibers (Figure 9–2). Appendages of the skin include hair, nails, sweat glands, and oil glands.

The skin of an average adult weighs 8–10 pounds and averages an area of about 22 square feet. It contains one-half to two-thirds of the blood in the body and one-half of the primary immune cells. Each inch of skin contains approximately:

- millions of cells
- 15 feet of blood vessels
- 12 feet of nerves
- 650 sweat glands

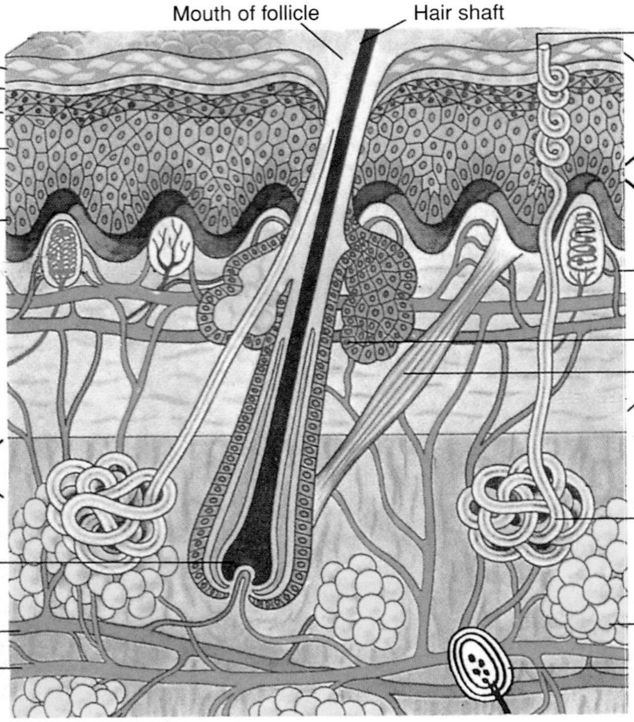
Mouth of follicle
Hair shaft
Sweat pore
Stratum corneum
Stratum lucidum
Stratum granulosum
Stratum spinosum
Epidermis
Stratum germinativum (Basal layer)
Papillary layer of dermis
Dermis (true skin)
Sebaceous (oil) gland
Arrector pili muscle
Reticular layer
Reticular layer of dermis
Sudoriferous gland
Subcutaneous tissue
Dermal papilla
Arteries
Adipose (fatty) tissue
Veins

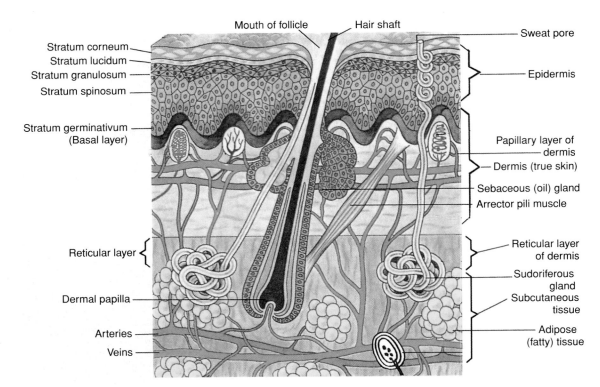

Figure 9–2 Layers of the skin.

- 100 oil glands
- 65 hairs
- 1,300 nerve endings
- 155 pressure receptors
- 12 cold and heat receptors

SKIN FUNCTIONS

The six primary functions of the skin are *protection, sensation, heat regulation, excretion, secretion,* and *absorption.*

Protection

The skin is a protective barrier to outside elements and microorganisms. It has many defense mechanisms to protect the body from injury and invasion. This outermost layer also traps water in the body. **Sebum** on the epidermis gives protection from external factors. The **acid mantle** is the protective barrier made up of sebum, lipids, sweat, and water that form a hydrolipidic film to protect the skin from drying out and from exposure to external factors. The acid mantle has an average pH of 5.5. The acid mantle is part of the skin's natural **barrier function,** a protective barrier on the epidermis. The barrier function protects us from irritation and intercellular **transepidermal water loss (TEWL),** the water loss caused by evaporation on the skin's surface. **Lipids** are substances that contribute to the barrier function of the epidermis. Lipids are protective oils; they make up

? Did You Know

Touch is one of the first senses to develop. Nerve fibers in the skin sense when we are touched. Sensations felt on our skin cause us to feel, react, or move, depending on the stimulation. Massage sends messages to the brain through nerve stimulation and lowers stress in the body. Studies have shown stress reduction in babies and older adults when they experience more touch and interaction with others.

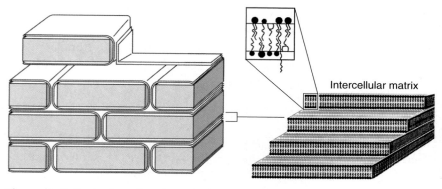

Figure 9–3 Barrier layer function—the brick-and-mortar concept.

the **intercellular cement** between epidermal cells. Damage to our barrier layer is the cause of many skin problems, including sensitivities, aging, and dehydration (Figure 9–3).

The skin's most amazing feature is the ability to heal itself. Skin can repair itself when injured, thus protecting the body from infection and damage from injuries. Through a hyperproduction of cells and blood clotting, injured skin can restore itself to its normal thickness. Our immune system kicks in when guard cells (Langerhans cells) sense unrecognized foreign invaders such as bacteria and produces T cells, the immune cells that protect us from infection. Another form of protection is **melanin,** the pigment that protects us from the sun.

Sensation

Sensory nerve endings in the dermis respond to touch, pain, cold, heat, and pressure (Figure 9–4). When the body senses touch, it is a stimulus that affects our body's functions. Massage and product application produce physiological

FYI

The epidermis is like a brick wall—the cells are the bricks, and the intercellular cement is the mortar between the bricks that holds everything together.

FYI

Hydro means "water." *Lipidic* means "oil." A *hydrolipidic film* is an oil–water balance on the skin's surface.

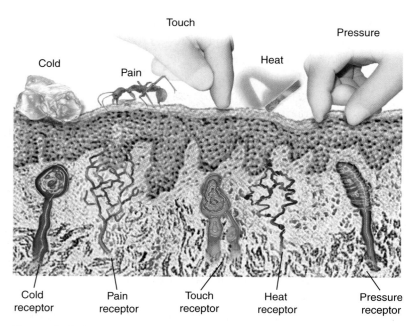

Figure 9–4 Sensory nerve endings.

benefits to the body. Millions of nerve end fibers on the surface of the skin detect stimuli. These sensations send messages to the brain as a protective defense mechanism or as a positive message that something is stimulating the surface. These signals also stimulate other nerves or muscles to react. Sensory nerve fibers are most abundant in the fingertips.

Heat Regulation

The average body's internal thermostat is set at 98.6° Fahrenheit (37° Celsius). When the outside temperature changes, the skin adjusts to warm or cool the body. Millions of hair follicles and sweat glands dissipate heat to keep us from overheating. We cool ourselves by evaporation through the sweat glands. Blood vessel dilation also assists in cooling the body. Conversely, we protect ourselves from the cold by constriction of the blood vessels and decreasing blood flow. The body's fat layers also help to insulate and warm the body.

When we are cold, the **arrector pili muscle** contracts and causes "goose bumps." Shivering is also an automatic response to cold and a way to warm up the body.

Excretion

The **sudoriferous** (soo-duh-RIF-uh-rus), **or sweat glands,** excrete perspiration and detoxify the body by excreting excess salt and unwanted chemicals through the pores. These gland functions are discussed later in the chapter. Sweat is also part of the acid mantle. Follicles are mistakenly called pores. **Follicles** are hair and hairless follicles with oil glands attached to them. **Pores** are openings for sweat glands. However, *pore* is used as a lay term for *follicle*, because both are openings on the top of the epidermis.

Secretion

Sebum is an oily substance that protects the surface of the skin and lubricates both the skin and hair. Oils produced by the **sebaceous glands** (sih-BAY-shus GLANZ) help keep the skin soft and protected from outside elements. The skin is approximately 50 to 70 percent water. Sebum coating the surface of the skin slows down the evaporation of water—also known as transepidermal water loss (TEWL)—and helps maintain water level in the cells. Emotional stress and hormone imbalances can increase the flow of sebum.

Absorption

Absorption of ingredients, water, and oxygen is necessary for our skin's health. The skin absorbs oxygen and discharges carbon dioxide. Vitamin D is produced in the skin upon exposure to the sun. Absorption occurs through the cells, follicles, and pores of the skin. The skin selectively absorbs topical products and creams through the hair follicles and sebaceous glands. While absorption is limited, some ingredients with a smaller molecular size can penetrate the skin. Penetration ability of the ingredient is determined by the size of the molecule and other characteristics of the product (Figure 9–5).

Absorption of select topical products helps keep skin moisturized, nourished, and protected. Technological advances are continually resulting in the

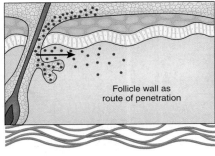

Follicle wall as route of penetration

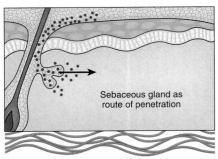

Sebaceous gland as route of penetration

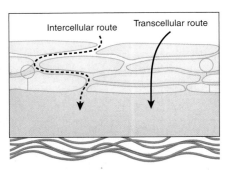

Intercellular route   Transcellular route

Figure 9–5 Primary routes of penetration.

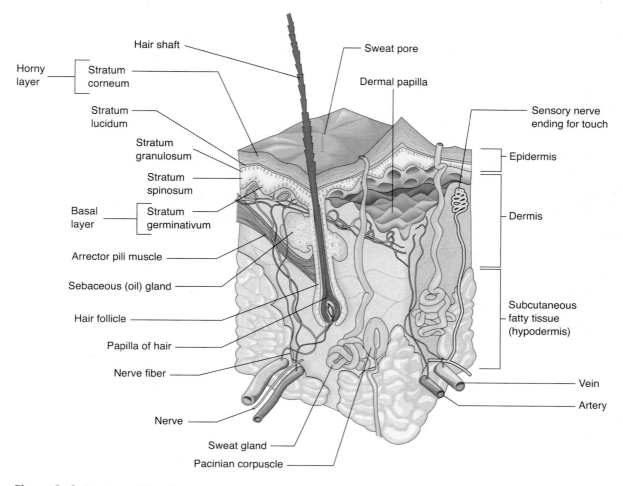

Figure 9–6 Structure of the skin.

creation of new products that are more readily absorbed by the skin, thus making them more effective. Many chemicals and prescription creams can penetrate the skin. This effect can be either harmful or beneficial, depending on the chemicals.

LAYERS OF THE SKIN

The skin is comprised of two parts, the epidermis and the dermis (Figure 9–6).

The Epidermis

The **epidermis** is the outermost layer of the skin. It is a thin, protective covering with many nerve endings. The epidermis is composed of the following five layers, called strata (singular: stratum): the uppermost layer is the stratum corneum, followed by the stratum lucidum, stratum granulosum, and stratum spinosum; the bottom layer is the stratum germinativum (basal layer).

Keratinocytes (keratin protein cells; kair-uh-TIN-oh-sytes) and epithelial cells protect the epidermis. Surrounding the cells in the epidermis are lipids, which protect the cells from water loss and dehydration. Understanding how the skin cell layers function is important in choosing ingredients and treatments. Estheticians are licensed to work only on the epidermis, not the dermis, unless they are working with a physician or another licensed medical practitioner.

The Stratum Corneum

The **stratum corneum** (STRAT-um KOR-nee-um) is the top, outermost layer of the epidermis. The esthetician is primarily concerned with this layer. The stratum corneum is very thin, yet it is waterproof, permeable, regenerates itself, detoxifies the body, and responds to stimuli. It is referred to as the *horny layer* because of the scale-like cells made primarily of soft keratin called **keratinocytes** (kair-uh-TIN-oh-sytes). **Keratin** (KAIR-uh-tin) is a fiber protein that provides resiliency and protection to the skin. Keratin is found in all layers of the epidermis. (Hard keratin is the protein found in hair and nails.) The "dead" protein cells known as keratinocytes comprise 95 percent of the epidermis. Keratinocytes are continually shed (*desquamation;* DES-kwuh-may-shun) and replaced by new cells coming to the surface. This process is known as *cell turnover.* The average cell turnover rate is every 28 days or longer depending on age.

In the stratum corneum, the keratinocytes harden and become corneocytes (KOR-nee-oh-sytes), the protective cells. As discussed earlier, cells and oil combine to form a protective barrier layer on the stratum corneum. *Desmosomes,* intercellular connections, provide strength to the cells. Also found here are squamous cells (flat cells) that protect other layers.

The Stratum Lucidum

The **stratum lucidum** (STRAT-um LOO-sih-dum) is a clear layer under the stratum corneum. It is a translucent layer made of small cells that let light pass through. This layer is found on the palms of the hands and soles of the feet. The keratinocytes in this layer contain clear keratin. The thicker skin on the palms and soles is composed of epidermal ridges that provide a better grip while walking and using our hands. This layer forms our unique fingerprints and footprints.

The Stratum Granulosum

The **stratum granulosum** (STRAT-um gran-yoo-LOH-sum) is composed of cells that resemble granules and are filled with keratin. The production of keratin and intercellular lipids takes place here. As these cells become keratinized, they move to the surface and replace the cells shed from the stratum corneum. Natural moisturizing substances such as triglycerides, ceramides, waxes, and other lipids form components of the skin's barrier function.

The Stratum Spinosum

The **stratum spinosum** (STRAT-um spy-NOH-sum) is a spiny layer above the basal layer. Cells continue to divide and change shape here, and enzymes are creating lipids and proteins. Cell appendages, which resemble prickly spines, become **desmosomes** (DEZ-moh-somes), the structures that assist in strengthening and holding cells together. Also found here are immune cells, which protect the body from infections by identifying foreign material (antigens). The immune cells help destroy these foreign invaders.

The Stratum Germinativum

The **stratum germinativum** (STRAT-um jur-min-ah-TI-vum) is also known as the basal layer of the epidermis. It is the live layer of the epidermis located above the papillary layer of the dermis, composed of basal cells. It is the lowest layer of the epidermis. **Cell mitosis** (cell division) occurs continuously in the basal cell layer. As cells divide, they migrate to the surface and become strong and protective. Cells here produce lipids that hold the cells together. The stratum germinativum also contains **melanocytes** (muh-LAN-uh-sytes), cells that produce melanin. Merkel cells—the sensory cells—are touch receptors also located here.

The Dermis

The **dermis** (DUR-mis) is the live layer of connective tissues below the epidermis. The dermis, which is about 25 times thicker than the epidermis, consists of two layers: the **papillary layer** (PAP-uh-lair-ee LAY-ur) and the **reticular layer** (ruh-TIK-yuh-lur LAY-ur). This live layer is a support structure and nourishes the lower epidermis. The dermis is comprised of connective tissues made of collagen protein and elastin fibers. The dermis contains blood and **lymph vessels,** which supply nourishment within the skin. Capillaries, sebaceous (oil) glands, sudoriferous (sweat) glands, nerves, additional receptors, and the arrector pili muscles are all located in the dermis.

The Papillary Layer

The papillary layer connects the dermis to the epidermis, forming the epidermal–dermal junction. Touch receptors, blood vessels, and capillaries are located here. The **dermal papillae** are membranes of ridges and grooves that attach to the epidermis. Attached to the dermal papillae are either looped capillaries that nourish the epidermis or tactile corpuscles, the nerve endings sensitive to touch and pressure. Note that dermal papillae are not the same as the **hair papillae** (puh-PILL-ay)—the small, cone-shaped structures at the bottom of hair follicles.

The Reticular Layer

The reticular layer, the deeper layer of the dermis, is comprised of the base of hair follicles, glands, blood and lymph vessels, nerve endings, collagen, and elastin. This layer supplies the skin with oxygen and nutrients. **Collagen** (KAHL-a-jen) is a protein substance that gives skin its strength and is necessary for wound healing. Collagen, produced by **fibroblasts** (FY-bro-blasts), makes up 70 percent of the dermis (Figure 9–7). Fibroblast cells aid in the production of collagen and elastin.

In contrast, the quantity of **elastin** (ee-LAS-tin) in the dermis is only about one-fifteenth of the collagen amount. Elastin is the fibrous protein that forms elastic tissue and gives skin its elasticity. Damage to these elastin

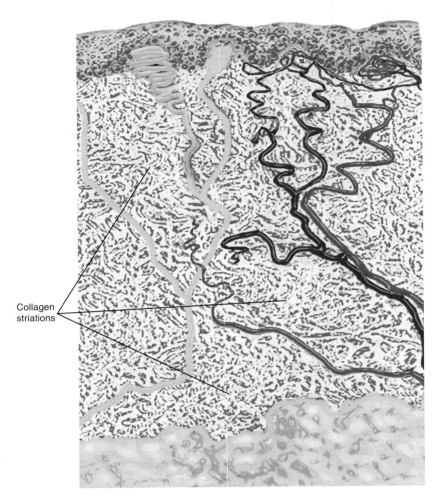

Figure 9–7 Collagen in the dermis.

Collagen
striations

fibers as they break down are the primary cause of sagging, wrinkles, and aging—loss of elasticity in the skin. Stretch marks are caused by damaged elastin fibers. Collagen and elastin are broken down by ultraviolet (UV) light damage and other factors.

In the dermis is a fluid matrix called the *ground substance*. Beneficial hydrating fluids such as **hyaluronic acid** (HY-uh-luhr-ahn-ik A-sid), a glycosaminoglycan (GAG: gly-KOSE-uh-mee-noh-GLY-kan), are found between the fibers in the reticular layer. Intercellular substances are comprised of water and other components to maintain water balance, and they aid in cell migration, metabolism, and growth. Ingredients that duplicate these natural intercellular fluids are important in esthetics and skin care products.

Subcutaneous Tissue

Below the reticular layer is a **subcutaneous layer** composed of **adipose** (AD-uh-pohs; fat) **tissue** or **subcutis** (sub-KYOO-tis) **tissue**. This tissue creates a protective cushion that gives contour and smoothness to the body, as well as providing a source of energy for the body. This subcutis layer below the skin decreases with age. Fat storage is also influenced by hormones.

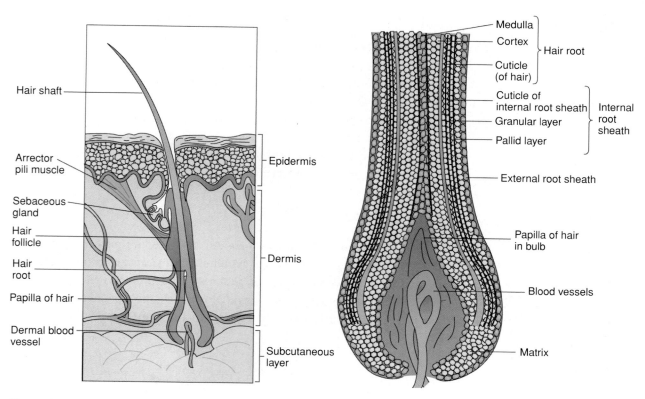

Figure 9–8 Hair follicle structure.

HAIR AND NAIL ANATOMY

Hair and the Skin

Hair is an appendage of the skin—it is a slender, threadlike outgrowth of the skin and scalp. Figure 9–8 shows the structure of the hair follicle. There is no sense of feeling in the hair, due to the absence of nerves.

Much of the hair on the body is invisible to the naked eye. The heavier concentration of hair is on the head, under the arms, around the genitals, and on the arms and legs. Due to hormonal influence, there are different male and female hair growth patterns. Genetics influence the distribution of each person's hair, its thickness, quality, color, rate of growth, and whether the hair is curly or straight.

The hair contains hard keratin, which has a sulfur content of 4 to 8 percent, a lower moisture and fat content, and is a particularly tough, elastic material. Keratin forms continuous sheets (fingernails) or long, endless fibers (hair). Hard keratin does not normally break off or flake away. It remains a continuous structure. The hair follicle structure is part of some skin disorders such as ingrown hairs or folliculitis (a bacterial infection).

Nails and the Skin

The nail, an appendage of the skin, is a hard translucent plate that protects fingers and toes. The nail is composed of hard keratin. Figure 9–9 shows the nail structure. *Onyx* (AH-niks) is the technical term for the nail. The hard, or horny, nail plate contains no nerves or blood vessels.

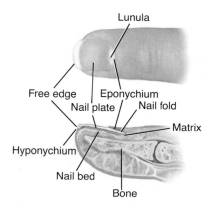

Figure 9–9 Nail structure.

NERVES

There are several notable classifications of nerves.

- *Motor nerve fibers* stimulate muscles, such as the arrector pili muscles attached to the hair follicles. **Arrector pili** muscles cause goose bumps when you are cold or frightened.
- *Sensory nerve fibers* send messages to the brain to react to heat, cold, pain, pressure, and touch.
- *Secretory nerve fibers* are dispersed to sweat and oil glands. They regulate excretion from the sweat glands and control sebum output to the surface of the skin.

SKIN COLOR

Melanocytes (muh-LAN-uh-sytes) are cells that produce pigment granules in the basal layer (Figure 9–10). These granules, called *melanosomes* (MEL- uh-noh-sohms), produce a complex protein, **melanin** (MEL-uh-nin), which determines skin and hair color. Every person has approximately the same number of melanocytes. Both internal and external factors affect melanin production.

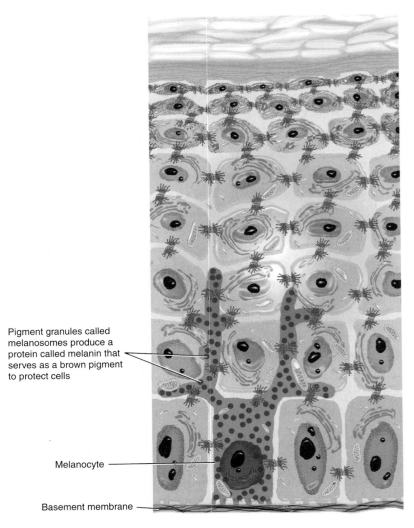

Pigment granules called melanosomes produce a protein called melanin that serves as a brown pigment to protect cells

Melanocyte

Basement membrane

Figure 9–10 Melanin production.

Differences in genetic skin color are due to the amount of melanin activated in the skin and the way it is distributed. Melanin is transferred into the cells through dendrites (branches) that move up to the skin's surface. Melanin is produced by exposure to sunlight and protects the cells below by absorbing and blocking UV rays. The body produces two types of melanin: pheomelanin (fee-oh-MEL-uh-nin), which is red to yellow in color, and eumelanin (yoo-MEL-uh-nin), which is dark brown to black. People with light-colored skin mostly produce pheomelanin, while those with dark-colored skin mostly produce eumelanin.

Products that suppress melanin production by interrupting biochemical processes are referred to as *brightening agents*. Some are called *tyrosinase inhibitors*. Tyrosinase (TY-ruh-sin-ays) is the enzyme involved in melanin production. Pigmentation disorders are discussed in Chapter 10, "Disorders and Diseases of the Skin."

GLANDS

The dermis of the skin contains two types of duct glands, each producing very different substances. The sebaceous (oil) glands secrete oil, while the sudoriferous glands excrete sweat (Figure 9–11).

The Sebaceous (Oil) Glands

Sebaceous glands are connected to the hair follicles and produce oil, which protects the surface of the skin. Glandular sacs open into the follicles through ducts. If the ducts become clogged, comedones (blackheads) are formed. The

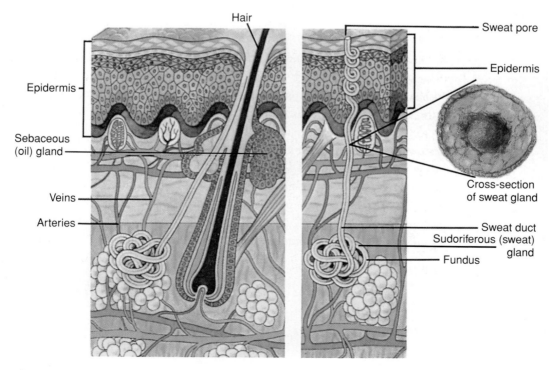

Figure 9–11 Oil and sweat glands.

> **? Did You Know**
>
> Glands in our skin produce chemicals known as *pheromones.* Pheromones are hormones that trigger biological reactions or send signals to others. This reaction is sometimes referred to as body chemistry.

oily secretions lubricate both the skin and hair. Sebaceous glands are larger on the face and scalp.

The Sudoriferous (Sweat) Glands

Sudoriferous (sood-uh-RIF-uh-rus) **or sweat glands** regulate body temperature and eliminate waste products by excreting sweat. They have a coiled base and duct openings at the surface, known as pores. Liquids and salts are eliminated daily through these pores. The excretion of sweat is controlled by the nervous system. Normally, one to two pints of liquids containing salts are eliminated daily through sweat pores in the skin.

There are two kinds of sweat glands—the apocrine and the eccrine.

The **apocrine glands** (AP-uh-krin GLANZ) are coiled structures attached to the hair follicles found under the arms and in the genital area. Their secretions are released through the oil glands. These are more active during emotional changes. Odors associated with these glands are due to the interaction of the secretions and bacteria on the surface of the skin.

The **eccrine glands** (EK-run GLANZ) are found all over the body, primarily on the forehead, palms, and soles. These glands are not connected to hair follicles. They have a duct and pore through which secretions are released. Eccrine glands are more active when the body is subjected to physical activity and high temperatures. Eccrine sweat does not produce an offensive odor.

SKIN HEALTH

Skin health and aging of the skin are both influenced by many different factors, including heredity, sun exposure, the environment, health habits, and general lifestyle. This topic is discussed thoroughly in Chapter 11, "Skin Analysis."

Skin Nourishment

Blood and lymph are the fluids that nourish the skin (Figure 9–12). Networks of arteries and lymphatics send essential materials for growth and repair throughout the body. Water, vitamins, and nutrients are all important for skin health. Blood supplies nutrients and oxygen to the skin. Nutrients are molecules from food such as protein, carbohydrates, and fats. Topical products also nourish the epidermis.

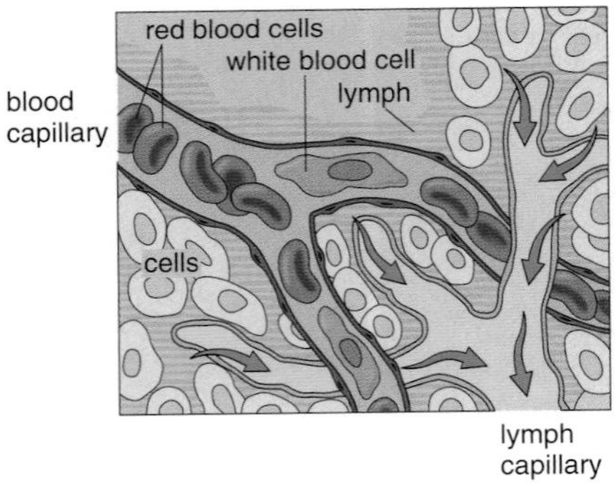

Figure 9–12 Nourishment through the blood and lymph systems.

Lymph, the clear fluids of the body that resemble blood plasma but contain only colorless corpuscles, bathe the skin cells, remove toxins and cellular waste, and have immune functions that help protect the skin and body against disease. Networks of arteries and lymph vessels in the subcutaneous tissue send their smaller branches to hair papillae, follicles, and skin glands.

Cells

Cells need these important elements to survive:

- nourishment
- protection
- function
- proliferation

The health of skin cells depends on the cellular membrane and the water-holding capacity of the stratum corneum. Phospholipids, glycolipids, cholesterol, triglycerides, squalene, and waxes are all lipids found in the stratum corneum and cell membranes. Intercellular lipids and proteins surround cells and provide protection, hydration, and nourishment to the cells. Glycolipids are responsible for cellular functions, and they are antigens. These **ceramides** are lipid molecules important to barrier function and water-holding capacity. Fatty acids are also components in the intercellular substances.

Lipids are reduced if the skin is dry, damaged, or mature. Topical products containing ceramides and other lipids benefit wrinkled skin and expedite healing. Exfoliation removes and depletes lipids, so topical reapplication is necessary to balance what was lost in exfoliation. Cell recovery depends on water to function properly.

Cell Replacement

The body replaces billions of cells daily. Organs such as the skin, heart, liver, and kidneys have their cells replaced every six to nine months. Cells of the bones are replaced every seven years. Unfortunately, elastin and collagen are not easily replaced by the body, and the skin does not regain its once pliable shape after being stretched or damaged by UV rays. However, research shows that certain procedures and ingredients such as vitamin A and alpha hydroxy acids (AHAs) stimulate cell turnover and reduce visible signs of aging.

Free Radical Damage

Free radicals are atoms or molecules with unpaired electrons. They steal electrons from other molecules, which damages the other molecules (Figure 9–13). The free radicals generated when the skin is exposed to sunlight will damage skin cells. When sunlight contacts the skin, it reacts with oxygen to create free radicals. These free radicals attack cell membranes. Free radicals are "super" oxidizers that not only cause an oxidation reaction but also produce a new free radical in the process. Normal oxidation deactivates the oxidizer and stops the oxidation from continuing, but the oxidation caused by free radicals continues in a chain reaction that can oxidize millions of other compounds. UV light can also kill cells by damaging their DNA.

The melanin pigment, produced by tanning, darkens the skin and absorbs UV rays to help keep cells from being damaged. Skin cells have built-in antioxidants to protect against sun damage, but their ability to protect cells deteriorates with sun exposure. Cell damage is cumulative, and photodamage causes photoaging. Pigment dysfunction, wrinkles, sagging, collagen and elastin breakdown, and skin cancer are the results of exposure to UV rays. Inflammation also causes free radical damage and leads to aging, pigmentation, and disease. Red and inflamed skin is an indication of free radical damage.

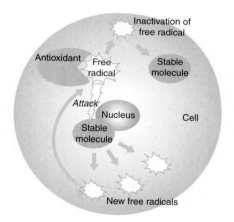

Figure 9–13 Free radicals.

The Environment

While the sun may play the predominant role in how the skin ages, changes in our environment also greatly influence this aging process. Pollutants in the air from factories, automobile exhaust, and even secondhand smoke can all influence the appearance and overall health of our skin. While these pollutants affect the surface appearance of the skin, they can also change the health of the underlying cells and tissues, thereby speeding up the aging process.

The best defense against these pollutants is the simplest one: follow a good daily skin care routine. Routine washing and exfoliating (removing dead surface skin cells) at night helps to remove the buildup of pollutants that have settled on the skin's surface throughout the day. Applying daily moisturizers, protective lotions, sunscreen, and even foundation products all help to protect the skin from airborne pollutants.

Lifestyle

What we choose to put into our bodies significantly affects our overall health. The impact of poor choices can be seen most visibly on the skin. Smoking, drinking, drugs, and poor dietary choices all greatly influence the aging process. It is the esthetician's responsibility to be aware of how these habits affect the skin and to point out (tactfully) these effects to clients without stepping outside the scope of practice.

Smoking and tobacco use may not only cause cancer but also have been linked to the premature aging and wrinkling of the skin. Nicotine in tobacco causes contraction and weakening of the blood vessels and small capillaries that supply blood to the tissues, causing decreased circulation. Eventually, the tissues are deprived of essential oxygen, and the skin's surface may appear yellowish or gray in color and can look dull (Figure 9–14).

Using prescription and illegal drugs affects the skin as much as smoking does. Some drugs have been shown to interfere with the body's intake of oxygen, thus affecting healthy cell growth. Some drugs can even aggravate serious skin conditions, such as acne. Others can cause dryness and allergic reactions on the skin's surface.

Consuming alcohol has an equally damaging effect on the skin. Heavy or excessive intake of alcohol dilates the blood vessels and capillaries. Over time, this constant over-dilation and weakening of the fragile capillary walls can cause them to expand and burst. This causes a constant flushed appearance of the skin and red splotches in the whites of the eyes. Alcohol can also dehydrate the skin by drawing essential water out of the tissues, making the skin appear dull and dry.

Both smoking and drinking contribute to the aging process on their own, but the combination of the two can be even more damaging to the tissues. The constant dilation and contraction of the tiny capillaries and blood vessels, as well as the constant deprivation of oxygen and water to the tissues, quickly makes the skin appear lifeless and dull. It is very difficult for the skin to adjust and repair itself. Usually, the damage done by these lifestyle habits is hard to reverse or even diminish.

SUN DAMAGE

The sun and its ultraviolet (UV) rays have the greatest impact on how our skin ages. Approximately 80 to 85 percent of our aging is caused by the rays of the sun. As we age, the collagen and elastin fibers of the skin naturally weaken. This weakening happens at a much faster rate when the skin is frequently

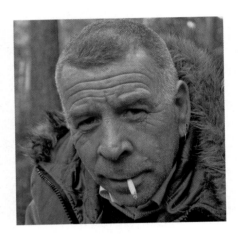

Figure 9–14 Smoking ages the skin.

exposed to ultraviolet rays. The UV rays of the sun reach the skin in two different forms, as UVA and UVB rays. Each of the rays influences the skin at a different level (Figure 9–15).

UVA rays, also called the "aging rays," contribute 90 to 95 percent of the sun's ultraviolet rays that reach the earth's surface. These longer rays penetrate deeper into the skin and cause cell death. They weaken the skin's collagen and elastin fibers, causing wrinkling and sagging in the tissues. UVA and UVB rays alter DNA and can cause skin cancer. UVA rays can penetrate glass.

UVB rays, also referred to as the burning rays, cause burning of the skin. Melanin is designed to help protect the skin from the sun's UV rays, but melanin can be altered or destroyed when large, frequent doses of UV light are allowed to penetrate the skin. Although UVB penetration is shorter than and not as deep as UVA, these rays are stronger and more damaging to the skin and can damage the eyes as well. On a positive note, UVB rays contribute to the body's synthesis of vitamin D and other important minerals.

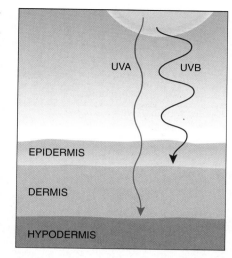

Figure 9–15 UV rays penetrate into the skin at different levels.

It is appropriate that you advise your clients about the necessary precautions to take when they are exposed to the sun. Sun protection does more than protect the skin; it defends cells from radiation, cell death, tissue breakdown, and aging.

Here are some helpful tips for using sunscreen:

- Wear a moisturizer or protective lotion with a sunscreen of sun protection factor (SPF) 30 on all areas of potential exposure. Apply 20 minutes before sun exposure.
- Avoid exposure during peak hours, when UV exposure is highest. This is usually between 10 A.M. and 3 P.M.
- Apply sunscreen liberally after swimming or any activities that result in heavy perspiration. Better yet, sunscreen should be reapplied every two hours or immediately after swimming.
- All sunscreen used for protection should be full- or broad-spectrum to filter out UVA and UVB rays. Check the expiration date printed on the bottle to make sure that the sunscreen has not expired.
- Avoid exposing children younger than six months of age to the sun.
- If you are prone to burning frequently and easily, wear a hat and protective clothing when participating in outdoor activities. Redheads are particularly susceptible to sun damage.
- Remember that sunlight comes through windows, and UV rays are even stronger through glass.
- Wear sunglasses to protect the eyes and the eye area.
- Avoid tanning beds. Research is showing more and more how damaging tanning beds are.

In addition to taking these precautions, clients should be advised to see a physician specializing in dermatology for regular skin checkups, especially if they detect any changes in coloration, size, or shape of a mole.

Home self-examinations can also be an effective way to check for signs of potential skin cancer between scheduled doctor visits. When performing a self-care exam, clients should be advised to check for any changes in existing moles and to pay attention to any new visible growths on the skin.

CAUTION!

Many medications and topical products are photosensitizers that make people more sensitive to sun exposure and can cause severe reactions such as burning, hyperpigmentation, and allergic reactions.

MATURE SKIN AND HORMONES

As we age, our skin changes significantly because of shifts in hormone balance. **Hormones** are the internal messengers for most of the body's systems and are significant internal factors in skin appearance, strength, and health. Estrogen (present in men and women, but predominantly in women) is the crucial hormone for good health and the appearance of skin. Estrogen is anti-inflammatory, an antioxidant, and a key factor in tissue repair. It is also responsible for maintaining health in several body functions such as coordination, balance, skin moisture, vision, bones, and even the nervous system. Estrogen has even been linked to memory and emotions.

Changes to the skin begin as women enter perimenopause in their forties, and they continue into menopause (fifties) and beyond, because of the decrease in estrogen. All tissues begin to thin and change the skin's protective barrier, epithelial (external) tissue, and dermis. The vascular and capillary walls begin to weaken, lipids are reduced, the lymphatic system is less efficient, glands slow down, and there are fewer fibroblasts, thus affecting the connective tissues collagen and elastin. Collagen loses its ability to respond to physical changes from aging and sun damage (Figure 9–16).

As estrogen is depleted, skin begins to lose its tone. Reduced glycosaminoglycans mean less moisture in the tissues; keratinocytes are reduced (slower cell mitosis); melanocytes are reduced (protective pigment lessens); and cellular exchanges are reduced. Testosterone levels become dominant as estrogen decreases, which can increase sebum production, pore size, and hair growth on the face. This explains the unwanted hair growth and unexpected adult acne.

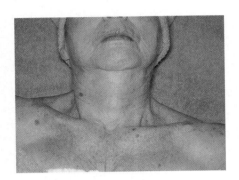

Figure 9–16 Aging of the skin.

Microcirculation

Hormonal changes are one cause of the microcirculation problems that are common in mature skin. One such problem is couperose (KOO-per-ohs) skin, or **telangiectasia** (tell-ann-jee-ek-TA-zhuh), the dilation of the capillary walls. As the endothelium (wall of the capillary) atrophies and loses its elasticity, the walls dilate and fill with blood, sometimes bursting.

Other causes of couperose or spider veins are heredity, alimentary (digestive) problems, alcohol, smoking, sun damage, harsh cosmetics, trauma, pregnancy, excess localized heat, topical corticosteroids, inflammation, and heat/cold fluctuations. These all lead to permanent dilation of the capillaries.

Rosacea (roh-ZAY-see-uh) is a chronic disorder characterized by couperose veins and congestion of the skin. Acne rosacea features all of the conditions found in rosacea, in addition to the presence of papules, pustules, and, in some cases, the fostering of parasitic microorganisms (mites).

Hormone Replacement Therapy

Hormone replacement therapy (HRT) is often suggested for women experiencing menopause. However, some HRT may be linked to breast cancer. These therapies may be derived from animal-source estrogens or plant-source estrogens. Estrogens from plants are called *phytoestrogens* (fy-toh-ES-tro-jins); they are about 400 times weaker than animal estrogens. Plants that provide phytoestrogens include Mexican wild yam, sage, hops, soy, Saint-John's-wort, licorice root, and butcher's broom. In addition to hormone balancing, maintaining good nutrition, skin care, lymphatic drainage massage, exercise, and a positive outlook will help keep skin looking radiant at any age. Do thorough research before choosing an HRT program.

REVIEW QUESTIONS

1. What are the six functions of the skin?

2. What does *barrier function* mean?

3. Why is sebum important?

4. In what ways does the skin protect itself?

5. What regulates the body's temperature?

6. How many layers of the skin are there?

7. Name the layers of the epidermis.

8. Name the layers of the dermis.

9. What is collagen?

10. Why is elasticity important?

11. What are melanocytes?

12. How does skin get its nourishment?

13. Name the three types of nerve fibers and describe what they do.

14. How often does the body replace cells?

15. How does skin get its color?

16. What are the two main glands associated with the skin?

17. What are the two types of sweat glands?

18. What are free radicals?

CHAPTER GLOSSARY

acid mantle: protective lipids and secretions on top of the skin.

adipose (fat) tissue: a protective cushion that gives contour and smoothness to the body.

apocrine glands: coiled structures attached to hair follicles found in the underarm and genital areas.

arrector pili muscle: the muscle that contracts and causes "goose bumps" when we are cold.

barrier function: the protective barrier of the epidermis; the corneum and intercellular cement protect the surface from irritation and dehydration.

cell mitosis: cell division; occurs continuously in the basal cell layer.

ceramides: lipid materials that are a natural part of the intercellular cement.

collagen: fibrous, connective tissue made from protein; found in the reticular layer of the dermis; gives skin its firmness. Topically, a large, long-chain molecular protein that lies on the top of the skin and binds water; derived from the placentas of cows or other sources.

dermal papillae: membranes of ridges and grooves that attach to the epidermis.

dermis: live layer of connective tissue below the epidermis.

desmosomes: the structures that assist in holding cells together.

eccrine glands: sweat glands found all over the body; not attached to hair follicles, do not produce an offensive odor.

elastin: protein fiber found in the dermis; gives skin its elasticity and firmness.

epidermis: the outermost layer of skin; a thin, protective layer with many nerve endings.

fibroblasts: cells that produce amino acids and collagen.

follicles: hair follicles and sebaceous follicles are tubelike depressions in the epidermis.

free radicals: oxygen atoms or molecules with unpaired electrons that cause oxidation. They steal electrons from other molecules, which damages the other molecules.

hair papillae: cone-shaped elevations at the base of the follicle that fits into the bulb. The papillae are filled with tissue that contains the blood vessels and cells necessary for hair growth and follicle nourishment.

histology: study of the structure and composition of tissue.

hormones: secretions produced by one of the endocrine glands and carried by the bloodstream or body fluid to another part of the body or a body organ to stimulate functional activity or secretion; the internal messengers for most of the body's systems.

hyaluronic acid: hydrating fluids found in the skin; hydrophilic agent with water-binding properties.

integumentary system: the skin and its extensions, such as the hair, nails, and glands.

intercellular cement: lipid substances between coreum cells that protect the cells from water loss and irritation.

keratin: fiber protein found in skin, hair, and nails; provides resiliency and protection to the skin.

keratinocytes: cells composed of keratin.

lipids: fats or fatlike substances. Lipids help repair and protect the barrier function of the skin.

lymph vessels: located in the dermis, these supply nourishment within the skin and remove waste.

melanin: skin pigment; a defense mechanism to protect skin from the sun.

melanocytes: cells that produce pigment granules in the basal layer.

papillary layer: the top layer of the dermis next to the epidermis.

physiology: study of the functions or activities performed by the body's structures.

pores: a tubelike opening for sweat glands on the epidermis.

reticular layer: the deeper layer of the dermis, containing proteins that give the skin its strength and elasticity.

sebaceous glands: sebaceous glands are connected to the hair follicles in the reticular layer; these produce sebum, which protects the surface of the skin.

sebum: provides protection for the epidermis from external factors and lubricates both the skin and hair.

stratum corneum: outermost layer of the epidermis, also called the horny layer.

stratum germinativum: first layer of the epidermis above the papillary layer of the dermis; also known as the basal layer.

stratum granulosum: layer of the epidermis composed of cells filled with keratin that resemble granules; replace cells shed from the stratum corneum.

stratum lucidum: clear layer of epidermis under the stratum corneum; found only on the palms of hands and soles of feet.

stratum spinosum: spiny layer of epidermis above the basal layer.

subcutaneous layer: subcutaneous adipose tissue located beneath the dermis.

subcutis tissue: subcutaneous tissue located beneath the dermis.

sudoriferous or sweat glands: excrete perspiration and detoxify the body by excreting excess salt and unwanted chemicals.

telangiectasia: describes capillaries that have been damaged and are now larger, or distended blood vessels. Commonly called *couperose skin*.

transepidermal water loss (TEWL): water loss caused by evaporation on the skin's surface.

UVA rays: longer, aging rays that penetrate deeper into the skin than UVB rays.

UVB rays: shorter, burning rays that are stronger than UVA rays.

CHAPTER 10

DISORDERS AND DISEASES OF THE SKIN

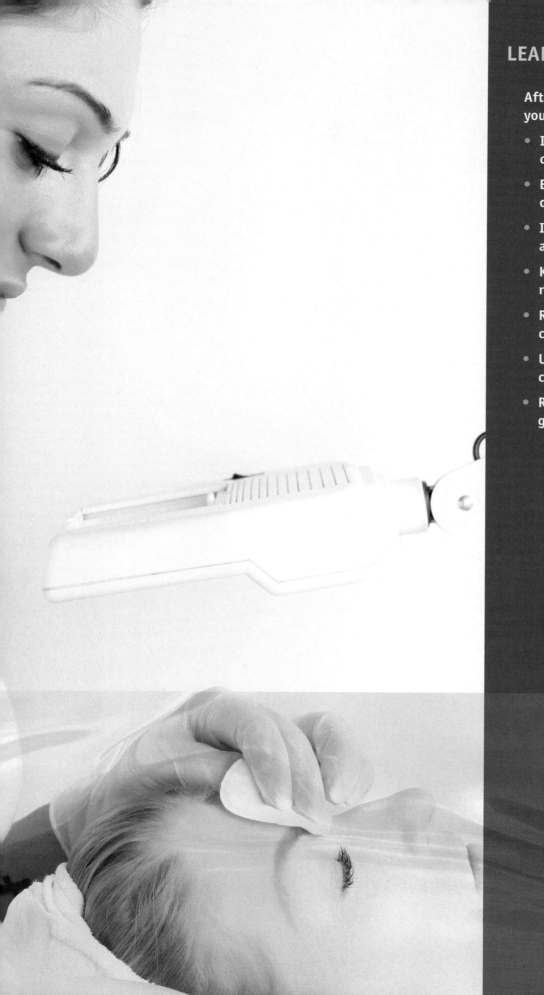

After completing this chapter, you will be able to:

- Identify common skin conditions and disorders.

- Explain the different types of skin lesions.

- Identify which disorders are contagious.

- Know which disorders to refer to a physician.

- Recognize potential skin cancer growths.

- Understand acne and the causes of the disorder.

- Recognize the different grades of acne.

KEY TERMS

Page numbers indicate where in the chapter each term is used.

Skin diseases and disorders are interesting and complex subjects. Estheticians need to be knowledgeable about skin disorders and diseases. Recognizing these conditions can help the esthetician work with clients effectively and safely. The medical field is progressing, and the treatment of skin disorders is becoming easier with advances in technology, ingredients, and medicine. Although there are hundreds of disorders, only the most common are discussed in this chapter. Knowledge of skin disorders takes years of experience and study, but reference books are helpful in identifying these diseases and disorders.

Estheticians can provide education and help clients with many of their skin concerns such as acne, rosacea, and hyperpigmentation. Never work on any skin condition you do not recognize. When in doubt, stop. Let clients know if you do not recognize a lesion, and they will appreciate your honesty and caution. Trying to extract a sebaceous hyperplasia mistaken for a comedone can lead to scarring and a potentially worse problem. Advanced classes are necessary to learn more about disorders. Treatments and products formulated for certain disorders are addressed in subsequent chapters.

DERMATOLOGY AND ESTHETICS

Dermatology is the branch of medical science that studies and treats the skin and its disorders and diseases. A **dermatologist** is a physician who treats these disorders and diseases.

Recognizing skin diseases and disorders is important for the protection of both the technician and the client. Estheticians may not perform services on clients who have contagious or infectious diseases. Any skin abnormality you do not positively recognize must be referred to a physician. Estheticians can help clients with many common disorders and conditions such as rosacea, minor acne, and sensitive skin. Dermatologists and physicians are qualified to treat skin problems, but estheticians may not diagnose or treat diseases and disorders of the skin beyond their scope of practice. Caution and strict sanitation practices are imperative when working with skin disorders. Knowledge of skin conditions that contraindicate a treatment is also necessary.

CAUTION!

Do not attempt to diagnose medical conditions. Estheticians are not licensed to diagnose skin conditions, disorders, or diseases. Refer clients to a physician if you think they have a disorder or disease that needs medical attention.

LESIONS

Lesions (LEE-zhuns) are structural changes in the tissues caused by damage or injury. Any mark, symptom, or abnormality is described as a lesion. The three types of lesions are primary, secondary, and tertiary. Some books refer to the tertiary, or third, type of lesions as *vascular lesions*. Vascular lesions involve the blood or circulatory system.

Primary Lesions

Primary lesions are lesions in the early stages of development or change. Primary lesions are characterized by flat, non-palpable changes in skin color—such as macules—or by elevations formed by fluid in a cavity, such as vesicles or pustules. **Primary lesions** of the skin include the following (Figure 10–1):

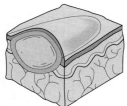

Bulla:
Same as a vesicle only greater than 0.5 cm
Example:
Contact dermatitis, large second-degree burns, bulbous impetigo, pemphigus

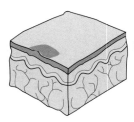

Macule:
Localized changes in skin color of less than 1 cm in diameter
Example:
Freckle

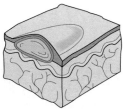

Tubercle:
Solid and elevated; however, it extends deeper than papules into the dermis or subcutaneous tissues, 0.5-2 cm
Example:
Lipoma, erythema, nodosum, cyst

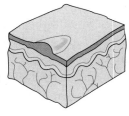

Papule:
Solid, elevated lesion less than 0.5 cm in diameter
Example:
Warts, elevated nevi

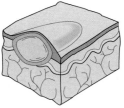

Pustule:
Vesicles or bullae that become filled with pus, usually described as less than 0.5 cm in diameter
Example:
Acne, impetigo, furuncles, carbuncles, folliculitis

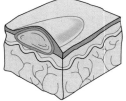

Vesicle:
Accumulation of fluid between the upper layers of the skin; elevated mass containing serous fluid; less than 0.5 cm
Example:
Herpes simplex, herpes zoster, chickenpox

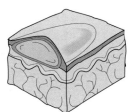

Nodule/Tumor:
The same as a nodule only greater than 2 cm
Example:
Carcinoma (such as advanced breast carcinoma); **not** basal cell or squamous cell of the skin

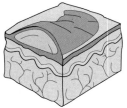

Wheal:
Localized edema in the epidermis causing irregular elevation that may be red or pale
Example:
Insect bite or a hive

Figure 10–1 Primary lesions of the skin.

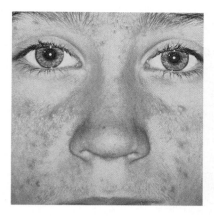

Figure 10–2 Papules.

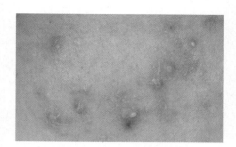

Figure 10–3 Pustules.

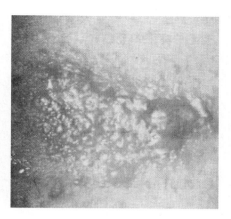

Figure 10–4 Vesicles.

Bulla (plural: bullae) A large blister containing watery fluid. It is similar to a vesicle, but larger.

Cyst A closed, abnormally developed sac containing fluid, infection, or other matter above or below the skin. An acne cyst is one type of cyst.

Macule A flat spot or discoloration on the skin, such as a freckle. Macules are neither raised nor sunken.

Nodules These are often referred to as tumors, but they are smaller bumps caused by conditions such as scar tissue, fatty deposits, or infections.

Papule A small elevation on the skin that contains no fluid, but may develop into a pustule (Figure 10–2).

Pustule An inflamed papule with a white or yellow center containing pus, a fluid consisting of white blood cells, bacteria, and other debris produced from an infection (Figure 10–3).

Tubercle An abnormal rounded, solid lump, larger than a papule.

Tumor A large nodule; an abnormal cell mass resulting from excessive cell multiplication, varying in size, shape, and color.

Vesicles A small blister or sac containing clear fluid. Poison ivy and poison oak produce vesicles (Figure 10–4).

Wheal An itchy, swollen lesion caused by a blow, insect bite, skin allergy reaction, or stings. Hives and mosquito bites are wheals. Hives are called **urticaria** (ur-tuh-KAYR-ee-ah) and can also be caused by exposure to allergens used in products.

Secondary Lesions

Secondary lesions of the skin develop in the later stages of disease (Figure 10–5).

Crust Dead cells formed over a wound or blemish while it is healing, resulting in an accumulation of sebum and pus, sometimes mixed with epidermal material. An example is the scab on a sore.

Excoriation (ek-skor-ee-AY-shun) A skin sore or abrasion produced by scratching or scraping.

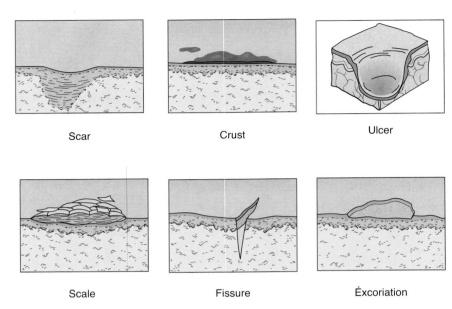

Figure 10–5 Secondary lesions.

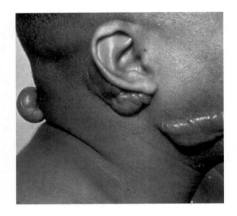

Figure 10–6 Keloids.

Acne excoriee (ak-nee ek-SKOR-ee) A disorder where clients purposely scrape off acne lesions, causing scarring and discoloration.

Fissure A crack in the skin that may penetrate into the dermis. Chapped lips or hands are fissures.

Keloid (KEE-loyd) A thick scar resulting from excessive growth of fibrous tissue (collagen). Keloids are usually genetically predisposed and may occur following an injury or surgery (Figure 10–6).

Scale Shredding of dead skin cells; flaky skin cells; any thin plate of epidermal flakes, dry or oily. An example is abnormal or excessive dandruff or psoriasis.

Scar Light-colored, slightly raised mark on the skin formed after an injury or lesion of the skin has healed. The tissue hardens to heal the injury. Thick, elevated scars are hypertrophic, like a keloid.

Ulcer An open lesion on the skin or mucous membrane of the body, accompanied by pus and loss of skin depth. A deep erosion or depression in the skin, normally due to infection or cancer.

SEBACEOUS (OIL) GLAND DISORDERS

Notable sebaceous gland disorders include the following:

Acne A chronic inflammatory skin disorder of the sebaceous glands characterized by comedones and blemishes. Also known as *acne simplex* or *acne vulgaris*. Skin disorder characterized by chronic inflammation of the sebaceous glands from retained secretions and *Propionibacterium acnes* (*P. acnes*) bacteria.

Asteatosis (as-tee-ah-TOH-sis) Dry, scaly skin from sebum deficiency; can be due to aging, body disorders, alkalies of harsh soaps, or cold exposure.

Comedone (KAHM-uh-dohn) A non-inflamed buildup of cells, sebum, and other debris inside follicles. An *open comedo* (KAHM-uh-doe) is a blackhead; when the follicle is filled with an excess of oil, a blackhead forms. It is dark because it is exposed to oxygen and oxidation occurs (Figure 10–7). A *closed comedo* is also referred to as a whitehead but should not be confused with the more hardened whitehead called milia.

Furuncle (FYOO-rung-kul) A subcutaneous abscess filled with pus. Also called boils, furuncles are caused by bacteria in glands or hair follicles.

Carbuncles (KAHR-bung-kuls) are groups of boils.

Milia (MIL-ee-ah) Also called *whiteheads;* whitish, pearl-like masses of sebum and dead cells under the skin with no visible opening. Hardened and closed over, milia are more common in dry skin types and may form after skin trauma, such as a laser resurfacing or exposure to UV radiation (Figure 10–8). They resemble small sesame seeds and are almost always perfectly round. They are usually found around the eyes, cheeks, and forehead.

Sebaceous hyperplasia (sih-BAY-shus hy-pur-PLAY-zhuh) Benign lesions frequently seen in oilier areas of the face. These overgrowths of the sebaceous gland appear similar to open comedones. They are often doughnut-shaped, with sebaceous material in the center. They cannot be removed by extraction, only surgically (Figure 10–9).

Seborrhea (seb-oh-REE-ah) Severe oiliness of the skin; an abnormal secretion from the sebaceous glands.

Seborrheic dermatitis (seb-oh-REE-ick derm-ah-TIE-tus) A skin condition caused by an inflammation of the sebaceous glands. It is often characterized by inflammation, dry or oily scaling or crusting, and/or itchiness. The red, flaky skin often appears in the eyebrows, in the scalp and hairline, the middle of the forehead, and along the sides of the nose. This condition is sometimes treated with cortisone creams. Severe cases should be referred to the dermatologist.

Steatoma (stee-ah-TOH-muh) A sebaceous cyst or subcutaneous tumor filled with sebum and ranging in size from a pea to an orange. It usually appears on the scalp, neck, and back; also called a *wen.*

DISORDERS OF THE SUDORIFEROUS (SWEAT) GLANDS

Disorders of the sudoriferous glands include the following:

Anhidrosis (an-hy-DROH-sus) A deficiency in perspiration due to failure of the sweat glands; often results from a fever or skin disease. Anhidrosis requires medical treatment.

Bromhidrosis (broh-mih-DROH-sis) Foul-smelling perspiration, usually in the armpits or on the feet. Bromhidrosis is caused by bacteria and yeast that break down the sweat on the surface of the skin.

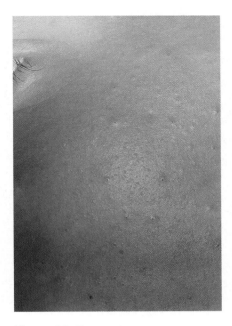

Figure 10–7 Comedones.

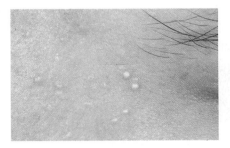

Figure 10–8 Milia.

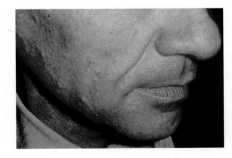

Figure 10–9 Sebaceous hyperplasia.

Hyperhidrosis (hy-pur-hy-DROH-sis) Excessive perspiration caused by heat, genetics or body weakness. Medical treatment is required.

Miliaria rubra (mil-ee-AIR-ee-ah ROOB-rah) Prickly heat; acute inflammatory disorder of the sweat glands; results in the eruption of red vesicles and burning, itching skin from excessive heat exposure.

INFLAMMATIONS OF THE SKIN

Inflammations of the skin include the following:

Atopic dermatitis Atopic dermatitis is a rash (*atopic* is "excess inflammation from allergies"). The redness, itching, and dehydration of the dermatitis make the condition worse. Use of humidifiers and lotion can help keep the skin more hydrated. Topical corticosteroids can relieve the symptoms.

Contact dermatitis An inflammatory skin condition caused by contact with a substance or chemical. (Contact dermatitis can be caused by either an allergic reaction or contact with an irritant.) Makeup, skin care products, detergents, dyes, fabrics, jewelry and plants can all cause this reaction and red, itchy skin. A*llergic contact dermatitis* is caused by exposure to allergens. Poison ivy is an example. *Irritant contact dermatitis* is caused by exposure to caustic irritants. Occupational disorders from ingredients in cosmetics and chemical solutions can cause contact dermatitis, or *dermatitis venenata*. Contact with allergens and caustic chemicals can also cause skin sensitivity or disorders. Allergies and skin eruptions are common (Figure 10–10). Wearing gloves or protective skin creams while working with chemicals or irritating substances can help prevent dermatitis venenata.

Dermatitis An inflammatory condition of the skin, various forms of which include lesions, such as eczema, vesicles, or papules.

Eczema (EG-zuh-muh) An inflammatory, painful, itching disease of the skin, acute or chronic in nature, with dry or moist lesions. This should be referred to a physician (Figure 10–11). A common form of eczema, **seborrheic dermatitis,** mainly affects oily areas. Avoid contact and skin care treatments if a client has eczema.

Edema (ih-DEE-muh) Swelling from a fluid imbalance in the cells or from a response to injury or infection.

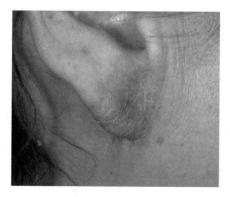

Figure 10–10 Contact dermatitis.

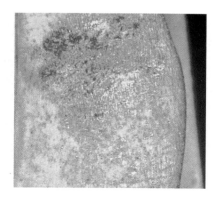

Figure 10–11 Eczema.

Erythema (er-uh-THEE-muh) Redness caused by inflammation.

Folliculitis (fah-lik-yuh-LY-tis) Hair grows under the surface instead of growing up and out of the follicle, causing a bacterial infection. These ingrown hairs are common in men, usually from shaving (Figure 10–12). Razor bumps without the pus or infection are called **pseudofolliculitis** (SOO-doe-fah-lik-yuh-LY-tis).

Perioral dermatitis (pair-ee-OR-ul derm-a-TIE-tuss) An acne-like condition around the mouth; consists mainly of small clusters of papules. It may be caused by toothpaste or products used on the face. It is not contagious. Antibiotics can help treat the condition.

Pruitis (proo-RYT-us) The medical term for itching.

Psoriasis (suh-RY-uh-sis) A skin disease characterized by red patches covered with white-silver scales. Caused by an overproliferation of skin cells that replicate too fast (Figure 10–13). Psoriasis is usually found in patches on the scalp, elbows, knees, chest, and lower back. If patches are irritated, bleeding can occur. Psoriasis is not contagious but can be spread by irritating the affected area.

Rosacea (roh-ZAY-see-uh) An inflammation of the skin characterized by redness, dilation of blood vessels, and in severe cases the formation of papules and pustules (Figure 10–14). It is chronic congestion primarily on the cheeks and nose. The cause and treatment of rosacea is a primary concern of skin care today. The cause is unknown, but may be due to heredity, bacteria, mites, or fungus. Certain factors are known to aggravate the condition. Vascular dilation **(vasodilation)** of the blood vessels makes it worse. Spicy foods, alcohol, caffeine, exposure to temperature extremes, heat, sun, and stress aggravate rosacea. Soothing and calming ingredients and treatments will help calm the skin and decrease the inflammation (see Chapter 12).

Telangiectasia (tel-an-jee-ek-TAY-zhuh) A vascular lesion; describes capillaries that have been damaged and are now larger, or distended blood vessels. Commonly called *couperose skin.*

Urticaria (ur-tuh-KAYR-ee-ah) An allergic reaction by the body's histamine production; also known as *hives.*

Allergic Contact Dermatitis

Allergic reactions are caused by repeated direct skin contact to an allergen. Normally the immune system protects us from pathogens and disease, but in an allergic reaction the immune system actually causes the problem by trying to do its job too well. An allergic reaction occurs when our immune system mistakes a harmless substance for a toxic one and mounts a major defense. Severe allergic reactions can result in high fever and anaphylactic (an-ah-fah-LAK-tik) shock, which can be life threatening.

An allergic reaction is caused by repeated exposure to an allergen. Initial exposure to an allergen does not always cause an allergic reaction. The development of hypersensitivity is the result of repeated exposure to an allergen over time. This process is called *sensitization* (SEN-sih-tiz-A-shun), and it may take months or years depending on the allergen and the intensity of exposure.

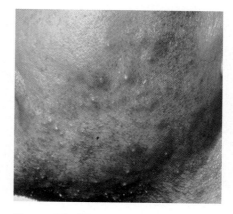
Figure 10–12 Folliculitis.

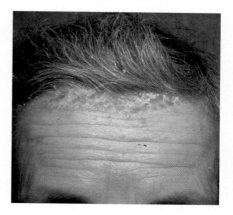
Figure 10–13 Psoriasis.

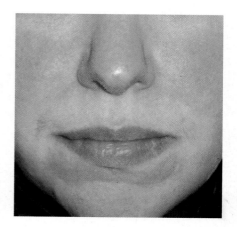
Figure 10–14 Rosacea.

Poison ivy is a common allergen. Although approximately 75 percent of the population is allergic to poison ivy, the remaining 25 percent will never have a reaction no matter how many times they are exposed. Individuals who are not predisposed never become sensitized and will not develop allergies. Also remember that different people develop allergies to different allergens. Individual predisposition may be inherited because sensitivity seems to run in families.

Here are some allergies from chemicals commonly seen in the salon:

- on practitioner's fingers, palms, or on the back of the hand
- on practitioner's face, especially the cheeks
- on client's scalp, hairline, forehead, or neckline

If you examine the area where the problem occurs, you can usually determine the cause. For example, hair colorists often use their bare fingers and hands to do strand tests of color. This is both prolonged and repeated contact! Sensitization is an increased or exaggerated sensitivity to products.

Irritant Contact Dermatitis

Irritant reactions affect everyone who comes in contact with an irritant, although the degree of irritation will vary depending on the individual. In acute cases symptoms are noticed immediately or within just a few hours. Chronic cases may take weeks, months, or years to develop. Symptoms range from redness, swelling, scaling, and itching to serious, painful chemical burns. Irritating substances will temporarily damage the epidermis. Caustic substances are examples of irritants. When the skin is damaged by irritating substances, the immune system springs into action. It floods the tissue with water, trying to dilute the irritant. This is why swelling occurs.

The immune system also tells the blood to release histamines, which enlarge the vessels around the injury. Blood can then rush to the scene more quickly and help remove the irritating substance.

The extra blood under the skin is quite easily visible. The entire area becomes red, warm, and may throb. Histamines cause the itchy feeling that often accompanies contact dermatitis. After everything calms down, the swelling will go away. The surrounding skin is often left damaged, scaly, cracked, and dry. Fortunately, irritations are not permanent. If you avoid repeated and/or prolonged contact with the irritating substance, the skin will usually quickly repair itself. However, continued or repeated exposure may lead to permanent allergic reactions and skin damage.

PIGMENTATION DISORDERS

The genetic background of a person influences pigmentation disorders. Abnormal pigmentation, referred to as *dyschromia* (diz-KRO-me-ah), can be caused by various internal or external factors. Sun exposure is the biggest external cause of pigmentation disorders and can make existing pigmentation disorders worse. Drugs also cause skin pigmentation abnormalities. **Hyperpigmentation,** overproduction of pigment, and **hypopigmentation,** lack of pigment, are the two types of pigmentation disorders. Causes and treatment are discussed in subsequent chapters.

Hyperpigmentation

Hyperpigmentation appears in the following forms:

Chloasma (klo-AZ-ma) Increased pigmentation; liver spots.

Hyperpigmentation An overproduction of pigment (Figure 10–15). Increased melanin causes excess pigment. Sun exposure, acne, medications, and post-inflammatory hyperpigmentation from skin damage can cause darkened pigmentation.

Lentigo/Lentigenes Lentigo (len-TY-goh) is one freckle. Lentigenes (len-tih-JEE-neez) are multiple freckles; small, yellow-brown spots. Lentigenes that result from sunlight exposure are actinic, or solar, lentigenes. Patches of freckles are referred to as large *macules*.

Melasma (muh-LAZ-muh) A term for hyperpigmentation. Pregnancy mask, often called melasma, is triggered by hormonal changes and may fade with time.

Nevus (NEE-vus) A birthmark or mole; malformation of the skin from abnormal pigmentation or dilated capillaries.

Stain Brown or wine-colored discoloration. Stains occur after certain diseases or after moles, freckles, or liver spots disappear. A *port wine stain* is a birthmark, which is a vascular type of nevus.

Tan Exposure to the sun causes tanning, a change in pigmentation due to melanin production as a defense against UV rays that damage the skin.

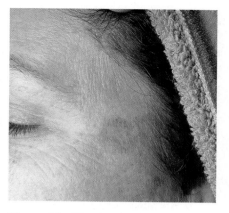

Figure 10–15 Hyperpigmentation.

Hypopigmentation

Hypopigmentation occurs in various forms.

Albinism (AL-bi-niz-em) The absence of melanin pigment in the body, including skin, hair, and eyes (Figure 10–16). The person is at risk for cancer development, is sensitive to light, and ages early without normal melanin protection. The technical term for albinism is *congenital leukoderma*.

Hypopigmentation Lack of pigment.

Leukoderma (loo-koh-DUR-ma) Light, abnormal patches caused by a congenital disease that destroys the pigment-producing cells. Vitiligo and albinism are leukodermas.

Vitiligo (vih-til-EYE-goh) White spots or areas on the skin from a lack of pigment cells (Figure 10–17); the condition can worsen with time and sunlight.

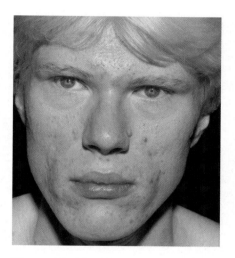

Figure 10–16 Albinism.

HYPERTROPHIES

Hyphertrophies include the following forms:

Hypertrophy (hy-PUR-truh-fee) An abnormal growth; many are *benign*, or harmless. However, some growths are premalignant or malignant and can be dangerous or cancerous. *Hypertrophic* is used to describe thickening of a tissue (the opposite of hypertrophy is *atrophy*, which means "wasting away or thinning").

Keratoma (kair-uh-TOH-muh) An acquired, thickened patch of epidermis. A callus caused by pressure or friction is a keratoma. If the thickening also grows inward, it becomes a corn.

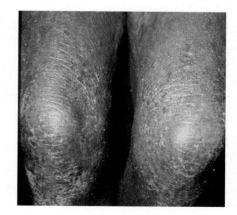

Figure 10–17 Vitiligo.

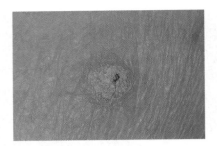

Figure 10–18 Actinic keratosis.

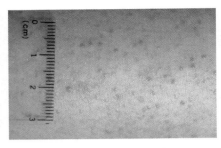

Figure 10–19 Keratosis pilaris.

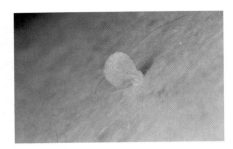

Figure 10–20 A skin tag.

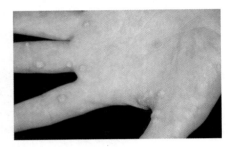

Figure 10–21 Verruca.

CAUTION!

Do not work on clients if you have a verruca or any other contagious conditions on any area that would touch or infect the client! Do not touch client's warts or planter's warts on the feet, because these are also contagious.

FYI

Benign means "not harmful"; *malignant* means "cancerous."

Keratoses (kair-uh-TOH-sees) An abnormally thick buildup of cells. **Hyperkeratosis** is a thickening of the skin caused by a mass of keratinized cells, **keratinocytes** (kair-uh-TIN-oh-cytes). **Actinic keratoses,** pink or flesh-colored precancerous lesions that feel sharp or rough, are a result of sun damage and should be checked by a dermatologist (Figure 10–18).

Keratosis pilaris (kair-uh-TOH-sis py-LAIR-us) Redness and bumpiness in the cheeks or upper arms; caused by blocked follicles. Exfoliation can help unblock follicles and alleviate the rough feeling (Figure 10–19).

Mole A brownish spot ranging in color from tan to bluish black. Some are flat, resembling freckles; others are raised and darker. Most are benign, but changes in mole color or shape should be checked by a physician. Hairs in moles are common and should not be removed unless by a physician because it may irritate or cause structural changes to the mole.

Skin tag Small outgrowths or extensions of the skin that look like flaps. They are benign and are common under the arms or on the neck (Figure 10–20).

Verruca (vuh-ROO-kuh) A wart; hypertrophy of the papillae and epidermis caused by a virus. *Infectious* and *contagious*, verrucas can spread. Wear gloves, and avoid contact with warts (Figure 10–21).

SKIN CANCER

Skin cancer risk increases with cumulative ultraviolet (UV) sun exposure and is found in three distinct forms that vary in severity. Each form is named for the type of cells that are affected. Skin cancer is caused by damage to DNA. Skin cancer tumors form when cells begin to divide rapidly and unevenly. See Table 10–1 for some facts on skin cancer.

If detected early, these abnormal growths can be removed. If not taken care of, they can be deadly. It is important for estheticians to recognize serious skin disorders so they can refer clients to physicians. Tactfully suggest that the client seek medical advice without diagnosing or speculating about the disorders. Annual exams are recommended to check for cancerous lesions. Sun damage and sunscreens are discussed in other chapters.

Table 10–1

FACTS ABOUT SKIN CANCER AND SUN EXPOSURE

- Melanoma is rising faster than any other cancer, and it causes 8,000 deaths every year.
- Death from skin cancer occurs at the rate of one death per hour in the United States.
- More than 1.3 million skin cancers are diagnosed annually in the United States.
- More than 90% of all skin cancers are caused by sun exposure.
- Only 33% of the population uses sunscreen.
- The risk of skin cancer doubles if a person has had five or more sunburns in their lifetime or even one severe sunburn as a child.
- Most parents do not correctly use sunscreen on their children or protect them with hats or clothing.
- Eighty percent of lifetime sun exposure occurs before age 18.
- Most of the people diagnosed with melanoma are white men over age 50.
- Skin cancer is the number one cancer in men over age 50.
- Men over age 40 spend the most time outdoors and have the most exposure to UV radiation.
- Skin cancer has tripled in women under age 40 in the past 30 years.
- Skin cancer kills more women in their late twenties and early thirties than breast cancer does.
- Nearly 30 million people in the United States tan indoors with UVA radiation exposure; 2.3 million are teens.
- The effects of photoaging from sun exposure or indoor tanning can be seen as early as age 20 or before.
- UV rays pass through clouds and window glass.
- There is no safe way to tan.

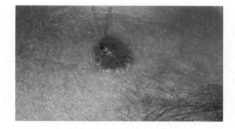

Basal Cell Carcinoma

Basal cell carcinoma (BAY-zul CEL kar-si-NOH-mah) is the most common and the least severe type of carcinoma (Figure 10–22). It often appears as light, pearly nodules. Sometimes blood vessels run through the nodules. Basal cells do not spread as easily as squamous or melanoma cells. They can be easily removed by surgery or other medical procedures.

Figure 10–22 Basal cell carcinoma.

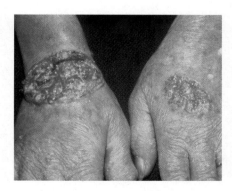

Squamous Cell Carcinoma

Squamous cell carcinoma (SKWAY-mus CEL kar-si-NOH-mah) is a more serious condition than basal cell carcinoma (Figure 10–23). It is characterized by red or pink scaly papules or nodules. Sometimes they are characterized by open sores or crusty areas that do not heal and may bleed easily. Squamous cell carcinoma can spread to other areas of the body.

Figure 10–23 Squamous cell carcinoma.

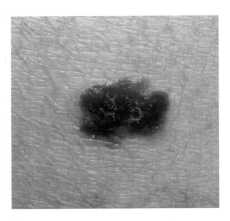

Figure 10–24 Malignant melanoma.

Malignant Melanoma

A **malignant melanoma** (muh-LIG-nent mel-ah-NOH-muh) is the most serious form of skin cancer. Black or dark patches on the skin are usually uneven in texture, jagged, or raised (Figure 10–24). It can be tan and even white. It is not always found on areas exposed to sunlight and is often found on feet, toes, and legs. Malignant melanoma is more deadly because it can spread throughout the body and to internal organs.

The ABCDE Cancer Checklist is a method of evaluating lesions; each letter corresponds to specific melanoma characteristics. Melanoma mole-like lesions are asymmetrical, have uneven borders, uneven color, are larger in diameter than a pencil eraser, and they change or evolve.

ABCDE'S OF MELANOMA DETECTION

The American Cancer Society recommends using the ABCDE Cancer Checklist to help make potential skin cancer easier to recognize. When checking existing moles, look for changes in any of the following:

- A—Asymmetry
- B—Border
- C—Color
- D—Diameter
- E—Evolution

Changes to any of these characteristics should be examined by a physician (Figure 10–25). For more information, contact the American Cancer Society at http://www.cancer.org or (800) ACS-2345.

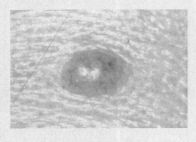
Benign mole-symmetrical

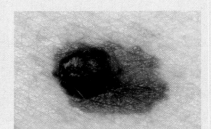
Melanoma-asymmetrical

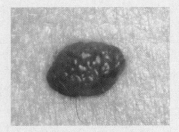
Benign mole-even edges

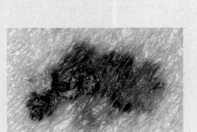
Melanoma-uneven edges

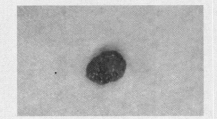
Benign mole-one shade

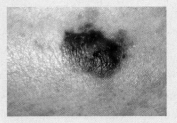
Melanoma-two or more shades

Figure 10–25 ABCDE checklist.

CONTAGIOUS DISEASES

The term *contagious disease* is used interchangeably with the terms *infectious* or *communicable* disease. Do not perform services on anyone with a contagious disease. Refer them to a physician.

The following are contagious diseases.

Bacterial conjunctivitis (bak-TEER-ee-ul kun-junk-tuh-VY-tus) Commonly called pinkeye; very contagious.

Herpes simplex virus 1 (HER-peez SIM-pleks VY-rus 1) Fever blisters or cold sores; recurring viral infection. A vesicle or group of vesicles on a red, swollen base. The blisters usually appear on the lips or nostrils. It is a contagious disease (Figure 10–26).

There are two types of herpes: herpes simplex virus 1 causes cold sores and lesions around the mouth; **herpes simplex virus 2** is genital herpes. Never work on clients with a current herpes lesion. Peels, waxing, or other stimuli may cause a breakout, even if the condition is not currently active. The virus can be spread to other areas of the person infected or to other people. Understanding a client's health history from his or her intake form may prevent problems.

Herpes zoster (HER-peez ZOHS-tur) Shingles, a painful skin condition from the chickenpox virus; characterized by groups of blisters that form a rash.

Impetigo (im-puh-TEE-go) A bacterial infection of the skin that often occurs in children; characterized by clusters of small blisters or crusty lesions filled with bacteria. It is extremely contagious.

Tinea (TIN-ee-uh) Fungal infections. Fungi feed on proteins, carbohydrates, and lipids in the skin. *Tinea pedis,* athlete's foot, is a fungal infection.

Tinea corporis (TIN-ee-uh KOR-pur-is) Highly contagious *ringworm*; it forms a ringed red pattern with elevated edges (Figure 10–27).

Tinea versicolor (TIN-ee-uh VUR-see-kuh-lur) Also called *pityriasis versicolor.* A fungal infection that inhibits melanin production. Hypopigmentation, or white patches, associated with this *sun fungus* can be treated with antifungal cream or medication. Selenium sulfide shampoos can also treat the condition. Tinea versicolor, while a fungal disease, is not contagious (Figure 10–28). High humidity and summer heat stimulates the condition.

Verruca (vuh-ROO-kuh) Warts. Hypertrophy of the papillae and epidermis caused by a virus. Infectious and contagious, verrucas can spread. Wear gloves and avoid contact with warts.

ACNE

Acne is a primary concern for many clients seeking skin care help from an esthetician. This severe skin problem can greatly affect a person's self-esteem. Acne, a skin disorder of the sebaceous glands, is characterized by comedones and blemishes and is a hereditary trait. It is usually triggered by hormonal changes. It begins to flare up when a person reaches puberty, but adult acne is becoming more prevalent.

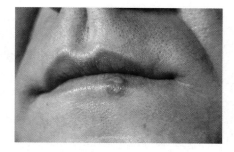

Figure 10–26 Herpes.

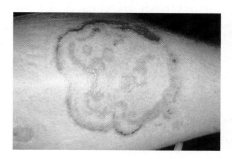

Figure 10–27 Tinea corporis (ringworm).

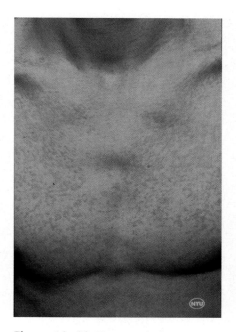

Figure 10–28 Tinea versicolor.

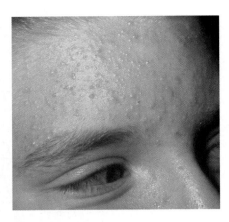

Figure 10–29 Acne.

Acne ranges from mild breakouts to disfiguring cysts and scarring (Figure 10–29). Acne can be controlled with proper medications, but medications have side effects and treatment may sometimes be a lifelong battle. Estheticians have a great opportunity to help people with less severe acne and make a difference in their lives. Acne can be a challenge to work with, but seeing visible improvement in a client's skin is very rewarding. Acne treatments and extractions are covered in Chapter 14, "Facials."

Causes of Acne

Causes of acne include the following:

- genetics/heredity
- clogged pores
- bacteria
- triggers including hormones, stress, cosmetics and skin care products, and foods

Genetics and Clogged Pores

Clogged pores are caused by a number of factors, including retention hyperkeratosis and sebaceous filaments.

Retention hyperkeratosis (ree-TEN-shun hy-pur-kair-uh-TOH-sis) is a hereditary factor in which dead skin cells do not shed from the follicles as they do on normal skin. Additionally, excessive sebum production can overtax the sebaceous follicles and cause further cell buildup. Sebum mixed with cells in the follicle become comedos—plugs in the follicles. Consequently, open and closed comedones are formed. While not inflamed, these comedones are the beginning of acne problems if they are not treated with proper skin care to alleviate the impaction. Another reason pores get clogged is that the opening, or *ostium* (AHS-tee-um), of the follicle may be too small to let impactions out.

There are two types of follicles or pores in the skin. One is a follicle, and the other is a sudoriferous pore. The pilosebaceous duct (py-loh-see-BAY-shus duct) is the term for the entire follicle that includes the hair, hair shaft (pilo), sebaceous gland, and the duct or canal to the surface. The hairless sebaceous follicle is the main type of follicle involved in acne (Figure 10–30).

Sebaceous filaments, similar to open comedones, are mainly solidified impactions of oil without the cell matter. These filaments also block the follicle and can cause an acne breakout. They are often found on the nose.

Bacteria

Bacteria in the follicles are *anaerobic*. This means they cannot live in the presence of oxygen. When follicles are blocked with sebum and dead skin buildup, oxygen cannot reach the bottom of the follicle. This results in *P. bacteria* (propionibacterium) proliferation. Sebum can irritate follicles and cause inflammation. As bacteria and inflammation grow, pressure is exerted on the follicle wall. If the wall ruptures, it becomes infected and debris spills out into the dermis. Redness and inflammation occur when a foreign object is detected in the skin, and white blood cells move in to fight the infection. Papules are red, inflamed lesions caused by this process.

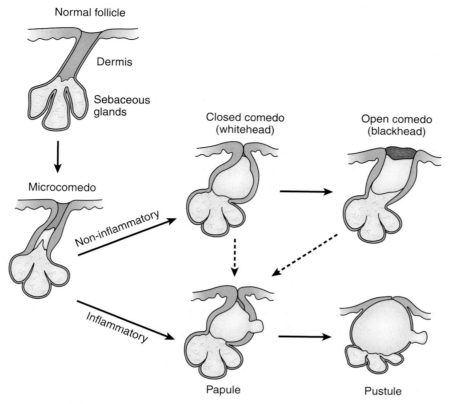

Figure 10–30 Acne and sebaceous follicles.

Papules may become more infected and pus develops, causing pustules that are filled with fluid from the dead white blood cells that fought the infection.

Cysts are nodules made up of deep pockets of infection. Skin forms hardened tissue around the infection to stop the spread of bacteria, which can lead to both depressed and raised scars from damage to the dermal tissue. Because it is in the dermis, this variety of acne—called *cystic acne*—can be treated only by a physician.

Acne Triggers

Hormonal changes, stress, products, and certain foods may aggravate acne. Climate, sun, friction, and medications also trigger skin flare-ups.

Hormones

Male hormones, known as *androgens* (AN-droh-jins), stimulate sebaceous glands. High levels of the male hormone testosterone (tes-TOSS-tur-own) cause an increase in oil production. These hormones increase during puberty, when teen acne is first evident. In females, acne is not as severe because there is less testosterone production. Adult acne is more common in females. Adrenal glands responding to stress also produce extra hormones. Hormonal fluctuations from birth control pills, premenstrual changes, pregnancy and menopause can all lead to acne inflammations in women. Hormonal acne is often seen on the chin. In the first trimester of pregnancy, women have more testosterone, making breakouts common. Changes are noticeable as the pregnancy progresses. Hormones also change with the seasons, and skin is also affected by the climate in other ways. Hormonal problems are becoming more evident in the effects they have on the skin.

Stress

Stress causes hormonal fluctuations and increased sebum production. The adrenal gland responds to stress and secretes adrenalin, which helps us cope with stressful events. The male hormone androgen is also produced by the adrenal gland and stimulates the sebaceous gland. Unfortunately, when we have a big event and want to look our best, blemishes may appear because of the increased stress level and sebum production.

Cosmetics and Products

Certain ingredients in products can aggravate acne. Fatty ingredients such as waxes and oils can clog pores or irritate follicles. These **comedogenic** ingredients can cause cells to build up. *Acnegenic* products also cause inflammation. Products rich in emollients and occlusive products are too heavy for problem skin types. Moisturizers and sunscreens should be oil-in-water (O/W) emulsions, not water-in-oil (W/O) emulsions. Many makeup products are comedogenic, especially foundations and powders that are made with solids and fatty ingredients. Other products for hair and skin can also trigger or irritate acne.

Foods

Foods blamed for triggering acne may not affect it directly, although our eating habits do affect our bodies' functions. Excessive iodides in salt, MSG, kelp, cheese, processed and packaged foods (especially fast foods), and minerals obtained from an ocean source found in vitamins can all irritate acne. The excess iodides are excreted through pores and irritate them. Eating fresh vegetables and fruits and increasing water intake seems to help those with acne experience fewer breakouts.

Many different opinions exist about whether our diet affects acne. Additional research may be needed. When researching topics, keep an open mind and determine the reliability of the source providing the information.

Other Irritations

Pressure or friction from rubbing or touching the face, phone use, or wearing hats can contribute to *acne mechanica* breakouts. Dirty pillows or makeup brushes can also transfer bacteria to the face. Keeping hands and items that touch the face clean can help reduce breakouts.

Prolonged pressure or heat will likely cause skin problems. Swelling from sweating or a moist, humid climate will close off pores rather than open them.

Various drugs such as steroids, birth control pills and patches, and marijuana will also affect the body and are known to irritate skin.

Grades of Acne

Acne is broken down into four grades (Table 10–2). The number of lesions, comedones, papules, pustules, or cysts present determines the severity of the acne.

Table 10–2

GRADES OF ACNE	
Grade I	Minor breakouts, mostly open comedones, some closed comedones, and a few papules (Figure 10–31).
Grade II	Many closed comedones, more open comedones, and occasional papules and pustules (Figure 10–32).
Grade III	Red and inflamed, many comedones, papules and pustules (Figure 10–33).
Grade IV	Cystic acne. Cysts with comedones, papules, pustules, and inflammation are present (Figure 10–34). Scar formation from tissue damage is common.

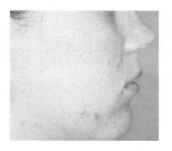

Figure 10–31 Grade I acne.

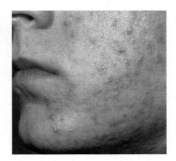

Figure 10–32 Grade II acne is characterized by many closed comedones and is difficult to treat.

Treating Acne

There are many ways to help clients control acne. Good skin care treatments and proper nutrition will help with skin problems. Estheticians can educate clients in caring for their skin and what causes acne flare-ups. Physicians may prescribe medications to treat Grade III and IV acne (Table 10–3).

Table 10–3

COMMON MEDICATIONS USED IN THE TREATMENT OF ACNE		
DRUG	**ACTIONS**	**SIDE EFFECTS**
Tretinoin (Retin-A®)	A topical vitamin A acid. A strong peeling agent that is drying and also flushes follicles.	Very drying, causes redness and irritation; photosensitivity.
Clindamycin	Topical antibiotic. Kills bacteria.	Very drying.
Adapalene (Differin®)	A topical peeling agent similar to retinoic acid. May be less irritating than tretinoin.	Drying, redness, and irritation; photosensitivity.
Tazarotene (Tazorac®)	Another retinoid, a topical peeling agent that may be less irritating than tretinoin.	Drying, redness, and irritation; photosensitivity.
Azelaic acid (Azelex®)	A topical acidic agent that flushes follicles.	Drying, redness, and irritation; photosensitivity.
Accutane	An oral medication similar to retinoic acid; used for severe acne.	Severe dryness, birth defects, other health problems; possible depression.

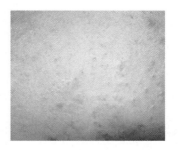

Figure 10–33 Grade III acne.

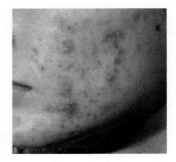

Figure 10–34 Grade IV acne.

REVIEW QUESTIONS

1. Name the nine primary lesions.

2. What is a comedone?

3. Name five secondary lesions.

4. Name six sebaceous gland disorders.

5. List six inflammations of the skin.

6. Define *rosacea*.

7. List three types of hyperpigmentation.

8. What is a hypertrophy?

9. Discuss the differences between the three types of skin cancer.

10. What system can be used to identify skin cancers?

11. Name four types of contagious diseases.

12. What are the causes of acne?

13. What may trigger an acne flare-up?

14. Describe the four grades of acne.

15. What contagious diseases contraindicate working on a client?

CHAPTER GLOSSARY

acne: a chronic inflammatory skin disorder of the sebaceous glands that is characterized by comedones and blemishes; also known as *acne simplex* or *acne vulgaris*.

acne excoriee: a disorder where clients purposely scrape off acne lesions, causing scarring and discoloration.

actinic keratoses: pink or flesh-colored precancerous lesions that feel sharp or rough, usually as the result of sun damage.

albinism: the absence of melanin pigment in the body, including skin, hair, and eyes; the technical term for albinism is *congenital leukoderma*.

anhidrosis: a deficiency in perspiration, often a result of a fever or skin disease, that requires medical treatment.

asteatosis: dry, scaly skin from sebum deficiency, which can be due to aging, body disorders, alkalies of harsh soaps, or cold exposure.

atopic dermatitis: dermatitis is genetically related to overreactive immune systems and is prevalent in people with nasal allergies and asthma.

bacterial conjunctivitis: pinkeye; very contagious.

basal cell carcinoma: the most common and the least severe type of skin cancer, which often appears as light, pearly nodules.

bromhidrosis: foul-smelling perspiration, usually in the armpits or on the feet.

bulla (plural: bullae): a large blister containing watery fluid; similar to a vesicle, but larger.

carbuncle: a large circumscribed inflammation of the subcutaneous tissue caused by staphylococci; similar to a furuncle (boil) but larger.

chloasma: increased pigmentation; liver spots.

comedogenic: a tendency to clog follicles and cause a buildup of dead skin cells, resulting in comedones.

comedone: an open comedo or blackhead; a mass of hardened sebum and skin cells in a hair follicle. When the follicle is filled with an excess of oil, a blackhead forms. It is dark because it is exposed to oxygen and oxidizes. Closed comedones do not have a follicular opening and are called *milia* or *whiteheads*.

contact dermatitis: an inflammatory skin condition caused by contact with a substance or chemical. Occupational disorders from ingredients in cosmetics and chemical solutions can cause contact dermatitis, or *dermatitis venenata*.

crust: dead cells form over a wound or blemish while it is healing, resulting in an accumulation of sebum and pus, sometimes mixed with epidermal material. An example is the scab on a sore.

cyst: a closed, abnormally developed sac containing fluid, infection, or other matter above or below the skin.

dermatitis: any inflammatory condition of the skin. Various forms of lesions, such as eczema, vesicles, or papules.

dermatologist: physician who treats skin disorders and diseases.

dermatology: branch of science that studies and treats the skin and its disorders.

eczema: an inflammatory, painful itching disease of the skin, acute or chronic in nature, with dry or moist lesions. This condition should be referred to a physician. Seborrheic dermatitis, mainly affecting oily areas, is a common form of eczema.

edema: swelling caused by a response to injury or infection.

erythema: redness caused by inflammation; a red lesion is erythemic.

excoriation: a skin sore or abrasion produced by scratching or scraping.

fissure: a crack in the skin that penetrates the dermis. Chapped lips or hands are fissures.

folliculitis: inflammation of the hair follicles.

furuncle: a subcutaneous abscess filled with pus; also called *boils,* furuncles are caused by bacteria in the glands or hair follicles.

herpes simplex virus 1: this strain of the herpes virus causes fever blisters or cold sores; it is a recurring, contagious viral infection consisting of a vesicle or group of vesicles on a red, swollen base. The blisters usually appear on the lips or nostrils.

herpes simplex virus 2: this strain of the herpes virus infects the genitals.

herpes zoster: shingles, a painful skin condition from the chickenpox virus; characterized by groups of blisters that form a rash.

hyperhidrosis: excessive perspiration caused by heat or body weakness. Medical treatment is required.

hyperkeratosis: a thickening of the skin caused by a mass of keratinized cells (keratinocytes).

hyperpigmentation: overproduction of pigment.

hypertrophy: an abnormal growth; many are benign, or harmless.

hypopigmentation: lack of pigment.

impetigo: a contagious bacterial infection often occurring in children; characterized by clusters of small blisters.

keloid: a thick scar resulting from excessive growth of fibrous tissue (collagen).

keratinocytes: cells composed of keratin.

keratoma: an acquired, thickened patch of epidermis. A callus caused by pressure or friction is a keratoma.

keratoses: abnormally thick buildups of cells.

keratosis pilaris: redness and bumpiness in the cheeks or upper arms; caused by blocked follicles.

lentigo/lentigenes: freckles; small yellow-brown colored spots. Lentigenes that result from sunlight exposure are actinic, or solar, lentigenes. Patches are referred to as *large macules.*

lesions: structural changes in tissues caused by damage or injury.

leukoderma: light, abnormal patches caused by a burn or

CHAPTER GLOSSARY

congenital disease that destroys the pigment-producing cells. Vitiligo and albinism are leukodermas.

macule: a flat spot or discoloration on the skin, such as a freckle. Macules are neither raised nor sunken.

malignant melanoma: the most serious form of skin cancer. Black or dark patches on the skin are usually uneven in texture, jagged, or raised.

melasma: term for hyperpigmentation; pregnancy mask is often called melasma. This condition is triggered by hormonal changes and may fade with time.

milia: also called whiteheads, milia are whitish, pearl-like masses of sebum and dead cells under the skin. Milia are more common in dry skin types and may form after skin trauma, such as a laser resurfacing.

miliaria rubra: prickly heat; acute inflammatory disorder of the sweat glands resulting in the eruption of red vesicles and burning, itching skin from excessive heat exposure.

mole: a brownish spot ranging in color from tan to bluish black. Some are flat, resembling freckles; others are raised and darker.

nevus: a birthmark or mole; malformation of the skin due to abnormal pigmentation or dilated capillaries.

nodules: also referred to as tumors, but these are smaller bumps caused by conditions such as scar tissue, fatty deposits, or infections.

papule: a pimple; small elevation on the skin that contains no fluid but may develop pus.

perioral dermatitis: an acne-like condition around the mouth. These are mainly small clusters of papules that could be caused by toothpaste or products used on the face.

primary lesions: primary lesions are characterized by flat, non-palpable changes in skin color such as macules or patches, or an elevation formed by fluid in a cavity, such as vesicles, bullae, or pustules.

pruitis: the medical term for itching.

pseudofolliculitis: often referred to as "razor bumps"; resembles folliculitis without the pus.

psoriasis: a skin disease characterized by red patches covered with white-silver scales. It is caused by an overproliferation of skin cells that replicate too fast. Immune dysfunction could be the cause. Psoriasis is usually found in patches on the scalp, elbows, knees, chest, and lower back.

pustule: an inflamed papule with a white or yellow center containing pus, a fluid consisting of white blood cells, bacteria, and other debris produced from an infection.

retention hyperkeratosis: hereditary factor in which dead skin cells do not shed from the follicles as they do on normal skin.

rosacea: inflammation of the skin; chronic congestion primarily on the cheeks and nose. Characterized by redness, dilation of blood vessels, and in severe cases, the formation of papules and pustules.

scale: flaky skin cells; any thin plate of epidermal flakes, dry or oily. An example is abnormal or excessive dandruff.

scar: light-colored, slightly raised mark on the skin formed after an injury or lesion of the skin has healed up. The tissue hardens to heal the injury. Elevated scars are hypertrophic; a keloid is a hypertrophic (abnormal) scar.

sebaceous filaments: similar to open comedones, these are mainly solidified impactions of oil without the cell matter.

sebaceous hyperplasia: benign lesions frequently seen in oilier areas of the face. An overgrowth of the sebaceous gland, they appear similar to open comedones; often doughnut-shaped, with sebaceous material in the center.

seborrhea: severe oiliness of the skin; an abnormal secretion from the sebaceous glands.

seborrheic dermatitis: a common form of eczema.

secondary lesions: skin damage, developed in the later stages of disease, that changes the structure of tissues or organs.

skin tag: small outgrowths or extensions of the skin that look like flaps. They are benign and are common under the arms or on the neck.

squamous cell carcinoma: more serious than basal cell carcinoma; characterized by scaly red papules or nodules.

stain: brown or wine-colored discoloration. Stains occur after certain diseases, or after moles, freckles, or liver spots disappear. A port wine stain is a birthmark, which is a vascular type of nevus.

steatoma: a sebaceous cyst or subcutaneous tumor filled with sebum; ranges in size from a pea to an orange. It usually appears on the scalp, neck, and back; also called a *wen*.

tan: an increase in pigmentation due to the melanin production that results from exposure to UV rays. Melanin is designed to help protect the skin from the sun's UV rays.

telangiectasia: describes capillaries that have been damaged and are now larger, or distended blood vessels. Commonly called *couperose skin*.

tinea: a fungal infection.

tinea corporis: a contagious infection that forms a ringed, red pattern with elevated edges. Also called *ringworm*.

tinea versicolor: yeast infection that inhibits melanin production.

tubercle: an abnormal rounded, solid lump; larger than a papule.

tumor: a large nodule; an abnormal cell mass resulting from excessive cell multiplication and varying in size, shape, and color.

ulcer: an open lesion on the skin or mucous membrane of the body, accompanied by pus and loss of skin depth. A deep erosion; a depression in the skin, normally due to infection or cancer.

urticaria: hives.

vasodilation: vascular dilation of blood vessels.

verruca: a wart; hypertrophy of the papillae and epidermis caused by a virus. It is infectious and contagious.

vesicles: a small blister or sac containing clear fluid. Poison ivy and poison oak produce vesicles.

vitiligo: white spots or areas on the skin from lack of pigment cells; sunlight makes it worse.

wheal: an itchy, swollen lesion caused by a blow, insect bite, skin allergy reaction, or stings. Hives and mosquito bites are wheals. Hives (urticaria) can be caused by exposure to allergens used in products.

CHAPTER **11**

SKIN ANALYSIS

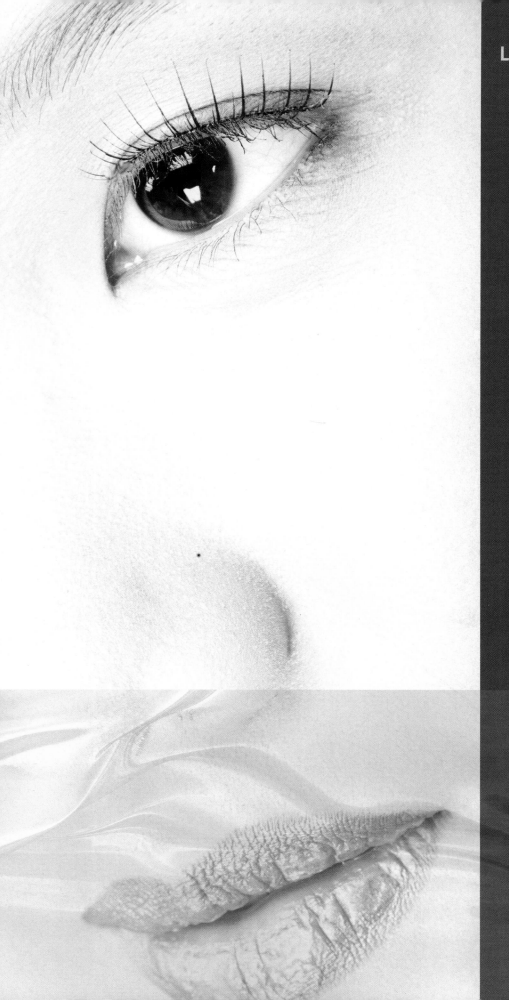

After completing this chapter, you will be able to:

- Identify skin types.

- Identify skin conditions.

- Be familiar with the causes of skin conditions.

- Explain the causes of skin conditions.

- Understand UV rays and how rays interact with skin.

- Explain healthy habits for the skin.

- Be aware of treatment contraindications.

- Perform a skin analysis.

- Conduct client consultations.

- Fill out skin analysis charts.

KEY TERMS

L earning about individual skin types and conditions is one of the most interesting aspects of skin care. It is never boring because every face is unique. Client skin analysis is an important part of an esthetician's skills, since recommending the appropriate skin care products and regime must be individualized to suit each person. Before performing services or selecting products, an individual's skin type and conditions must be analyzed correctly.

People want to know what their skin conditions are and what they can do to improve their skin's appearance. They rely on estheticians for information and education. Clients need to be educated about the benefits of professional skin care treatments. Skin analysis and consultations are also good marketing tools to introduce services and products to prospective clients. The first-time client may have specific skin concerns, or may want to experience a relaxing spa service. Be sure to let the client know what services are offered. This is an opportunity to promote all services in the spa.

The consultation and skin analysis will help determine which products to use and recommend. It is also a guide to determine the type of service to perform (Figure 11–1). A client chart is used to record the analysis and consultation notes, an important part of record keeping. Additionally, estheticians need to know which services and products are contraindicated. These **contraindications** are factors that prohibit a treatment due to a condition. Treatments could cause harmful or negative side effects to those who have specific medical or skin conditions.

Skin conditions may be caused by both internal and external factors and are unique to each individual. Ethnic skin also has unique conditions and challenges. Products are formulated for different **skin types** and conditions, and the number of new product lines grow annually. Skin care products and treatments are discussed in the following chapters. The consultation, health screening questions, and client chart are all used as part of an in-depth skin analysis.

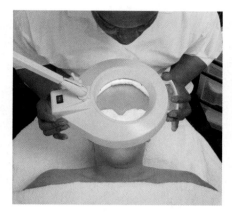

Figure 11–1 Conducting a skin analysis with a magnifying light.

SKIN TYPES ARE GENETICALLY DETERMINED

People are born with their skin type, which is determined by their genetics and ethnicity. Like everything else, skin can change over time. An individual's skin type is based primarily on how much oil is produced in the follicles from the sebaceous glands and on the amount of lipids found between the cells. The **T-zone** is the center area of the face, corresponding to the "T" shape formed by the forehead, nose, and chin (Figure 11–2). How large the pores are in the T-zone and throughout the face can usually determine the skin type. Generally, an individual's skin becomes drier over time. Our cellular metabolism and oil/lipid production slow down as we age.

Skin types include dry, normal, combination, oily, or sensitive. Sensitive skin is discussed more now as a skin type; but it can also be a condition, depending on the causes. Acne is considered a disorder, as explained in Chapter 10, "Disorders and Diseases." All skin types need proper cleansing, exfoliating, and hydrating. Finding the right care for each individual can be challenging, and this makes the esthetician's job even more interesting.

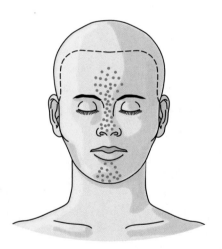

Figure 11–2 The T-zone area of the face.

FYI

Skin types are categorized as follows:

- dry
- normal
- combination
- oily
- sensitive (both a skin type and a condition)

Dry Skin

Dry skin does not produce enough oil. **Alipidic** (al-lah-PID-ik) skin lacks oil (lipids). The follicles are usually small and the sebum is minimal. If you can barely see the follicles or they are small, this indicates a dry skin type.

The natural oil secretions in our follicles help protect us from environmental damage and aging. Dry skin needs extra care because it lacks this normal protection.

Dry skin is more sensitive because the acid mantle and barrier function are not as healthy due to the lack of lipids. Skin texture can be slightly rough and feel tight. Stimulating oil production and protecting the surface is imperative to taking care of dry skin. **Occlusive** (uh-KLOO-sive) products can reduce transepidermal water loss (TEWL) to help hold in moisture and protect the skin's top barrier layer, which helps to combat dryness.

Dry Versus Dehydrated Skin

While common for someone with dry skin, **dehydration** is a condition that can be seen with all skin types. Dehydrated skin lacks water. This is different from dry skin that lacks oil. It is important to remember the difference, because even oily skin can be dehydrated and needs to be hydrated.

Dehydrated skin can look thin or flaky and can feel tight and dry. Skin that needs moisture tends to absorb products quickly. Dehydrated skin can be caused by internal and external factors such as medications and products. Drinking plenty of water and hydrating the skin with moisturizers and humectants can help minimize the negative effects of dryness and dehydration.

Normal Skin

Normal skin has a good oil–water balance. It can fluctuate and sometimes will be a little more dry or oily. The follicles are a normal size, and the skin is usually free of blemishes. If you can see the follicle size change from smaller to medium just on the edge of the T-zone by the nose, measuring outward from the center of the face, this is a normal skin type. Maintenance and preventative care are the goals for this type of skin.

Combination Skin

Combination skin can be both oily and dry, or both oily and normal, at the same time. The T-zone through the middle of the face on the forehead, nose, and chin is oilier. This area has more sebaceous glands and larger pores. The outer areas of the face can be either normal or dry and can even appear flaky from either dehydration or buildup of dead skin cells. At the center of the face, if you can see the pore size change from medium to larger just outside the T-zone on the cheeks next to the nose, this is a combination skin type.

Combination skin needs to be balanced and requires more care than normal skin does. To care for combination skin, the oil–water balance can be achieved by treating both the oily and dryer areas of the face. Deep cleansing and regular exfoliation help to keep skin clear and blemishes minimal. Water-based products for combination skin work best.

Oily Skin

Oily skin is characterized by excess sebum (oil) production. The follicle (pore) size is larger and contains more oil. If the pore size is visible or larger over most of the face, this indicates an oily skin type. Oily skin requires more cleansing and exfoliating than other skin types do. It is prone to blemishes because the pores get clogged with oil and buildup of dead skin cells. This excess oil and buildup on the surface can make the skin appear thicker and sallow. Blemishes and comedones are common.

Balancing the oil production through treatments and products is important. Over-cleansing can make matters worse by stripping the skin's acid mantle and irritating it. If skin is stripped of oil, it is unbalanced. This causes the body's protection mechanism to produce additional oil to compensate for the dryness on the surface. Remember: no matter what the skin type, the goal is to balance the barrier function.

Educating clients (especially teenagers with hormonal flare-ups) on how to care for their skin will help them tremendously. Proper exfoliation and a water-based hydrator will help keep oily skin clean and balanced. The positive side to having oily skin is that it ages more slowly because of the protection provided by oil secretions. However, oily skin is more prone to acne, so people with this skin type may need professional treatments more often than those with normal skin. After a deep-cleansing facial and good home care, visible improvements are noticeable (Figure 11–3).

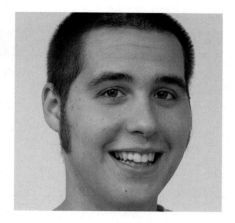

Figure 11–3 Taking care of oily skin brings visible improvements.

Sensitive Skin

Sensitive skin is increasingly common. We are constantly bombarded by environmental stimuli, stress, sun exposure, and other unhealthy elements. Sensitive skin is a condition, but it is also genetically predisposed. This skin type or condition is characterized by fragile, thin skin and redness. It is easily irritated by products and by exposure to heat or sun (Figure 11–4). Telangiectasia, or couperose conditions, are noticeable.

Sensitive skin needs to be treated very gently with nonirritating, calming products. Many companies now have product lines designed specifically for sensitive skin. Fragile or thin skin can also be the result of age or medications. Sensitive skin can be difficult to treat because of its low tolerance to products and stimulation. Avoid irritating products and procedures. For example, excessive rubbing, heat, and strong exfoliation or extractions can cause damage and increase redness. Soothing and calming the skin are usually the primary treatment goals.

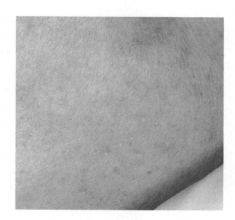

Figure 11–4 Sensitive skin is characterized by redness and is easily irritated.

THE FITZPATRICK SCALE

Developed by Dr. Thomas Fitzpatrick, the **Fitzpatrick Scale** is used to measure the skin type's ability to tolerate sun exposure (Table 11–1). It is important to be familiar with this method when determining treatments and products for your clients. Everyone's tolerance level is different for peels and treatments. Lighter skin types are generally more sensitive and reactive. Individuals with darker skin types have more melanin, which gives more protection from the sun, but they have other sensitivities and concerns.

Table 11–1

THE FITZPATRICK SCALE		
SKIN TYPE	**APPEARANCE**	**REACTION TO SUN EXPOSURE**
Type I	Very fair; blond or red hair; light-colored eyes; freckles common	Always burns, never tans
Type II	Fair skinned; light eyes; light hair	Burns easily
Type III	Very common skin type; fair; eye and hair color vary	Sometimes burns, gradually tans
Type IV	Mediterranean Caucasian skin; medium to heavy pigmentation	Rarely burns, always tans
Type V	Mideastern skin; rarely sun sensitive	Tans
Type VI	Black skin, rarely sun sensitive	Tans easily

ETHNIC SKIN

Ethnic skin types contain more melanin than Caucasian skin types do. Black, Hispanic, Asian, and Native American skin types all have different amounts of melanin. The number of melanocytes is the same, but the melanin transferred to keratinocytes by the **melanosome** (MEL-uh-noh-sohm), is greater in dark skin. Melanosomes are pigment granules of melanocyte cells that produce melanin in the basal layer. While ethnic skin types are considered oilier and thicker, they can also be fragile. Reactions are hard to see on darker skin, but they may be just as intense as those on lighter skin (Figure 11–5).

Black skin is prone to hyperkeratosis—excessive cell turnover and dead skin cell buildup—so it needs more exfoliation and deep pore cleansing. Abnormal hypertrophic scarring (keloids) is also problematic for black skin.

Black skin does not age as quickly, because it is thicker and has more melanin for additional sun protection. However, dark skin still needs protection from sun damage.

Hyperpigmentation is a greater problem for darker skin types. Pigmentation disorders also include hypopigmentation such as vitiligo. Post-inflammatory hyperpigmentation can result from hormones, trauma, extractions, sun damage, or exfoliation. Hyperpigmentation can be caused by peels and lightening agents, so use caution when applying these products and treatments.

Asian skin is considered to be one of the most sensitive skin types. It has great elasticity and firmness, and it does not show signs of aging as quickly as Caucasian skin does. However, Asian skins can become hyperpigmented from exfoliating agents such as alpha hydroxy acids (AHAs). Gentler exfoliating products such as enzymes are recommended. Sunscreens are also necessary to slow down hyperpigmentation.

Caution clients that receiving lightening treatments for their age spots (dark areas) can actually make things worse; if their exfoliated areas produce melanin in an uneven pattern, lightening treatments can lead to splotchiness. Avoiding sun exposure and wearing sunscreen daily is a must for anyone prone to hyperpigmentation. A good skin care routine will keep your client's skin looking beautiful for years to come.

Care and precautions for other ethnic skin types including Native American, Indian, and Hispanic skin are the same as for other ethnic skin types. Thicker skin is usually characterized by more oil production and needs more deep-cleansing treatments. Additionally, individuals with thicker hair and roots in the follicle can make waxing more difficult. If you want to specialize in ethnic skin care, investigate the educational resources and advanced classes addressing this area of study. No matter what the skin type or ethnic background, everyone needs an individualized skin care consultation and program to maintain healthy skin.

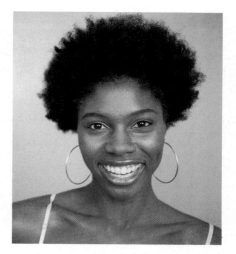

Figure 11–5 Ethnic skin is more fragile than it looks.

SKIN TYPES VERSUS SKIN CONDITIONS

Many internal and external factors affect the condition of a person's skin. Skin conditions are not just a result of our genetic makeup. These conditions are what the esthetician is most concerned about, and they are the focus of skin treatments. The most common skin conditions estheticians see today are adult acne, **actinic** (ak-TIN-ik) aging from sun damage, and problems from hormonal fluctuations.

Dehydration, pigmentation disorders, and rosacea are also significant concerns to clients. Other skin conditions include comedones, hyperkeratinization, redness, sensitivities, and of course aging. We can improve some of these conditions through routine facials, by using specialized products, and by avoiding the factors that affect the conditions. On the client's chart, you will want to note other skin abnormalities that you learn about here and in Chapter 10 ("Disorders and Diseases of the Skin") that may not be listed as a condition in Table 11–2.

ACTIVITY

What do you think your skin type is? What skin conditions do you have? After doing your skin analysis in class, see how closely the analysis matches your answers to these questions.

Table 11–2

A TABLE OF SKIN CONDITIONS AND DESCRIPTIONS	
SKIN CONDITIONS	**DESCRIPTION**
Actinic keratosis	A rough area resulting from sun exposure, sometimes with a layered scale or scab that sometimes falls off. Can be precancerous.
Adult acne	Acne breakouts from hormonal changes or other factors.
Asphyxiated	Smokers have asphyxiated skin from lack of oxygen. Characterized by clogged pores and wrinkles; dull and lifeless-looking. Can be yellowish or gray in color.
Comedones	Open comedones are blackheads and clogged pores caused by a buildup of debris, oil, and dead skin cells stuck in the pores. Closed comedones are not open to the air or oxygen. They are trapped by dead skin cells and need to be exfoliated and extracted. Also called whiteheads if hardened.
Couperose skin; Telangiectasia	Redness; distended capillaries from weakening of the capillary walls; internal or external causes.
Cysts	Fluid, infection, or other matter under the skin.
Dehydration	Lack of water (also caused by the environment, medications, topical agents, aging, or dehydrating drinks such as caffeine and alcohol).
Enlarged pores	Larger pores due to excess oil and debris trapped in the follicles or expansion due to elasticity loss or trauma.
Erythema	Redness caused by inflammation.
Hyperkeratinization	An excessive buildup of dead skin cells/keratinized cells.
Hyperpigmentation	Brown or dark pigmentation; discoloration from melanin production due to sun, other factors, or irritation.
Hypopigmentation	White, colorless areas from lack of melanin production.
Irritation	Usually redness or inflammation; from a variety of causes.
Keratosis/**Keratoses**	A buildup of cells; a rough texture.
Milia	Hardened whiteheads. Oil and dead skin cells trapped beneath the surface of the skin. These are not exposed to oxygen and have to be lanced to open and remove them.
Papules	Raised lesions; also called *blemishes*.
Poor elasticity	Sagging. Loose skin from damage, the sun, and aging.
Pustules	An infected papule with fluid inside.
Rosacea	A vascular disorder. Chronic redness. Papules and pustules may be present.
Sebaceous hyperplasia	Benign lesions seen in oilier areas of the face. Described as looking like doughnut holes. Cannot be extracted.
Seborrhea	Oiliness of the skin.
Sensitivities	Reactions from internal or external causes.
Solar comedones	Large blackheads, usually around the eyes, due to sun exposure.
Sun damage	UV damage to the epidermis and dermis; primary effects are wrinkles, collagen, and elastin breakdown, pigmentation, and cancer.
Wrinkles/Aging	Lines and damage from internal or external causes.

FACTORS THAT AFFECT THE SKIN

Habits, diet, and stress all play a part in our health, which in turn is reflected in our skin's appearance. Skin conditions can be caused by allergies/reactions, genetics/ethnicity, medications, medical conditions, and many other internal or external factors. Being aware of what can affect the skin will help the esthitician determine why the client may be experiencing problems. Knowledge of healthy habits and "enemies" of the skin will give you a better understanding of how to help the client with his or her concerns.

Internal Factors

Our body's health affects how we feel as well as how our body and skin looks. Stress, our lifestyle, even our attitude can contribute to our skin's health. Free radicals in the body, dehydration (lack of water), vitamin deficiency, improper nutrition, alcohol, caffeine, hormones, and menopause all affect our skin's well-being. Unfortunately, sun damage shows up at the same time as menopause—a double attack on a woman's outermost layer. Hormonal imbalances can lead to sensitivity, dehydration, hyperpigmentation, and microcirculation problems that affect our capillaries. Additionally, lack of exercise, lack of sleep, smoking, medications, and drugs will have negative effects both inside and out (Table 11–3).

External Factors

Sun damage is the main external cause of aging (Figure 11–6). Environmental exposure, pollutants, air quality, and humidity also affect the skin's health (Table 11–4). Poor maintenance and home care can also contribute to skin problems. Misuse of products or poor facial treatments can be detrimental to maintaining a healthy and attractive complexion. This is another reason why correct skin analysis and product recommendations are important.

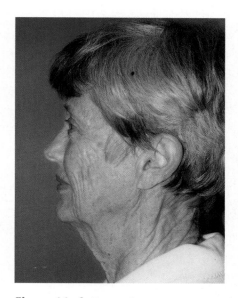

Figure 11–6 Photoaging.

ACTIVITY

What are some examples of contraindications you may see as a skin care specialist? Write down any medications, contagious diseases, skin disorders, medical conditions, and skin irritations you can think of that would contraindicate a service.

Table 11–3

INTERNAL EFFECTS ON THE SKIN
• Genetics and ethnicity-influenced conditions
• Stress, lifestyle, negative attitude
• Free radicals
• Dehydration
• Vitamin deficiency
• Improper nutrition, alcohol, caffeine
• Hormones and menopause
• Lack of exercise
• Lack of sleep
• Smoking
• Medications, drugs
• Medical conditions

Table 11–4

EXTERNAL EFFECTS ON THE SKIN
• Sun damage
• Environmental exposure, pollutants, and air quality
• Environment and humidity
• Poor maintenance and care
• Misuse of products or treatments
• Allergies and reactions to environmental factors or products

Sunlight and Interaction with the Skin—UV Rays

Sunlight is energy. Both UVA and UVB rays are absorbed, scattered, and reflected by the skin. See Table 11–5 for a comparison on UVA and UVB rays. UVC rays are even shorter and more energetic but are mainly absorbed by the ozone layer. The amount of energy organisms get from sunlight depends on how much exposure and how strong or intense the exposure is. This is referred to as the dosage. *Minimal erythemal dose* (MED) is the term used to describe how long it takes to become red (erythema) from sun exposure. The dosage is the intensity of the sun multiplied by the time exposed: Dosage = Intensity × Time. Erythema is the result of cell damage and blood vessel dilation in the dermis. It can appear hours after exposure and last for several days.

Table 11–5

ULTRAVIOLET LIGHT COMPARISONS	
UVA RAYS (320–380 NM)	**UVB RAYS (280–320 NM)**
UVA rays have longer wavelengths that penetrate deeper into the dermis than UVB rays.	UVB rays have shorter wavelengths and are stronger than UVA rays because they deliver more energy.
UVA rays are less energetic because of the lower frequency.	UVB have more energy because the wavelengths have a higher frequency.
UVA rays are absorbed by the epidermis and dermis. Rays above 320 nm penetrate more readily into the dermis.	UVB penetrate less because the shorter wavelengths are scattered or reflected more by the epidermis.
Long wavelengths have low energy, or frequency, so the cell damage is not as severe.	Short wavelengths have higher energy. The higher energy from UVB rays causes more interaction and has a greater effect on DNA, molecules, and cells.
UVA rays affect the dermis, collagen, and elastin. They can also cause DNA damage, leading to skin cancer.	UVB are the main cause of sunburns and skin cancers.
UVA rays cause tanning, wrinkling, and premature aging.	
Tanning beds use UVA light.	

HEALTHY HABITS FOR THE SKIN

Preventative measures for skin care include avoiding the sun and wearing sunscreen, which is the best protection for our skin. Proper home care, skin treatments, and ingredients such as **antioxidants, peptides,** lipids, and **AHAs (alpha hydroxy acids)** are all beneficial (see Chapter 12 for a discussion of product selection and ingredients). A good diet, vitamins, water intake, exercise, and other healthy practices all have a positive effect on our health and our complexion. Some authorities even believe positive thinking can decrease premature aging.

CONTRAINDICATIONS

Contagious diseases, skin disorders, medical conditions, medications, and skin irritation can all *contraindicate* a service (Table 11–6). Legally, you may not ask clients about contagious diseases, but they may list them on the client questionnaire. Recognizing diseases is vital to avoid causing harm to clients or to yourself. Medications such as Accutane® or topical peeling agents can make the skin too sensitive for facials or waxing.

FOCUS ON . . .

HEALTHY FOOD

Examples of foods with antioxidants include berries and citrus fruits. Polyphenols are plant chemicals; a family of polyphenol antioxidants includes foods such as green tea, red grapes, strawberries, and pomegranates.

Table 11–6

CONTRAINDICATIONS FOR SKIN TREATMENTS

- Use of Accutane® or any skin-thinning or exfoliating drug, including Retin-A®, Renova™, Tazorac®, Differin®, and so on. Avoid waxing, any exfoliation or peeling treatment, or stimulating treatments.
- Pregnancy—The client should not have any electrical treatments, or any questionable treatment, without her physician's written permission. Some pregnant clients also experience sensitivities from waxing.
- Metal bone pins or plates in the body—Avoid all electrical treatment.
- Pacemakers or heart irregularities—Avoid all electrical treatment.
- Allergies—Any allergic substances listed should be strictly avoided. Clients with multiple allergies should use fragrance-free products designed for sensitive skin.
- Seizures or epilepsy—Avoid all electrical and light treatments.
- Use of oral steroids like prednisone—Avoid any stimulating or exfoliating treatment, or waxing.
- Autoimmune diseases such as lupus—Avoid any harsh or stimulating treatments.
- Diabetes—Be aware that due to their poor blood circulation, many diabetics heal very slowly and may not readily feel pain, especially in the feet. If you are in doubt, get approval from the client's physician before treatment.
- Blood thinners—No extraction or waxing.

Medical conditions and illnesses may contraindicate any stimulation to the face or body. Additionally, allergies to products and ingredients are common. Electrical contraindications are listed in Chapter 16, Facial Machines. Clients who have obvious skin abnormalities such as open sores, fever blisters (herpes simplex), or other abnormal-looking conditions should be referred to a physician for treatment.

CONSULTATIONS, CLIENT CHARTS, AND HEALTH SCREENING

A thorough consultation is important for many reasons. The most important is to know about any contraindications that the client may have. Contraindications include any disorder, medical condition, medication, allergy, or sensitivity to products. A consultation will help you to determine why a client may be experiencing skin problems. Their health, lifestyle, occupation, and product use will all affect their skin. Sometimes estheticians are like detectives, trying to determine why the client is having a certain skin problem. The more you know about your client, the more you discover what they need.

Ask questions relating to skin conditions and the client's personal health. You may have three forms for a client: a questionnaire, a release form, and a client chart that includes their skin analysis. Have clients fill out a confidential questionnaire. See form in Chapter 3, Figure 3–5. A *client release form* is also highly recommended. A client release form is a document that a client reads and signs, releasing you from liability before you perform services. A *client chart* is a record all of your notes from the skin analysis, what you used in the treatment, and your home care recommendations (Figure 11–7).

Questions to ask during the consultation include the following:
- Do you have allergies to products or scents?
- Why are you here? (What brought the client in? Is it for deep cleansing or just relaxation?)
- What are your skin concerns? (What does he or she care about?)
- What products do you use? (What is the client's home care routine? What are the ingredients, and how often are they used?)
- Have you had treatments before? (Is this the client's first facial?)
- Is this a normal state for your skin? (Is it normally more clear? Is it usually less irritated?)
- How does your skin feel during different times of the day? (What is degree of oiliness or dryness?)

Think about how you can help the client through treatments, home care suggestions, and preventative measures. Conduct the consultation, discuss what you see with the client, and give advice during the analysis or after the treatment. Use a client chart to record the analysis, the type of treatment performed, and the consultation notes.

ACTIVITY

Analyze the faces of your friends and family to determine their skin type. Ask questions and fill out the client charts. Consult with them about taking care of their skin. They might be your best clients!

CAUTION!

Contraindications such as medications, contagious diseases, skin disorders, medical conditions, and skin irritation can all make a service inadvisable.

CONSULTATION CARD

Name	Date of Consultation
Address	Age ___ Sex ___
City ___ State ___ Zip ___	Known allergies
Tel. (Home) ___ (Business) ___	
Ref. by	Medication
(Person, advertising, etc.)	

SKIN CLASSIFICATION

Facial Area	Facial Area
Normal	Acne ___ How many years
Dry	Vulgaris ___ Chronic
Dehydrated	Cystic ___ Rosacea
Aging	Scars (acne, etc.)
Thin, sensitive skin	Wrinkles
Oily	Superficial lines
Open pores	Deep lines
Comedones (blackheads)	Relaxed elasticity
Milia (whiteheads)	Good elasticity
Asphyxiated	Couperose (capillaries)
	Discolorations

Remarks

Rec. Treatment

FACIAL RECORD

Date	Type of treatment	By	Products purchased
2/14	Cleansing, Peel - Relaxing Massage	Mary	Moisturizer with sunscreen
3/16	Cleansing, Peel - Modelage Mask	Mary	Cleanser, Toner
4/5	Cleansing, Peel - High Frequency indirect	Mary	Moisturizer, Foundation # 1
4/26	Cleansing, Peel - Massage - Alginate Mask	John	
5/13	Cleansing, Peel - Iontophoresis - Paraffin Mask Skin is showing marked improvement.	Mary	Night cream for dry skin Lipstick # 43
6/1	Cleansing, Peel - Relaxing Massage	Mary	Eye contour mask

Figure 11–7 A client consultation form and skin analysis chart.

PERFORMING A SKIN ANALYSIS

Knowing how to analyze skin is the first step in providing skin care. Identifying conditions and contraindications, as well as providing thorough consultations and charting client notes, are all elements of good facial treatments.

Educating clients on healthy habits and the causes of skin conditions is part of the service. Products, ingredients, different types of facials and a home-care regime for preventative maintenance are all beneficial in caring for the skin. A series of treatments may be necessary to effectively help the client's conditions. Twenty years of sun damage cannot be helped overnight. Realistically, it could take weeks or months to see a visible difference in the skin for some conditions, such as hyperpigmentation.

Beneath the surface, however, treatments have positive benefits and do make a difference, even if the effects are not instantly visible. (Information on choosing products for treatments and home care is presented in Chapter 12.) While at first skin analysis seems difficult, practice and experience will build confidence in using this important skill. Soon you will automatically notice skin conditions.

Knowing about skin types, conditions, and the factors affecting the skin's health enables you to give an accurate skin analysis. The best tool for analyzing the skin is a magnifying lamp/light. A Wood's lamp can also be useful (see Chapter 16). Note the following details in a skin analysis: the client's skin type, any skin conditions, and the skin's visible appearance and texture (Table 11–7).

After cleansing, observe the skin. First determine the skin type and the conditions present. Besides making a visual analysis, use your fingers to touch the skin (Figure 11–8). Does the texture feel rough or smooth? Try to determine the factors that may contribute to the individual's skin conditions. The more faces you see, the better you will be at recognizing different types and conditions.

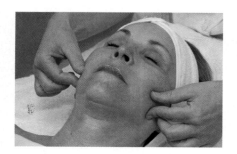

Figure 11–8 Checking elasticity in the skin.

Table 11–7

A SKIN ANALYSIS CHECKLIST

1. Skin type: Check the pore size and oil distribution.
2. Conditions present: Note the comedones, capillaries, pigmentation, sun damage, and other conditions. Refer to the client chart and Table 11–2 for a list of conditions.
3. Appearance: Is the skin dry, clear, oily, red, irritated? What else do you notice?
4. Texture: Is the texture rough, smooth, dehydrated, firm? Record your observations on the client's chart.

PROCEDURE 11–1

PERFORMING A SKIN ANALYSIS: STEP BY STEP

SUPPLIES (This list will be used for all cleansing procedures.)
- disinfectant or sanitizer
- hand sanitizer or antibacterial soap
- covered trash container
- bowl
- spatula
- hand towels
- headband
- clean linens
- bolster

DISPOSABLES
- gloves
- cotton pads
- cotton rounds
- cotton swabs
- plastic bag
- paper towels
- tissues

PRODUCTS
- eye makeup remover or cleanser
- facial cleanser
- toner
- moisturizer

Preparation

1 Prepare the bed and room.

2 Set out the supplies and products on a sanitary maintenance area (SMA).

3 Prepare the client and cover the hair.

Procedure

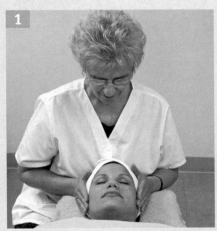

Look at the client's skin before starting the treatment. *(Figure P-11–1-1)*

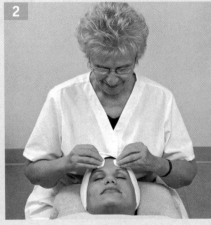

Cleanse the skin. *(Figure P-11–1-2)*

1 *Look* briefly at your client's skin with your naked eye or a magnifying light. (Figure P-11-1-1). You cannot do an accurate analysis if your client is wearing makeup.

2 *Cleanse* the skin (a client's normal state of dryness or oiliness may not be as visible after cleansing) (Figure P-11-1-2).

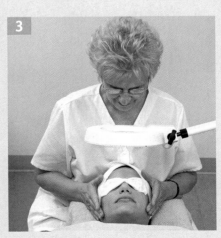

Use the magnifying lamp for a skin analysis. *(Figure P-11–1-3)*

3 Use a *magnifying* light to examine the skin more thoroughly (Figure P-11–1-3). *Cover the eyes* with eye pads. (In addition to the magnifying light, a Wood's lamp can be used here.)

PROCEDURE 11–1, CONT.

Procedure (cont.):

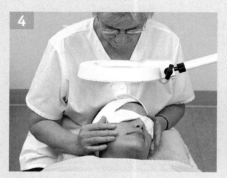

Feel the texture of the skin.
(Figure P-11–1-4)

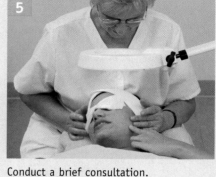

Conduct a brief consultation.
(Figure P-11–1-5)

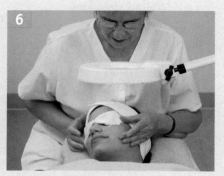

Ask questions during the analysis.
(Figure P-11–1-6)

4 *Look* closely at the client's skin type, the conditions present and the appearance; also *touch* the skin with the fingertips to feel its texture (Figure P-11-1-4).

5 *Listen*: Conduct a brief *consultation* while continuing to analyze with the magnifying lamp (Figure P 11-1-5). (A Wood's lamp can be used here to see conditions not visible with the naked eye.)

6 *Ask questions* relating to the skin's appearance and the client's personal health. Discuss what you see with the client; also recommend products and a home care routine (Figure P 11-1-6).

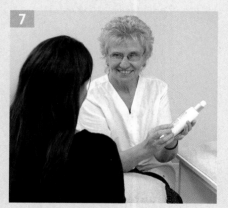

Choosing products for treatment and home care. *(Figure P-11-1-7)*

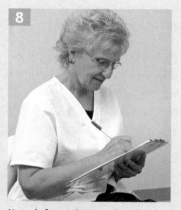

Note information on the client chart. *(Figure P-11–1-8)*

FYI

The four components of skin analysis are *look, feel, ask,* and *listen.*

7 *Choose products* for treatment and home care (Figure P 11-1-7).

8 *Record* the information on the client chart at the appropriate time—usually after the treatment is completed (Figure P-11-1-8).

Clean-Up

9 Follow the aseptic procedure to avoid contamination. You will follow the same clean-up and sanitation steps as presented in the Basic Facial Procedure (see Procedure 14–4).

REVIEW QUESTIONS

1. Are all skin types genetic?

2. List the five skin types.

3. What is the difference between dry and dehydrated skin?

4. What is the Fitzpatrick Scale?

5. List six common skin conditions.

6. How are skin conditions different from skin types?

7. List four intrinsic, or internal, factors affecting the skin.

8. List four extrinsic factors that affect the skin.

9. What are five healthy habits for the skin?

10. What is the main cause of premature extrinsic aging?

11. What is the difference between UVA and UVB rays?

12. List five contraindications.

13. Describe the steps in a skin analysis.

CHAPTER GLOSSARY

actinic: damage or condition caused by sun exposure.

AHAs (alpha hydroxy acids): acids used to exfoliate the skin.

alipidic: lack of oil.

antioxidants: free radical scavengers, vitamins, and ingredients.

contraindications: a factor that prohibits a treatment due to a condition; treatments could cause harmful or negative side effects to those who have specific medical or skin conditions.

couperose skin: redness; distended capillaries from weakening of the capillary walls.

dehydration: lack of water.

Fitzpatrick Scale: a scale used to measure the skin type's ability to tolerate sun exposure.

keratoses: abnormally thick build-ups of cells.

melanosome: pigment granules of melanocyte cells that produce melanin in the basal layer.

occlusive: products that reduce transepidermal water loss (TEWL) to help hold in moisture and protect the skin's top barrier layer.

peptides: chains of amino acids; used to treat wrinkles and elasticity.

skin types: classification that describes a person's genetic skin type.

T-zone: the center area of the face; corresponds to the "T" shape formed by the forehead, nose, and chin.

SKIN CARE PRODUCTS: CHEMISTRY, INGREDIENTS, AND SELECTION

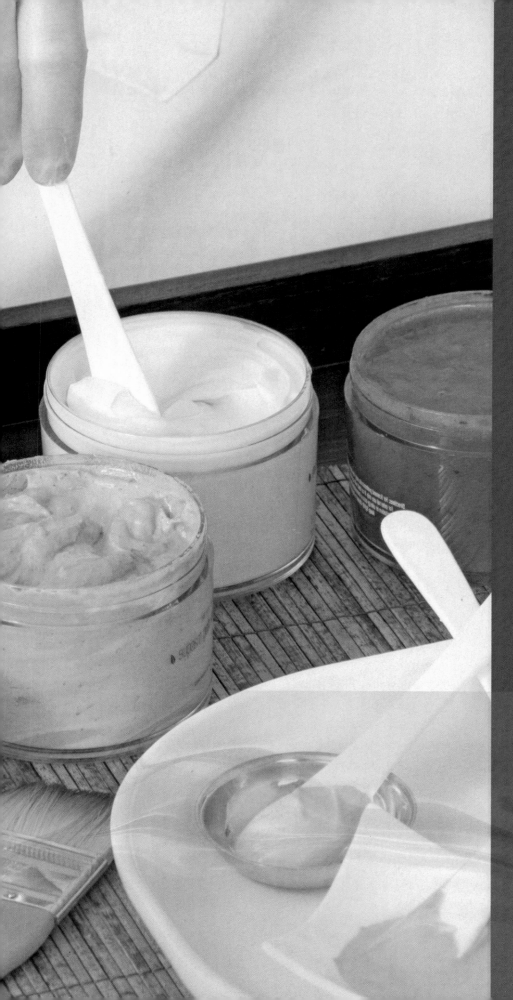

KEY TERMS

Page numbers indicate where in the chapter each term is used.

T

he products the esthetician uses are the lifeblood of the facial treatment (Figure 12–1). The performance ingredients in products do the actual work of cleansing, normalizing, moisturizing, or otherwise treating the skin. Products come in many forms and types: solids, liquids, gases, or combinations of these. They may be formulated as cleansers, moisturizers, exfoliants, or other types of products. Within each category they are further differentiated by skin type.

In addition to understanding basic chemistry and cosmetic ingredients, you will need to know about new, more advanced ingredients and treatments, particularly those to which "antiaging" benefits are ascribed. While estheticians may not yet be allowed to claim the actual benefits of these products, you should understand them.

The cosmetics industry is continually developing new products to improve the appearance of the skin. Products used in treatments and for home care can make a significant difference in the skin's health and appearance. The effectiveness of skin care formulations has increased as our knowledge of the biology of the skin expands. Both natural and clinical approaches are advancing. From **phytotherapy** to clinical formulations, product ingredients are one of the most exciting subjects in skin care. The chemistry of ingredients can be studied at the molecular level, but product chemistry and biochemistry are complex subjects you can learn more about when researching ingredients and the effects on the skin.

As an esthetician, you will need to know what a wide spectrum of skin care products do, how they work, and how they are used. You will need to make decisions about products that will best suit your client's skin type and current condition. A person's skin care needs can change depending upon the season or life's activities. Be sure to check with clients to see if changes in their products are necessary. Educate them about the product or ingredient that is being used, what it does for them, and why it is effective.

Product ingredients are derived from a variety of sources including herbs, essential oils, plants, and synthetic performance ingredients. You should be familiar with each ingredient in the product and know its potential side effects. Read the manufacturer's literature and follow their instructions. This extensive chapter covers three main topics: chemistry, ingredients, and product selection.

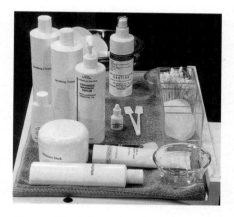

Figure 12–1 Treatment products are the esthetician's most important tools.

COSMETIC CHEMISTRY AND INGREDIENTS

The Food and Drug Administration (FDA) views cosmetics according to the Cosmetic Act of 1938, which distinguishes between drugs and cosmetics. **Cosmetics** are defined by the FDA as "articles that are intended to be rubbed, poured, sprinkled or otherwise applied to the human body or any part thereof for cleansing, beautifying, promoting attractiveness or altering the appearance." In contrast, drugs are products (other than food) intended to affect the structures and/or function of the body of humans or other animals. These definitions are important because they state that estheticians cannot make claims that a product or treatment can affect the structure or function of the skin. Estheticians focus on improving the skin's cosmetic appearance.

Every ingredient employed in cosmetic chemistry has some function in the finished product. These ingredients are divided into two basic types: functional ingredients and performance ingredients.

Functional ingredients make up the majority of a product. They allow products to spread, give them body and texture, and give them a specific form such as a lotion, cream, or gel. These ingredients do not affect the appearance of the skin but are necessary to the product formulation. A preservative is an example of an inactive functional ingredient.

Performance ingredients cause the actual changes in the appearance of the skin. Examples include glycerin, which hydrates the skin's surface; alpha hydroxy acids (AHAs), which exfoliate the corneum; and lipids, which help patch the skin's barrier. Performance ingredients are sometimes referred to as active agents—or erroneously called "active ingredients," which is an official term reserved for use in the drug industry to indicate ingredients that chemically cause physiological changes.

A third category has been proposed: **cosmeceuticals,** which are products intended to improve the skin's health and appearance. Cosmeceuticals are stronger performance ingredients that may cause biochemical reactions and physiological effects to the skin. This category is not yet recognized by the FDA.

PRODUCT INGREDIENTS

Ingredients can be derived from plants, vitamins, or animals. They are also synthesized from chemicals in a lab. The terms *natural* and *organic* are often used in referring to skin product ingredients, but these terms have no specific definition. *Hypoallergenic* describes ingredients that may be less likely to cause allergic reactions. *Noncomedogenic* describes ingredients that will not clog pores or cause comedones. Many of the terms used in relation to products used by estheticians are descriptive and are for consumer marketing purposes. Research or testing of products varies, and product chemistry is complicated, so it may be difficult to predict how a certain product will work for an individual.

Water

Water makes up a large part of the skin. It is also the most frequently used cosmetic ingredient—it is both a vehicle and a performance ingredient. As a vehicle, it helps keep other cosmetic ingredients in solution and helps spread products across the skin. As a performance ingredient, water replenishes moisture in the surface of the skin. Almost all skin care products are a mixture of oil and water, or emulsions. Products that do not contain any water are called **anhydrous** (an-HY-drus). These include oil serums, petrolatum-based products such as lip balm, and silicone serums (Figure 12–2). Generally, anhydrous products are designed for very dry skin.

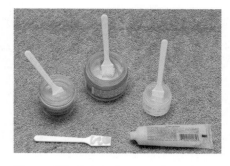

Figure 12–2 Anhydrous products do not contain water.

Emollients

Emollients are fatty materials used to lubricate and moisturize the skin. They can act as either vehicles or performance ingredients. As vehicles, emollients help place, spread, and keep other agents on the skin. For example, emollients in sunscreen cream help spread the sunscreen agents across the skin and hold it in place. Emollients in loose powder help the powder slip evenly across and adhere to the skin.

As performance ingredients, emollients lubricate the skin's surface and set up a guard for the barrier function. Emollients lie on top of the skin and prevent dehydration by trapping water and decreasing transepidermal water loss (TEWL), which increases moisture in the epidermis. This technique of moisturization is called occlusion (Figure 12–3). Silicones and oils are both emollients.

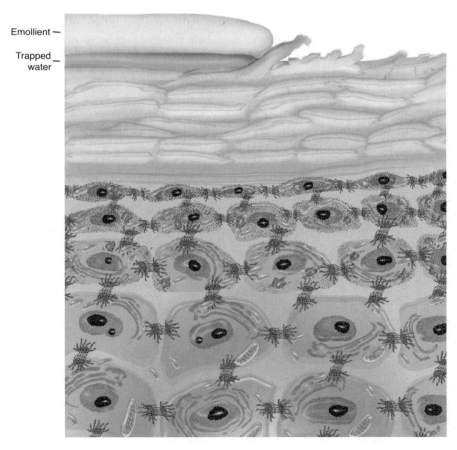

Emollient —

Trapped water

Figure 12–3 Emollients trap moisture in the skin by the process of occlusion.

ACTIVITY

Did you know that you can easily and safely test the pH of a solution? pH test papers (litmus papers and pH papers) can be used to indicate the pH of any aqueous solution. You can test any skin care product. You will need pH test papers, several small open containers, bottled drinking water, stirring sticks, and some white towels. Place the product you want to test in a small, open cup or bowl. If the product is a powder or is extremely thick, add a small amount of bottled water and stir thoroughly. Dip the test paper into the product. Immediately place the paper on a white towel, and compare the color obtained to the color chart on the package to determine the pH level. Test anything you can think of. Be creative! What you discover may surprise you.

Oils

Many oils are used in skin care. They vary in density, fat content, and heaviness. They also vary in their tendency to cause comedones in oily or acne-prone skin. Different oils are appropriate for different degrees of dryness in the skin. Oils come from many sources.

Oils from the Earth. Mineral oil and petrolatum come from the earth, specifically from petroleum sources. Both emollients are time tested, offer excellent protection against dehydration, and help prevent irritant skin contact. They are completely nonreactive and biologically inert, which means that they do not react with other chemicals involved in the skin's function. They can be combined with water and blended with an emulsifier into a cream, lotion, or fluid, which makes them much less oily. Classic cold cream, one of the first moisturizers ever made, was blended with mineral oil. Mineral oil and petrolatum can be used with no added preservatives because they do not harbor bacteria or other organisms. Mineral oil is also a lubricant. **Lubricants** coat the skin and reduce friction.

Oils from Plants. Dozens of plant oils are used in skin care products. Most plant oils are used for their emollient properties; but some, such as aromatic essential oils, are used for their fragrances. Plant oils contain fatty acids, which are beneficial for skin that does not produce enough sebum. The oils help keep the skin from dehydrating. Plant oils vary in fatty acid content and heaviness. Coconut oil and palm oil are two of the fattiest and heaviest oils. Some lighter and less comedogenic natural oils are safflower, sunflower, canola, and jojoba (huh-HOH-buh) oil.

Other Emollients

Literally hundreds of emollients exist. Some come from natural sources, and others are synthesized in a laboratory or derived from other oils or fatty materials.

Fatty acids are lubricant ingredients derived from plant oils or animal fats. Although these ingredients are acids, they are not irritating. Fatty acids are actually more like oils. Common fatty acids that you will see are oleic acid, stearic acid, and caprylic acid.

Fatty alcohols are fatty acids that have been exposed to hydrogen. They are not drying; they have a waxlike consistency and are used as emollients or spreading agents. Examples of fatty alcohols are cetyl alcohol, lauryl alcohol, and stearyl alcohol.

Fatty esters are produced from fatty acids and fatty alcohols. Esters are easily recognized on labels because they almost always end in *–ate,* such as octyl palmitate. They often feel better than natural oils and lubricate more evenly. Frequently used fatty esters are isopropyl myristate, isopropyl palmitate, and glyceryl stearate.

Silicones are a group of oils that are chemically combined with silicon and oxygen and leave a noncomedogenic protective film on the surface of the skin. They also act as vehicles in some products, including makeup foundations. They are excellent protectants, helping to keep moisture trapped in the skin yet allowing oxygen in and out of the follicles. Silicones also add an elegant, nongreasy feel to products. Examples of silicones are dimethicone, cyclomethicone, and phenyl trimethicone. These ingredients are frequently used in sunscreens, foundation, and moisturizers.

Emollients and Comedogenicity

Many emollient ingredients can cause or worsen the development of comedones in the skin. These emollients are said to be comedogenic, which means they block pores. **Comedogenicity** (kahm-uh-do-jen-IS-suh-tee) is the tendency of any topical substance to cause or to worsen a buildup of dead cells in the follicle, leading to the development of a comedo (blackhead).

Emollients that are comedogenic are generally not intended for clog-prone or acne-prone skin. Oilier skin produces enough of its own emollient, as sebum, and does not need more. Dry skin that does not produce enough sebum may need heavier emollient ingredients to protect the skin from dehydration. This type of skin does not clog easily and is not acne prone.

Surfactants

One of the biggest categories of cosmetic ingredients is **surfactants.** Surfactants reduce the surface tension between the skin and the product, and increase the spreadability of cosmetic products.

Detergents

The main types of surfactants used in skin-cleansing products are **detergents.** These are not the type of detergents you associate with washing clothes, but they are from the same chemical family. Detergents are used primarily in cleansing products. They reduce the surface tension of the dirt and oil on the skin's surface and form an emulsion to lift them from the skin (Figure 12–4). They are also the agents that cause cleansers to foam. However, detergents that are too strong can remove too much sebum and actually damage the lipid barrier function of the skin. Some common detergent examples are sodium lauryl sulfate, sodium laureth sulfate, and ammonium lauryl sulfate.

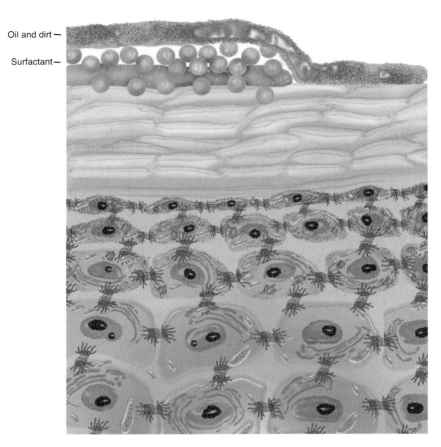

Oil and dirt —

Surfactant —

Figure 12–4 Detergents reduce the surface tension of dirt and oils and lift them from the skin.

Cleansers are soaps and/or detergents that clean the skin. Soaps may be combined with detergents to make cleansers.

Emulsifiers

Emulsifiers are another category of surfactants. In fact, some detergents can also act as emulsifiers. **Emulsifiers** are surfactants that cause oil and water to mix to form an emulsion. Without emulsifiers, oil and water would separate into layers. Emulsifiers surround oil particles, allowing them to remain evenly distributed throughout the water (Figure 12–5). When skin care products are mixed, materials that are compatible with oil are mixed in with the oil. These substances are called **oil soluble,** and they are mixed into the oil phase of the product during manufacturing. Substances that are mixable with water are known as **water soluble** and are mixed in the water phase.

Gellants and Thickeners

Gellants are agents that are used to give a product a gel-like consistency. Certain vehicle ingredients are added to thicken products or to help suspend ingredients that are hard to mix into a product. One example is **carbomers** (KAHR-boh-murz), which are used to thicken creams and are frequently used in gel products.

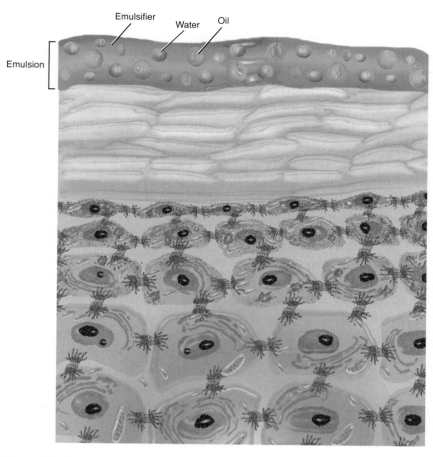

Figure 12–5 In an emulsion, an emulsifier is added to the oil and water process.

Fragrances

Consumers love wonderful scents, especially in products they associate with relaxation, such as bath oils and bath salts. **Fragrances** can come from plant, animal, or synthetic sources, but plant oils are especially popular. These perfumes give products their scent. Essential oils are often used for their natural fragrance.

Aromatherapy is the therapeutic use of plant aromas and **essential oils** for beauty and health treatment purposes. Essential oils are highly concentrated plant oils with properties that can have various effects on the skin. Essential oils are also used to relax, stimulate, or balance the psyche (Figure 12–6). Aromatherapy has been used medically for thousands of years, and it is still used today in treatment and skin care products.

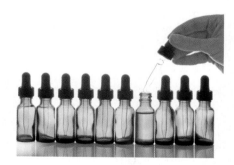

Figure 12–6 Essential oils are frequently used in skin care products.

Preservatives

Preservatives are an important functional ingredient in many skin care and cosmetic products. Preservatives prevent bacteria and other microorganisms from living in a product. Without preservatives, products could easily be contaminated with bacteria, fungi, molds, or other microorganisms that could cause disease in the person using the product. Examples of preservatives used in skin care products are chelating agents.

FOCUS ON . . .

AROMATHERAPY

Essential oils are the fragrant soul of the plant.

A **chelating agent** (CHE-layt-ing A-junt) is a chemical that is added to cosmetics to improve the efficiency of the preservative. Chelating agents work by breaking down the cell walls of bacteria and other microorganisms. Common chelating ingredients are disodium EDTA, trisodium EDTA, and tetrasodium EDTA. EDTA is an acronym for the chemical name ethylenediaminetetraacetic acid. These ingredients are usually on the bottom of the ingredient list because they are used in small quantities. Parabens, quaternium (kwah-TAYR-nee-um) 15, and urea are all preservatives.

Besides fighting bacteria, preservatives help protect products from chemical changes that can adversely affect the product. **Antioxidants** are substances that inhibit oxidation reactions. They are used to help the condition of the skin as well as stop the oxidation that causes products to turn rancid and spoil.

Color Agents

Color agents serve several purposes. In skin care products, they add color, which mainly enhances a product's visual appeal. In color cosmetics, of course, the color agents are responsible for most of the product's cosmetic effects. They give color to products such as eye shadows, lipsticks, and foundations (also called base makeup). Vegetable, pigment, or mineral dyes give products color.

The FDA closely regulates color agent ingredients. There are two types of color ingredients: certified colors and noncertified colors.

Certified colors are synthetic, inorganic, and are known as metal salts. These **colorants** that have been batch certified and approved by the FDA. **Noncertified colors** are organic, meaning that they come from animal or plants extracts and can also be natural mineral pigments. Noncertified colors are less irritating than certified colors, making them more useful for cosmetics applied to the eye area, for example. They are listed on ingredient labels as "D&C," which stands for "drug & cosmetic" or "FD&C," which stands for "food, drug & cosmetic." **Lakes** are insoluble pigments made by combining a dye with an inorganic material and are commonly used in colorful cosmetics. These colorants can be blended to produce many different colors for skin care products and makeup.

Exempt colors, those that do not require certification, include zinc oxide, iron oxides, carmine, mica, and the ultramarine colors. They are less intense in color than certified colors. Nonetheless, zinc oxide and iron oxide help with opacity, meaning that they provide a solid color that is not transparent. They are used extensively in coverage makeup products such as foundations.

Other Product Components

pH adjustors-Substances called pH adjusters are acids or alkalis (bases) used to adjust the pH of products. Buffering ingredients prevent changes in pH. Sodium hydroxide and citric acid are often used as pH adjusters.

Solvents—These are substances, such as water or alcohol, that dissolve other ingredients.

Botanicals—Ingredients derived from plants. Ingredients used in phytotherapy are derived from plants.

Healing agents—These are substances, such as chamomile, licorice, azulene, and aloe, that heal the skin.

Hydrators and Moisturizers

Hydrators, also known as **humectants** (hyoo-MEK-tents), are ingredients that attract water to the skin's surface. They can lock water on the skin, improving dehydration. Many humectants are available, including glycerin, sodium PCA, sorbitol, seaweed extracts, algae (AL-jee) extract, hyaluronic acid (HY-uh-lur-AHN-ik A-sid), and propylene glycol.

Most moisturizing products are combinations of emollients and humectants. Thousands of possible combinations exist. These combinations determine the differences between moisturizers as well as the differences between creams, lotions, and fluids. Creams usually have more emollients than lotions or fluids.

Lipids

Lipids are used to improve hydration, plumpness, and smoothness of the skin. They can also reduce sensitivity by making the skin more resistant to irritants and dehydration. Common lipid ingredients are sphingolipids, phospholipids, and glycosphingolipids. These lipids or ceramides are all known to improve the barrier function of the skin.

Exfoliating Ingredients

Exfoliation (eks-foh-lee-AY-shun), or the removal of dead corneum cells, can improve the look of most skin types. Mechanical exfoliating ingredients are added to products, often cleansers, to physically scrape dead cells from the skin's surface. The ingredients include polyethylene and jojoba beads, ground nuts such as almonds, and various seeds.

Exfoliation can also be achieved through chemical action (Figure 12–7). **Alpha hydroxy acids (AHAs)** and **beta hydroxy acids (BHAs)** include glycolic, lactic, malic, tartaric, citric, and salicylic (sal-uh-SIL-ik) acids.

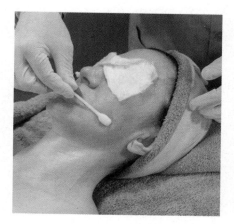

Figure 12–7 Applying an AHA peel.

These exfoliants work by loosening the bond between cells in the surface of the corneum. They can also help to lighten pigmented areas, soften rough skin, and heal areas that are prone to breakouts. Any of these exfoliants can be added to gels, lotions, serums, or creams. Acids come in a variety of concentrations and pH levels that affect the irritancy of a given product. A product with the same concentration of hydroxy acid is more irritating at a lower pH. A concentration of 10 percent or less at a pH of 3.5 or greater is recommended for over-the-counter sales and home use.

Enzymes

Enzymes such as papain, bromelain, and pancreatin are also used in exfoliating products. These ingredients are designed to dissolve keratin proteins on the surface of the skin to make it softer and smoother and thus help maintain the hydration level of the epidermis. Once the dead skin cells are gently removed, the skin is clearer and can absorb products more easily. This is true for all types of exfoliants.

Lighteners and Brighteners

Lighteners and brighteners are ingredients that are used in the bleaching or lightening of the skin, actually "lifting" a darker pigmented area to a lighter

---

? Did You Know

The chemical difference between alpha hydroxy acids and beta hydroxy acids is the location of the hydroxy group on the carbon chain of the acid. *Alpha* indicates that the group is on the first carbon atom, whereas *beta* indicates that the group is on the second carbon atom. Glycolic acid has the smallest molecular structure so it can penetrate between cells more easily than all of the other hydroxy acids.

color. Commonly used ingredients are hydroquinone, kojic acid, arbutin, vitamin C, licorice root, bearberry, green tea extract, and alpha hydroxy and beta hydroxy acids. These ingredients work either by bleaching the upper layers of the epidermis or by slowing down the pigment factories in the skin, known as melanocytes, thus blocking the production of melanin. These ingredients are also known as tyrozinase inhibitors. Tyrozinase (TY-ruh-sin-ays) is the enzyme that converts tyrosine, an amino acid, into melanin. When using these products, it is important for clients to wear sunscreen to protect the skin and to prevent the pigmented areas from returning.

Delivery Systems

Delivery systems are chemical systems that deliver ingredients to specific tissues of the epidermis. Vehicles, liposomes, and polymers are types of delivery systems.

Vehicles are spreading agents and carrying bases necessary to the formulation of a cosmetic. Water and emollients are both vehicles. Vehicles carry or deliver other ingredients into the skin and make them more effective.

Liposomes (LY-puh-zohms) are closed lipid bilayer spheres that encapsulate ingredients, target their delivery to specific tissues of the skin, and control their release. The bilayer structure of liposomes mimics cell membranes and is therefore compatible with cells—in contrast to standard micelle emulsions, which disrupt and damage cell membranes.

Polymers (PAHL-uh-murs) are chemical compounds formed by a number of small molecules. Another use of polymers is in delivery systems. They are used as advanced vehicles that release substances onto the skin's surface at a microscopically controlled rate. They are also referred to as microsponges.

Ingredients That Improve Cell Metabolism and Oxygenation

A major goal in advanced skin care treatments is to help the skin function at its maximum capacity at any age. Improvements in cell turnover that emulate younger skin, together with nutrients to facilitate this process, can slow the appearance of aging. While it is impossible to reverse major damage, a well-planned skin care program can reduce the signs of aging. A number of high-tech ingredients serve as antioxidants and actually stimulate metabolic processes.

Antioxidants, applied topically, neutralize free radicals before they can attach themselves to the cell membrane and destroy the cell. Antioxidants are also added to cosmetic formulations to prevent the oxidation that causes a product to turn rancid and spoil. Vitamins C and E, green tea, and DMAE are examples of antioxidants.

Polyglucans (PAHL-ee-glue-kans) and **beta-glucans** (BAY-tuh GLUE-kans) are thought to help strengthen the immune system and stimulate the metabolism. They are normally derived from yeast cells and have a natural affinity for the skin. In addition, polyglucans are hydrophilic and therefore help preserve and protect collagen and elastin. Beta-glucans help reduce the appearance of fine lines and wrinkles by stimulating the formation of collagen.

Tissue respiratory factor (TRF) is also derived from yeast cells. TRF functions as an anti-inflammatory and moisturizing ingredient.

Glycoproteins (gly-koh-PRO-teens; also called glycopolypeptides), another yeast cell derivative, have been found to enhance cellular metabolism, which boosts oxygen uptake in the cell. This revitalizing capacity strengthens the skin's natural ability to protect itself against damaging environmental influences. Glycoproteins are especially beneficial to skin that appears unhealthy, is dull from smoking, has diffused redness, or has environmental damage.

Peptides and Collagen Stimulants

Peptides are chains of amino acids used in skin care products to produce changes in the skin's appearance. Peptides have been shown to help aging skin by stimulating the fibroblasts, the cells that produce **collagen** (KAHL-uh-jen), to improve skin firmness and soften wrinkles. Two of the more common peptide ingredients are palmitoyl pentapeptide-3 and palmitoyl oligopeptide. Peptides are less irritating than some of the other ingredients for aging skin, and they are often used along with other ingredients such as hydrators and antioxidants.

Retinol and Retinoic Acid (Retin-A®)

A natural form of vitamin A, **retinol** (RET-in-all) stimulates cell repair and helps to normalize skin cells by generating new cells. It has been used in serums, creams, and lotions and varies in concentration when used in a cosmetic and a drug. As with many cosmetic ingredients, more than a trace amount is necessary to be effective, but high concentrations of vitamin A can be irritating to sensitive skin. As discussed previously, vitamin A is an antioxidant.

Retinoic acid (Retin-A®, Renova®, Tazorac®) is also a form of vitamin A, and is approved as an active drug ingredient. It is of the keratolytic (kair-uh-tuh-LIT-ik) group, meaning that it causes peeling of the skin. It is used for skin problems such as acne and sun-damaged skin as well as for wrinkles. Because many people have moderate to severe reactions to retinoic acid, a physician must be treating anyone using retinoids.

Vitamins and Other Antioxidants

Vitamins such as vitamin C and vitamin E have been used in skin care products as antioxidants for many years. It is believed that they work by interfering with inflammation, thus reducing the production of enzymes that injure and destroy skin cells. Other antioxidants include alphalipoic acid, idebenone, stearyl glycyrrhizinate, green tea, and grapeseed. When used in combinations, these formulas are called broad-spectrum antioxidants.

Coenzyme Q10 protects and revitalizes skin cells. It is often formulated with other natural protective ingredients to strengthen the capillary network and increase energy to epidermal cells. It is considered a powerful antioxidant. It seems to fortify the skin's immune function and activate metabolic functions. Use of CoQ10 often results in visible reduction of wrinkles and fine lines.

Vitamin K has been used in products for blood coagulation. It is helpful for clients with telangiectasias and spider veins.

FYI

Federal Food and Drug Administration regulations do not allow the term *sunblock* to be used in products, because no product blocks 100 percent of UVA and UVB rays.

CAUTION!

If a client has an allergic reaction to a product that requires medical treatment, the manufacturer of the product is responsible—unless the product was purchased in bulk, repackaged by the salon in smaller containers, and resold, in which case the salon is at fault. If the product is made in the salon, the salon is also responsible. Malpractice insurance does not generally cover products formulated or repackaged in the salon.

Sunscreen Ingredients

There are two types of active sunscreen ingredients. Chemical sunscreens are organic (carbon) compounds that chemically absorb ultraviolet rays. Physical sunscreens are inorganic (without carbon) compounds that physically reflect ultraviolet rays.

Examples of organic chemical sunscreens are:

- octinoxate (octyl methoxycinnimate)
- octisalate (octyl salicylate)
- oxybenzone (benzophenone)

Examples of inorganic physical sunscreens are:

- titanium dioxide
- zinc oxide

NATURAL VERSUS SYNTHETIC INGREDIENTS

Some of the most effective cosmetic ingredients are not derived from plants. Synthetically produced ingredients can be just as effective and may have certain advantages over ingredients derived naturally from plants.

Natural and synthetic ingredients can both have drawbacks. Natural ingredients may cause allergies in people who are sensitive, while synthetic versions of the same ingredients may not. Moreover, certain synthetic ingredients are effective cell renewal stimulants.

Sometimes it can be difficult to know when to choose natural ingredients or synthetic ones. Both make tremendous contributions to skin care formulations. Manufacturers do extensive research and development to bring the latest technologies into cosmetic formulations. For example, hyaluronic acid, an ingredient used to bind moisture in formulations, was initially derived from roosters' combs. Synthetic production of this ingredient was developed, and today it is derived from synthetic sources for use in cosmetics. The synthetic version is more stable and has more effective water-binding properties.

To make informed choices, estheticians must stay current with developments in cosmetic chemistry. Combining both natural and synthetic ingredients is effective in product formulations. The quality and the sources of ingredients are both important factors to consider when choosing products.

PRODUCT SAFETY

The FDA does not require approval of cosmetics before their manufacture and sale. The FDA does require that all drugs be proven safe and effective before their manufacture and sale. The FDA regulates cosmetics only in the areas of safety, labeling, and the claims made for a product. If a cosmetic product makes a drug claim, is not properly labeled, or has been reported as unsafe, the FDA can take legal action against the manufacturer. Drugs may claim to change a function of the body. Cosmetics may claim only to change the appearance of the body.

FDA regulations for cosmetic labeling state that cosmetic companies must list the company's name, location, or distribution point as well as all the ingredients in the product. This allows consumers to check for ingredients they may be allergic to. Ingredients must be listed in descending order of predominance, starting with the ingredient having the highest concentration and ending with the ingredient having the lowest concentration. Ingredients with a concentration of less than 1 percent may be listed in any order. A fragrance must be listed as "fragrance," but the ingredients need not be listed.

Allergic Reactions

Many ingredients used in skin care products—including fragrances, essential oils, and preservatives—may cause adverse skin reactions. Being aware of a client's allergies and the ingredients being used in treatments is very important to avoid problems or reactions. Sometimes a product or treatment will cause a reaction. If the skin becomes excessively red or the client complains of burning, immediately remove the product and rinse the skin with cold water. Having a cortisone cream available and products to calm skin reactions is a good precaution. Before the treatment, it is a good idea to conduct a patch test on clients with reactive skin. Try the product on the inside of the arm, near the elbow, or on a small area of the face.

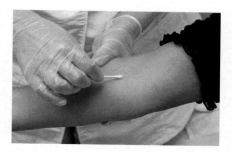

Figure 12–8 A patch test is the best way to determine if a client is allergic to a product.

Fragrances and some preservatives are among the most common allergens. Allergic reactions may not be detected until several days later. Symptoms may include inflammation of the skin, burning or itching, blisters, blotches, or rashes. The eyes may swell, puff, or produce tears.

The best way to guard against allergic reactions is to pretest a small quantity of the product with a test patch (Figure 12–8). If there is any reaction within 24 hours, the product should not be used. If the reaction is serious, the product should be taken to a physician who can determine what has caused the problem and can treat the condition appropriately. The manufacturer of the product should be notified immediately.

Always follow strict sanitary procedures in treatment areas and elsewhere in the salon. Products must be kept sanitary and be stored properly. Close containers when not in use. Do not share cosmetics with anyone else. Never use saliva to moisten eye makeup or other cosmetics; use only fresh, clean water. Discard outdated, rancid, or stale products. Products stored in dark containers and in cooler temperatures will last longer.

INGREDIENTS

We have discussed why choosing products and ingredients that are effective for a person's individual needs are the most important part of any treatment and for home care. When products are used correctly, results are more noticeable. The next section includes a partial list of ingredients used in skin care and beauty products. Their definitions and properties are included in Tables 12–1 through 12–4.

Many products are made synthetically rather than from plants or animal products. It is important to know the source of the ingredient, particularly if clients have a preference for one type over another.

ACTIVITY

Why are some products better than others? Take this opportunity to do some research. Go to a drugstore and compare its product prices and ingredients to those of a professional line. Comparing ingredients often reveals the answer to this question. Use a cosmetic ingredients dictionary to look up ingredients.

Table 12–1

COMMON PRODUCT COMPONENTS AND INGREDIENTS	
INGREDIENT	**DESCRIPTION**
alcohol	Used as an antiseptic and solvent in perfumes, lotions, and astringents. There are many types of alcohols; not all are drying.
alum	A compound made of aluminum, potassium, or ammonium sulfate. An astringent, antiseptic, and stimulating. Good for oily skin; also stops bleeding.
benzyl peroxide	A drying ingredient with antibacterial properties commonly used for blemishes and acne. It can be a skin allergen and irritant.
ceramides	Lipid materials found in skin's intercellular cement; a natural moisturizing factor; products help lipid replacement and combat dryness, aging, and dehydration.
collagen	Protein derived from animals or synthetically manufactured. Plumps the surface of the skin and prevents water loss.
essential oils	Oils derived from plants and herbs; they have many different properties and effects on the skin and psyche.
glycerin	Formed by a decomposition of oils or fats, glycerin is an excellent skin softener and humectant as well as a very strong water binder.
herbs	These, along with plant extracts, contain phytohormones. Hundreds of different herbs are used in skin care products and cosmetics to help heal, stimulate, soothe, and moisturize. Herbs are also used as astringents.
hyaluronic acid	A hydrophilic agent with excellent water-binding properties.
lanolin	An emollient with moisturizing properties, lanolin is a sheep's wool derivative formed by a fatlike, viscous secretion of the sheep's sebaceous glands.
liposomes	Closed lipid bilayer spheres that encapsulate ingredients, targeting their delivery to specific tissues of the skin, and controlling their release.
methylparaben	One of the most frequently used preservatives because of its very low sensitizing potential; one of the oldest preservatives in use to combat bacteria and molds. It is noncomedogenic.
mineral oil	An emollient that dissolves dirt trapped in pores; mineral oil is a clear, odorless substance derived from petroleum. It is not known to cause allergic reactions.
mucopolysaccharides	Carbohydrate–lipid complexes; good water **binders.**
parabens	One of the most commonly used groups of preservatives in the cosmetic, pharmaceutical, and food industries, parabens provide antibacterial and antifungal activity against a diverse number of organisms.
petroleum jelly	An occlusive agent that restores the barrier layer by holding in water. It is used after laser surgery to protect the skin as it heals.
potassium hydroxide	A strong alkali used in soaps and creams.
propylene glycol	A humectant often used in dry or sensitive skin moisturizers.

continues on next page

Table 12–1 *(continued)*

INGREDIENT	DESCRIPTION
quaternium 15	An all-purpose preservative active against bacteria, mold, and yeast, this ingredient is probably the greatest formaldehyde releaser among cosmetic preservatives and causes dermatitis and allergies.
retinoic acid	A vitamin A derivative, retinoic acid has demonstrated an ability to alter collagen synthesis. It is used to treat acne and visible signs of aging. Side effects are irritation, photosensitivity, skin dryness, redness, and peeling.
salicylic acid	A beta hydroxy acid with exfoliating and antiseptic properties, its natural sources include sweet birch, willow bark, and wintergreen. Check for client allergies to this acid.
silicone	Oil that is chemically combined with silicon and oxygen and leaves a noncomedogenic, protective film on the surface of the skin.
sodium bicarbonate	Baking soda; an inorganic salt used as a buffering agent, neutralizer, and a pH adjuster.
sorbitol	A humectant that absorbs moisture from the air to prevent skin dryness. If the skin's moisture content is greater than the atmosphere, sorbitol will draw moisture out of the skin. It is obtained from the leaves and berries of mountain ash. It also occurs in other berries, cherries, plums, pears, apples, seaweed, and algae.
sphingolipids	Ceramides—lipid materials that are a natural part of the intercellular cement. Glycosphingolipids and phospholipids are also natural lipids found in the barrier layer.
squalane	Derived from olives, squalane is an emollient, desensitizing, and nourishing.
squalene	Originally from shark-liver oil, squalene occurs in small amounts in olive oil, wheat germ oil, and rice bran oil. It is also found in human sebum. Insoluble in water, it is a lubricant and perfume fixative.
sulfur	Sulfur reduces oil-gland activity and dissolves the skin's surface layer of dry, dead cells. This ingredient is commonly used in acne products. It can cause allergic skin reactions in some sensitive people.
titanium dioxide	An inorganic sunscreen that reflects UVA rays. When applied, it remains on the skin surface, basically scattering UV light. Used in sunscreen, makeup bases, and daytime moisturizers; also used to give cosmetic preparations a white color.
urea	Properties of urea include enhancing the penetration abilities of other substances. It is anti-inflammatory and an antiseptic; its deodorizing action allows it to protect the skin's surface and help maintain healthy skin. It does not induce photoallergy, phototoxicity, or sensitization.
zinc oxide	An inorganic sunscreen that reflects UVB rays. Also used to protect, soothe, and heal the skin. Zinc oxide is somewhat astringent, antiseptic, and antibacterial. It is obtained from zinc ore and is nonallergenic.

Table 12–2

INGREDIENTS FROM NATURE		

Some of the following natural ingredients are derived from plants (phytotherapy), and some are also produced synthetically.

INGREDIENTS	DESCRIPTION	PRIMARY BENEFITS
algae	Derived from seaweed; contains minerals	Moisturizing, nourishing
allantoin	Derived from the comfrey plant or uric acid; used in soothing products	Healing, promotes healthy tissue growth
almond meal	Ground almonds; commonly used in scrubs	Soothing and exfoliating
aloe vera	A plant used in many products	Healing, soothing, hydrating, anti-inflammatory
arnica	Healing; great for sore muscles, bruising	Anti-inflammatory
avocado	An emollient; contains vitamins A and C	Moisturizing, soothing
azulene	Derived from the chamomile plant; used for sensitive skin and calming	Anti-inflammatory, soothing
bayberry	Root bark; good for oily skin	Antiseptic, astringent
birch leaf	Good for oily skin	Antiseptic, stimulating
calendula	From the marigold plant; good for itching, swelling, and acne	Healing, soothing, anti-inflammatory
carrot	Used in creams and masks; rich in vitamin A	Antioxidant, moisturizing, soothing
chamomile	Plant extract; used for sensitive skin	Calming, anti-inflammatory
cocoa butter	From the cocoa tree	Moisturizing
coconut	Commonly used for oils, soaps, and creams	Lathers, cleanses, lubricates
comfrey	Has many beneficial qualities	Healing, moisturizing, antioxidants
coneflower	**Echinacea** (ek-uh-NAY-shah) is from the coneflower; used internally to support the immune system	Healing, preventing infection
cucumber	Commonly used for masks and the eye area to reduce puffiness	Antiseptic, soothing
eucalyptus	From the gum tree; used for acne and oily skin	Antiseptic, antimicrobial, astringent; stimulating
evening primrose	Known to help women's menstrual pain	Treats dry skin, flakiness; healing
geranium	Used to calm irritation	Astringent, anti-inflammatory
grapeseed extract	A soothing antioxidant derived from grapes	Healing, moisturizing, antiaging
green tea	Known for its health benefits	A strong antioxidant and anti-inflammatory
horsechestnut	A plant extract with bioflavonoids (vitamin P); strengthens capillary walls	Good for couperose skin and redness

continues on next page

Table 12–2 *(continued)*

INGREDIENTS	DESCRIPTION	PRIMARY BENEFITS
jojoba	A widely used noncomedogenic oil derived from a desert shrub	A soothing emollient, moisturizer, and lubricant
kojic acid	Usually derived from mushrooms	A skin-brightening agent for hyperpigmentation
lavender	A popular herb and oil used for calming	Soothing, anti-inflammatory; antiseptic properties
licorice	An anti-irritant good for sensitive skin; also inhibits melanin production	Soothing; used to lighten surface hyperpigmentation
mint	An herb good for circulation	Stimulating; also an antiseptic
oatmeal	Good for skin irritation, rashes, and sunburns	Soothing, anti-inflammatory, healing
olive	Olive tree extracts are used for many beauty products	Moisturizing and calming
orange	An aromatic, fresh, uplifting scent	An antioxidant and an astringent
papaya	Contains papain, an enzyme used in enzyme peels	Exfoliating; softening, moisturizing
peppermint	Cools skin and constricts capillaries; has refreshing properties	Reduces irritation and itching
pineapple	Contains bromelain, an enzyme with stimulating and antiseptic properties	Good for exfoliation and treating blemishes
pomegranate	A powerful antioxidant; treats sun damage	Healing; fights free radicals
rose	One of the most common ingredients in skin care products; used for dry, aging skin	Soothing and moisturizing
sandalwood	An exotic scent used for aromatherapy; good for skin irritations	Soothing and antiseptic properties
seaweed	Derivatives such as algae have many nourishing minerals and properties; detoxifies, stimulates metabolism (May be an allergen if allergic to seaweed or iodine.)	Humectant and moisturizing properties, firming
sesame	Used in massage and moisturizing products	Moisturizing
shea butter	A heavier moisturizer; native to Africa	Moisturizing and healing
soy	A protein and a source of vitamins	Anti-inflammatory, moisturizing
tea tree	Good for oily skin and scalp treatments	Germicidal, healing antifungal, antiseptic
witch hazel	From the hamanelis shrub; good for toning the skin	An astringent and antiseptic

Table 12–3

ESSENTIAL OILS AND HERBS

Here are some common essential oils or herbs used for their aromatherapeutic properties as well as skin benefits.

INGREDIENTS	PRIMARY PROPERTIES	SKIN BENEFITS
benzoin	astringent	oily skin; acne
bergamot	soothing	oily skin; acne
birch leaf	stimulating	moisturizing
eucalyptus	stimulating	increases circulation
evening primrose	soothing	moisturizing
frankincense	soothing	healing, rejuvenating
geranium	stimulating	antiseptic, healing
jasmine	soothing	moisturizing
lavender	soothing	healing
lemon	stimulating	antiseptic for acne, oily skin
lemongrass	stimulating	antiseptic for acne, oily skin
melissa (lemon balm)	soothing	soothes irritation
myrrh	healing	soothes irritation, acne
neroli	soothing	antiseptic for acne, oily skin
orange	stimulating	astringent
patchouli	soothing	moisturizing
peppermint	stimulating	increases circulation
rose	soothing	moisturizing
rosemary	stimulating	increases circulation
rosewood	stimulating	healing, dry skin
sandalwood	soothing	anti-inflammatory
tea tree	stimulating	antiseptic; acne
ylang-ylang	soothing	antiseptic, enhances circulation

Herbs and Plant Properties

Another classification system is to list ingredients by the category or properties. The following is a partial list of plant and herbal properties that have astringent, stimulating, calming and/or soothing, healing, and hydrating properties. Many of the plants or herbs listed have more than one property or effect on the skin or senses. Check out aromatherapy and herb books for more information on this intriguing subject.

Table 12–4

NATURAL FOOD INGREDIENTS AND THEIR BENEFITS

- avocado—rich in vitamins and oil; beneficial for dry and sensitive skin
- cucumber—soothing and healing; commonly used as a mask or for eye pads
- eggs—egg whites tone and tighten the skin
- herbs—many herbs and teas such as chamomile are used for masks and compresses
- honey—hydrating, toning, and tightening effects
- oatmeal—used in face and body masks
- papaya—exfoliating with enzymatic properties; papaya enzyme peels are popular
- potatoes—used for oily skin or to reduce puffiness in the eye area
- yogurt—cleansing and mildly astringent

- *aromatic:* lavender, mint, rose, orange, eucalyptus
- *antiseptic:* peppermint, tea tree, clove
- *astringent:* comfrey root, witch hazel, alum root, lemon
- *stimulating:* eucalyptus, wintergreen, spearmint
- *calming:* comfrey root (allantoin), chamomile (azulene), almond
- *cleansing:* lemongrass, aloe
- *healing:* chamomile, comfrey, aloe
- *moisturizing:* rose, chamomile

AROMATHERAPY

Aromatherapy is an ancient healing practice. Essential oils and aromas from plants are used to treat the body, mind, and spirit (Figure 12–9 A,B). These plant components have medicinal and healing properties. The practice is used therapeutically for physical ailments and for mental balancing. Essential oils can affect the brain and emotions. The psychological benefits from essential oils depend on the oil chosen. Aromatherapy incorporated in esthetic services can make a treatment even more relaxing and effective.

FYI

A necessary book for estheticians to have on hand is an ingredients dictionary, which lists the properties of hundreds of natural and synthetic ingredients. One example is Milady's Skin Care and Cosmetic Ingredients Dictionary.

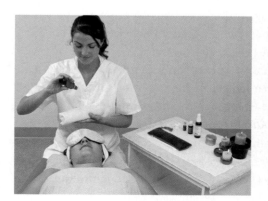
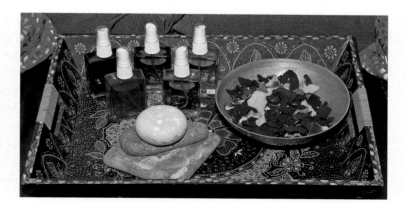

Figure 12–9 A,B Aromatherapy is used to treat the body, mind, and spirit.

To retain the plant's natural living properties, it must be extracted properly. Synthetically produced oils do not have the therapeutic value that natural oils retain. **Phytotherapy** is the use of plant extracts for therapeutic benefits. The different parts of the plants used for making products from oils and essences are the roots, bark, stem, seeds, and flowers. The extraction process can be expensive, and the way essences are extracted determines their strength and quality.

Aromatherapy, a form of phytotherapy, must be used with caution. The oils are powerful and can irritate the skin or the senses if overused. One or two drops of a pure oil are usually enough. Some people are allergic to certain fragrances, and a wonderful facial could turn into an unpleasant experience if that oil is used. Study aromatherapy and the contraindications before using oils on clients.

The Olfactory System

The body's **olfactory system** gives us our sense of smell, which is the strongest of the five senses. Scents have a strong effect on our reactions to places, products, and other people. Memories are also brought on by familiar scents. Aromatherapy scents can affect us because of the sensitive olfactory system. Fragrances are a large part of our everyday life, from food scents to our perfume. Notice how fragrance influences our moods and how much more relaxed we are when the room diffuses the scent of a favorite candle. Different blends have different effects, both physically and mentally.

The benefits of aromatherapy oils for the skin are many. Oils can moisturize, stimulate, cleanse, soothe, and nourish. Plant extracts, teas, flowers, and fruits have therapeutic value when applied as compresses, masks, sprays, oils, or lotions.

Essential oils can be used in a variety of ways. Lighting a cinnamon candle in the winter can give the salon a cozy feeling, cheering up both clients and the staff. You can use a spray bottle to diffuse well-diluted essential oils in the treatment room, or spray it on the sheets and towels. You can create your own aromatherapy massage oil by adding a few drops of essential oil to a massage oil, cream, or lotion.

FREE RADICALS

Antioxidants are included in many skin care formulas designed to combat **free radicals.** Free radicals are aggressive, unstable, oxygen-containing molecules. They have lost an electron and need to steal other electrons from other molecules, thereby damaging the cells they steal from.

Free radicals are "super" oxidizers that not only cause an oxidation reaction but also produce a new free radical in the process. Normal oxidation deactivates the oxidizer and stops the reaction from continuing, but the oxidation reaction caused by free radicals continues in a chain reaction that can go on forever. One free radical can oxidize millions of other compounds.

Free radicals damage cell membranes and normal cellular metabolism systems. They can also damage DNA and RNA, and they contribute to the hardening of collagen and elastin cells. This all leads to premature aging and increases skin sensitivity, irritation, age spots, and dryness.

> **CAUTION!**
>
> Essential oils are powerful. To prevent allergic reactions, they should be used with caution and only after proper training.

Antioxidants

Antiaging products and treatments are a main focus of the skin care industry. Antioxidants are one of the most effective treatments for the skin. Antioxidants are vitamins, amino acids, and other natural substances that neutralize the damaging effects of free radicals and help skin cope with the damaging effects of environmental influences. Vitamins C, E, and A; minerals; green tea; and grapeseed extract are all examples of antioxidants that help protect the body from free radicals. Aging or sun-damaged skin needs antioxidants topically and orally.

Antioxidants are also used to stabilize skin care products by preventing oxidation that causes a product to turn rancid and spoil. Antioxidants play a vital role in maintaining the quality, integrity, and safety of cosmetic products. Typical cosmetic antioxidants include reducing agents and free radical scavengers.

Here are some of the most widely used antioxidants:

- **Vitamin C** (L-ascorbic acid) is a water-soluble antioxidant. It strengthens the white blood cells and immune system and is essential for producing collagen.
- **Ester Vitamin C,** also called **Ester C** joined by a chemical ester bond with a fatty acid derived from palm oil (palmitic acid). It is oil soluble and is absorbed into the skin much more easily than are water-soluble ingredients. It is highly stable and keeps its effectiveness when mixed with other ingredients. Vitamin C ester stimulates fibroblasts, the cells that produce collagen and elastin.
- Alpha lipoic acid is a natural molecule found in every cell in the body. It is a powerful antioxidant and is soluble in water and oil. This antioxidant increases cellular metabolism and the effects of other antioxidants. Alpha lipoic acid is also anti-inflammatory and reduces redness.
- **DMAE (dimethylaminoethanol)** is an antioxidant that stabilizes cell membranes. It also boosts the effects of other antioxidants. DMAE increases chemicals that control muscle tone, thus improving the appearance of sagging skin.

A combination of alpha lipoic acid, vitamin C ester, DMAE, and glycolic acid is one of the most effective formulas to combat premature aging. Topical ingredients need to have high-tech delivery systems to carry or deliver the ingredients effectively into the skin.

Antioxidants can help prevent wrinkles, promote skin healing, and reduce the formation of scar tissue (pre- and post-surgery). Vitamins A and E (fat soluble) protect the phospholipid structure of the cell membrane. Vitamin C (water soluble) guards the inside of cells and DNA.

MATURE SKIN

In addition to peptides and other antioxidants, the following ingredients are proven to have a positive effect on mature skin and rosacea:

- green tea
- dipotassium glycyrrhizate (licorice root)
- squalane oil (vegetable oil from green olives)—rich in vitamins A, D, and E

- seaweed
- chamomile
- micronized vitamin E
- panthenol—vitamin B_5
- allantoin
- guarana (from the Amazon, an anti-inflammatory and decongestant)
- rose essential oil

Green tea (from China and Japan) is an excellent everyday source of help for microcirculation problems. It contains polyphenols (strong antioxidants); essential oils; salts; calcium; potassium; manganese; copper; zinc; fluoride; vitamins A, B, and C; and caffeine. It is one of the best antioxidants available and provides effective lipid protection. Green tea is an anti-irritant and anti-bacterial and provides UV protection.

Licorice root is 50 to 100 times sweeter than sugar and contains sugar, flavonoids (found in plants with yellow pigment), estrogens, amino acids, and polysaccharides. It is anti-inflammatory and a natural replacement for hydrocortisone (used to reduce rashes and redness). Licorice root also inhibits histamine release in allergic reactions. An antioxidant, licorice root lightens skin because it inhibits tyrosinaze activity.

When working with mature skin, estheticians would be wise to inform their clients of the cause of the changes to their skin. Knowledge of hormone replacement, diet, and lifestyle influences is useful. Suggest home-care products suitable for clients' needs, and use care when selecting treatments. Many ingredients are now available to support the needs of mature skin.

PRODUCT SELECTION

All products are formulated for different skin types and conditions. A product for dry skin contains ingredients to nourish dry skin. A product for oily skin is designed to treat the oiliness. The most important step in recommending products is determining which ingredients are best for an individual's needs. Learning about ingredients is necessary, and it takes time. Before applying a product, be sure to ask the client discreetly about any allergies he or she may have. No matter what the skin type, using the correct ingredients and following the proper steps in a home-care routine are essential for healthy skin.

Most facial skin care products (Figure 12–10) can be grouped into the following main categories:

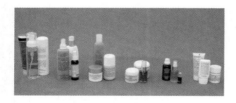

Figure 12–10 A variety of facial products.

- cleansers
- toners
- exfoliants
- masks
- hydrators and moisturizers
- serums and ampoules
- sunscreens

Cleansers

Cleansers come in many forms and should be used twice a day as the first step in a skin care routine. Cleansers that rinse clean with water and do not strip the skin's natural acid mantle are the best choices. Different skin types require different ingredients to achieve this balance. All cleansers should leave the skin pH-balanced. Soap is not usually recommended; it can leave a film on the skin and can be quite alkaline, causing dryness and other problems.

Cleanser Benefits

Skin cleansers have the following benefits:
- Cleansers dissolve makeup and dirt to keep pores clean and prepare the skin for other products.
- Cleansers may have emollients that soften dry skin.
- Cleansers may contain ingredients to counteract various skin problems.
- Additional ingredients can help certain skin conditions such as sensitivity, dehydration, or capillary problems.

Types of Cleansers

Cleansers for all skin types and conditions come in three basic forms: gels, lotions, and creams. All products are unique and depend on the ingredients in that particular product. Keep this in mind when reading about each product category. These are general categories, not absolutes.

A *cleansing gel* is a detergent-type "foaming" cleanser with a neutral or slightly acidic pH. Foaming cleansers are designed to dissolve more oil. Many people are accustomed to the foaming type of bar soap and want that "squeaky clean" feeling. Gels leave the skin feeling clean, but often a little tight. Clients with oily or combination skin like these foamy cleansers.

For acne-prone skin, an antimicrobial agent may be added to kill bacteria. Recommend gel cleansers with caution because they can dry out the skin. This often leads to irritation, stimulates an overproduction of oil in the skin, and can exacerbate acne.

A *cleansing lotion* is a water-based emulsion for normal and combination skin. For dry skin, "milky" lotion cleansers containing more oils or emollients that soften the skin are recommended. These cleansers do not strip the skin's natural oil or pH balance. Additional ingredients can be added to cleansers to suit certain skin conditions such as sensitivity, dehydration, or capillary problems.

A *cleansing cream* is a water-in-oil emulsion used primarily to dissolve makeup and dirt. It is suitable for very dry and mature skin. Cleansing creams are heavier than cleansing lotions. Actors and other performers use these products to remove heavy stage makeup. Remember that like dissolves like, so oil dissolves oil. Cleansing cream should be removed with a sponge or a soft cloth; otherwise, a residue may be left on the skin. Cleansing creams may be followed by a toner or another cleanser to remove any residue.

Makeup removers are special cleansers designed primarily to remove eye makeup or heavier makeup. Makeup removers are generally oil based. Most cleansers will remove makeup without needing an additional product. Some makeup removers need to be rinsed off because they can leave a residue on the skin or in the eye area.

Toners

Toner Benefits

Toners, fresheners, tonics, and astringents are all essentially the same type of product; these terms are sometimes used interchangeably. Here are some benefits of using toners.

- Toners and similar products remove residue left behind by cleansers or other products.
- Fresheners restore the skin's natural pH after cleansing, and they hydrate the skin.
- Astringents have a temporary tightening effect on both the skin and follicle openings.
- Some products can help certain skin conditions, depending on the ingredients.

Types of Toners

Toners, fresheners, and astringents have different properties and vary in alcohol content. These are watery liquids, used after cleansing in the skin care routine and generally before a moisturizer is applied. Toners can be applied to the face with a cotton pad or can be sprayed directly onto the skin.

- **Fresheners,** or skin freshening lotions, often have the lowest alcohol content and are beneficial for dry and mature skin as well as for sensitive skin.
- **Toners** usually have a higher alcohol content and are designed for use on normal and combination skin. They tone, or tighten, the skin.
- **Astringents** may have the highest alcohol content and are used for oily and acne-prone skin. They help oily and acneic conditions and remove excess oil on the skin, but some are too drying and should be used carefully or with caution.

Exfoliants

Exfoliation Benefits (Mechanical or Chemical)

Removing dead epidermal cells benefits the skin in many ways:

- Skin texture is smoother and softer.
- Follicle openings are cleaner.
- Deep pore cleansing and extraction are easier.
- The cell turnover rate is increased, bringing new cells to the surface more rapidly.
- The skin's ability to retain moisture and lipids is improved.
- Product penetration is improved, and delivery of ingredients into the epidermis is more effective.
- Blood flow and circulation are stimulated.
- Makeup application is smoother and more even.

Exfoliation is beneficial for the following conditions:

- oily, clogged skin with blackheads, whiteheads, and minor acne breakouts
- dry or dehydrated skin with cell buildup, flaking, and a tight, dry surface
- dull, lifeless-looking skin (this skin condition actually has a tremendous buildup of dead cells that produces a slight gray color on the surface)

The term *exfoliation* refers to the peeling or sloughing of the horny (outer) layer of the skin, also known as the corneum. **Exfoliants** (eks-FOH-lee-unts) are ingredients that exfoliate the skin. Many different types of peeling and exfoliation treatments are available, ranging from brushing treatments and light enzyme peels to strong surgical peels that can be administered only by dermatologists and plastic surgeons.

Alpha hydroxy acids (AHAs), gentle scrubs, and peeling creams all exfoliate dead skin cells that clog pores. Exfoliating the skin can treat a variety of skin problems and is necessary for healthy skin.

Use caution when exfoliating the skin. It is important to note that the esthetician's domain is the superficial epidermis, not treatments that involve the live layers of the skin below the epidermis. There are two basic types of exfoliation treatments: mechanical and chemical.

Mechanical Exfoliants

Mechanical exfoliation is a method of physically rubbing dead cells off of the skin. Examples of mechanical peeling treatments include granular scrubs, such as those made with almond meal or jojoba beads, or treatments that use a brushing machine. The movement of the brushes or scrubs removes cells from the surface of the corneum.

Granular scrubs are usually used after cleansing from one to two times per week and are rinsed with water. Frequency of use depends on the skin conditions. Exfoliation should be avoided if someone has sensitive or irritated skin. Microdermabrasion, a strong type of mechanical exfoliation, is covered in Chapter 18, "Advanced Topics and Treatments."

Chemical Exfoliants

In **chemical exfoliation,** dead skin cells and the intercellular "glue" that holds them together (desmosomes), are dissolved by chemical agents such as AHAs (Figure 12–11). AHAs penetrate into the skin and dissolve the intercellular glue.

> **CAUTION!**
>
> As a student, you should always receive hands-on training from your instructor before attempting exfoliation procedures. Exfoliation can cause irritation and damage to the skin and capillaries if overused or used incorrectly.

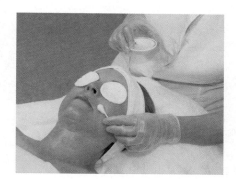

Figure 12–11 Chemical exfoliation with AHAs.

> **CAUTION!**
>
> To avoid damaging skin, do not use brushing machines, scrubs, or any harsh mechanical peeling techniques on these skin conditions:
> - sensitive skin
> - skin with many visible capillaries
> - thin skin that reddens easily
> - older skin that is thin and bruises easily
> - acne-prone skin with inflamed papules and pustules
> - skin being medically treated with tretinoin (retinoic acid or Retin-A®), Accutane,® azelaic acid, adapalene (Differin®), alpha hydroxy acids (AHAs), or salicylic acid (found in many common skin products)

Unlike AHAs, enzymes digest only the dead cells on the surface. Superficial enzyme peels are very gentle. You might consider using them when mechanical exfoliation is not appropriate. AHAs are much stronger peels than enzymes.

Enzyme Peels. Enzyme peels involve the use of keratolytic enzymes, which help speed up the breakdown of keratin, the protein in skin. One enzyme often used is papain, which is derived from the papaya. Another frequently used enzyme is pancreatin (derived from beef by-products). Pineapple, or bromelain, is another good enzyme.

There are two basic types of enzyme peels. The most popular type of enzyme peel uses a powdered form of enzyme that is either mixed by the esthetician with warm water or can be purchased premixed in a base similar to a treatment mask. Other ingredients are combined in the peel formula to address different skin types and conditions. This type of enzyme treatment generally produces a more even peeling of the cell buildup and helps to dilate the follicle openings slightly.

A second type of enzyme peel is in a cream form that is applied and then massaged or "rolled" off the skin. This cream may contain paraffin or oatmeal. Products of this type are often called **gommage** (French: go-MAHJ). This treatment is actually a combination of an enzyme and a mechanical peeling (Figure 12–12).

The enzyme peel is an exfoliating treatment for clients who are Retin-A users and for "ultrasensitive" clients who have skin that is too sensitive for glycolic acid peels. Many acne clients (when first starting treatments) fall into this category. These peels digest keratinized epidermal cells, dislodge "sebaceous filament" (sebum and other cellular wastes accumulated in the follicles), prepare the skin for extraction, and help fade and even out superficial irregular skin tone.

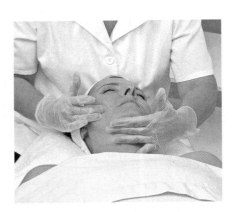

Figure 12–12 Gommage is used for exfoliation.

Masks

Mask Benefits

Masks and **packs** provide many benefits for the skin. Depending on their ingredients, they can do the following:

- tighten and tone the skin
- draw impurities out of the pores
- clear up blemishes
- hydrate
- nourish
- calm and soothe
- rejuvenate the skin
- brighten the complexion

Types of Masks

A good **mask** can do wonders for the skin, and like most beauty treatments, the benefits of masks have been known for thousands of years. Mask ingredients include herbs, vitamins, and oils, which can be combined in clay, seaweed, or hydrating bases. Masks come in powder form or

Did You Know

THE INFLAMMATION CASCADE

Inflammation can be caused by too much irritation from exfoliation or other factors and leads to premature aging. Stimulating the body's histamine activity that reacts to irritants and allergens causes the enzyme collagenase to break down collagen, and the enzyme elastase to break down elastin. Natural hydrators in the skin, such as hyaluronic acid, are also lost when the skin is excessively irritated. Over-exfoliating can break down our natural protection and impede normal cellular functions. This is an example of "too much of a good thing."

premixed. Masks allow an esthetician to treat a variety of skin conditions at the same time.

There are two types of mask categories: *setting and non-setting.* Setting masks harden or dry, and non-setting masks do not dry or "set up."

Masks that harden often include setting ingredients, which dry and provide a complete barrier on top of the skin. Ingredients such as clay, alginate, paraffin wax, and gypsum (a kind of plaster) generally account for this effect. Keep in mind that some of these ingredients do not always set up, depending on the formulation and the purpose of the product.

Non-setting masks, such as cucumber or aloe, are designed to stay moist and are more hydrating. For home care, masks are usually applied once a week, after exfoliation for best results and penetration.

Non-Setting Masks. Also referred to as cream masks or gel masks, non-setting masks are not formulated to dry, but to nourish or treat the skin rather than deep-cleanse it. They remain soft and are highly beneficial for sensitive, couperose, aging, or dry skin because ingredients such as collagen, aloe, and seaweed have excellent hydrating properties.

Cream masks, which do not dry on the skin like clay masks do, are often used for dry skin. They often contain oils and emollients as well as humectants, and they have a strong moisturizing effect.

Gel masks can be used for sensitive or dehydrated skin. They often contain hydrators and soothing ingredients and thus help plump surface cells with moisture, making the skin look more supple and hydrated.

Collagen masks are another great mask choice with many benefits, such as plumping and diminishing wrinkles.

Clay Masks. **Clay masks** draw impurities to the surface of the skin as the mask dries and tightens. Clay also stimulates circulation and temporarily contracts the pores of the skin. These masks contain clay, kaolin, bentonite, or silica for their tightening and sebum-absorbing effects. Stronger clay masks are used on oily and combination skin. Clay-based masks with sulfur have healing and antiseptic properties and have a beneficial effect on acne.

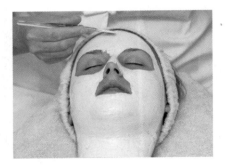

Figure 12–13 Applying a clay mask.

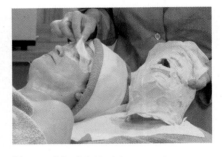

Figure 12–14 Modelage mask.

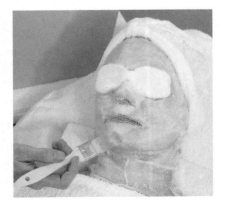

Figure 12–15 The paraffin wax mask.

Clay masks are applied with a mask brush or the fingers and are allowed to set for about 10 minutes (Figure 12–13). After they are fully dried, clay masks are often softened with towels or steam and then removed with cotton pads or towels.

Algae and Seaweed Masks. Alginate masks (AL-jun-ate) are often seaweed based. They come in powder form and are mixed with water or sometimes serums. After mixing, they are quickly applied to the face and then dry to form a rubberized texture. A treatment cream or serum is generally applied under them. The alginate mask forms a seal that encourages the skin's absorption of the serum or cream underneath. These masks are generally used only in the salon, not at home.

Algae (derived from seaweed) is also used in other types of masks and products for its moisturizing properties, ability to smooth wrinkles, and detoxification. Seaweed is high in mineral content and therapeutic ingredients.

Modelage Masks. **Modelage masks** (MA-dell-ahj), also known as thermal masks, contain special crystals of gypsum, a plaster-like ingredient. Modelage masks are used with nourishing products underneath. When mixed with water immediately before application and applied about 1/4 inch (.6 cm) thick, the modelage mask hardens (Figure 12–14). The chemical reaction that occurs when the plaster and the crystals mix with water produces a gradually increasing temperature that reaches approximately 105°F. Left on the skin, the mask gradually cools. The setting time for modelage masks is approximately 20 minutes.

Like other heat-creating treatments that increase circulation, modelage masks are very beneficial for dry, mature skin or dull-looking skin. This type of mask is not typically recommended for use on sensitive skin, skin with capillary problems, oily skin, or skin with blemishes. Massage is not recommended either before or after a modelage mask application, because blood circulation will already be increased from the mask. These masks can become heavy on the face and should not be applied to the lower neck or to clients who suffer from claustrophobia.

Paraffin Wax Masks. **Paraffin wax masks** are used to warm the skin and promote penetration of ingredients deeper into the skin through the heat trapped under the paraffin. The heat increases blood circulation and is beneficial for dry, mature skin or skin that is dull and lifeless. It has a plumping and softening effect.

Paraffin wax masks are specially prepared facial masks containing paraffin and other beneficial ingredients. They are melted at a little more than body temperature before application. When applied, the paraffin quickly cools to a lukewarm temperature and hardens to a candle-like consistency (Figure 12–15). Paraffin masks are used with a treatment cream because the paraffin, which has no treatment properties of its own, allows for deeper penetration of the cream's ingredients into the skin. The paraffin mask procedure is presented in Chapter 14, "Basic Facials."

Custom-Designed Masks. Homemade masks derived from fresh fruits, vegetables, milk, yogurt, or eggs have been used for years. Ingredients such as honey and almond meal or oatmeal can be mixed with milk into a paste for use as a mask. These masks are generally beneficial unless the person is allergic to a particular substance. Custom-designed masks can be fun to experiment with, but they are usually done at home rather than in a professional setting. Sanitation, regulations, and convenience precludes the use of homemade masks in the salon. Additionally, products not packaged by the manufacturer may not be covered under your employer's insurance. While problems are unlikely, there are insurance liability issues about any skin reactions to homemade products.

A client may ask about homemade products. It is important for estheticians to be familiar with these ingredients and to know why the quality of prepackaged professional products gives more predictable results. However, some product lines are designed to custom-blend products and add ingredients to various products. This is a good way to customize treatments.

> **CAUTION!**
>
> Paraffin and thermal masks are not recommended for use on sensitive skin, skin with capillary problems, oily skin, or skin with blemishes. These masks are designed for dry and mature skin; the heat is too stimulating for other skin conditions and may cause redness or irritation.

Serums and Ampoules

Serums and ampoules are concentrated and specialized ingredients designed for effective penetration into the skin. These products are applied under a moisturizer or massage cream.

Types of Serums and Ampoules

Serums (SIR-ums) are concentrated ingredients that target specific skin conditions. Serums are chemically formulated with smaller molecules that are able to penetrate further into the skin and thus are extremely effective. Serums are thin liquids made with performance ingredients such as vitamins, lipids, and antioxidants.

Ampoules (AM-pyools) are small, sealed vials containing a single application of highly concentrated extracts in a water or oil base. They are designed for a wide variety of skin types and problems. The advantage of ampoules is that they deliver highly concentrated performance ingredients in a premeasured amount. The extract is applied to the client's face with light massage movements until it has been completely absorbed.

Eye Creams
Benefits

Eye creams have several benefits, including the following:
- protecting thin, delicate tissue
- firming
- reducing lines
- decreasing puffiness

Types of Eye Creams

Eye creams are usually thicker to protect thin, delicate tissue. Products made for the eye area include ingredients for firming and reducing lines. Eye masks, tea bags, or compresses are beneficial for the eye area and can be used in facial treatments. Products formulated for the eye area are similar to concentrated specialty creams.

Lip Treatments

Lip treatments include moisturizing balms and products. Some contain collagen derivatives to plump up the lips. Exfoliating and healing ingredients are also used in lip conditioners.

Moisturizers and Hydrators

Benefits

The following are some benefits of using moisturizers and hydrators:
- protecting skin from the elements
- nourishing skin through ingredients
- balancing oil–water content of skin
- treating various skin conditions such as redness, aging, or dryness

Types of Moisturizers

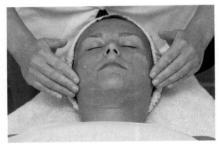

Figure 12–16 Applying a moisturizer.

Moisturizers are products formulated to add moisture to the skin. Lotions, hydrators, and creams are all referred to as moisturizers, the products we put on the skin twice a day after cleansing to protect and nourish it. They are applied at the end of the facial and are ideal for daily use as a day cream or makeup base. *Moisturizer* is a good general term to use with clients, even though technically there are differences in the products. Moisturizers are available for various skin types and conditions, from acne-prone skin to dry and mature skin (Figure 12–16).

The performance ingredients of moisturizers depend on the skin type they are intended for. Treatment creams and massage lotions are also different forms of moisturizers. Moisturizers usually contain an ingredient that helps retain water within the surface layers of the skin. Hydrators are formulated with humectants that attract water to the skin.

Oil-based moisturizers contain emollients and are heavier and occlusive, designed to protect the surface and trap water under the cream. It is important to use a moisturizer to hydrate and balance the oil–water moisture content of the skin. Water-based moisturizers are lighter emulsions for combination to oily skin that are absorbed quickly and leave no residue on the skin's surface. Even oily skin needs hydration and protection from a hydrator; if not hydrated, this skin type will try to overcompensate for dryness and produce more oil, or it will become dehydrated.

A valuable ingredient included in some day creams is sunscreen. Sunscreen guards against premature aging of the skin and helps prevent skin cancer. These creams are good only for incidental sun exposure. For direct sun exposure, stronger sunscreens must be used and reapplied often.

Treatment Creams. Treatment creams, also referred to as nourishing creams, are designed to moisturize and condition the skin—especially during sleep, when normal tissue repair is taking place. Treatment creams are often heavier in consistency and texture than moisturizers are, and they contain more emollient and active ingredients. However, the amount of emollient in a treatment cream depends on the skin type it is designed for. Treatment creams for oily skin usually have very little or no emollient.

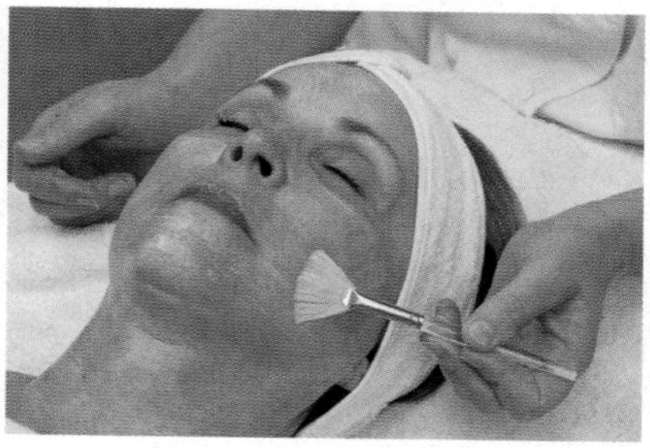

Massage Creams. Massage creams, lotions, or oils have a variety of bases and ingredients. These are designed to provide slip (gliding ability) for massage while also nourishing and treating skin conditions. Massage lotions are also blended with aromatherapy oils to use during the treatment (Figure 12–17). Choose the appropriate massage blend for the skin type.

Figure 12–17 Applying massage cream.

Sunscreens

Daily sunscreen is imperative to protect skin from UV rays. An important part of an esthetician's job is to recommend sunscreen. Estheticians should stress to clients that sun exposure leads to skin cancer as well as to aging, hyperpigmentation, capillary damage, free radical damage, and collagen and elastin deterioration. Daily sunscreen can be in moisturizer form and comes in all weights and formulas. Oil-free, light lotions that will not clog pores are available for oily skin.

Sunscreen Ingredients

UVA rays are longer rays that cause aging. UVB rays are shorter rays that cause sunburns. Full-spectrum sunscreens protect the skin from both UVA and UVB rays. Sunscreens absorb or reflect ultraviolet rays. Sunscreens that protect the skin from UVB rays include octyl salicylate, octyl methoxycinnamate, oxybenzone, octylhomosalate, and titanium dioxide. Some of the sunscreens that protect the skin from UVA rays are oxybenzone, avobenzone, benzophenone-3, zinc oxide, and butyl methoxydibenzoylmethane.

SPF refers to the sun protection factor in sunscreens. An SPF 2 sunscreen blocks 50 percent of UVB rays, allowing you to stay in the sun twice as long as you could with no sun protection. Increasing the SPF increases the protection. An SPF 15 sunscreen blocks 93.3 percent of UVB rays; and an SPF 30 sunscreen blocks 96.9 percent of UVB rays. But notice that doubling the SPF from 15 to 30 does not double the protection. In this case it increases UVB protection by only 3.6 percent, and at higher SPFs the increase is even less. Although doubling the SPF does not double the protection, the higher SPF increases the potential for sensitivity due to the increase in the concentration of active ingredients.

Self-Tanners

Self-tanning lotions are formulated with dihydroxyacetone (DHA), an ingredient that reacts with the proteins (keratin) on the surface cells of the skin and turns them darker. Most self-tanners have no sunscreen protection; sunscreen should still be applied. Looking tan does not mean the skin has protection from sunburns or photoaging.

Here's a Tip

With all product usage, choose the right formulas for your client's skin. Be sure to apply the appropriate amount of product; using too much can have adverse affects on the skin and wastes money on products.

ACTIVITY

Choose products and ingredients for different skin types and conditions according to your product line. Write in ingredients and product types you think you would use. Use the ingredient tables in this chapter or a cosmetic ingredients dictionary to research your products.

PRODUCT TYPE AND INGREDIENTS FOR DIFFERENT SKIN TYPES AND CONDITIONS	MATURE	SENSITIVE	DRY	NORMAL	COMBO	OILY	ACNE
cleansers	(Example: cleansing cream with antioxidants)						
exfoliants		enzyme peel					
masks	collagen						
massage lotions							
additives and oils		Calming— chamomile					
toners							
serums							
moisturizers and sunscreen	ceramides						
eye and lip care products							

HOME-CARE PRODUCTS

Products the client can use at home are as important as those you use during the facial. The same principles that you use in determining products for treatments apply here. Give clients simple, precise instructions as to how and when to use the product. It is a good idea to give a home-care sheet to those clients who may not remember what you told them. Your product line and specific treatments will determine what to recommend. Explaining instructions, precautions, and realistic expectations will be beneficial to both you and your clients.

Use Table 12–5 as a general home-care guideline for clients. Giving out samples saves money for you and your clients: they help you determine what works best, and your clients will appreciate being able to try a product

Table 12–5

CLIENT HOME-CARE INSTRUCTION SHEET. WRITE IN RECOMMENDATIONS FOR CLIENTS FROM THE PRODUCT LINE YOU CARRY. MOST PRODUCT COMPANIES PROVIDE HOME-CARE SHEETS TO GIVE OUT TO CLIENTS			
DAY	**NIGHT**	**WEEKLY**	**PRODUCT RECOMMENDATIONS**
1. Cleanser	1. Cleanser	1. Cleanser	
2. Toner	2. Toner	2. Exfoliation—1–2×/week	
3. Serums/eye cream	3. Serums/eye cream	3. Masks 1–2×/week	
4. Moisturizer	4. Moisturizer	4. Toner	
5. Sunscreen		5. Serums/eye cream	
		6. Moisturizer	

without investing a lot of money. A product guarantee and refund policy will depend on the place where you work. Satisfied clients are good for business and will be loyal if you take care of them.

Retail sales are not just about making money. You are helping your clients take care of their skin. When you are familiar with clients' needs and their skin, as well as the various ingredients and products, you are in the best position to recommend products. Professional products sold only by licensed professionals (estheticians) are generally better formulated for individual needs. While professional products may cost more initially, they are usually more effective due to a higher concentration of performance ingredients—and this means less product is needed. With proper products chosen just for them, clients will see better results in their home care. This saves your clients money in the long run because they will avoid wasting money in trying different products that might not be suited to their individual needs (Figure 12–18).

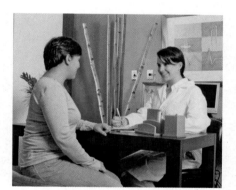

Figure 12–18 The home-care consultation.

CHOOSING A PRODUCT LINE

Deciding what product lines to use and retail can be one of the biggest business decisions an esthetician can make. Whether a technician is self-employed or involved in choosing product lines for a salon owner, the product line and retail sales affect the success of the business. If the staff like the product and use it at home, it will be easy to use in treatments. It will also be easier to promote and sell.

When choosing a product line, take into consideration the following selling points:
* Are the ingredients high quality and beneficial?
* Are the products versatile—that is, effective for all skin types?
* Are the wholesale cost and the retail pricing affordable?
* Is the product name recognizable and reputable? Many clients choose a product based on its name and how it is marketed.
* How are the products packaged?
* What fragrances are used?

Here's a Tip

To save time and be ready for the post-consultation, pull home-care products while the client is getting dressed after a facial.

Here's a Tip

A good way to determine product cost is to break down the costs into daily or weekly amounts. This gives clients a better idea of how affordable the product is and how much they are spending on the recommended products, which is usually not more than a cup of coffee per day.

- What can clients in your area afford?
- What support can you anticipate from the company or supplier? (The costs of samples and brochures, return policies, and marketing promotions affect your business.)
- What educational opportunities and training are provided by the supplier? These can help you become more knowledgeable and successful.

There are countless skin care ingredients and hundreds of product lines for the esthetician to choose from. Researching the different product options will help estheticians become familiar with these choices. Knowing the daily skin care steps for maintaining healthy skin is necessary in making product recommendations. Choosing the correct product formulas for clients is important to effectively and safely treat the skin. Understanding what ingredients do for the skin will make it easier to recommend and choose products. Ingredient and product technology is an exciting part of esthetics. It is an area demanding continuous attention and review, but it is also one of the most interesting aspects of the industry.

Product Prices and Costs

Pricing and costs of products are a consideration for both you and your client. Product costs can be expensive if you do not choose wisely. Generally, the markup for retail products is 100 percent, or doubled from the wholesaler cost. Let your client know why professional products available only from licensed estheticians cost more than those they can purchase over the counter. Consider the quality of the ingredients and the concentration of performance ingredients in the products when comparing prices. When comparing skin care product lines, determine what you and your clientele like. Use Table 12–6 to compare and rate product lines. Make a copy of the chart, or create your own and fill in the blanks while sampling and testing different products.

Table 12–6

CHART FOR COMPARING AND RATING PRODUCT LINES

Use your own rating system—for example, rate products from 1 to 5 or from excellent to fair.

PRODUCT LINE	CLEANSER	TONER	MOISTURIZER	EXFOLIANT	MASK	OTHER
skin types						
main ingredients						
cost						
quality						
texture						
scent						
color						
packaging						
overall rating						

REVIEW QUESTIONS

1. How does the FDA define *cosmetics*?

2. What is the difference between functional and performance ingredients?

3. What functions does water serve in cosmetic formulations?

4. What are emollients?

5. What are the two basic categories of oils used in skin care products?

6. Describe three emollients other than oil that are used in skin care products.

7. Define *comedogenicity*.

8. What are essential oils?

9. Why are preservatives necessary in cosmetic products?

10. What is the function of humectants in skin care products?

11. Name and describe four products that slow the appearance of aging in the skin.

12. What are the two basic types of sunscreen products?

13. What is the FDA's role in the regulation of cosmetic products?

14. Describe the symptoms of an allergic reaction to cosmetic products.

15. What two main product components cause the most allergic reactions?

16. Give five examples of antioxidant ingredients.

17. List four ingredients beneficial for mature or aging skin.

18. List two ingredients beneficial for acne.

19. List two ingredients beneficial for sensitive skin.

20. What are the main categories of professional skin care products?

21. What are the benefits of astringents and toners?

22. List the two categories of exfoliants. Give examples of each type, and explain what they do.

23. What are the benefits of exfoliation?

24. List the benefits of a mask.

25. What is the difference between a physical sunscreen and a chemical sunscreen?

26. What does *SPF* refer to?

27. Why is sunscreen important?

28. List the steps in a good daily skin care routine.

29. Why are moisturizers necessary?

30. What considerations are important in choosing product lines?

CHAPTER GLOSSARY

AHAs (alpha hydroxy acids): AHAs are naturally-occuring mild acids; glycolic, lactic, malic, and tartaric acid. AHAs exfoliate by loosening the bonds between dead corneum cells and dissolve the intercellular cement. Acids also stimulate cell renewal.

alcohol: antiseptic and solvent used in perfumes, lotions, and astringents. SD alcohol is a special denatured ethyl alcohol, also known as *ethanol.*

algae: derived from minerals and phytohormones; remineralizes and revitalizes the skin.

allantoin: used in cold cream, hand lotion, hair lotion, aftershave, and other skin-soothing cosmetics because of its ability to help heal wounds and skin ulcers and to stimulate the growth of healthy tissue.

aloe vera: the most popular botanical used in cosmetic formulations; emollient and film-forming gum resin with hydrating, softening, healing, antimicrobial, and anti-inflammatory properties.

alum: compound made of aluminum, potassium, or ammonium sulfate with strong astringent action.

ampoules: small, sealed vials containing a single application of highly concentrated extracts in a water or oil base.

anhydrous: describes products that do not contain any water.

antioxidants: free radical scavengers; vitamins, and ingredients. Antioxidants also inhibit oxidation. They are used both to help the condition of the skin and to stop the oxidation that causes products to turn rancid and spoil.

aromatherapy: the therapeutic use of plant aromas and essential oils for beauty and health treatment purposes.

astringents: liquids that help remove excess oil on the skin.

azulene: derived from the chamomile plant and characterized by its deep blue color; has anti-inflammatory and soothing properties.

benzyl peroxide: drying ingredient with antibacterial properties commonly used for blemishes and acne.

beta-glucans: ingredients used in antiaging cosmetics to help reduce the appearance of fine lines and wrinkles by stimulating the formation of collagen.

BHAs (beta hydroxy acids): BHAs are exfoliating organic acids; salicylic and citric acids. BHAs are milder than AHAs. BHAs dissolve oil and are beneficial for oily skin.

binders: substances such as glycerin that bind, or hold, products together.

botanicals: ingredients derived from plants.

calendula: anti-inflammatory plant extract.

carbomers: ingredients used to thicken creams; frequently used in gel products.

carrot: rich in vitamin A, commonly derived from seeds and as an oil; also used as product coloring.

ceramides: lipid materials that are a natural part of the intercellular cement.

certified colors: inorganic color agents also known as metal salts; listed on ingredient labels as D&C (drug and cosmetic).

chamomile: plant extract with calming and soothing properties.

chelating agent: a chemical added to cosmetics to improve the efficiency of the preservative.

chemical exfoliation: chemical agent that dissolves dead skin cells.

clay masks: masks that draw impurities to the surface of the skin as they dry and tighten.

cleansers: soaps and detergents that clean the skin. Alkalines and fatty acids of oils or soaps are combined to make soaps.

coenzyme Q10: powerful antioxidant that protects and revitalizes skin cells.

collagen: typically, a long-chain molecular protein that lies on the top of the skin and binds water, also plumps the surface of the skin and prevents water loss. A topical protein derived from animals or synthetically manufactured. Collagen is the protein fiber in the dermis.

colorants: substances such as vegetable, pigment, or mineral dyes that give products color.

comedogenicity: tendency of any topical substance to cause or to worsen a buildup in the follicle, leading to the development of a comedo (blackhead).

cosmeceuticals: products intended to improve the skin's health and appearance.

cosmetics: as defined by the FDA, "articles that are intended to be rubbed, poured, sprinkled or otherwise applied to the human body or any part thereof for cleansing, beautifying, promoting attractiveness or altering the appearance."

delivery systems: chemical systems that deliver ingredients to specific tissues of the epidermis.

detergents: type of surfactant used as cleansers in skin care products.

DMAE (dimethylaminoethanol): antioxidant that stabilizes cell membranes and boosts the effect of other antioxidants.

echinacea (purple coneflower): prevents infection and has healing properties. Used internally to support the immune system.

emollients: ingredients that lubricate, moisturize, and prevent water loss.

emulsifiers: surfactants that cause oil and water to mix and form an emulsion.

enzyme peels: enzyme products that dissolve keratin proteins (dead skin cells) and exfoliate the skin.

essential oils: oils derived from herbs; have many different properties and effects on the skin and psyche.

exfoliants: mechanical and chemical products or processes used to exfoliate the skin.

exfoliation: the peeling or sloughing of the outer layer of skin.

fatty acids: lubricant ingredients derived from plant oils or animal fats.

fatty alcohols: fatty acids that have been exposed to hydrogen.

fatty esters: emollients produced from fatty acids and alcohols.

fragrances: these give products their scent.

free radicals: oxygen atoms or molecules with unpaired electrons that cause oxidation. They steal electrons from other molecules, which damages the other molecules.

fresheners: skin-freshening lotions with a low alcohol content.

functional ingredients: ingredients in cosmetic products that allow the products to spread, give them body and texture, and give them a specific form such as a lotion, cream, or gel.

glycerin: formed by a decomposition of oils or fats; excellent skin softener and humectant; very strong water binder.

glycoproteins: yeast cell derivatives that enhance cellular metabolism, which boosts oxygen uptake in the cell.

gommage: peeling cream that is rubbed off the skin.

grapeseed extract: powerful antioxidant with soothing properties.

CHAPTER GLOSSARY

green tea: powerful antioxidant and soothing agent. Antibacterial, anti-inflammatory, and a stimulant. Helpful for couperose skin.

healing agents: substances such as chamomile or aloe that help to heal the skin.

herbs: along with plant extracts, herbs contain phytohormones. Hundreds of different herbs are used in skin care products and cosmetics; they heal, stimulate, soothe, and moisturize.

horsechestnut: extract containing bioflavonoids; also known as vitamin P. Helps strengthen capillary walls; used for couperose areas or telangiectasia.

humectants: ingredients that attract water. Humectants draw moisture to the skin and soften its surface, diminishing lines caused by dryness. Glycerin is a humectant used in creams and lotions.

hyaluronic acid: hydrating fluids found in the skin; hydrophilic agent with water-binding properties.

hydrators: ingredients that attract water to the skin's surface; also known as *humectants* or *hydrophilic agents*.

jojoba: oil widely used in cosmetics; extracted from the beanlike seeds of the desert shrub. Used as a lubricant and noncomedogenic emollient and moisturizer.

kojic acid: skin-brightening agent.

lakes: the common term for certified colors.

lanolin: emollient with moisturizing properties; also an emulsifier with high water absorption capabilities.

lavender: all-purpose oil having many properties. Antiallergenic, anti-inflammatory, antiseptic, antibacterial, balancing, energizing, soothing, healing, and, conversely, stimulating.

licorice: anti-irritant used for sensitive skin.

lipids: fats or fatlike substances. Lipids help repair and protect the barrier function of the skin.

liposomes: closed lipid bilayer spheres that encapsulate ingredients, target their delivery to specific tissues of the skin, and control their release.

lubricants: coat the skin and reduce friction. Mineral oil is a lubricant.

mask: ingredients such as herbs, vitamins, and oils combined with clay, seaweed, or hydrating bases that treat the skin.

mechanical exfoliation: method of rubbing dead cells off of the skin.

methylparaben: one of the most frequently used preservatives because of its very low sensitizing potential. Combats bacteria and molds; noncomedogenic.

mineral oil: a lubricant derived from petroleum.

modelage masks: thermal heat masks.

moisturizers: products formulated to add moisture to the skin.

mucopolysaccharides: carbohydrate–lipid complexes that are also good water binders.

noncertified colors: colors that are organic, meaning they come from animal or plant extracts; they can also be natural mineral pigments.

oil soluble: compatible with oil.

olfactory system: gives us our sense of smell, which is the strongest of the five senses.

packs: cream masks or gel masks that nourish rather than deep-cleanse the skin.

papaya: natural enzyme used for exfoliation and in enzyme peels.

parabens: one of the most commonly used groups of preservatives in the cosmetic, pharmaceutical, and food industries; provide bacteriostatic and fungistatic activity against a diverse number of organisms.

paraffin wax masks: mask used to warm the skin and promote penetration of ingredients deeper into the skin through the heat trapped under the surface of the paraffin.

peptides: chains of amino acids used to treat wrinkles and elasticity.

performance ingredients: ingredients in cosmetic products that cause the actual changes in the appearance of the skin.

petroleum jelly: an occlusive agent that restores the barrier layer by holding in water. Used after laser surgery to protect the skin while healing.

phytotherapy: the use of plant extracts for therapeutic benefits.

pH adjusters: acids or alkalis (bases) used to adjust the pH of products.

polyglucans: ingredients derived from yeast cells that help strengthen the immune system and stimulate the metabolism; they are also hydrophilic and help preserve and protect collagen and elastin.

polymers: chemical compounds formed by a number of small molecules; advanced vehicles that release substances onto the skin's surface at a microscopically-controlled rate.

potassium hydroxide: a strong alkali used in soaps and creams.

preservatives: chemical agents that inhibit the growth of microorganisms in cosmetic formulations. These kill bacteria and prevent products from spoiling.

propylene glycol: a humectant often used in dry or sensitive skin moisturizers.

quaternium 15: an all-purpose preservative active against bacteria, mold, and yeast. It is probably the greatest formaldehyde releaser among cosmetic preservatives, causing dermatitis and allergies.

retinoic acid: a vitamin A derivative. It has demonstrated an ability to alter collagen synthesis and is used to treat acne and visible signs of aging. Side effects are irritation, photosensitivity, skin dryness, redness, and peeling.

retinol: a natural form of vitamin A, stimulates cell repair and helps to normalize skin cells by generating new cells.

rose: credited with moisturizing, astringent, tonic, and deodorant properties; found in the forms of rose extracts, oil, or water.

salicylic acid: a beta hydroxy acid with exfoliating and antiseptic properties; natural sources include sweet birch, willow bark, and wintergreen.

seaweed: seaweed derivatives such as algae have many nourishing properties. Specifically, seaweed is known for its humectant and moisturizing properties, vitamin content, metabolism stimulation and detoxification, and aiding skin firmness.

serums: concentrated liquid ingredients for the skin designed to penetrate and treat various skin conditions.

silicones: an oil that is chemically combined with silicon and oxygen and leaves a noncomedogenic, protective film on the surface of the skin.

sodium bicarbonate: baking soda; an alkaline inorganic salt used as a buffering agent, neutralizer and a pH adjuster.

solvent: substances that dissolve another substance to form a solution.

sorbitol: humectant that absorbs moisture from the air to prevent skin dryness.

sphingolipids: ceramides, or lipid material, that are a natural part of the intercellular cement. Glycosphingolipids and phospholipids are also natural lipids found in the barrier layer.

squalane: derived from olives; desensitizes and nourishes; an emollient.

squalene: originally from shark-liver oil; also occurs in small amounts in olive oil, wheat germ oil, and rice bran oil; also found in human sebum. A lubricant and perfume fixative.

sulfur: sulfur reduces oil-gland activity and dissolves the skin's surface layer of dry, dead cells. This ingredient is commonly used in acne products. It can cause allergic skin reactions in some sensitive people.

surfactants: surface active agents that reduce surface tension between the skin and the product to increase product spreadability; also allow oil and water to mix; detergents and emulsifiers.

tea tree: soothing and antiseptic; antifungal properties.

tissue respiratory factor (TRF): ingredient derived from yeast cells that functions as an anti-inflammatory and moisturizing ingredient.

titanium dioxide: an inorganic physical sunscreen that reflects UVA rays.

toners: liquids that tone and tighten the skin.

urea: properties include enhancing the penetration abilities of other substances. Anti-inflammatory, antiseptic, and deodorizing action allow urea to protect the skin's surface and help maintain healthy skin. Does not induce photoallergy, phototoxicity, or sensitization.

vehicles: spreading agents and ingredients that carry or deliver other ingredients into the skin and make them more effective.

vitamin C (ascorbic acid): an antioxidant vitamin needed for proper repair of the skin and tissues.

vitamin K: vitamin responsible for the synthesis of factors necessary for blood coagulation.

water soluble: mixable with water.

witch hazel: extracted from the bark of the hamanelis shrub; can be a soothing agent or, in higher concentrations, an astringent.

zinc oxide: an inorganic physical sunscreen that reflects UVA rays. Also used to protect, soothe, and heal the skin; is somewhat astringent, antiseptic, and antibacterial.

PART

4

ESTHETICS

CHAPTER **13**

THE TREATMENT ROOM

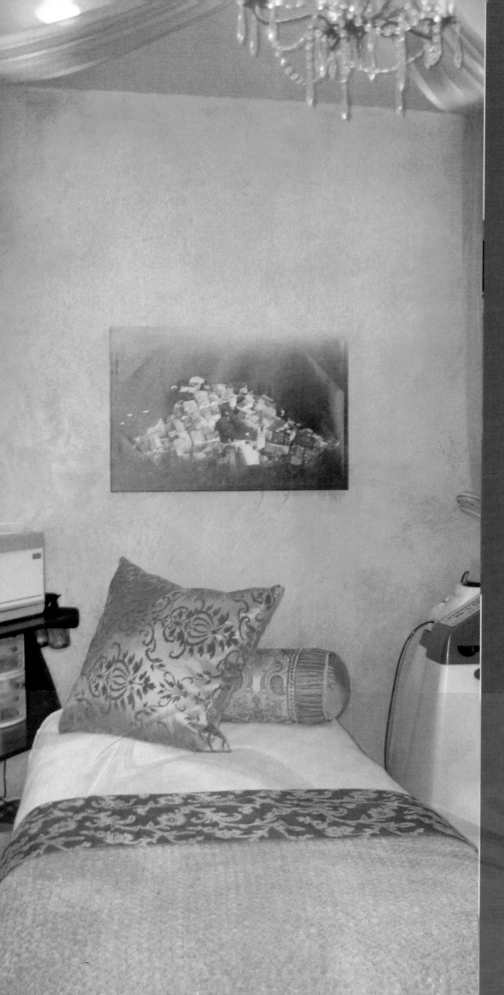

After completing this chapter, you will be able to:

- Understand the components of creating a professional atmosphere.

- Describe what equipment and supplies are needed for facials.

- Explain why the room setup should be comfortable for the esthetician.

- Prepare and set up the treatment room for services.

- Disinfect and clean the treatment room.

KEY TERMS

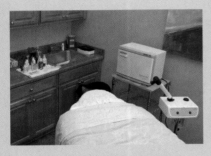

Figure 13–1 A prepared treatment room.

This chapter is designed to help the esthetician learn to prepare the treatment room for services. Included are easy-to-use checklists and advice for setting up, cleaning, and keeping the room well stocked. Just about everything needed for room preparation is listed in this chapter. Treatment room setup and preparation are integral parts of giving treatments (Figure 13–1). Creating a professional atmosphere involves many details. After the facial service, clean-up and sanitation are needed to prepare the room for the next client. Treatment room setup includes choosing furniture, equipment, supplies, and products.

THE ESTHETICIAN'S PRESENTATION

Making a good first impression is important in any business setting. Your success depends on many factors, including your image and attitude. An esthetician's appearance and professionalism reflect on the business. Practicing good hygiene, dressing professionally, and having a neat appearance all convey a polished image (Figure 13–2). Additionally, employers, coworkers, and clients appreciate working with someone who has a positive attitude. This positive attribute will contribute favorably to the team.

Being dependable and providing excellent customer service is imperative. Professionalism includes being a self-starter and taking the initiative to prepare the treatment room. Plan enough time to set up the room before the day begins. You will project a calm, confident image if you are prepared.

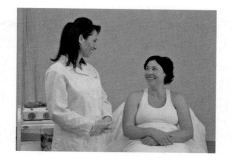

Figure 13–2 The technician's presentation.

CREATING A PROFESSIONAL ATMOSPHERE

Planning and preparing the treatment room for clients is the first step in performing services (Figure 13–3). The setup and supplies will vary, depending on the school or business. Whether you are an employee or self-employed, a well-stocked and organized room is necessary to function efficiently. You can provide services with minimal equipment, if necessary. A clean, comfortable, and relaxing atmosphere is part of your service. A pleasant ambiance also improves the work environment. A facility needs to be professional looking and clutter-free. Stations must be spotless. Consider the clients' comfort and yours when choosing equipment. The goal is to give quality service in a nice, quiet atmosphere. In this service-oriented business, the primary focus is the client and their entire experience while they are in your care.

FURNITURE, EQUIPMENT, AND ROOM SETUP

Treatment room furnishings can range from the basics to high-end designer equipment. A spa environment is usually more relaxing than a clinical one. Relaxing colors, music, and décor are preferable in a spa (Figure 13–4). When setting up a room for treatments, think about the services you will perform

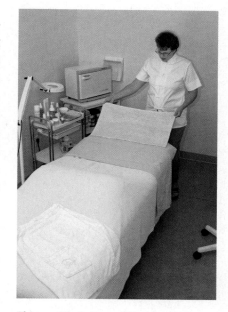

Figure 13–3 Preparing the facial room.

> **CAUTION!**
>
> A workstation that is uncomfortable for the body and posture could cause neck, back, and hand problems over time.

Figure 13–4 A beautifully appointed treatment room.

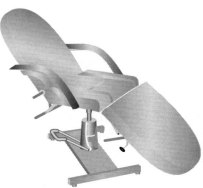

Figure 13–5 An adjustable facial bed.

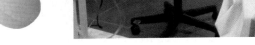

Figure 13–6 The esthetician's stool.

and how you will work at the station. Another consideration is how comfortable the client will be in the facial chair (be sure to consider the needs of the male client). State board sanitation regulations and client safety are the most important considerations before, during, and after treatments.

A Checklist of Furniture and Equipment

Equipment for the facial treatment consists of the following items:

- *Facial bed,* also called a facial chair or table. The facial bed can be a massage table or an esthetician's table. Make sure it is large enough to accommodate clients comfortably and is suitable for body waxing (Figure 13–5).
- *Esthetician's chair,* or operator's stool (Figure 13–6). The technician's stool needs to be **ergonomically correct:** healthy for the body and spine. Make sure it is comfortable for you while you perform services and that it can roll around easily. Back support is preferable.
- *Towel warmer,* or "hot cabbie." A towel warmer keeps towels warm and can also be used to warm products and cotton pads (Figure 13–7). Plastics will melt in a towel warmer, so use glass or ceramic dishes for warming products. Professional product warmers are also available.
- *Magnifying lamp or light.* A "mag" lamp is used to analyze the skin and to perform detail work such as tweezing (Figure 13–8).
- *Steamer* (Figure 13–9). Steamers are great tools for warming and softening the skin. Use steam in moderation. Steam is part of a standard facial procedure. See Chapter 16 for more on electrotherapy equipment and facial machines.

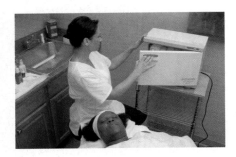

Figure 13–7 The towel warmer.

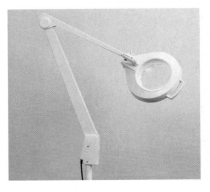

Figure 13–8 The magnifying lamp.

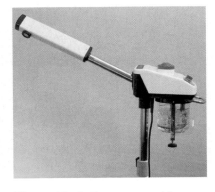

Figure 13–9 The steam machine.

- *Step stool.* A step stool helps clients get on and off the bed safely. Make sure the stool is stable. Assist clients if they need help.
- *Utility cart.* A cart holds tools, supplies, and products. This can be a stationary table or roll cart.
- *Galvanic, high-frequency, brush, vacuum and spray machines* (Figure 13–10). These can either be individual machines or multifunctional machines all on one stand.
- *Sanitizer.* An ultraviolet (UV), wet, or dry **sanitizer** should be located in each treatment room for disinfecting tools and equipment (Figures 13–11 A, B and C). An autoclave is a sterilizer.
- *Wax heater.* The wax heater is an electric warming device used for soft-wax, paraffin, or hard-wax application (Figure 13–12). They are usually kept activated during the day for walk-ins or unexpected requests. Waxing is discussed in Chapter 17, "Hair Removal."
- Closed, covered *waste container*
- Closed, covered *laundry hamper*
- *Sharps container.* A **sharps container** is a biohazard container for disposal of lancets. It is red, labeled, and puncture-proof (Figure 13–13). Follow OSHA and state regulations for proper disposal. Not all facilities perform services that require a sharps container.

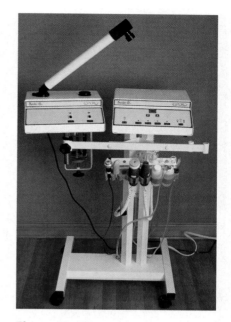

Figure 13–10 Multifunctional machines.

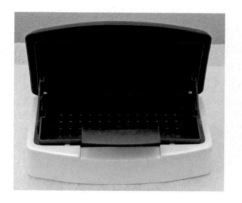 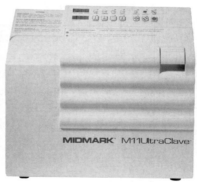 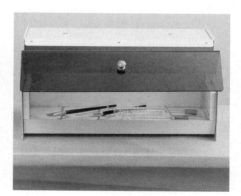

Figure 13–11 13–11A) Wet sanitizer 13–11B) Autoclave and 13–11C) Ultraviolet (UV) sanitizer.

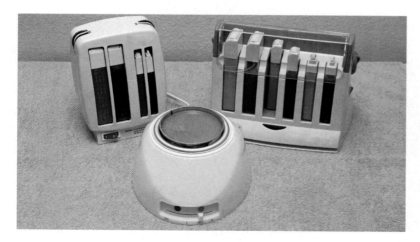

Figure 13–12 Wax heaters.

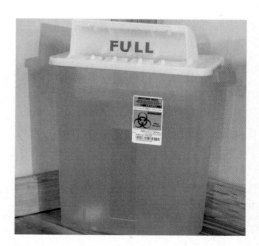

Figure 13–13 A sharps container.

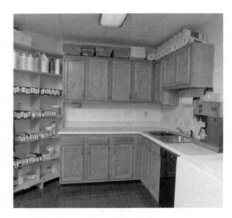

Figure 13–14 A neat dispensary helps maintain and control inventory.

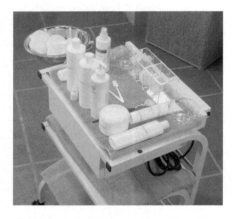

Figure 13–15 Proper setup of supplies helps the treatment go smoothly.

TREATMENT ROOM SUPPLIES, DISPOSABLES, AND PRODUCTS

The Dispensary

If supplies and products are not kept in the treatment room or at the workstations, then they are kept in a **dispensary,** which is a separate room for mixing products and storing supplies (Figure 13–14). Supplies are kept in clean, covered, labeled containers. Proper storage is necessary to keep items from being contaminated. The amount of supply usage depends on the facility. Different setups require different numbers of towels or cotton supplies. Each instructor or manager will have a special setup procedure to follow (Figure 13–15). The following section presents an example of what is needed for a basic facial. Refer to the waxing and makeup chapters to set up for those services.

Facial Supplies

Facial supplies include the following (Figure 13–16):

- hand cleanser or antibacterial *soap* for hand washing
- face and hand *towels*
- *astringent* or witch hazel for the skin and to use on cotton pads for extractions
- *disinfectant* cleanser to clean surfaces
- fan and mask *brushes* to apply masks or massage lotions
- *bowls* to warm or mix product in; also used to hold cotton pads or other supplies
- *spatulas* to disperse products from jars
- client *headband* to protect the hair and hold it out of the way
- client *gown/wrap* for the client to change into
- clean *sheets/linens/bath towels* (depending on the setup, use either sheets or towels)
- *blankets* to cover the client
- distilled *water* for the steamer
- client *chart*
- relaxing *music*
- *implements*: tweezers, an extraction tool
- a bed *warmer*/electric blanket
- a *bolster* for back support, placed under the knees
- a *pillow or rolled hand towel* for neck support

CAUTION!

Do not put an electric blanket beneath the bed linens. This is a fire hazard and can scorch the facial bed. Use only specified bed warmers made for this purpose. Electric blankets must go on top of the blankets.

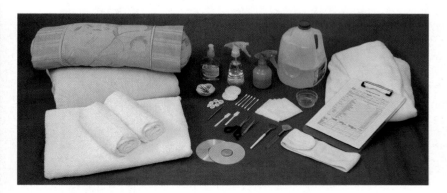

Figure 13–16 Facial supplies.

Disposables

Disposable supply usage depends on your facility and may include the following:

- *paper towels*
- cotton 4" × 4" *pads* or disposable sponges to remove product from the skin (sponges are porous and cannot be sanitized or reused)
- *gauze squares* for use with certain facial treatments
- *cotton* or round cotton pads for toner application, to make eye pads and cleansing pads
- *tissues* for blotting the face
- cotton *swabs* for product application, removing eye makeup, or performing extractions
- one pair of disposable vinyl *gloves* (latex is not recommended, as many people are allergic to latex and oil can break down the latex, compromising the protection of the gloves)
- a sealable *plastic bag* for putting all used disposables into
- *extraction supplies:* cotton, swabs, lancets/needles, or extraction tool (see state regulations for extraction rules)

Products

Products are the main ingredients in performing services. Chapter 12 addresses the guidelines for choosing products. Have the correct products for all client services on hand. Basic products used in facials include the following (Figure 13–17):

- cleanser
- exfoliant
- mask
- face massage cream or lotion
- toner
- moisturizer
- sunscreens
- optional: serums, eye cream, lip balm

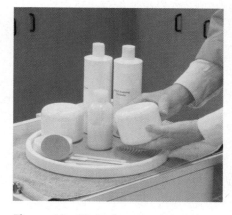

Figure 13–17 Gather all products to be used before beginning the service.

ROOM PREPARATION

Before setting up the room, refer to the setup checklist that the facility uses. Look at your schedule to see what supplies are needed. If specified, put the clean laundry away. Have the client's chart notes ready, and review the retail consultation forms if applicable. After practicing for a while, you will find that setting up becomes easier. The following guidelines are for a standard facial setup. It takes approximately 15 minutes to set up for a service and 15 minutes to clean up after a service. A checklist of equipment, supplies, and disposables is summarized in Chapter 14, "Basic Facials." Once you have gathered all you need for treatments, you can start setting up.

Equipment Preparation

To prepare equipment, use the following guidelines:

1. Turn on the waxer. Check and adjust the temperature.
2. Preheat the hot cabbie, and put in wet towels and cotton cleansing pads to warm.

> ### Here's a Tip
>
> When setting up for a facial, preheat your towel warmer, towels, and steamer first. They take the longest to heat up.

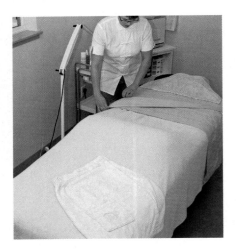

Figure 13–18 Prepare the facial bed properly.

3. Preheat the steamer. First check the steamer water level (it should be just slightly below the red fill line). If necessary, refill the steamer—using only distilled water. Follow the manufacturer's directions for care.

Prepare the Bed

Procedures for preparing the facial bed are as follows (Figure 13–18).
1. Place clean linens on the facial bed.
2. Place a blanket on top of the linens to keep the client warm and comfortable.
3. Lay out one hand towel to place under the head and one for placement over the décolleté (day-call-TAY; upper chest area), if applicable.
4. Have a clean headband and gown or wrap ready for the client.
5. Have a bolster and pillow available.

Setting Up Supplies

Follow these procedures for setting up supplies:
1. Wash your hands with antibacterial soap before setting up and touching clean items.
2. Check to make sure the sanitizer is ready. Wet sanitizers are filled and changed according to manufacturer's instructions (check to see that the strength is maintained by regular refilling).
3. Place supplies on a **sanitary maintenance area (SMA).** This is a clean towel (paper or cloth) on the clean workstation. Put out supplies in the order used, lined up neatly, and cover with another towel until you are ready to use them. Place any used or soiled items away from the SMA.

Setting Out Disposables

Disposables are kept in clean, covered containers or closed cupboards to prevent contamination. After washing your hands, dispense only the amount needed for the service. Use clean forceps or tongs to retrieve additional supplies during a service.

The proper procedure for setting out disposables include the following:
1. Set out disposable supplies on an SMA (a clean towel).
2. Do not put clean or soiled supplies on bare counter surfaces. Dirty items must be disposed of properly.

Arranging the Products

Set out the treatment products in order of the procedure application: cleanser, massage cream or lotion, masks, toner, moisturizer, and other products as determined by the client's skin analysis.

Setting Up the Dressing Area

Set up the dressing area for the client, if appropriate. Arrange a place for the client to sit while changing. Get water or tea ready for the client, and have a client chart and release form prepared.

Remember to explain to the client where to put their personal belongings and how to put on the spa wrap. Explain how to get into the bed and where to position their head (if you leave the room for them to change). Some clients have not had a facial or wax service and do not know exactly what they are expected to do.

Ergonomics

Ergonomics is the study of adapting work conditions to suit the worker. The equipment and the positions we use should be healthy for the spine and body. Adjust the facial chair height, if possible. When setting up, remember to align the stool with the facial chair for the correct height and position for performing services. The technician's feet should be flat on the floor, and hands should be below chest level. Do not overstretch your back to reach something (Figure 13–19).

Arrange the supply cart or counter as close to the facial chair as possible. When reaching for a product or implement, or to adjust equipment, get up out of the chair. Be aware of the position of your back, and remind yourself to sit up straight. Pay attention to your posture. Stretching and loosening up the hands before and after working is helpful in maintaining the health and flexibility of the wrists and hands.

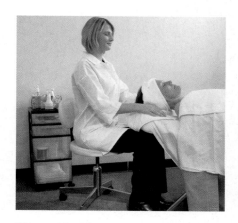

Figure 13–19 Correct sitting posture for an esthetitican.

FOCUS ON . . .

EXERCISES FOR STRENGTHENING THE HANDS AND WRISTS

1. Hold the hands at chest level with fists clenched. Make a fist, squeezing as hard as you can, while holding for a count of five. Release the hands, spreading the fingers wide for a count of five. Repeat 10 to 20 times. This exercise is excellent for strengthening the hands and wrists (Figure 13–20).

2. Place both hands, palms down, on a flat surface. Tap each finger, beginning with the thumbs, and count each finger from thumb to little finger, as it is tapped in rhythm. Count 1, 2, 3, 4, 5. Then, starting with the little finger, tap each finger to the count of 5, 4, 3, 2, 1. This exercise is similar to playing the piano and is especially good for building coordination and hand control (Figure 13–21).

3. Place the palms together at chest level. Keep them together as you bend the left wrist as far back as it will go, and then do the same with the right wrist. Keep bending the wrists in rhythm for 20 counts. This exercise strengthens the hands and wrists and makes them more flexible (Figure 13–22).

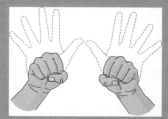

Figure 13–20 Strengthening hands and wrists.

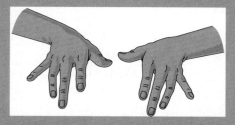

Figure 13–21 Building coordination and hand control.

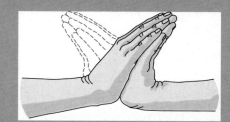

Figure 13–22 Increasing flexibility of the hands and wrists.

PROCEDURES 13–1 AND 13–2

MAKING CLEANSING PADS AND EYE PADS

SUPPLIES
- roll of cotton
- bowl
- water
- disinfectant
- sanitary maintenance area
- covered container or zip-lock plastic bag for storage

Preparation of Cotton Pads and Compresses

If prepackaged 4" × 4" esthetic wipes or sponges are not available, cotton pads can be made from a roll of cotton. You can prepare all cotton cleansing pads, eye pads, and the cotton compress pads that are used in a facial before the treatment begins. In a busy salon, the esthetician should check the appointment book at the beginning of each work day to see how many appointments are booked for that day. To save time, enough pads and compresses can then be made for the entire day if they are kept sanitary. Store pads and compresses in a covered container.

Remove enough pads from the container before each treatment, and place them in a plastic, steel, or glass bowl that is kept within easy reach during the facial treatment. For each client, you may need a minimum of one pair of eye pads, one cotton compress mask, and four to six cleansing pads. The pads and compresses that are not used on the day they are made can be stored safely in an airtight, covered container, or placed in a zip-lock plastic bag and refrigerated for use the next day.

Procedure 13–1: Making Cleansing Pads

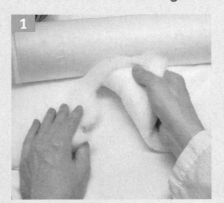

Divide cotton. *(Figure P13–1-1)*

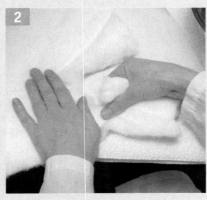

Tear cotton. *(Figure P13–1-2)*

1 Divide a roll of cotton into strips approximately 4" wide. This is about the width of the average hand. Tear the cotton (do not cut) so that the edges are frayed and the cleansing pads are less lumpy when the edges are folded under (Figure P13–1-1).

2 To make cleansing pads, hold one of the cotton strips in one hand and pull downward with the hand until the cotton tears, making a cotton square approximately 4" wide by 5" long. Four to six of these pieces will be needed for each facial treatment (Figure P13–1-2).

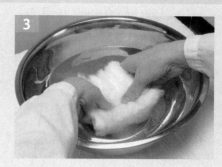

Submerge in water. *(Figure P13–1-3)*

3 Submerge the cotton in water while supporting the pad with your fingers (Figure P13–1-3).

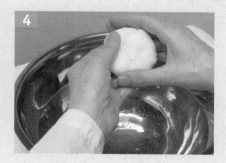

Tuck edges. *(Figure P13-1-4)*

4 Tuck the edges of the cotton under while turning it in your hands (Figure P13–1-4). Place the round pad in the palm of your hand, placing the other palm over the pad. Squeeze out excess water from the pad.

Eye pads can be made from either 4" × 4" cotton squares, prepackaged round cotton pads, or pieces of cotton. There are two types of eye pads: round and butterfly. Both styles of eye pads are correct, and the choice of which to use is up to the esthetician. The pads should be large enough to cover the entire eye area, but not so large that they interfere with product application or treatment. The advantage of the butterfly pad over the round pad is that it will not fall off of the eyes as easily. Round eye pads are made following the same procedure as for round cleansing pads, but the cotton piece should measure about 2½" × 2½".

Procedure 13–2: Making Butterfly Eye Pads

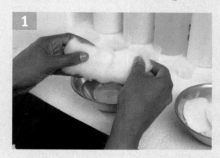

Dip cotton into water. *(Figure P13–2-1)*

1 Dip a piece of cotton measuring approximately 2" × 6" into the water (Figure P13–2-1).

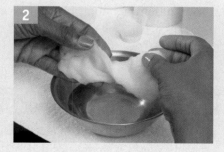

Twist. *(Figure P13–2-2)*

2 Twist the cotton in the center with a one-half turn (Figure P13–2-2).

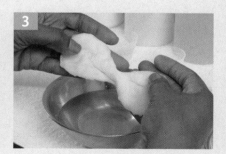

Butterfly pads. *(Figure P13–2-3)*

3 Fold the pad in half and squeeze out the excess water (Figure P13–2-3).

Optional: Take a square 4" × 4" pad, unfold lengthwise, and twist it in the middle.

Clean-Up

Follow aseptic procedures after the service.

AFTER THE FACIAL: CLEAN-UP PROCEDURES AND SANITATION

Since we have just reviewed the facial setup, this is a good time to discuss the clean-up procedures, even though the facial procedure has not been performed yet. It is helpful to learn and practice each phase of a service before moving on to the next step. This way you can focus on the procedure since you will already be familiar with the pre- and post-service steps. After completing the post-consultation with the client, be sure to record the client chart notes and write up retail sales. Then prepare the room for the next client, or clean the room in preparation for the end of the day. Remember that the order of the clean up varies with each facility's guidelines and that sanitation procedures improve as laws and technology evolve.

Cleaning and Disinfecting Implements

Appropriate cleaning and disinfecting involves the following:
- Wash and disinfect all brushes, tweezers, and other non-disposable **implements.** Implements are non-disposable items and tools such as brushes, tweezers, and comedone extractors.
- Wash implements thoroughly with antibacterial soap, and dry them off first before placing in the disinfectant. This process is important to maintain the wet disinfectant strength and keep it from becoming dirty or diluted.
- Be sure all implements remain in the disinfectant for the appropriate amount of time according to the manufacturer's instructions. Then rinse, dry, and put them away. Store them in a covered container in a drawer or cupboard when not in use.
- Clean and disinfect bowls and other reusable items. Dry and store properly.
- Change the disinfectant to comply with manufacturer's directions and sanitation regulations. If required, record on a dated log when the disinfectant is changed (Table 13–1).

Table 13–1

DISINFECTANT LOG

Change the high-level disinfectant solution in the container according to the manufacturer's directions or if it is cloudy and seems to require changing. Record when it is changed.

DATE CHANGED	YOUR INITIALS

Table 13–2

DETERMINING THE COSTS OF SETTING UP A TREATMENT ROOM	
ITEMS	**ESTIMATED COSTS**
facial bed/chair	
esthetician stool	
steamer	
hot cabinet/towel warmer	
step stool	
utility cart	
waxers	
sink/water supply	
magnifying lamp	
optional electrical equipment	
furniture	
linens	
products	
supplies	
disposables	
stereo/music	
	Total Cost: $

ACTIVITY

It is interesting to find out what setting up a treatment room might cost. On your own, make a list of suppliers that carry the tools and supplies you need. Check out beauty supply houses, Internet sites, trade journals, and trade shows to get an idea of what is available. Research supplies and equipment costs to determine what you would need to spend to set up your own room (Table 13–2).

Equipment and Room Sanitation

Sanitizing the equipment and facial room involves the following procedures:
- Clean the wax machine, and turn it off at the end of the day.
- Disinfect the steamer.
- Disinfect the equipment used, and turn it off.
- Clean all containers, and wipe off dirty product containers with a disinfectant.
- Clean all counters, sinks, surfaces, and floor mats with disinfectant.
- Properly dispose of used supplies.
- Turn off the facial chair warmer or electric blanket, if used.

Laundry and Linens

Clean-up procedures for laundry and linens:
- Remove dirty linens, and remake the facial chair for the next client or leave it unmade.
- Place the used linens, towels, and sheets in the appropriate covered container or laundry hamper.
- Fasten the Velcro™ on the headbands and client wraps before putting them in the laundry to keep lint from sticking to the Velcro.

Disposables

Appropriate handling of disposables involves the following:

- Soiled items such as gloves and extraction supplies must be placed in a sealable plastic bag and then in a covered waste container or biohazard container. While in use, disposables must be placed on surfaces that can be disinfected or disposed of, such as a paper towel.
- Keep the clean supplies separate from the used ones. Take out only what is needed for each service.
- Disposable extraction lancets and needles go in a biohazard/sharps container. (Check OSHA and state rules for proper handling.)

End-of-the-Day Clean-Up

In most facilities, esthetiticians/students are responsible for the cleanliness of the treatment rooms. Technicians must be prepared to clean up areas they use. Be sure to alert the manager about areas of the facility that may need repair or deep cleaning. Clean-up procedures are regulated by state laws, so be aware of these regulations.

End-of-the-Day Checklist

At the end of the day, be sure to follow these procedures:

- Prepare the room, and check the schedule for the next shift or workday.
- Use a clean-up checklist to make sure you did not forget anything.
- Turn off all equipment.
- Refill all containers, wax supplies, and the steamer.
- Check floors; sweep or mop as required. Check for wax spills.
- Empty waste containers. Replace with clean trash liners.
- Remove personal items from the area.
- Leave the hot cabbie door open to dry, and empty the tray underneath before sanitizing it.
- Clean anything that has not been cleaned after the last service, including the bed, counters, and doorknobs.

You now have a good idea about how much work goes into preparing for services. Once you have a good setup and all of the tools needed, it is easy to stay organized and work efficiently. A clean, sanitary environment is necessary for client safety and to comply with the laws of your state board Health Licensing Agencies. Clients will be confident in your ability and feel safe in your hands when they know your facility is sanitary. Keeping the room clean and organized is necessary for a smooth operation. Now you are ready to welcome clients. The next chapters will cover facial, waxing, and makeup procedures.

REVIEW QUESTIONS

1. What type of salon atmosphere is it important to create?

2. Why are room esthetics important?

3. What are the two most important considerations in preparing and cleaning the room?

4. What essential equipment do you need for facials?

5. How long does it take to set up for a facial?

6. What does *ergonomically correct* mean?

7. Where do you put soiled disposable items when you have completed the service?

8. How do you disinfect implements?

9. What steps are involved in cleaning the room or workstation at the end of the day?

10. What is an SMA?

CHAPTER GLOSSARY

dispensary: a room used for mixing products and storing supplies.

ergonomically correct: furniture and body positions healthy for the body and spine.

ergonomics: the study of adapting work conditions to suit the worker.

implements: tools used by estheticians.

sanitary maintenance area (SMA): an area kept clean for setup of procedure implements and supplies; for example, an SMA can be a towel (paper or cloth) on the workstation.

sanitizer: an ultraviolet (UV), wet, or dry sanitizer is used for disinfecting tools and equipment. An autoclave is a sterilizer.

sharps container: plastic biohazard containers for disposable needles and anything sharp. The container is red and puncture-proof and must be disposed of as medical waste.

CHAPTER 14

BASIC FACIALS

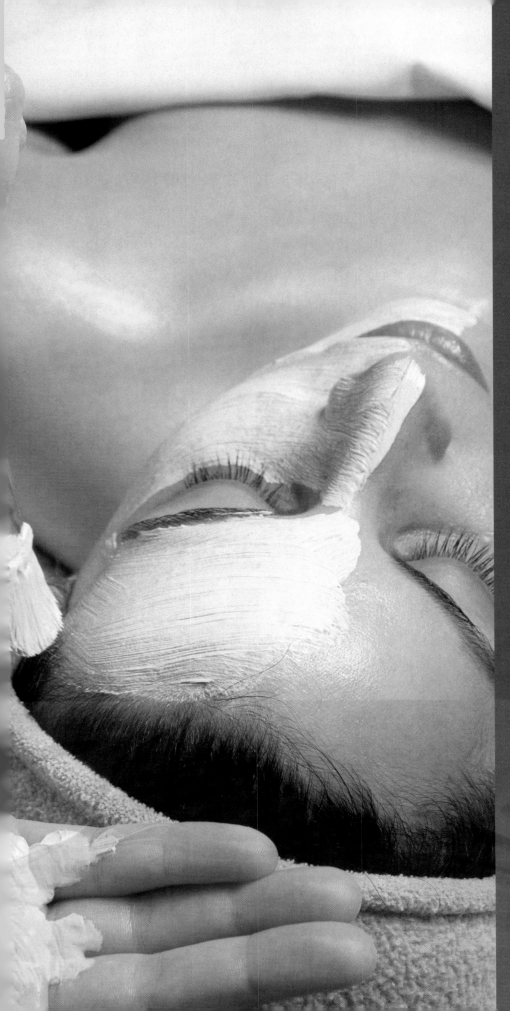

LEARNING OBJECTIVES

After completing this chapter, you will be able to:

- Describe the benefits of each step in a facial treatment.

- Explain the key elements of the basic facial treatment.

- List and describe the products used in a facial treatment.

- Recognize different facial treatment philosophies and methods.

- Perform the step-by-step facial treatment.

- Perform sanitation procedures and provide a safe environment for clients.

- Understand extraction methods.

- Describe acne facials and home care.

- Understand the treatment needs for oily, dry, dehydrated, sensitive, and mature skin.

- Discuss men's skin care and treatments.

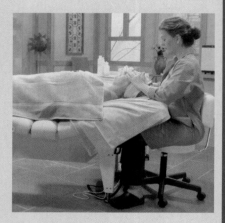

Figure 14–1 Facials improve and
rejuvenate the skin.

The skin care field has advanced rapidly in recent years due to the growing interest in health and beauty. This increase in the popularity of skin care has brought the field of esthetics to the forefront of the beauty and spa industry. Once considered luxuries, regular facials and skin care maintenance are now regarded as necessities by many (Figure 14–1). Facial treatments are also welcome breaks from the stresses of life in today's fast-paced society.

Stress reduction and caring for our health go hand in hand. Facials offer both benefits at the same time: they improve the skin's health while offering a relaxing service. Regular treatments result in noticeable improvements in the skin's texture and appearance. Clinical esthetics and technological advances in light therapy and lasers are constantly expanding the skin care industry (Chapter 18).

Facial treatments are the core treatments that estheticians perform. Giving a facial is both interesting and enjoyable. You were probably attracted to esthetics because you wanted a rewarding career that allowed you to give to others. This is the perfect job to help others feel good and make a positive impact on their self-image. After a treatment, clients are rejuvenated and feel good when they walk out the door to face the world again.

The basic facial treatment procedure is covered here; however, there are many different types of facials and methods. It is best to get a basic routine memorized before implementing new steps or changing the routine. For example, the steps, the products, the focus of corrective treatments, and the massage methods can all be varied. Once you are comfortable with routine procedures, your creativity will begin to flow naturally as you incorporate new ideas into your treatments.

FACIAL TREATMENT BENEFITS

What is a facial treatment? A **facial** is a professional service designed to improve and rejuvenate the skin. What can a facial/skin treatment do for your client? A skin treatment has many benefits. Facials help maintain the health of the skin and correct certain skin conditions through deep cleansing, massage, the use of masks and other products, and various treatment methods. Clinical services in a medical office usually focus more on corrective skin treatments, whereas spa treatments may focus more on the relaxation experience. Blending a results-oriented treatment with a relaxing experience leads to the best overall service (Figure 14–2).

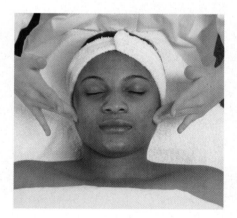

Figure 14–2 A facial treatment is one of the most relaxing services in a salon.

Providing education and consultations are also part of a facial. The benefits of the facial procedure are outlined below. Understanding what the benefits are gives you confidence that you are making a difference in the client's skin. This knowledge also helps you communicate those benefits to your clients.

Facial treatments include the following benefits:

- deep cleanses
- exfoliates
- increases circulation and detoxifies
- relaxes the senses, nerves, and muscles
- stimulates the skin functions and metabolism
- slows down premature aging
- treats conditions such as dryness, oiliness, or redness
- softens wrinkles and aging lines
- helps clear up blemishes and minor acne

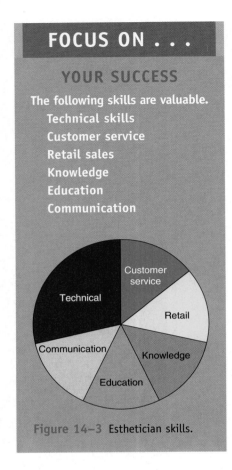
ESTHETICIAN SKILLS AND TECHNIQUES

What skills are needed to be successful at giving facials? Knowledge of skin histology, skin analysis, and skin care products is essential for an esthetician to make informed decisions for the client. Additionally, knowledge of contraindications, technological advances, and facial equipment is important. Client-relation skills are another facet of being an esthetician. Connecting with the client and knowing how to communicate with him or her will partially determine your success. Massage techniques and your touch, pressure, and flow in the facial are also a valuable part of your skills. Retailing and client consultations are another part of the job.

Some of these skills may seem to come more naturally to you, but as you get more experience, you will improve in all of these areas. Pay attention to little details that make the client comfortable. Knowing how to communicate well will also help build client loyalty. Educated, well-trained technicians are the best promotion for the esthetics industry. Facials are a valuable service with wonderful benefits. The market will continue to expand as more people discover these benefits.

Continuing your education with advanced classes and attendance at conferences and trade shows will keep you informed, excited, and motivated. It is invaluable to continue your education annually. A true professional will not miss these opportunities for growth. Make a commitment to yourself to attend at least one esthetics class or trade show every year: this will make a difference in your potential career success.

Facial Treatment Protocol

To be successful and to maintain client loyalty, follow these guidelines:
- Help the client to relax by speaking in a quiet and professional manner.
- Explain the benefits of the products and service you offer, and answer any questions the client may have.
- Provide a skin analysis and educational consultation.
- Provide a quiet atmosphere, and work quietly and efficiently.
- Maintain neat, clean, and sanitary conditions in the facial work area. Have your supplies arranged in orderly fashion.
- If your hands are cold, warm them before touching the client's face.
- Keep your nails smooth and short to avoid scratching the client's skin.
- Remove rings, bracelets, and other jewelry that may injure the client or get in the way during the treatment.
- Follow systematic procedures.
- Be moderate in all applications. Too much of a good thing can counteract the benefits.
- Be aware of your touch and the amount of pressure you apply to the face.
- Massage and apply or remove products in a smooth, consistent pattern. What you do for the right side, do for the left, using the same order and for the same number of times.

- Apply and remove products neatly, avoiding getting it in the eyes, mouth, and nostrils.
- Do not let water or products drip down the client's neck or in the eyes or ears.
- Be genuine in your concern for your client and focus on her or his needs.
- Give the client your full attention at all times.

TREATMENT AND CLIENT PREPARATION

Use the following resources to prepare for client treatments:
- Refer to the treatment room setup checklist in Table 14–1.
- Refer to the room setup information in Chapter 13.
- Review the contraindication information in Chapter 11.
- Use the client charts and consultation information in Chapter 11.

Meeting and Greeting Clients

One of the most important communications you will have with a client occurs the first time you meet (Figure 14–4). Be polite, friendly, and inviting. Remember that your clients are coming to you for services for which they are paying hard-earned cash. That means you need to give great service every time they come to see you; otherwise, you may lose them to another esthetician. The following are good customer service practices:
- Always approach a client with a smile.
- Even if you are having a difficult day or have a problem of some sort, keep it to yourself. The time you are with your client is for your client and her needs, not yours.
- Always introduce yourself to new clients, and greet return clients by name. A brief, yet warm handshake will make the client feel welcome.

> **FOCUS ON . . .**
>
> **BUILDING YOUR BUSINESS**
>
> Share the benefits of your facial services with others as you meet new contacts or clients. Many people are not aware of these benefits!

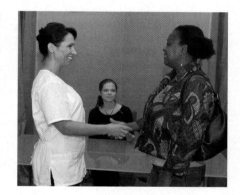

Figure 14–4 Greeting the client.

Table 14–1

THE FACIAL SUPPLY CHECKLIST			
SUPPLIES		**DISPOSABLES**	**PRODUCTS**
disinfectant/sanitizer	implements	paper towels	cleanser
hand sanitizer/antibacterial soap	hand towels	gloves/finger cots	exfoliant
covered trash container	client gown or wrap	cotton pads	mask
bowls	clean linens	cotton swabs	massage lotion
spatulas	blanket	cotton rounds	toner
fan and mask brushes	headband	baggies	moisturizer
distilled water	sharps container	tissues	sunscreen
Equipment: Choose as needed	bolster	extraction supplies	optional: serums, eye cream, lip balm

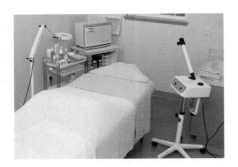

Figure 14–5 An efficient workstation is organized.

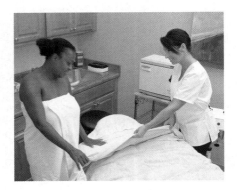

Figure 14–6 Help the client prepare for the facial.

- Set aside a few minutes to take new clients on a quick tour of the facility. Introduce them to the receptionist and other coworkers. This helps clients to feel comfortable and at home.
- Be yourself. Your clients can sense when you are being genuine and open, and they will have more confidence in you and in your expertise.

Setup, Products, and Supplies Checklist

It is important to assemble supplies in an organized, efficient manner (Figure 14–5).

Preparing the Client for the Facial Treatment

After warmly greeting the client, put her at ease by assisting her in preparing for the facial (Figure 14–6). Show the client where to change and store any belongings. Clients can change into their gown and remove their shoes in a changing room or the treatment room. Instruct the client how to prepare for the treatment and how to put on the facial wrap. There are many styles of wraps and gowns; for example, men wear a kimono-type robe or a wrap around the waist. Show the client how to get on the facial bed safely and where to position the head. Assist her or him in getting comfortable.

Adjust the head drape, towels, and linens, following your instructor's method. Place a towel across the client's chest and a cover over the body as directed. Drape the hair with a towel or headband. Check to make sure the headband is not too tight and that all of the hair is covered. Consider efficiency and laundry costs when determining what to use for draping. A bolster under the knees and a neck pillow are also used for the client's comfort.

KEY ELEMENTS OF THE BASIC FACIAL TREATMENT

Each step in the facial process is described below. A more thorough explanation of the steps is given before the actual steps of the procedure are listed. This way, you can become familiar with the steps before having to perform the procedure. As you practice facials, follow the chart (Table 14–2) to memorize the steps. Adapt this basic procedure to fit your local facility and regulations.

The Initial Consultation and Analysis

The initial consultation and skin analysis determine the products and procedures to be used and give you time to discuss the client's home-care needs. Before cleansing, inspect the skin type and conditions to see if it is dry, normal, or oily; if the skin texture is smooth or rough; if fine lines or creases exist; if blackheads or acne are present; if dilated capillaries are visible; and if the skin color is even.

You want to see the skin's natural state before cleansing and then again after cleansing, especially if the client is wearing makeup. Complete a thorough analysis with a magnifying lamp after cleansing (Table 14–3). Check for any other conditions or contraindications prohibiting a facial (Table 14–4).

Table 14-2

THE FACIAL PROCEDURE CHECKLIST

The facial procedure is divided into the following steps:
1. Client consultation, including review of contraindications and initial skin analysis
2. Client draping
3. Warm towels and cleansing
4. In-depth skin analysis (refer to Table 14–3)
5. Exfoliation product or mask
6. Softening with steam or warm towels
7. Extractions (and/or brow waxing, if applicable)
8. Massage (massage and mask steps can be reversed)
9. Mask
10. Toner
11. Moisturizer and/or sunscreen

Table 14-3

SKIN ANALYSIS CHECKLIST: LOOK, TOUCH, ASK, LISTEN

Analyze the skin using a magnifying lamp. If the client's eyes are sensitive to light, place eye pads on the eyes. Try not to cover what you need to look at around the eye.
1. Look for any obvious skin conditions and note the skin type.
2. Touch the skin, noting its elasticity, softness, texture, skin condition, and so on.
3. Continue the consultation, asking questions while analyzing.
4. Choose the products.
5. Note the information on the client chart. (This can be done before, during, or after the facial.)

Table 14-4

FACIAL CONTRAINDICATIONS

- contagious diseases such as HIV, herpes or hepatitis, pinkeye, or ringworm
- skin disorders
- medical conditions, including pregnancy
- medications: use of Accutane® or other topical peeling agents
- skin irritation
- allergies to products and ingredients
- electrical contraindications as listed in Chapter 16, "Facial Machines"

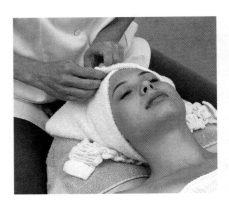

Figure 14–7 Draping the hair with a towel.

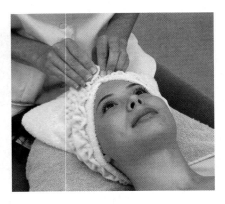

Figure 14–8 Make sure the headband is comfortable.

Draping the Hair

Drape client's head: fasten a clean headband, towel, or other head covering around the client's head to protect the hair.

To drape the head with a towel, follow these steps:

1. Place the towel on the headrest. Fold the towel lengthwise from one of the top corners to the opposite lower corner, and place it over the headrest with the fold facing down.
2. When the client is in a reclined position, the back of the head should rest on the towel, so that the sides of the towel can be brought up to the center of the forehead to cover the hairline (Figure 14–7).
3. Use a headband with a Velcro™ closure or a fastener to hold the towel in place (Figure 14–8). Make sure that all strands of hair are tucked under the towel, that the earlobes are not bent, and that it is not wrapped too tightly.

Removing Eye and Lip Color

Make sure the client is not wearing contacts. Before starting the cleansing procedure, the client's eye and lip color can be removed. If it is appropriate to remove the eye makeup, use a wet, soft cotton pad to gently rub from the brow line to the top lash line stroking downward. Then to remove mascara or other makeup from under the eye always work from the outside in. Do not use too much cleanser because it can run into the eye. Some clients prefer to leave their eye makeup on, and it is appropriate to work around it.

To remove lip color, use cotton or fold a tissue into about three folds and apply a small amount of cleanser or makeup remover. Be careful not to apply too much cleanser because it can get into the client's mouth. Hold the skin taut next to the side of the lips. Start cleansing the lips at the outside corner of the lips, and slide the tissue to the center of the lips. Alternate the strokes on both sides of the mouth. Turn the tissue to the clean side, and repeat the procedure until all cleanser is removed and the lips are clean.

Cleansing and Analysis

After the initial dry skin analysis, apply warm towels for a few minutes. Warm towels are used before cleansing to prepare the client for your touch, to warm and moisten the skin, and to make cleansing more effective and enjoyable.

> **CAUTION!**
>
> If any product gets into the eyes, have the client rinse and flush the eyes immediately at the sink. Then resume the procedure. If they wear contacts, they may need to remove them before receiving a treatment.

Cleanse to remove impurities and makeup before the in-depth skin analysis and facial treatment (Figure 14–9). Use a milky or creamy cleanser that rinses easily. During a facial, it is hard to remove foam or gel cleansers. Avoid over rubbing or stimulating the skin and thoroughly, but efficiently, complete the cleansing. If there is makeup residue, do a double cleansing—once before using the towels and once after. Some estheticians use a toner between facial steps to remove any makeup or product residue. Most facial products can be applied with fingertips and removed with cotton pads or sponges.

Exfoliation

Exfoliation can be achieved by using products such as peels, or you can use the brush machine to remove dead skin cells that make the skin feel rough and clog the pores. Exfoliation makes the skin smoother, helps product penetration by unblocking the surface, and promotes stimulation, which increases the cell turnover rate (Figure 14–10). A clay-lifting mask or enzyme mask can also help exfoliate the skin. This step can be performed before steam, extractions, or a mask. It is most effective in the beginning of the treatment after cleansing. Exfoliation was discussed in Chapter 12, "Skin Care Products."

Steam or Warm Towels

Warmth softens the pores, promotes more effective cleansing, prepares the skin for extractions or product penetration, softens superficial lines, and increases circulation (Figure 14–11). Towels or steam should never be too warm or used too long because they can damage capillaries and cause overstimulation, redness, and irritation. Always check the towel temperature on the inside of your wrist before applying. Keep towels away from the nostrils. Warm towels can be used in place of steam or for product removal during treatments.

Steam is typically used before deep pore cleansing. The steamer nozzle is placed approximately 18 inches away from the client. Check to make sure the client is comfortable and does not feel claustrophobic. The nozzle can be positioned above or below the client's face.

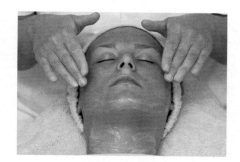

Figure 14–9 Cleansing the skin is the first step in the facial process.

Here's a Tip

To remove makeup from under the eye, try to use light, inward strokes around the eye area under the lower lashes to avoid tugging outward on the delicate skin when applying or removing products.

FYI

There are many different variations of a facial procedure. The order of steps can be changed. This will depend on what you are trying to achieve in the facial, the client's needs, the product line, the facility where you work, or your school's individual training program. Be flexible and enjoy the variety.

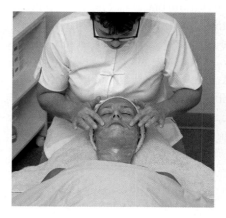

Figure 14–10 Exfoliating the skin can be achieved by a number of methods.

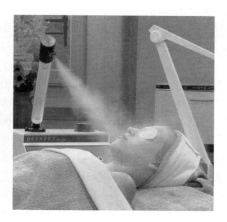

Figure 14–11 Steam softens the pores.

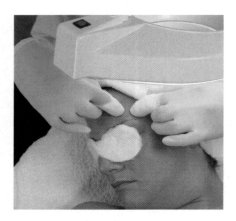

Figure 14–12 Extractions remove impurities and refine the pores.

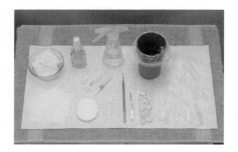

Figure 14–13 Extraction supplies.

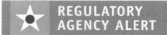

REGULATORY AGENCY ALERT

Check with your local regulating agencies for the extraction regulations.

Extractions and/or Deep Pore Cleansing

Manually removing impurities and comedones helps unblock clogged areas and refines pores (Figure 14–12). Cleaning out the debris that expands them allows the pores to contract. Manual extraction is often the only way to expel impurities and clean out the pores. It is also necessary to remove papules and pustules in order to release bacteria and fluids so they can heal more rapidly. Training and caution are needed before performing extractions. The skin must be exfoliated and warmed before performing **extractions.** It is also imperative that the esthetician wear gloves during extractions, and it is recommended that gloves remain on the hands throughout the rest of the procedure. Protective eyewear is also recommended in some instances. Proper extraction procedures are necessary to safely extract oil and debris from the follicles. Do not practice extractions without prior instruction or training.

There are three methods to use for extractions: the forefingers wrapped with finger gloves and cotton, known as "finger cots"; cotton swabs, and comedone extractors (Figure 14–13).

- Finger cots are individual finger "gloves" that are used with thin, dampened cotton wrapped around the gloved index fingers.
- Comedone extractors are metal tools used for open comedones and sebaceous filaments.
- Cotton swabs are smaller than fingertips and are especially useful around the nose area.

For all methods, press gently around the lesion.

Extraction of Open Comedones (Blackheads)

Desincrustation procedures such as the galvanic current, enzyme peels, or lifting masks must be used before an extraction to soften sebaceous material. The follicles must also be prepared by using either the steam machine or warm, moistened towels to facilitate extractions. If the skin is dry and tight, extractions will be ineffectual and damage the skin. The blackheads can usually be coaxed from the follicle with a minimum amount of pressure.

Wrap fingertips with wet cotton strips that have been lightly saturated with astringent. The fingertips are used to exert firm pressure on the skin directly surrounding the blackhead and to lift the blackhead from the follicle. Concentrating on one blackhead at a time, the esthetician must work gently and carefully so as not to bruise the tissue. Never use the fingernails on the skin or for extractions.

When extracting blackheads from the nose, it is important not to press down on the cartilage that forms the semiflexible part of the bridge of the nose.

To use the comedone extractor, place the loop over the lesion so that the lesion is inside the loop. Be aware that the pressure exerted can traumatize tissues. The follicle walls can rupture, spilling sebum, keratin, and bacteria into the dermis. This debris can cause infection and irritation that leads to the start of even more blemishes. Never force extractions.

Most clients will tolerate 10 minutes of extractions. Check to make sure they are comfortable with the procedure if you intend to work longer. Once the skin becomes dry and resistive, it is time to stop the procedure. At the end of your service, rebook the client's next appointment to be able to continue their extractions during their next treatment.

Extraction of Closed Comedones, Whiteheads, and Other Blemishes

Closed lesions are removed in the same manner as blackheads except that an opening in the dead cell layer must first be made. This is done by placing a lancet almost parallel to the surface of the skin and pricking the dead cell layer to make an opening for the debris to pass through. The lesion is then removed by applying gentle pressure. It is necessary to open closed lesions. The lancet is a small, sharp, pointed surgical blade with a double edge used to pierce or prick the skin. Each lancet is sterilized and comes in a separate, sealed envelope. If the envelope is open, the lancet cannot be guaranteed to be sterile. A fresh lancet must be used for each client.

In treating acne or blemished skin, the most important step for the esthetician is the effective removal and cleansing of blemishes. When the follicles are properly cleansed, the client's skin will begin to show marked improvement. It is important to explain to the client that you cannot always remove all blemishes during one treatment.

To achieve optimum success when performing extractions, you must put pressure on the skin surrounding the follicular wall so that you can extract the impaction with the least trauma to the surrounding tissue. Understanding the angle of the various pores in the different locations on the skin will enable you to perform extractions easily and effectively.

All areas of the forehead, the top of the nose, the chin, and the jawline have follicular walls perpendicular to the surface of the skin. The follicles are positioned this way on all flat surfaces. All other areas of the skin, such as the nose and cheeks, have slanted follicular shafts.

Before extractions, the use of desincrustation fluid or an enzyme peel will help to prep the skin by softening the plug of dead cells, sebum, and debris from the follicular shaft. After extractions, a calming, healing mask is beneficial. Antibacterial products and the high-frequency machine kill bacteria and help heal the skin. Cool water or skin globes can also calm irritated skin and redness.

Massage

Massage promotes physiological relaxation, increases circulation and metabolism, and increases product penetration (Figure 14–14). Additionally, the products used for massage have many benefits. Refer to Chapter 15 for facial massage steps and protocol. Memorize all steps of the massage or procedure before doing a complete facial. This way you will not have to memorize everything at the same time. The massage can be performed at different times during treatments, depending on the order of your procedures. Massage products are applied warm, with fingertips or a fan brush.

> ### CAUTION!
>
> To avoid spreading infection elsewhere on the skin, it is important to follow proper cleansing procedures when extracting blemishes.

> ### ★ REGULATORY AGENCY ALERT
>
> Using a lancet in the extraction procedure may be illegal in some regions. Check your local regulations to determine whether you may use this procedure.

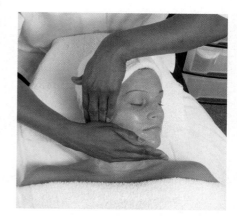

Figure 14–14 The most soothing and relaxing part of the facial is the massage.

Application of Treatment Masks

As discussed previously, masks can draw impurities out of the pores, clear up blemishes, tighten and tone the skin, and hydrate, calm, or rejuvenate the skin.

Depending on their function, masks are applied at different times during a treatment (Figure 14–15). If you are drawing impurities out of the skin, it may be beneficial to apply the mask before using steam and doing extractions. If it is a calming, hydrating mask, then it is applied at the end of a facial to calm the skin and leave it hydrated.

Towels, sponges, or cotton 4" × 4" pads are used to remove products. The cotton compress mask has also been used for removing the treatment mask.

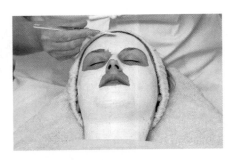

Figure 14–15 The mask is applied with a brush or the fingers.

Application of Toners

Toners hydrate and finish the cleansing process by removing any products left on the skin and balancing the skin pH (Figure 14–16). Different formulas can also help skin problems such as dehydration or acne. Toners can be misted onto the face or applied with a soft cotton pad.

Serums, Eye and Lip Treatments

Serums are concentrated ingredients used for specific corrective treatments. Serums or ampoules are applied with fingertips under a mask or moisturizer. These are also used with facial equipment in a variety of treatments. Eye and lip creams are usually thicker and are applied with fingertips or cotton swabs.

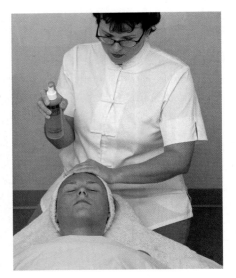

Figure 14–16 Toners can be applied with a cotton pad or sprayed on.

Application of Moisturizers

Depending on the formula, moisturizers can seal in moisture and protect the barrier layer of the skin. They can also hydrate and balance the oil–water moisture content of the skin. Products with performance ingredients will be even more effective when applied at the end of a treatment.

Sunscreens

Daily application of sunscreen is imperative! After finishing a stimulating, nourishing facial, do not send your client out with a newly exfoliated face without sun protection. Sunscreens are often in a moisturizing base (Figure 14–17).

Completing the Service

After completing the facial service, quietly and slowly let the client know you are finished. Tell her to take her time sitting up, offer to assist her in getting off the bed and then leave the room so she can change.

* Explain to the client what to do next—for example, meet you outside in the reception area or other appropriate instructions. Offer her some water to rehydrate after the service.

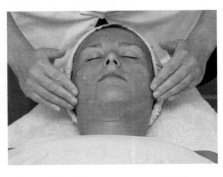

Figure 14–17 Sunscreen application.

- The client consultation after the service includes recommending products and rebooking their next appointment. Show the client which products you recommend, and write them down on a home-care instruction sheet for her to keep (Figure 14–18).
- Explain that you will also record the products you recommend on her file. Recommend that she reschedule once a month for a facial and any other services you believe would benefit her, such as a brow wax.
- Ask her what products she would like to take home with her, and recommend a time for scheduling the next appointment.
- Thank her for coming, and let her know you enjoyed meeting her.
- Make your chart notes and file them away. Clean up the room and prepare yourself for the next client.

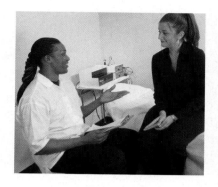

Figure 14–18 After the facial, discuss home-care products with your client.

FACIAL PHILOSOPHIES AND METHODS

There are many different types of facials. Some incorporate different massage philosophies, and others focus on specific results from a product manufacturer. Some facials have specific goals, such as stimulating or calming the skin, body, and mind. Philosophies range from holistic ayurvedic treatments to Chinese face-mapping. Using different facial zones to target treatments has also become more popular. Machines such as microdermabrasion and light therapy are another type of treatment focus.

Different nations also practice different methods. It is interesting to learn about European techniques, such as those practiced by the French and Germans, who have been instrumental in developing skin care for hundreds of years. European-trained beauty therapists learn many aspects of skin and beauty care beyond basic esthetics. The American industry tends to be oriented toward the newest technology available, with a focus on advanced ingredients. Regions such as Bali, Hawaii, and Japan have their own fascinating methods and products, bringing their native philosophies and ingredients to the skin care world. These different philosophies and methods offer many choices to incorporate into the treatment menu (Figure 14–19).

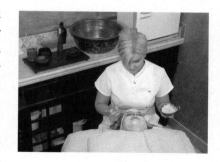

Figure 14–19 An exotic facial treatment.

VARIATIONS OF THE BASIC FACIAL

Remember that the steps of the facial procedure will vary depending on the focus of the facial. Sometimes the massage is the last step after the mask, and sometimes two masks are used. Sometimes steam or massage is omitted. The procedure used depends on what you are trying to achieve. Are you trying to hydrate and calm the skin, or deep-cleanse and stimulate it? For example, if the client needs hydrating, you may choose to omit the cleansing mask and the extractions. Do not be too concerned about utilizing different methods or procedures right now. As you continue your practice, you can vary the treatments you offer.

PROCEDURE 14–1

EYE MAKEUP AND LIPSTICK REMOVAL

SUPPLIES

(Use this list for all cleansing procedures.)
- disinfectant/sanitizer
- hand sanitizer/antibacterial soap
- covered trash container
- bowl
- spatula
- hand towels
- headband
- clean linens
- bolster

DISPOSABLES
- gloves
- cotton pads
- cotton rounds
- cotton swabs
- plastic bag
- paper towels
- tissues

PRODUCTS
- eye makeup remover or cleanser
- facial cleanser

Preparation

1 Prepare the bed and room.

2 Set out supplies and products on an SMA (sanitary maintenance area).

3 Prepare the client and cover the hair.

Procedure
Eye Makeup Removal

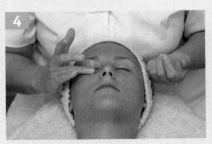
Cleanse the eyelid and lashes. *(Figure P14–1-1)*

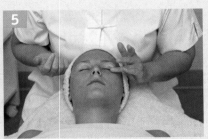
Apply the product to the eyelid with downward strokes. *(Figure P14–1-2)*

4 Bring the left hand over and lift the right eyebrow with the middle and ring fingers. With the middle and ring fingers of the right hand, apply the product to the eyelid with downward strokes (Figure P14-1-1). Use downward movements with the cleansing pad to cleanse the eyelid and lashes. Gently rinse with cotton pads.

5 Move the middle and ring fingers of the right hand over to the left side of the face and lift the left eyebrow. With the middle fingers of the left hand, apply the product to the left lid with downward strokes (Figure P14-1-2). If the client is wearing contacts, do not remove the eye makeup.

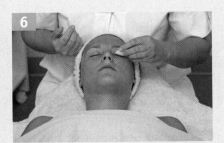
Repeat cleansing. *(Figure P14–1-3)*

6 Repeat this step as necessary to remove eye makeup. While cleansing the eyes, rotate the pad to provide a clean, unused surface (Figure P14-1-3).

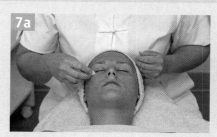

Remove mascara under the eyes. *(Figure P14–1-4)*

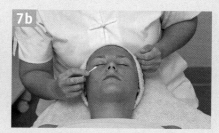

Make a complete circular pattern. *(Figure P14–1-5)*

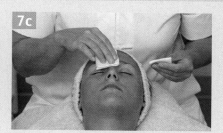

Rinse with water. *(Figure P14–1-6)*

7a Place the edge of the pad under the lower lashes at the outside corner of the eyes, and slide the pad toward the inner corner of the eyes. The mascara will gradually work loose and can be wiped clean. Be especially gentle when cleansing the eyes because the skin around the eyes is very sensitive and can become irritated (Figure P14–1-2). Remove any makeup underneath the eyes. Always be gentle around the eyes; never rub or stretch the skin, as it is very delicate and thin.

7b Use the cotton pad or a cotton swab to wipe inward under the eye toward the nose and then outward on the top of the eyelid (Figure P14–1-5). Making a complete circular pattern.

7c Rinse the eye area with plain water to remove the eye makeup remover (Figure P14–1-6). Make sure the remover is rinsed off thoroughly.

Lipstick Removal

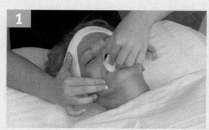

Remove lipstick. *(Figure P14–1-7)*

2 With the index and middle finger (either the left or right side) of one hand, hold on next to the outside edge of the lips to keep the skin tight so it does not move around; then remove with even strokes from the corners of the lips toward the center.

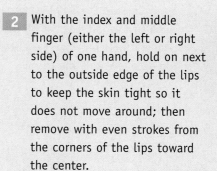

Repeat on other side. *(Figure P14–1-8)*

1 To remove lipstick, apply eye makeup remover or a cleanser to a damp cotton pad or tissue and gently remove the client's lipstick (Figure P14–1-7).

3 Repeat the procedure on the other side until the lips are clean (Figure P14–1-8).

Clean-Up and Sanitation

Follow the clean-up procedure described in the basic facial (Procedure 14–4).

PROCEDURE 14-2

APPLYING CLEANSING PRODUCT

SUPPLIES
- disinfectant/sanitizer
- hand sanitizer/antibacterial soap
- covered trash container
- bowl
- spatula
- hand towels
- headband
- clean linens
- bolster

DISPOSABLES
- gloves
- cotton pads
- cotton rounds
- cotton swabs
- plastic bag
- paper towels
- tissues

PRODUCTS
- eye makeup remover or cleanser
- facial cleanser
- toner
- moisturizer

The following method of application is used when applying cleansers, massage creams, treatment creams, and protective products. Most product removal requires rinsing each area at least three times. If possible, use both hands at the same time. The hands must be clean before touching the client's face.

Preparation

1 Prepare the bed and room.

2 Set out supplies and products on an SMA.

3 Prepare the client and cover the hair.

Procedure

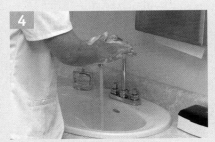

Sanitize hands. *(Figure P14-2-1)*

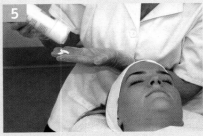

Apply product to fingers. *(Figure P14-2-2)*

4 Cleanse and sanitize the hands before touching the client's face. (Figure P14-2-1). Apply warm towels. After checking the temperature, apply one towel to the décolleté and one to the face.

5 Apply approximately one-half teaspoon of the product to the fingers or palms of the hand. Water-soluble cleansing lotion is preferred when cleansing the face because it can be easily removed with moistened cotton pads or sponges (Figure P14-2-2).

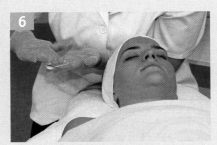

Use circular motion to distribute product. *(Figure P14-2-3)*

6 Use circular motions to distribute the product onto the fingertips. You are now ready to apply the product to the client's décolleté, neck, and face (Figure P14-2-3).

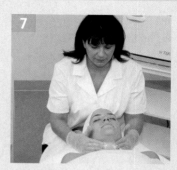

Apply product on neck. *(Figure P14–2-4)*

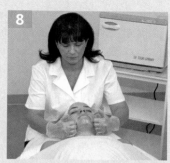

Slide fingers along jawline. *(Figure P14–2-5)*

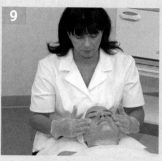

Slide fingers over cheeks. *(Figure P14–2-6)*

7 Start applying the product by placing both hands, palms down, on the neck. Slide hands back toward the ears until the pads of the fingers rest at a point directly beneath the ear-lobes (Figure P14–2-4). While applying the product, do not lift your hands from the client's face until you are finished.

8 Reverse the hand, with the back of the fingers now resting on the skin, and slide the fingers along the jawline to the chin (Figure P14–2-5).

9 Reverse the hands again and slide the fingers back over the cheeks until the pads of the fingers come to rest directly in front of the ears (Figure P14–2-6).

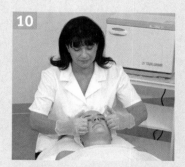

Slide fingers over cheekbones to the nose. *(Figure P14–2-7)*

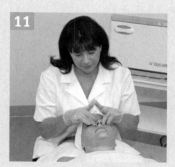

Make small, circular motions on the flare of the nostrils. *(Figure P14–2-8)*

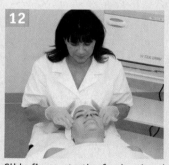

Slide fingers to the forehead and out toward the temple. *(Figure P14–2-9)*

10 Reverse the hands again, and slide the fingers forward over the cheekbones to the nose (Figure P14–2-7).

11 With the pads of the middle fingers, make small, circular motions on the top of the nose and on each side of the nose (Figure P14–2-8). Avoid pushing the product into the nose.

12 Slide the fingers up to the forehead and outward toward the temples, pausing with a slight pressure on the temples. Slide fingers across the forehead using circles or long strokes from side to side (Figure P14–2-9).

Clean-Up and Sanitation

Follow the clean-up procedure described in the basic facial (Procedure 14–4).

PROCEDURE 14-3   REMOVING PRODUCT

Rinse each area at least three times. Some estheticians prefer to use wet cotton pads or disposable facial sponges when removing product. Others prefer to use towels. Both methods are correct and equally professional, and many estheticians use both methods. For example, an esthetician who usually uses the sponges will use cotton pads when working on acne skin. Even when using sponges, an esthetician may need some cotton during the treatment for eye pads or extracting blackheads.

Movements are generally done in an upward and outward direction from the center to the edges of the face. Under the eyes, it is usually inward to avoid tugging on the eye area.

Procedure

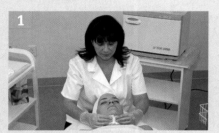

Cleanse the neck. *(Figure P14-3-1)*

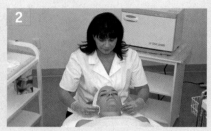

Slide pad along the jawline. *(Figure P14-3-2)*

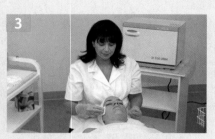

Use upward movements to cleanse the cheeks. *(Figure P14-3-3)*

1 Starting at the décolleté, cleanse sideways and up to the neck. Cleanse the neck using upward strokes. To keep the pad from slipping from the hand, pinch the edge of the pad between the thumb and upper part of the forefinger. It is important that most of the surface of the pad remain in contact with the skin. Do not exert pressure on the Adam's apple (Figure P14-3-1).

2 Place the pad directly under the chin and slide the pad along the jawline, stopping directly under the ear. Repeat the movement on the other side of the face. Alternate back and forth three times on each side of the face, or do the movement concurrently by using both hands at the same time (Figure P14-3-2).

3 Starting at the jawline, use upward movements to cleanse the cheek (Figure P14-3-3).

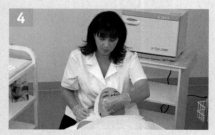

Cross over the chin to the other cheek. *(Figure P14-3-4)*

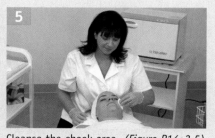

Cleanse the cheek area. *(Figure P14-3-5)*

4 Continuing the upward movement, cross over the chin to the other cheek (Figure P14-3-4).

5 Continue the cleansing movement with approximately six strokes on each cheek (Figure P14-3-5).

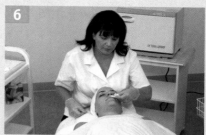

Cleanse underneath the nose. *(Figure P14–3-6)*

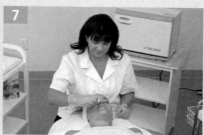

Cleanse the sides of the nose. *(Figure P14–3-7)*

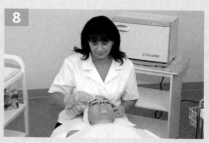

Cleanse the forehead. *(Figure P14–3-8)*

6 Cleanse the area directly underneath the nose by using downward and sideways strokes. Start at the center and work outward toward the corners of the mouth. Alternate the movements back and forth three times on each side of the face (Figure P14-3-6).

7 Starting on the bridge of the nose, cleanse the sides of the nose and the area directly next to it. Use light, outward movements (Figure P14-3-7).

8 Place the pads flat on the center of the forehead, and slide them outward to the temples. Apply a slight pressure on the pressure points of the temples. Repeat the movement three times on each side of the forehead (Figure P14-3-8).

Clean-Up and Sanitation

Follow the clean-up procedure described in the basic facial (Procedure 14–4).

PROCEDURE 14-4

THE BASIC STEP-BY-STEP FACIAL

EQUIPMENT
- facial equipment (towel warmer, steamer, mag light)

SUPPLIES
- disinfectant/sanitizer
- hand sanitizer/antibacterial soap
- covered trash container
- bowls
- spatulas
- fan and mask brush
- implements
- distilled water
- sharps container
- hand towels
- clean linens
- blanket
- headband
- client gown or wrap
- bolster
- client charts

DISPOSABLES
- cotton pads
- cotton rounds
- cotton swabs
- paper towels
- tissue
- gloves/finger cots
- baggies

PRODUCTS
- cleanser
- exfoliant
- masks
- massage lotion
- toner
- moisturizer
- sunscreen
- optional: serums, eye cream, lip balm, extraction supplies

Now that you have practiced the preliminary steps and cleansing, it is time to put it all together in a complete facial. The steps for performing a basic facial treatment are listed here. Some procedures may vary, however, so be guided by your instructor.

Preparation

1 Set up the room.

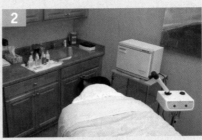

Prepare the treatment room. *(Figure P14–4-1)*

Help the client prepare for the service. *(Figure P14–4-2)*

2 Prepare the bed, equipment, and workstation (Figure P14–4-1).

3 Help the client prepare for the service (Figure P14–4-2).

4 Put on headband (Figure P14–4-3).

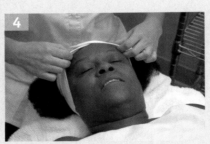

Put on the headband. *(Figure P14–4-3)*

Procedure

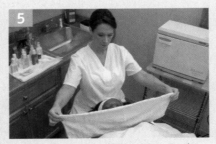

Apply warm towels. *(Figure P14–4-4)*

5 **Cleanse your hands and apply warm towels.** After checking the temperature, apply one towel to the décolleté and one to the face (Figure P14–4-4).

Optional: Remove eye makeup and lipstick. If your client has no makeup, skip this part and proceed to step 2. Remember to ask about contact lenses before putting product on the eyes. If the client is wearing contacts, do not remove the eye makeup.

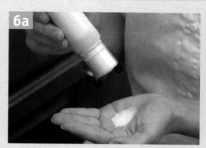

Apply cleanser to fingertips. *(Figure P14–4–5)*

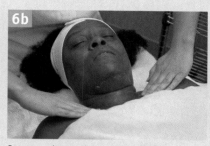

Start at the neck or décolleté. *(Figure P14–4–6)*

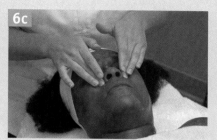

Make small, circular movements with fingertips. *(Figure P14–4–7)*

6 **Cleanse.**

a. Remove about one-half tea-spoon of cleanser from the container (with a sanitized spatula if it is not a squirt-top or pump-type lid). Place it in the palm and then apply a small amount to your fingertips (Figure P14–4–5). This conserves the amount of product you use.

b. Starting at the neck or décol-leté and with a sweeping movement, use both hands to spread the cleanser upward and outward on the chin, jaws, cheeks, and temples (Figure P14–4–6). Spread the cleanser down the nose and along its sides and bridge.

c. Make small, circular movements with the fingertips around the nostrils and sides of the nose (Figure P14–4–7). Continue with upward-sweeping move-ments between the brows and across the forehead to the temples.

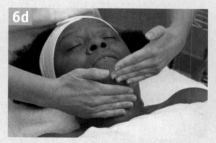

Apply more cleanser with long strokes. *(Figure P14–4–8)*

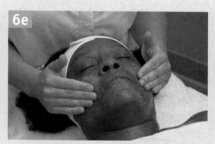

Continue moving up toward the fore-head. *(Figure P14–4–9)*

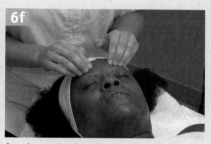

Continue circular pattern out to tem-ples. *(Figure P14–4–10)*

d. Apply more cleanser to the neck and chest with long, even strokes (Figure P14–4–8). Cleanse the area in small, cir-cular motions from the center of the chest and neck toward the outside, moving upward. Try to use both hands at the same time on each side when applying or removing product.

e. Visually divide the face into left and right halves from the center. Continue moving upward with circular motions on the face from the chin and cheeks, and up toward the forehead using both hands, one on each side (Figure P14–4–9).

f. Starting at the center of the fore-head, continue with the circular pattern out to the temples (Figure P14–4–10). Move the fingertips lightly in a circle around the eyes to the temples and then back to the center of the forehead. Lift your hands slowly off of the face when you finish cleansing.

Note: Remember that procedures vary. In cleansing, the instructor may have you use mainly long strokes, rather than circles.

PROCEDURE 14-4, CONT.

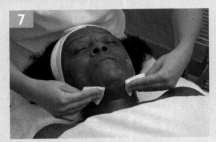

Remove the cleanser. *(Figure P14-4-11)*

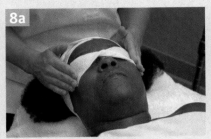

Place eye pads on client. *(Figure P14-4-12)*

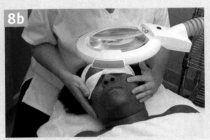

Use the magnifying light to determine skin type and condition. *(Figure P14-4-13)*

7 **Remove the cleanser.** Using moist cotton pads or disposable facial sponges, start at the neck or forehead and follow the contours of the face. Move up or down the face in a consistent pattern, depending on where you start according to the instructor's procedures (Figure P14-4-11). Remove all the cleanser from one area of the face before proceeding to the next. (Under the nostrils, use downward strokes when applying or removing products to avoid pushing product up the nose. This is uncomfortable and will make the client tense.) Blot your hands on a clean towel, and touch the face with dry fingertips to make sure there is no residue left.

8 **Analyze the skin.** Cover the client's eyes with eye pads (Figure P14-4-12). Position the magnifying light where you want it before starting the facial, so that you can swing it over easily to line up over the face (Figure P14-4-13). Note the skin type and condition, and feel the texture of the skin.

Optional: Cleanse the face again. Some treatment protocols do not include this second cleansing. Be guided by your instructor.

Optional: If exfoliation is part of the service, it could be done at this time before steaming. If eyebrow arching is needed, it could be done either at this time or following the steam and extractions to avoid irritation from the steam. Be careful what you apply to waxed areas.

9 Steam the face (Figure P14-4-14).

a. Preheat the steamer before you need it. Turn it on, wait for it to start steaming, and then turn on the ozone button if applicable.

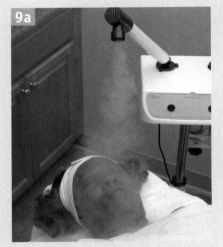

Steam the face. *(Figure P14-4-14)*

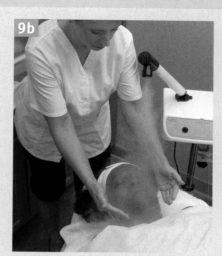

Check that steam reaches both sides of face. *(Figure P14–4-15)*

b. Check to make sure the steamer is not too close to the client (approximately 18 inches away) and that it is steaming the face evenly. If you hold your hands close to the sides of the client's face, you can feel if the steam is reaching both sides of the face (Figure P14–4-15). Steam for approximately 5 to 10 minutes.

c. Turn off the steamer immediately after use. (Review the section on steamers in Chapter 16 for steamer cautions.)

If using towels, remember to test them for the correct temperature. Ask the client if she is comfortable with the temperature. Towels are left on for approximately 2 minutes. Steam or warm towels should be used carefully on couperose skin.

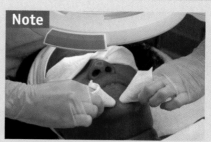

Performing extractions. *(Figure P14–4-16)*

Note Extractions are done immediately after the steam, while the skin is still warm (Figure P14–4-16). Refer to the extractions section of this chapter to incorporate this step into your basic facial procedure if it is applicable to your facility.

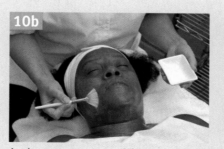

Apply massage cream. *(Figure P14–4-17)*

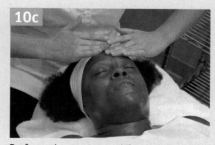

Perform the massage. *(Figure P14–4-18)*

10 **Massage the face.** Use the facial manipulations described in Chapter 15.

a. Select a water-soluble massage cream or product appropriate to the client's skin type.

b. Use the same procedure as you did for product application to apply the massage cream to the face, neck, shoulders, and chest. Apply the warmed product in long, slow strokes with a brush, moving in a set pattern (Figure P14–4-17).

c. Perform the massage as directed (Figure P14–4-18).

PROCEDURE 14–4, CONT.

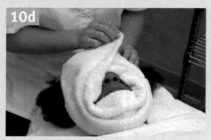

Remove massage cream. *(Figure P14–4-19)*

d. Remove the massage cream. Use warm towels or cleansing pads and follow the same procedure as for removing other products or cleanser (Figure P14-4-19).

11 **Apply a treatment mask.**

a. Choose a mask formulated for the client's skin condition. Remove the mask from its container, and place it in the palm or a small mixing cup. (Use a clean spatula, if necessary, to avoid contamination.) Warming the mask is recommended.

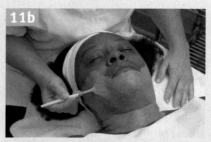

Applying a mask. *(Figure P14-4-20)*

b. Apply the mask with fingers or a brush, usually starting at the neck. Use long, slow strokes from the center of the face, moving outward to the sides (Figure P14-4-20).

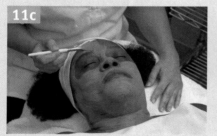

Apply mask from the center outward. *(Figure P14–4-21)*

c. Proceed to the jawline and apply the mask on the face from the center outward (Figure P14-4-21). Avoid the eye area unless the mask is appropriate for that area.

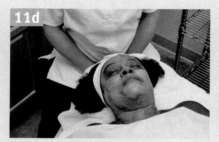

Leave mask on for 7–10 minutes. *(Figure P14-4-22)*

d. Allow the mask to remain on the face for approximately 7 to 10 minutes (Figure P14-4-22).

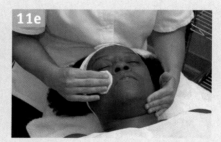

Remove the mask. *(Figure P14–4-23)*

e. Remove the mask with wet cotton pads, sponges, or towels (Figure P14-4-23).

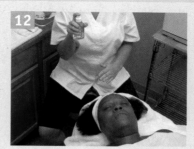

Apply toner. *(Figure P14–4-24)*

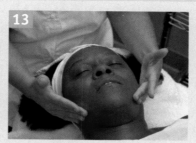

Apply moisturizer and sunscreen. *(Figure P14–4-25)*

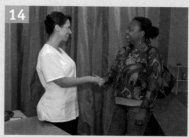

Discuss home-care products and regime. *(Figure P14–4-26)*

12 Apply the toner product appropriate for the skin type (Figure P14-4-24).

Note: Serums as well as eye and lip creams are optional for application before the final moisturizer.

13 Apply a moisturizer and an additional sunscreen if applicable (Figure P14-4-25).

14 End the facial by washing your hands and quietly letting the client know you are finished. Give the client instructions for getting dressed. Have her come out to the reception area when ready to discuss the home-care products and regime (Figure P14-4-26).

Clean-Up and Sanitation

15 Discard all disposable supplies and materials.

16 Close product containers tightly, clean them, and put them away in their proper places. Return unused cosmetics and other clean items to the dispensary.

17 Place used towels, coverlets, head covers, and other linens in a closed, covered laundry hamper.

18 Disinfect your workstation, including the facial table.

19 Wash your hands with soap and warm water.

CAUTION!

For sanitary reasons, never remove products from containers with your fingers. Always use a spatula. Do not touch fingertips to lids or openings of containers.

FOCUS ON . . .

CLIENTS

The importance of following proper hygiene and sanitation guidelines when giving facials cannot be overemphasized. As much as possible, wash your hands in the presence of your clients. When they see you doing this, they will have more confidence in your sanitation procedures.

> **CAUTION!**
>
> To avoid damage to capillaries, do not use strong steam or hot towels on couperose skin.

Consultation and Home Care

Home care is probably the most important factor in a successful skin care program. The key word here is *program*. Clients' participation is essential to achieve results. A program consists of a long-range plan involving home care, salon treatments, and client education.

Every new client should be thoroughly consulted about home care for his or her skin conditions. After the first treatment, block out about 15 minutes to explain proper home care for the client.

After the treatment is finished, have the client sit in the facial chair, or invite her to move to a well-lit consultation area. A mirror should be provided for the client, so that she can see conditions you will be discussing.

Explain, in simple terms, the client's skin conditions, informing her of how you propose to treat the conditions. Inform her about how often treatments should be administered in the salon, and very specifically explain what she should be doing at home.

Set out the products you want the client to purchase and use. Explain each one, and tell her in which order to use them. Make sure to have written instructions for the client to take home.

It is important to have products available for the client that you believe in and that produce results. Retailing products for clients to use at home is important to the success of your treatments and to your business.

CLEAN-UP/SANITATION CHECKLIST

After the facial, complete the clean-up procedures and sanitation steps (Table 14–5).

Table 14–5

THE CLEAN-UP CHECKLIST

Facial Sanitation and Clean-Up Checklist

SANITATION AND POST-FACIAL	EQUIPMENT/ROOM	SUPPLIES	DISPOSABLES
• Wash your hands.	• Clean the wax machine and turn it off at the end of the day.	• Wash and disinfect brushes, spatulas, tweezers, and other nondisposable implements used during the process.	• Soiled items such as gloves and extraction supplies must be placed in a sealable plastic bag and then in a covered waste container.
• Say good-bye to the client after the post-consultation.	• Disinfect the steamer. Refill with distilled water.	• Clean and disinfect bowls and other reusable items. Dry and store properly.	• Disposable extraction lancets go in a bio-hazard sharps container.

Table 14–5 (*continued*)

SANITATION AND POST-FACIAL	EQUIPMENT/ROOM	SUPPLIES	DISPOSABLES
• Make the client chart notes.	• Wipe and disinfect the equipment used.	• Remove the dirty linens and remake the bed.	
• Write up retail sales.	• Clean all containers and wipe off dirty product containers with a disinfectant.	• Turn off the bed warmer if used. • Put the linens, towels, and sheets in the appropriate covered laundry hamper.	
• Prepare the room for the next client or carry out end-of-the-day clean-up tasks.	• Clean all counters, sinks, surfaces, and floor mats with disinfectant.	• Change the disinfectant in the sanitizer to comply with sanitation regulations.	
		• Change towels on the workstation tables.	
		• Put away the supplies.	

PROCEDURE 14–5

APPLYING THE COTTON COMPRESS

SUPPLIES
- cotton roll
- scissors
- basin of warm water
- product

Preparation

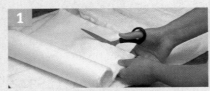

Prepare cotton. *(Figure P14–5-1)*

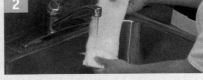

Wet and unfold the cotton strip. *(Figure P14–5-2)*

1   Prepare the cotton on an SMA (Figure P14-5-1).

2   Wet and unfold the cotton strip, and carefully divide it length-wise into three separate strips (Figure P14-5-2). Try to keep the thickness of each strip as even as possible.

Procedure

The steps for applying a cotton compress alone or over a mask are as follows:

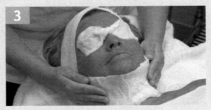

Take the strip that feels the thinnest and mold it to the client's neck. *(Figure P14–5-3)*

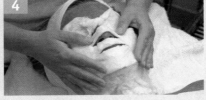

Apply the cotton under the jaw, chin, and lower part of the cheeks. *(Figure P14–5-4)*

3   Secure eye pads on the client's eyes. Take the strip that feels the thinnest and mold it to the client's neck. Be sure the strip does not overlap on the under-side of the chin and jawline (Figure P14-5-3).

4   Place the center of the second strip of cotton (saving the thickest piece for last) on the chin, under the lower lip. Mold the cotton under the jaw, chin, and lower part of the cheeks. Leave breathing access by mold-ing the strips around the tip of the nose (Figure P14-5-4).

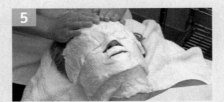

(Figure P14–5-5)

5   Place the third and thickest cotton strip over the upper por-tion of the face (eye pads remain in place). Carefully stretch the cotton (Figure P14-5-5).

PROCEDURE 14–6   REMOVING THE COTTON COMPRESS

1 *Optional step:* Massage over the surface of the compress mask with an ice cube or cool face globes if available, using circular movements. The ice will feel refreshing and will firm the skin. As the ice melts, the water seeps into the compress, helping to soften the mask underneath.

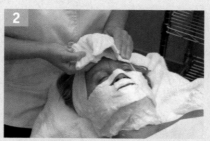

Slide the compress slowly toward the side of the face, picking up as much of the treatment mask as possible. *(Figure P14–6-1)*

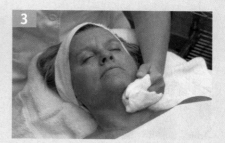

Use cotton mitts to further remove remaining traces of the mask. *(Figure P14–6-2)*

2 Starting on the upper part of the face, place the hands, palms down, on each side of the face. With one hand, slide the compress slowly toward the side of the face, picking up as much of the treatment mask as possible (Figure P14–6-1). The eye pads will come off at the same time and should be discarded. Fold the strip in half, so that the side of the compress that has the treatment mask on it is inside and the compress strip has two clean surfaces. Squeeze the cotton over a waste container to remove any excess water.

3 Tear a separate strip of wet cotton in half, wrapping around the first three fingers of the hand to form a cotton mitt. Use the cotton mitts to further remove remaining traces of the mask (Figure P14–6-2). If necessary, cotton pads, rather than finger mitts, can be used to cleanse the face.

When all traces of the treatment mask have been removed, move down to the next cotton compress strip and repeat the same steps. Repeat again on the neck strip.

PROCEDURE 14–7

EXTRACTIONS

SUPPLIES

- basin of water
- cotton pads
- gloves
- astringent
- zip-lock plastic bag
- other appropriate facial supplies, products, and equipment

Preparation

Preparing the Fingers for Comedone Extractions

If you are using 4" × 4" or 2" × 2" premade pads, apply astringent to pads (without oversaturating them) and wrap around fingers. If you are not using 4 premade pads, prepare cotton as follows.

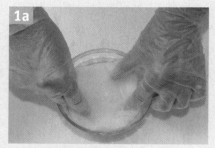

Wet cotton. *(Figure P14–7-1)*

1 Dip strips of clean cotton in water and squeeze out the excess (Figure P14–7-1 a, b).

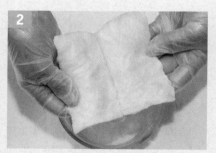

Divide pad in half. *(Figure P14–7-2)*

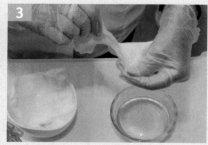

Tear strips. *(Figure P14–7-3)*

2 Unfold the pad and divide it in half (Figure P14–7-2). Place one-half of the pad back in the bowl that holds the cleansing pads. With astringent, lightly saturate the half of the pad you are holding. Squeeze out the excess astringent.

3 Tear small strips from the astringent-saturated cotton (Figure P14–7-3).

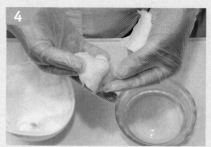

Wrap strips around index fingers.
(Figure P14–7-4)

4 Put on gloves, and wrap fingers with dampened pads. Wrap the strips smoothly around the end of each index finger. Repeat this step until the fingertips are well padded (Figure P14–7-4).

Performing Extractions

Prepare the client's skin. Extractions are performed during a treatment after the skin is warmed and prepared/softened with product. Never extract on unprepared dry, cold skin. Extraction procedures for different facial areas follow:

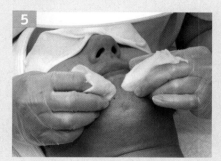

Extractions on the chin. *(Figure P14–7-5)*

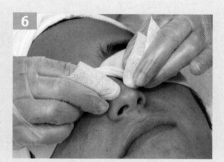

Extractions on the nose. *(Figure P14–7-6)*

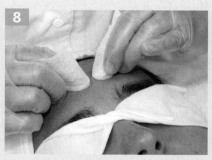

Extractions on the forehead.
(Figure P14–7-7)

5 **Chin.** On a flat area, press down, under, and up. Work around the plug, pressing down, in, and up (Figure P14–7-5). Bring fingers in toward each other around the follicle without pinching.

6 **Nose.** Slide fingers down each side of the nose, holding the nostril tissue firmly, but do not press down too firmly on the nose. The fingers on top do the sliding, while the other one holds close to the bottom of the follicle. Do not cut off the air flow to the nostrils (Figure P14–7-6).

7 **Cheeks.** Slide fingers down the cheek, holding the skin as you go. The lower hand holds and the other hand slides toward the lower hand.

8 **Forehead; upper cheekbones.** Extract as on the chin: press down, in, and up (Figure P14-7-7).

Clean-Up

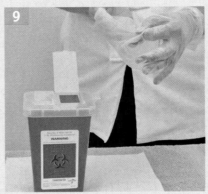

Change gloves. *(Figure P14–7-8)*

9 Dispose of gloves and supplies properly. Change gloves to continue the treatment (Figure P14–7-8).

10 After completing the treatment, perform the clean-up steps following a service. It is important to follow thorough sanitation procedures after doing extractions or an acne facial.

FYI

LANCETS

When a lesion is sealed over, as in old blackheads and closed comedones, a small-gauge needle or lancet is used for extraction. The lancet should be inserted at a 35-degree angle or parallel to the surface of the skin. Slowly insert the needle just under the top of the plug, lift the top off, and open it gently. Never put the needle down into the follicle because it is painful and could damage it. Extract in the appropriate direction to release sebum (Figure 14–20). Lancets are disposed of in biohazard containers.

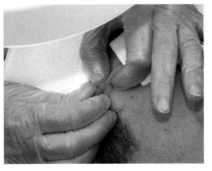

Figure 14–20 Using a lancet.

THE MINI-FACIAL

The main differences between a mini-facial and a basic facial are the time and the number of steps. Mini-facials may take only 25 minutes and do not include all the steps of a full, 60-minute facial. Omitted steps may include the comprehensive skin analysis, massage, or extractions. Deep cleansing and masking are the most important elements of the mini-facial because they produce the most visible results.

The mini-facial gives clients a treatment that can be completed quickly if they are pressed for time. It will introduce them to a light, refreshing facial that may lead to rebooking for a more in-depth, relaxing facial to address specific skin concerns and conditions.

MINI-PROCEDURE

THE MINI-FACIAL

1. Perform a quick cleansing to remove makeup. Rinse well.
2. Analyze with a magnifying lamp.
3. Perform a second quick cleansing with an exfoliant or a deep pore cleanser. Rinse thoroughly. A brush machine can be used as a quick exfoliating method.
4. Apply a mask.
5. Remove the mask.
6. Apply a toner appropriate to the client's skin type.
7. Apply day cream or moisturizer and sunscreen.
8. Recommend a treatment for the client's next visit.
9. Recommend initial home-care products and complete the home-care chart.

TREATMENTS FOR DIFFERENT SKIN TYPES AND CONDITIONS

Skin conditions and products have been covered in previous chapters, so review ingredients and the factors influencing the skin's health to choose treatments for the individual client. The following treatments incorporate the same basic procedures as the basic facial, but certain steps and products are added or omitted, based on the condition and skin type being treated. Too many choices can be overwhelming to clients, so it is appropriate to offer a basic facial with ingredients designed for a normal skin type. This service can be effective for almost any client.

Dry Skin

Skin is often dry due to inactivity of the sebaceous glands, which produce the sebum (oil) that lubricates the skin. Dry skin may appear to be thin, and in some cases small capillaries can be seen near the surface of the skin. Dry skin can appear to be fine in texture but coarse to the touch. Facial treatments and home maintenance can help minimize dryness and stimulate the production of sebum.

The skin may have dry and oily areas that can be treated separately. Serums and creams for dry skin are important. Occlusive products are necessary to protect and balance dry skin. Conversely, there is a theory that using a heavy cream or oil on dry skin may inhibit its production of natural oils, so moderation is the key. When discussing the client's dry skin condition, the esthetician can explain that the excessive application of heavy creams may in some cases interfere with the production of sebum and that stimulating the natural oil of the skin is far more beneficial than just applying heavy oils or creams. Balance and protect skin with the appropriate products and in the proper amounts.

Treatments for Dry Skin

For dry or mature skin, the treatment goals are similar: to hydrate and nourish the skin. The purpose of the treatment is to stimulate the cell metabolism by using performance ingredients. Protecting the barrier function and keeping dry skin well lubricated is important.

Follow the facial steps using products designed for dry skin. Complete procedures and facial steps are not included here—only the additions to the facial.

1. Use a gentle enzyme peel, or a gentle alpha hydroxy acid peel, to exfoliate the skin.
2. For a mask, a collagen, hydrating, paraffin wax, or thermal mask can be used.
3. The galvanic machine or the massage can be used to assist in the penetration of a hydrating serum or nourishing product.
4. A moisturizing cream with an oil base, antioxidants, and a sunscreen finish the treatment.

Dry Skin That Lacks Moisture (Dehydrated)

A skin may have enough oil, but still feel dry and flaky due to lack of water in the skin. The skin may become dehydrated from drying products, too much sun, wind, harsh soaps, a poor diet, and aging. Limited water intake, excessive steaming of the face, the use of drying packs and masks, the use of drying cosmetics, medication taken internally or applied externally, or other environmental factors all contribute to dehydration. A dehydrated skin is prone to fine lines and wrinkles.

If the client's skin seems to be dehydrated from factors that require medical attention (such as diet, lack of fluids, or medication), the esthetician should recommend that the client seek the advice of his or her physician or dermatologist. In the meantime, facial treatments to improve the general health of the skin and to help it to retain moisture will be beneficial.

Dehydration of the skin may be a temporary condition, varying from season to season and due to various factors in the environment. Use a treatment similar to the one for dry, mature, or sensitive skin. The goal is to hydrate and nourish the skin. Adapt the products for the individual's needs.

Treatments for Mature or Aging Skin

Dry skin is often due to the natural aging process of the body. As a person advances in years, the body's processes slow down, and cells are not replaced as rapidly as they were when the person was younger. It is not difficult to diagnose aging skin, but skin ages at different rates due to the following factors:

- The skin ages due to neglect and the external treatment it has received.
- Exposure to extreme climates; too much sun, wind, or polluted air will hasten the aging process.
- Physiological disease, poor health, and psychological (emotional) problems can cause the skin to appear older.
- Extreme weight loss can result in loss of muscle tone and lined and sagging skin, which in turn gives the skin an aged appearance.
- Medications, lack of proper diet, smoking, and the misuse of alcoholic beverages affect the skin's appearance.

The mature client's skin can be improved; but the natural aging process cannot be reversed, nor will the skin be restored to the same vital condition of youth. The client should be advised that treatments can make the skin look and feel better, but there are no miracle treatments that restore aging skin.

Elasticity of the Skin

Aging skin often lacks elasticity. The skin is tested for elasticity by taking a small section of the facial skin or neck between the thumb and forefinger and giving the skin a slight outward pull. When the skin is released, and if the elasticity is good, the skin will immediately return to its normal shape. If the skin is slow to resume its normal shape, it is lacking elasticity. Firming ingredients and treatments are beneficial for skin's elasticity.

Ingredients for Mature Skin

Aging or sun-damaged skin needs antioxidants topically and orally. Antioxidants such as vitamins C, E, and A; minerals; green tea; and grape-seed extract all help protect the body from free radicals. Other beneficial care for aging skin includes protecting the barrier function of the skin and wearing sunscreen. Additionally, alpha hydroxy acids can help combat the signs of aging and sun damage. Hydrating ingredients such as hyaluronic acid, sodium hyaluronate, sodium PCA, and glycerin all bind water to the skin and retain the moisture that is essential to maturing skin. Peptides, lipids, polyglucans, coenzyme Q10, and liposomes are all beneficial performance ingredients.

Treatment goals are to hydrate and soften the skin. Stimulating the metabolism and firming the skin are also part of an antiaging facial. Facial treatments are wonderful rejuvenators for clients with mature, aging, or sun-damaged skin. Remember all of the benefits derived from each of the facial steps.

Mature Skin Treatment

Here are some suggestions for treating mature skin:
- Use procedures similar to those designed for dry skin, adapting the ingredients.
- Massage with a deep-penetrating serum and cream.
- Collagen or hydrating masks are both beneficial in a facial treatment for mature skin.
- A thermal or paraffin mask will also plump and force-feed nutrients into the skin.
- Firming products can also be effective in visibly tightening the skin.

PROCEDURE 14–8

APPLYING THE PARAFFIN MASK

EQUIPMENT
- paraffin wax and heater

SUPPLIES
- paraffin wax brush
- covered trash container with plastic bag
- bowl
- spatula
- bolster
- disinfectant/sanitizer
- hand sanitizer/antibacterial soap

LINENS
- hand towels
- client gown or wrap
- clean linens
- blanket
- headband

DISPOSABLES
- gauze
- paper towels
- gloves
- cotton pads
- cotton rounds
- tissues

PRODUCTS
- cleanser
- serum
- mask
- toner
- eye cream
- moisturizer
- sunscreen
- lip balm

Preparation

1 Prepare the room and station for a facial.

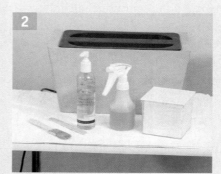

(Figure P14–8-1)

2 Melt the paraffin in a warming unit to a little more than body temperature (Figure P14-8-1). This may take an hour to heat up.

Procedure

3 Place eye pads on client.

4 Apply an appropriate product, such as a serum or hydrating mask, under the paraffin mask.

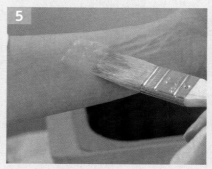

Test the temperature on the wrist.
(Figure P14–8-2)

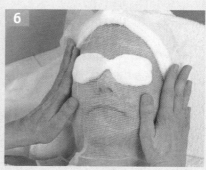

Place the gauze on the face.
(Figure P14–8-3)

5 Test the temperature of the paraffin on the wrist (Figure P14-8-2).

6 Cut the gauze to the desired size, and place it over the face and neck (Figure P14–8-3). It is not usually necessary to cut holes for the eyes and nose, because the gauze is woven very loosely. Occasionally, however, a client may feel claustrophobic. In that case, make slits in the gauze for the eyes, nose, and mouth. Precut gauze pads are available and are more efficient for this use.

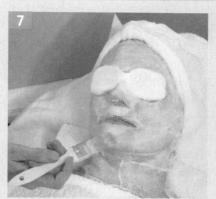

Apply the first coat of paraffin with a brush. *(Figure P14–8-4)*

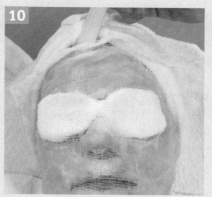

Use a wooden spatula to work the mask loose. *(Figure P14–8-5)*

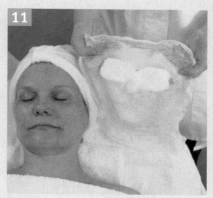

Carefully remove the mask. *(Figure P14–8-6)*

7 Apply the first coat of paraffin over the gauze with a brush, beginning at the base of the neck and working up to the forehead (Figure P14–8-4).

8 Continue adding layers of paraffin to the top of the gauze until the application is approximately 1/4" thick. The application of wax will take several minutes.

9 After the wax application is completed, have the client relax until the wax is hardened and ready to remove (approximately 15 minutes).

10 When ready to remove the mask, use a wooden spatula to work the edges of the mask loose from the face and neck (Figure P14–8-5).

11 Carefully lift the mask from the neck in one piece (Figure P14–8-6).

12 Finish the service with the appropriate products (toner, moisturizer).

Clean-Up

13 Remove the head covering and show the client to the dressing room, offering assistance if needed.

14 Discard all disposable supplies and materials.

15 Close product containers tightly, clean them, and put them away in their proper places. Return unused cosmetics and other clean items to the dispensary.

16 Place used towels, head covers, and other linens in a closed, covered laundry hamper.

17 Disinfect supplies, equipment, and the workstation, including the facial table. Turn off the equipment.

18 Wash your hands with soap and warm water.

Treatments for Sensitive Skin or Rosacea

For sensitive skin, the primary goal is to calm and cool the skin. Increasing the skin's barrier function is another important part of treating sensitive skin. Rosacea is treated much the same because it is also characterized by red, couperose, and sensitive conditions. Calming ingredients such as aloe vera, chamomile, allantoin, azulene, and licorice extracts are all effective on sensitive or irritated skin.

Individuals with sensitive skin should avoid stimulating, drying products and heat. Advise these clients to avoid vasodilators that dilate capillaries: heat, the sun, spicy foods, and stimulating products. Irritants and sensitizing ingredients can be essential oils, exfoliants, fragrances, color agents, and preservatives. All of these may cause allergies and irritation. Home-care product recommendations should be designed for sensitive skin, but that is no guarantee they will not irritate the skin.

Rosacea

Rosacea, like seborrhea, can be characterized by excessive oiliness of the skin. The nose and cheeks are the most frequently affected. The face will have a flushed appearance and, if neglected, the skin can become lumpy where the papules and pustules are formed. Although sometimes referred to as "acne rosacea," this skin condition is not to be confused with acne. Rosacea is not the same type of skin condition that appears during adolescence, because it usually does not appear before the age of 35. Rosacea is more common in adult females than in males. However, when a male develops rosacea, it usually becomes quite severe. Rosacea can be aggravated by alcohol and heavily spiced foods. The client should be advised to avoid squeezing or picking lumps that appear on any area of the face. In ordinary cases, soothing treatments will be helpful. In recent years rosacea has been treated successfully by dermatologists. The client should be encouraged to consult a dermatologist for medication when experiencing severe flairs.

Sensitive Skin Treatment

Follow the facial procedure and incorporate the following guidelines:

1. To soothe irritation, a gentle cleanser is the best type of cleanser. Foaming, detergent-based cleansers can strip the skin's lipids and barrier protection.
2. Less steam and heat should be used. Make sure warm towels are not hot, or skip them altogether. Cold towels are **vasoconstricting**, which means they constrict capillaries and blood flow.
3. An enzyme peel formulated for sensitive skin gently exfoliates the skin.
4. A soothing gel mask is great for calming and toning down redness. Freeze-dried collagen masks are also excellent for sensitive skin.
5. Lipids protect the skin, and a serum or moisturizer with lipids is essential for treating sensitive and dry skin. Moisturizers with calming ingredients are also beneficial.

Treatments for Hyperpigmentation

Hyperpigmentation is a condition that affects many people. Sun exposure causes dark pigmentation areas on the skin that clients often want to diminish. Advise clients that the best preventative measures are to stay out of the sun and wear sunscreen daily. Peels and brightening agents can be effective in reducing some of these hyperpigmented areas. Melanin-suppressant agents are also used for this condition. Hydroquinone is the only FDA-approved agent, but it thins the skin. It is not a bleaching agent, but a melanin suppressant. Brighteners such as kojic acid, mulberry, licorice root, bearberry, and azaleic acid are known to reduce pigmentation. These affect melanin production and are more effective when used with AHAs, BHAs, and peels. Remember that over-exfoliating can make hyperpigmentation worse—or conversely, cause hypopigmentation.

Treatments for Oily Skin

Oily and combination skins need water-based products. Facial goals are focused on deep cleansing. Use products for oily skin, not heavy creams or oils. This skin can usually tolerate more stimulation and stronger products, but be careful not to overdo it or overdry the skin. Aggressive products and treatments may make it worse. The trick is to apply the right products without irritating the skin. Machines work well on oilier skin that is not irritated or red. Treatment for oily skin can be similar to the following acne treatments.

ACNE FACIALS

Acne facial treatments can significantly affect the skin's appearance. Extractions and a good mask can improve the skin, and clients will be greatly relieved to have clearer, smoother skin. A gentle, cautious approach is best, especially for first-time clients. Extractions must be done gently and without pain to the client. If it hurts, it is probably too rough and forceful. Treatment care and client education regarding acne can be challenging, but the results are rewarding for clients and the esthetician (Figure 14–21).

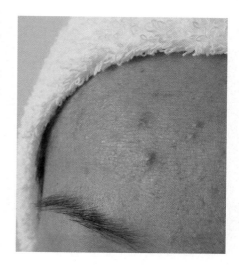

Figure 14–21 Acne can be challenging to work with.

Acne Treatment Care

The esthetician can outline a treatment plan to balance the skin. Treatments focus on clearing the follicles by deep cleansing and extractions. Physicians will prescribe medications that will work to suppress acne flare-ups. However, medications can have adverse side effects and, even with medication, acne can return. Working with problem skin is a continuous process, and clients need to follow regular skin care programs.

Acne treatments may include clay, oxygen, sulfur, or anti-inflammatory masks. **Desincrustation** (des-in-krus-TAY-shun), steam and extractions are all part of an acne facial. Glycolic acid peels are also effective. Each client is treated individually according to her or his needs.

Here are some products and vitamins recommended for acne:

* *Beta hydroxy acids (salicylic acid, citric acid).* These products work synergistically with AHAs to slough old cells and keep pores open. BHAs

CAUTION!

Some minerals in multivitamins aggravate acne because of iodides from sea-sourced products.

are not as strong as AHAs, but they are effective when used alone, especially for sensitive skin (Check for aspirin allergies before using salicylic acid).

- *Sulfur masks.* These products exfoliate skin, and heal and dry blemishes. (Check for sulfur allergies).
- *Vitamins.* These should include zinc (60 ml, twice daily with food) and B complex vitamins.
- *Increased vitamin C.* This vitamin has antioxidant value and healing effects.
- *AHAs (glycolic, lactic, malic, and tartaric acids).* These products are used in different percentages and pH factors to dissolve the desmosomes between cells to keep skin cells exfoliated. Exfoliation also softens acne impactions and stimulates cell production.
- *Vitamin A.* This vitamin benefits the skin in several ways; it stimulates new cell production and clears up acne impactions and the skin in general.
- *Benzoyl peroxide.* This product releases free radical oxygen that kills the bacteria, sterilizes the follicle, and stops the irritating effects of the bacteria; it also irrigates and sloughs out acne impactions.
- *Healing creams.* These products encourage new cell growth.
- *Oxygen therapy treatments.* These products reduce bacteria; they also oxygenate and open impacted pores for easier extractions.
- *Spot blemish treatments.* These include products such as tea tree oil and benzoyl peroxide.

Acne Care Tips

Here are some suggestions for clients with acne.

- *Eliminate comedogenic products. Oil-free* does not mean "noncomedogenic." Examine the ingredients on product labels to determine if they are correct for problem skin (refer to Chapter 12 for ingredient information).
- *Control oil through proper product usage.* Do not irritate the skin with harsh products.
- *Exfoliate the follicles.* Keep follicles clean and exfoliated to keep sebum and cells from building up. Benzoyl peroxide or alpha hydroxy acids are beneficial. Do not overuse these products. Sometimes once a day is too much.
- *Avoid environmental aggravators* such as dirt, grease, sun, humidity, and pollution.
- *Practice stress reduction and good nutrition.*
- *Have regular facials* once a month or as needed.

Home Care for Acne

Proper home care can usually help keep acne under control. However, when clients cannot achieve results with their home care, they may seek the aid of the esthetician or a physician. After the skin is analyzed, suggestions are given to the client specific to his or her needs. It is important for clients to

MINI-PROCEDURE

THE ACNE TREATMENT PROCEDURE

The following general procedure can be used for problem skin. Most of the facial focuses on deep-cleansing and extracting impactions from the follicles. Some steps may be omitted or rearranged, depending on the treatment goals and the client's needs. See the facial machine procedures (Chapter 16) for details.

1. Cleanse with an acne-appropriate cleanser that rinses clean.
2. Exfoliate with an enzyme peel, an AHA or BHA peel, or an exfoliating mask. (Scrubs and brushes are too irritating on inflamed skin.)
3. Steam (can reverse steps 2 or 3, depending on the products and methods of choice).
4. *Optional desincrustation:* Use the galvanic machine with a desincrustation fluid to soften the follicles. (Alternate method: A desincrustation fluid can be used while steaming.)
5. Perform extractions.
6. After extractions, use an astringent/toner to kill bacteria.
7. *Optional:* Use the high-frequency mushroom electrode to spark blemishes to help kill bacteria and heal the lesions. An acne serum can also be applied after extractions to treat the skin.
8. *Optional:* Use light acupressure massage with less friction on non-inflamed areas.
   Note: Massage is irritating to inflamed acne and is usually not part of the acne facial.
9. Apply a clay or soothing mask after extractions.
10. Apply benzoyl peroxide on blemishes, if the client is not allergic to it. (If in doubt, send clients home with a sample for patch testing.)
11. Finish the treatment with a light, soothing, hydrating gel and any other appropriate product.

follow the recommended home-care routine as outlined by the esthetician. Treatments must be accompanied by a real commitment from the client to maintain their home-care regimen.

It is important to ask clients not to "pick" at their blemishes. Explain to them that the internal membrane is delicate, and picking will cause the infection to go deeper and spread more rapidly. Picking also is the cause of external bacterial infections and scarring, both under the skin and on the surface. When the skin shows signs of infection, it is important to treat the area as you would any inflamed area. A cold compress or towel will calm the infection by constricting blood flow to the area. Calm the skin down with anti-inflammatory products, and ice the lesions when necessary.

Home care will include a cleanser, an exfoliant, a mask, a toner, and a light calming hydrator:

- A foaming cleanser with an exfoliant (AHA, salicylic acid, or benzoyl peroxide) is the best choice if it is not irritating or the individual is not allergic to the ingredients.
- Use a soothing or antibacterial toner to calm skin, control oil, or kill bacteria.
- Use an AHA gel or benzoyl peroxide (BP) gel. Alternate using AHAs and BP. Use these at different times or on alternate days to avoid reactions or overdrying the skin.
- Apply a light, hydrating, oil-free moisturizer and sunscreen for balance and protection.
- A clay mask is recommended twice per week. A sulfur mask works well for acne.

All home care includes an analysis of lifestyle to help the client better understand what some of her or his triggers might be (Chapter 10). By understanding the causes, the client is better prepared to follow a program.

MEN'S SKIN CARE

Men's skin care needs are just as important as women's. It is becoming more common for men to use spa services and to take care of their skin. Estheticians need to take a simple, direct approach when discussing skin care with their male clients. Men need the same skin care programs that women do, but most men will want to use only a few products.

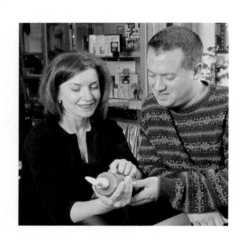

Figure 14–22 The male client market continues to grow.

Male clients are willing to follow suggestions and want a basic, consistent routine. They tend to be loyal customers. Male clients represent 15–20 percent of a spa's business, and this percentage is expected to grow.

The challenge is to attract male clients to make the initial visit in the first place. Using the term *skin treatment* rather than *facial* is a better way to promote men's services. One way to attract male clientele is to offer special services designed just for them. Make them feel comfortable, and tactfully assure them that it is normal for men to have spa services and practice good skin care habits. Conduct consultations privately, without discussing products and treatments out in the reception area where other clients may be present. Some salons and spas cater to men only. The male client market will continue to grow as men feel more comfortable about receiving services (Figure 14–22).

Men's Skin Care Products

To build the market, your salon or spa could carry a specific line of men's skin care products. Most unisex product lines will work as long as packaging or fragrance is not overly feminine. Men typically have larger sebaceous glands and oilier skin. They also need sun protection. They may tend to neglect their skin care because it is not considered masculine or a priority. Clients who are especially pleased with treatment results are more willing to try a home maintenance program.

When considering a men's skin care line, keep in mind several key points. Be sure the products are basic and the routines are simple. Men do not want highly fragranced, fluffy products. For example, lotions need to be light, without fragrance, highly absorbent, and with a matte finish. Most men do not like the greasy feeling of some products.

Men prefer simple routines and multipurpose products. They would rather have a combined cleanser and toner. They also like the foaminess of soaps, so a foaming cleanser is a good choice. They can use a toner just like they would an aftershave lotion. They should then apply a light moisturizer with sunscreen. Give male clients specific instructions on how and when to use products.

Keep the following tips in mind when working with male clients:

- Tubes and pumps are more male-friendly than jars.
- His home care regimen should begin with only two products: a cleanser and a hydrating lotion. If he wants three, add the sunscreen.
- As he grows accustomed to the regimen and sees favorable results, he will most likely add to his regimen by purchasing a toner, eye cream, and a mask.
- Educate him on sun protection and skin cancer facts, even if he chooses not to purchase sunscreen.
- Estheticians should teach male clients to shave in a downward direction—in the direction of the hair growth pattern—because it is less irritating.
- Once he is accustomed to receiving treatments and using products, your male client will use an eye cream if he is taught how. While men may be conscious of lines and wrinkles around their eyes, they seldom request an eye product. Estheticians should point out the benefits of these and other products.

Professional Treatments for Men

Depending on the client's skin conditions, you can offer various treatments. Most men love steam and the brush machine (Figure 14–23). Even if a client's skin is slightly sensitive, he will prefer the assertiveness of a brush and foamy cleanser. A firmer touch and deeper massage are also needed on male skin.

There are some other important aspects of men's facials. First, sponges and towels are more appropriate for a man's face. Cotton pads or gauze will grab the beard hair, leaving particles clinging to the face. Shaving before a facial actually makes the skin more sensitive. On freshly shaven skin, exfoliating products or techniques, including strong sensitizing agents such as alpha hydroxy acids and microdermabrasion, may be contraindicated.

Professional movements during a man's facial should flow with the hair growth. For example, most massage movements in the beard area should move downward, not upward (Figure 14–24). This goes against the typical esthetic procedure of lifting movements up the neck and face. Overall, the beard area tends to be relatively sensitive due to shaving lotions that

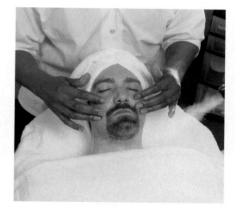

Figure 14–23 Most men love steam and the brush machine.

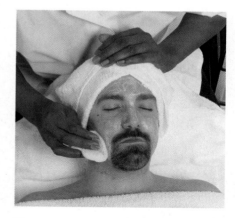

Figure 14–24 Most movements for the beard and moustache area should follow the hair-growth pattern.

contain perfume, alcohol, or other similar substances. Shaving itself is also quite abrasive to the skin, so men need more calming and healing products.

Folliculitis

Folliculitis (fah-lik-yuh-LY-tis; inflammation of the hair follicles) can be a problem for many men, especially if they have very coarse or curly beard hair (Figure 14–25). Folliculitis is an infection characterized by inflammation and pus. Improper shaving may also cause **folliculitis barbae** (fah-lik-yuh-LY-tis BAR-bay), where the hair grows slightly under the skin and is trapped there, causing a bacterial infection. The treatment goal for this condition is to alleviate the irritation, dry up and disinfect the pustules, and desensitize the area. A soothing gel mask is probably the most comfortable product for a male client to use in this area.

Pseudofolliculitis (SOO-doe-fah-lik-yuh-LY-tis), often referred to as "razor bumps," resembles folliculitis without the infection. This condition also results from improper shaving techniques.

There are products on the market for ingrown hairs that help exfoliate and keep the follicles clean. Exfoliating is necessary to keep the follicles open. A foaming cleanser will also help a man's beard area. Estheticians can help clients by keeping them informed of how to take care of their skin on a regular basis.

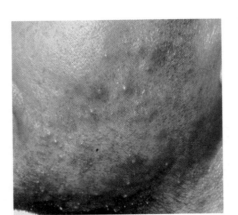

Figure 14–25 Folliculitis can be a problem for many men.

REVIEW QUESTIONS

1. Name six benefits of a facial.

2. List the steps in a basic facial.

3. How does a mini-facial differ from the basic facial?

4. What are three contraindications for facials?

5. What are three important guidelines to follow in order to be successful and to maintain client loyalty?

6. How long is a mask left in place?

7. List four ingredients that are beneficial for mature skin.

8. What are the treatment contraindications for sensitive skin?

9. List four ingredients that are used for acne.

10. What are the key points to consider when choosing skin care products for men?

CHAPTER GLOSSARY

desincrustation: process used to soften and emulsify grease deposits (oil) and blackheads in the hair follicles.

extractions: the manual removal of impurities and comedones.

facial: a professional service designed to improve and rejuvenate the skin.

folliculitis: an infection of the hair follicles characterized by inflammation and pus.

folliculitis barbae: hair is trapped under the skin, causing a bacterial infection; from improper shaving.

pseudofolliculitis: often referred to as "razor bumps"; resembles folliculitis without the infection.

vasoconstricting: vascular constriction of capillaries and blood flow.

CHAPTER 15

FACIAL
MASSAGE

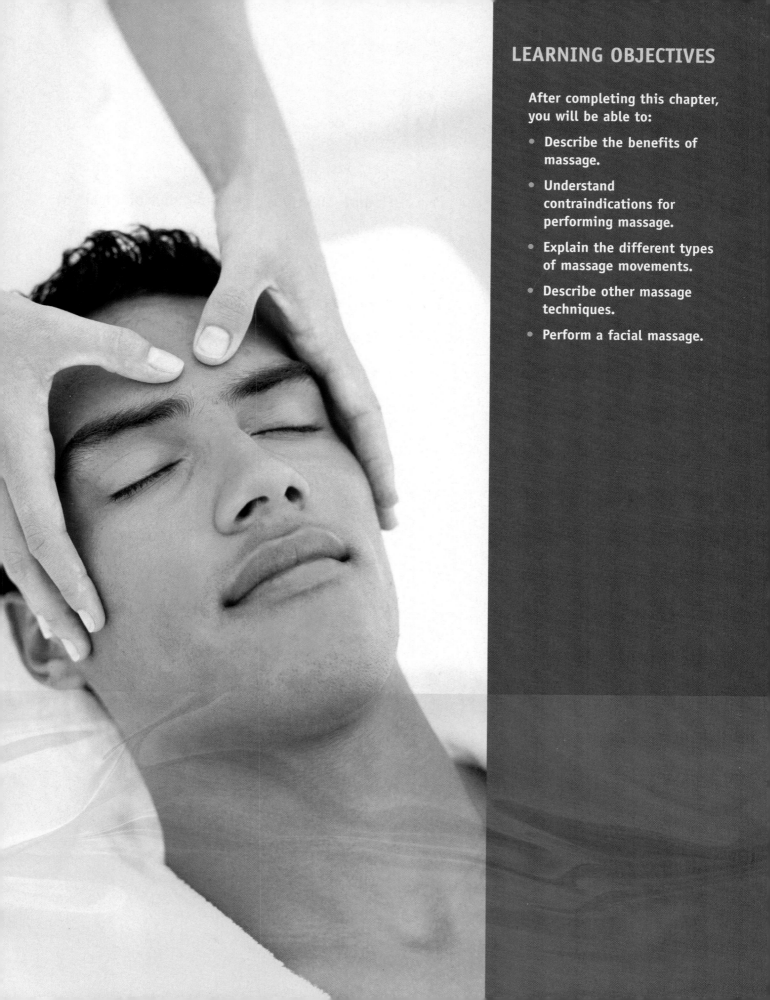

LEARNING OBJECTIVES

After completing this chapter, you will be able to:

- Describe the benefits of massage.

- Understand contraindications for performing massage.

- Explain the different types of massage movements.

- Describe other massage techniques.

- Perform a facial massage.

KEY TERMS

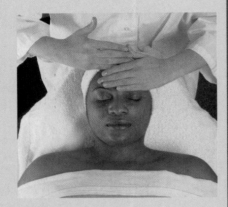

Figure 15–1 Massage is one of the oldest therapeutic methods.

Massage is one of the oldest therapeutic methods, dating back thousands of years (Figure 15–1). It has many physiological and psychological benefits. When the body senses touch, reflex receptors respond by increasing blood and lymph flow. The central nervous system is affected, resulting in a state of relaxation. **Massage** (muh-SAHZH) is defined as a manual or mechanical manipulation by rubbing, kneading, or other methods that stimulate metabolism and circulation. Massage also assists in product absorption and relieves pain. A thorough knowledge of muscles, nerves, connective tissues, and blood vessels is vital to performing a correct massage.

THE BENEFITS OF MASSAGE

Massage during facials benefits the client in many ways. A variety of techniques can be used to give the best massage for the client's individual needs. Massage should never be given too long or too deeply. Be mindful of the results you are trying to achieve when giving a facial massage. Stimulating muscle and nerve motor points will both contract muscles and relax the client. Massage is an enjoyable part of the facial that keeps clients coming back. It is very relaxing and stress relieving. Most new clients are surprised at how relaxing a facial can be, and they enjoy the benefits of skin rejuvenation as well as an overall feeling of well-being (Figure 15–2).

The following are benefits of massage:

- It relaxes the client and the facial muscles.
- It stimulates blood and lymph circulation.
- It improves overall metabolism and activates sluggish skin.
- It helps muscle tone.
- It helps cleanse the skin of impurities and softens sebum.
- It helps slough off dead skin cells.
- It reduces puffiness and sinus congestion.
- It helps product absorption.
- It relieves muscle tension and pain.
- It provides a sense of physiological and psychological well-being.

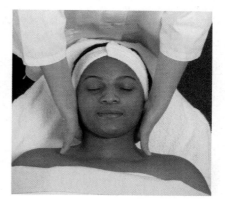

Figure 15–2 The facial massage has numerous benefits.

INCORPORATING MASSAGE DURING THE FACIAL TREATMENT

This chapter contains general guidelines that vary according to each specialized treatment. The massage procedure and when it is performed in the facial depends on many factors. A facial massage routine will change depending on the training or protocols established by the facility or product manufacturer. A facial massage is performed for approximately 10 to 15 minutes during a facial. Some treatments incorporate more massage, and others do not include a massage. Massage techniques also depend on the client's skin analysis and what you are focusing on in the treatment.

Technical Skills

A professional facial massage is one of the major differences between a professional treatment in a salon or spa and a home-care regimen. When performed correctly, massage is relaxing and healthy. Massage movements need to flow and be consistent. Hand movements should be smooth and glide easily from one area to the next. Mental focus is important when giving a massage (Figure 15–3). Do not let mental distractions reduce your focus on the massage and your client.

Communicate with clients, and adjust the touch according to their preferences. Remember: estheticians are not massage therapists (unless they are licensed) and cannot do deep tissue work. Too much pressure on the face can weaken elastin fibers and break down elasticity. Always massage from muscle insertion to origin. Know the correct direction to massage to avoid breaking

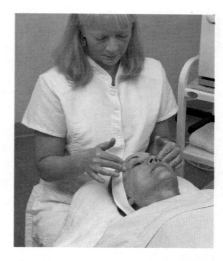

Figure 15–3 Mental focus is important when giving a massage.

FYI

To maintain soft skin, keep hands moisturized and exfoliated. Frequent washing and sanitizing hands is drying, so routinely nourish them with lotion.

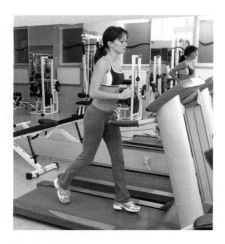

Figure 15–4 Take care of yourself by exercising and stretching.

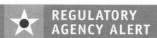

CAUTION!

Do not massage a client who has certain health problems or contraindications, including:

- high blood pressure, heart conditions, or cancer.
- open lesions, acne, or other disorders on the skin.
- rosacea, severe couperose conditions, erythema, or sunburn.
- sensitive or deeply peeled skin.
- contagious diseases.

★ REGULATORY AGENCY ALERT

Refer to licensing regulations regarding your scope of practice regarding massage services that are legal to perform under your license.

down tissue and potentially causing premature aging. Educate your clients so they understand that excessive or deep massage is too rough for facial tissue and couperose skin. Massage pressure, the direction of movements, and the duration will vary accordingly. It is helpful to explain to clients what you are trying to achieve with your facial massage techniques.

Hand Mobility

A technician's hands need to be flexible and have a controlled and firm touch. Hands should be soft with short, well-filed nails. Hand mobility is important in maintaining a smooth rhythm and regulating the massage pressure. Both the left and right hands need to be synchronized using equal pressure on both sides. The correct balance comes with practice and being attentive to your touch.

Hand exercises can help strengthen hands and prevent repetitive motion problems, such as carpal tunnel syndrome. Therapists are susceptible to problems because of repetitive movements, muscle and tendon strain, and fatigue due to improper or poor posture (refer to Chapter 13 for hand-strengthening exercises). Skin care therapists have a physical job, and stretching the body maintains flexibility and can help alleviate aches and pains. Remember to take care of yourself with exercise and self-care maintenance, such as massage (Figure 15–4). They are necessary parts of a healthy lifestyle.

MASSAGE CONTRAINDICATIONS

Certain health problems and skin conditions contraindicate a massage. If you cannot perform a massage, you can alter your service by substituting another step or leaving a mask on longer. It is appropriate to improvise in your facials. Contraindications include contagious diseases, inflamed acne, sunburn, or sensitive skin. Do not massage a client who has certain health problems such as high blood pressure or cancer, because massage increases circulation and may be harmful to clients with medical conditions. If necessary, have the client consult a physician first. If a client has arthritis or other pain, be very careful to avoid vigorous massage. If a client is sick, the massage may be too stimulating and make the client feel worse. Of course, if the client has a cold and is contagious, it is not a good idea to work on them anyway.

Scope of Practice

An esthetician's massage services are limited to certain areas of the body: the face, neck, shoulders, and décolleté. Therapeutic massage, such as deep tissue massage and **manual lymph drainage,** should be performed only by therapists who specialize in these areas. Therapeutic body massage requires special training and, in most cases, licensure. If the client wants a full body massage, refer her or him to a licensed massage therapist. Although skin treatments such as back facials and body treatments are part of esthetics services, massage is not being performed—only the application of products. Refer to licensing regulations regarding your scope of practice and services that are legal to perform under your license.

TYPES OF MASSAGE MOVEMENTS

Classical Swedish massage movements include effleurage, petrissage, friction, tapotement, and vibration.

Effleurage

Effleurage (EF-loo-rahzh) is a soft, continuous stroking movement applied with the fingers (digital) and palms (palmar) in a slow and rhythmic manner (Figure 15–5). The gliding movement is soothing and relaxing. The fingers are used on smaller surfaces such as the forehead or face, and the palms are used on larger surfaces such as the back or shoulders. Effleurage is often used to begin and end most massage sessions. It is used on the forehead, face, scalp, back, shoulders, neck, chest, arms, and hands.

To correctly position the fingers for stroking, slightly curve the fingers with just the cushions of the fingertips touching the skin. Do not use the ends of the fingertips, because fingertips cannot control pressure and may scratch the client. To correctly position the palms for stroking, hold the whole hand loosely. Keep the wrist and fingers flexible, and curve the fingers to conform to the shape of the area being massaged. Effleurage, the most important of the five movements, is used in conjunction with other types of massage such as **shiatsu** (shee-AH-tsoo), a form of acupressure.

Petrissage

Petrissage (PEH-treh-sahzh) is a kneading movement that stimulates the underlying tissues (Figure 15–6). The skin and flesh are grasped between the thumb and forefinger. As the tissues are lifted from their underlying structures, they are squeezed, rolled, or pinched with a light, firm pressure. Petrissage is performed on the fleshier parts of the face, shoulders, back, and arms. The pressure should be light but firm, and the movements should be rhythmic. Petrissage can stimulate sebum production and activate sluggish skin.

Fulling is a form of petrissage in which the tissue is grasped, gently lifted, and spread out. It is used mainly for massaging the arms. With the fingers of both hands grasping the arm, apply a kneading movement across the flesh, with light pressure on the underside of the client's forearm and between the shoulder and elbow.

Friction

Friction (FRIK-shun) is a rubbing movement. Pressure is maintained on the skin while the fingers or palms are moved over the underlying structures (Figure 15–7). Friction stimulates the circulation and glandular activity of the skin. Circular friction movements are usually used on the scalp, arm, and hands. Lighter circular friction movements are used on the face and neck.

Chucking, rolling, and *wringing* are variations of friction movements used mainly on the arms or legs:

- *Chucking.* Grasp the flesh firmly in one hand, and move the hand up and down along the bone while the other hand keeps the arm in a steady position (Figure 15–8).

> ### Here's a Tip
>
> To keep the relaxing flow and connection, do not remove your hands from the client's face once you have started the massage. Choose instrumental music with a slow, even tempo.

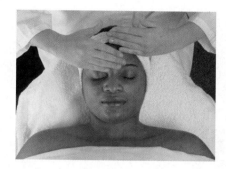

Figure 15–5 Effleurage.

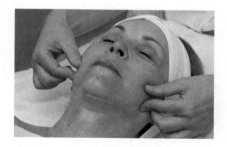

Figure 15–6 Petrissage

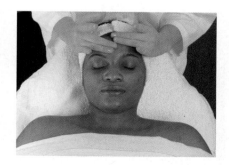

Figure 15–7 Friction.

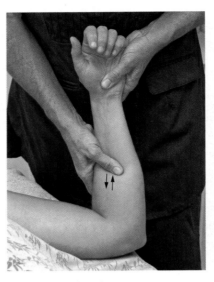

Figure 15–8 Chucking.

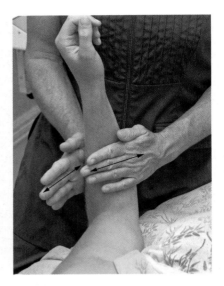

Figure 15–9 Rolling.

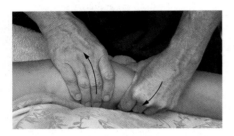

Figure 15–10 Wringing.

- *Rolling.* Used on the arms and legs to apply pressure to the tissues; press the tissues firmly against the bone, and roll your hands around the arm or leg with a rapid back-and-forth movement. Move both hands at the same time, opposite to each other, while rolling the flesh up and down the bone (Figure 15–9).
- *Wringing.* This is a vigorous movement with the hands placed a small distance apart on both sides of the arm. While the hands are working downward, the flesh is twisted against the bones in opposite directions (Figure 15–10).

Tapotement

Tapotement (tah-POT-ment), or *percussion,* consists of fast tapping, patting, and hacking movements (Figure 15–11). This form of massage is the most stimulating and should be applied carefully and with discretion. It is good for toning and is beneficial to sluggish skin. Only light, digital tapping should be used on the face. The fingertips are brought down against the skin in rapid succession. This movement is sometimes referred to as a "piano movement."

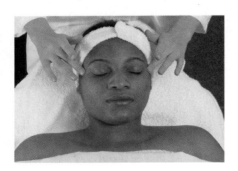

Figure 15–11 Tapotement.

Slapping and hacking movements are used by massage therapists on the back, shoulders, and arms. In slapping movements, keep the wrists flexible so that the palms come in contact with the skin in light, firm, and rapid strokes. One hand follows the other. With each slapping stroke, lift the flesh slightly. Hacking is a chopping movement with the wrists and outer edges of the hands. Both the wrists and fingers move in fast, light, firm, flexible motions against the skin in alternate succession.

Vibration

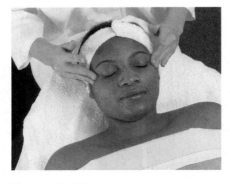

Figure 15–12 Vibration.

Vibration (vy-BRAY-shun) is a rapid shaking movement in which the technician uses her or his body and shoulders—not just the fingertips—to create the movement. It is accomplished by rapid muscular contractions in the arms (Figure 15–12). The balls of the fingertips are pressed firmly on the point of application. Vibration is a highly stimulating movement, but it should be used sparingly and never for more than a few seconds on any one spot.

CAUTION!

The Dr. Jacquet movement must be done with care because the pressure of the movement can cause pain, and too much kneading can stretch the skin. Do not use the movement in the eye area. If used close to the eye area, keep pressure to a minimum. Do not perform stimulating massage on couperose areas, or the capillaries could be damaged.

Do not perform the Dr. Jacquet movement over areas of the skin that are infected or irritated. Too much pressure will rupture follicle walls and cause tissue damage.

Here's a Tip

Whatever movements you use, be consistent on the number of passes you make for each step. If you repeat a step three times or six times, repeat all of your steps the same amount of times. Always perform the same routine on both the left and right sides of the area being massaged.

DR. JACQUET MOVEMENT

Some years ago in Europe, the famous dermatologist, Dr. Jacquet (zha-KETT), introduced a massage method that is especially effective in the treatment of oily skin and acne-blemished skin.

To perform this method, gather a small section of the skin between the thumb and forefinger and squeeze gently. At the same time, give the skin a slight twisting or kneading movement. This helps to empty the oil ducts. The movement is somewhat similar to squeezing the peel of an orange until a fine spray of oil is expelled, but it is much more subtle. The **Dr. Jacquet movement** keeps the sebum moving forward and out of the follicles. When the movement is done as part of a facial treatment, it should follow the desincrustation step that prepares the skin for extractions.

The following movements combine the Dr. Jacquet method with variations on the original technique, so that the client will receive the maximum benefits.

1. Start with a slight twisting or kneading movement on the chin (Figure 15–13).
2. Continue with a kneading movement on the cheeks.
3. When the skin on the forehead is too tight to twist between the thumb and forefinger, place the tips of the fingers parallel to one another approximately 3/4 inch apart on the forehead. Push the fingertips toward one another, so that the skin is pinched gently between the fingers. Continue this movement across the entire forehead.

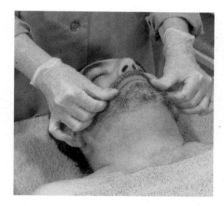

Figure 15–13 The Dr. Jacquet massage is a form of kneading similar to petrissage.

FYI

For your male clients, use downward movements in the area of beard growth. It feels uncomfortable when you massage against hair growth. Pressure point massage in the beard area works well.

OTHER MASSAGE TECHNIQUES

Different types of massage are based on body structure and energy flow within the body. Most massage techniques are based on classical, or Swedish, massage movements. There are many additional advanced techniques that stimulate and detoxify the body. Massage techniques require additional training and study. A combination of techniques can be used in treatments.

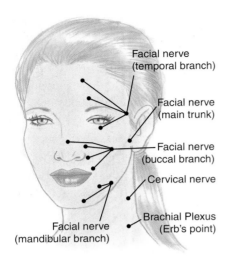

Figure 15–14 Motor points of the face.

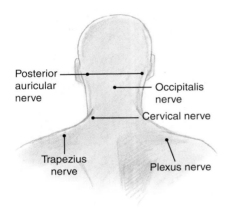

Figure 15–15 Motor points of the neck.

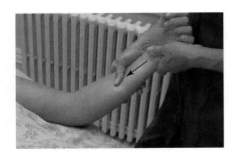

Figure 15–16 Massage from muscle insertion to origin.

Some of these are discussed more thoroughly in Chapter 18, "Advanced Topics and Treatments."

- *Acupressure* is an Oriental technique of applying pressure to specific points of the body (acupressure points) to release muscle tension and *chi* (CHEE; life force). *Shiatsu* is a Japanese technique using acupressure massage points. Many of the motor points on the face and neck are acupressure points (Figures 15–14 and 15–15).

- *Pressure point massage*—on each acupressure point, the movement is repeated three to six times. Pause for three to six seconds on each point, moving from either top to bottom on the face, using light inward pressure at each point and then lifting the pressure to slide to the next point. Training is necessary to perform this movement correctly. Techniques and patterns vary with different methods.

- *Aromatherapy massage* uses essential oils applied to the skin during massage movements. These oils are often used during the facial massage to promote mental relaxation and to treat the skin in numerous ways.

- **Manual lymph drainage** massage uses gentle, rhythmic pressure on the lymphatic system to detoxify and remove waste materials from the body more quickly. It reduces swelling and is used before and after surgery for pre- and post-op care. It is a very light touch.

- Another interesting technique is **reflexology** (re-flexs-AHL-uh-jee), which is similar to acupressure, manipulating areas on the hands and feet. It is very relaxing for the entire body.

Estheticians are not usually trained in reflexology, so be aware of your scope of practice.

BASIC FACIAL MASSAGE TECHNIQUE

Different massage movements may be used on the various parts of the face, chest, and shoulders. Massage may be started on the chin, décolleté, or forehead. Most movements are repeated three to six times before moving on to the next one. Use both hands at the same time, or alternate hands with a flowing rhythm, depending on the steps. Slide the hands back down to each starting point to repeat the movements in each step.

When performing facial massage, keep in mind that an even tempo, or rhythmic flow, promotes relaxation. Do not remove the hands from the client's face once you have started the massage. Should it become necessary to lift the hands from the client's face, feather them off (slowing down the movement is often called "feathering"), then gently replace them with feather-like movements. When coming back to the face, gently make contact on the side of the face or top of the head to avoid startling the client.

Keep one hand on the client's body at all times if it is necessary to take one hand away (if you need to apply more product, for example). Remember that to avoid damage to muscular tissues, massage movements are generally directed from the insertion toward the origin of a muscle (Figure 15–16). Massage toward the heart on the extremities in order to move the blood flow toward the heart. The sequence of massage movements permits a smooth and graceful flow of one movement into another.

One type of massage is a cleansing massage. The main purpose of a cleansing massage is to continue the cleaning process, help remove dead surface cells, and stimulate the skin to help increase blood circulation. These "massage" movements are more vigorous than those used for a slower, relaxing massage. Massage or cleansing cream that is not formulated to penetrate the skin is used for this cleansing massage technique. Deep-penetrating creams should not be used in this massage procedure, because they would act as vehicles to carry dirt and makeup deeper into the pores. Other massage products are designed to penetrate into the skin and are applied to clean skin. These products range from serums to oils, lotions, and creams.

Massage is the most relaxing part of the facial and has many benefits. Various massage techniques can be incorporated into facial treatments. Classical massage movements include effleurage, petrissage, friction, tapotement, and vibration. Appropriate massage movements are based on the anatomy of the facial structure, nerves, and muscles (Figure 15–17). Using the proper techniques is important. It is also necessary to know the contraindications for massage. Once the basic massage flows smoothly, other movements can be added to the routine. Many estheticians find that giving a facial massage is also relaxing to them and one of the most enjoyable parts of their job.

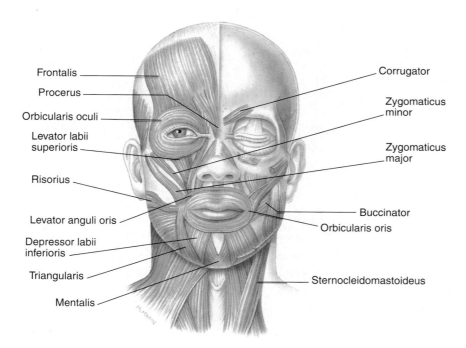

Figure 15–17 Facial structure and muscles.

PROCEDURE 15–1

THE FACIAL MASSAGE

SUPPLIES
- disinfectant/sanitizer
- hand towels
- hand sanitizer/antibacterial soap
- covered trash container
- bowls
- spatulas
- fan brush
- bolster
- blanket
- headband
- clean linens
- client gown or wrap

DISPOSABLES
- paper towels
- gloves/finger cots
- cotton pads/4" × 4" pads
- tissues
- cotton rounds
- plastic baggie

PRODUCTS
- cleanser
- massage lotion
- toner
- moisturizer
- sunscreen

EQUIPMENT
- facial bed/table
- towel warmer (as needed)

The following procedure is a standard relaxing massage.

- Use a product that will easily glide across the skin. Warm the product before applying.
- A good rule of thumb is to repeat all movements consecutively three to six times.
- The number of movements to perform for each step may vary—these are only suggestions.
- Each instructor may have developed her or his own routine. Follow your instructors' lead.

Preparation

1 Set up the room.

2 Prepare the table, equipment, and workstation.

3 Help the client prepare for the service.

Procedure

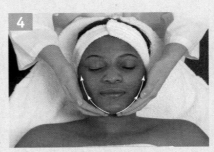

Apply the massage product with relaxing strokes. *(Figure P15–1-1)*

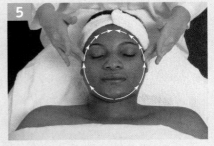

Move up to the forehead. *(Figure P15–1-2)*

4 With clean, warm hands, evenly apply the warmed massage product to the décolleté and face by using the hands or a soft brush (Figure P15–1-1). One teaspoon should be enough product for the facial area.

5 Start with hands on the décolleté (Figure P15–1-2). Move slowly up the sides of the neck and face to the forehead.

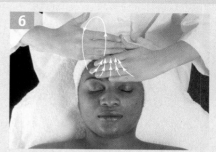

Begin upward strokes in the middle of the forehead and at the brow line. *(Figure P15–1-3)*

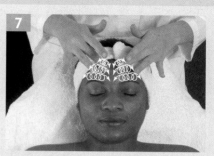

Begin a circular movement in the middle of the forehead along the brow line. *(Figure P15–1-4)*

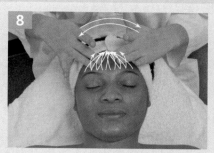

Start a crisscross stroking movement at the middle of the forehead, starting at the brow line. *(Figure P15–1-5)*

6 With the middle and ring fingers of each hand, start upward strokes in the middle of the forehead and at the brow line. Working upward toward the hairline, one hand follows the other as the hands move toward the right temple, move back across the forehead to the left temple, and then move back to the center of the forehead (Figure P15–1-3). Repeat the movements three to six times.

7 With the middle finger of each hand, start a circular movement in the middle of the forehead along the brow line. Continue this circular movement while working toward the temples. Bring the fingers back quickly to the center of the forehead at a point between the brow line and the hairline. Each time the fingers reach the temple, pause for a moment and apply slight pressure to the temple (Figure P15–1-4). Repeat three to six times.

8 With the middle and ring fingers of each hand, start a crisscross stroking movement at the middle of the forehead, starting at the brow line and moving upward toward the hairline. Move toward the right temple and back to the center of the forehead. Now move toward the left temple and back to the center of the forehead (Figure P15–1-5). Repeat three to six times.

PROCEDURE 15–1, CONT.

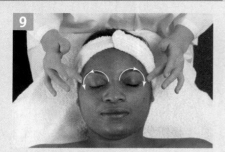

Slide the fingers to the outer corner of the eye, lifting the brow at the same time. *(Figure P15–1-6)*

9 Place the ring fingers under the inside corners of the eyebrows and the middle fingers over the brows. Slide the fingers to the outer corner of the eye, lifting the brow at the same time (Figure P15-1-6). This movement continues with step 7.

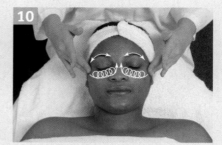

Start a circular movement at the outside corner of the eye, on the cheekbone to under the center of the eye. *(Figure P15–1-7)*

10 Start a circular movement with the middle finger at the outside corner of the eye. Continue the circular movement on the cheekbone to the point under the center of the eye, and then slide the fingers back to the starting point (Figure P15-1-7). Repeat six to eight times. The left hand moves clockwise, and the right hand moves counterclockwise.

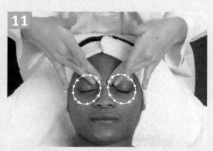

Tap lightly around the eyes. *(Figure P15–1-8)*

11 Start a light tapping movement with the pads of the fingers. Tap lightly around the eyes as if playing a piano. Continue tapping, moving from the temple, under the eye, toward the nose, up and over the brow, and outward to the temple. Do not tap the eyelids directly over the eyeball (Figure P15–1-8). Repeat six times.

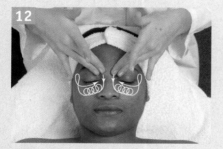

Begin a circular movement down the nose and continuing across the cheeks to the temples. *(Figure P15–1-9)*

12 With the middle finger of each hand, start a circular movement down the nose and continuing across the cheeks to the temples. Slide the fingers under the eyes and back to the bridge of the nose (Figure P15-1-9). Repeat the movements six times.

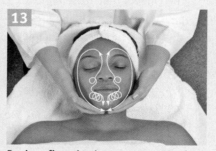

Begin a firm circular movement on the chin. *(Figure P15–1-10)*

13 With the middle and ring fingers of each hand, slide the fingers from the bridge of the nose, over the brow (lifting the brow), and down to the chin. Start a firm circular movement on the chin with the thumbs. Change to the middle fingers at the corner of the mouth. Rotate the fingers five times, and slide the fingers up the

sides of the nose, over the brow, and then stop for a moment at the temple. Apply slight pressure on the temple. Slide the fingers down to the chin, and repeat the movements six times. The downward movement on the side of the face should have a very light touch to avoid dragging the skin downward (Figure P15-1-10).

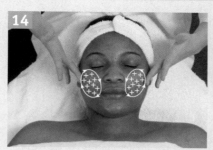

Begin a light tapping movement on the cheeks. *(Figure P15–1-11)*

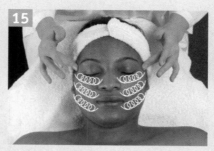

Begin a circular movement at the center of the chin and move up to the earlobes. *(Figure P15–1-12)*

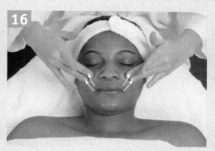

Begin the "scissor" movement. *(Figure P15–1-13)*

14 With the pads of the fingertips, start a light tapping movement (piano playing) on the cheeks, working in a circle around the cheeks (Figure P15–1-11). Repeat the movements six to eight times.

15 With the middle finger of each hand, start a circular movement at the center of the chin and move up to the earlobes. Slide the middle fingers to the corner of the mouth and then continue the circular movements to the middle of the ears. Return the middle fingers to the nose and continue the circular movements outward across the cheeks to the top of the ear (Figure P15–1-12). Repeat three to five times.

16 With the index and middle fingers of each hand, start the "scissor" movement, gliding from the center of the mouth, upward over the cheekbone, and stopping at the top of the cheekbone. Alternate the movement from one side of the face to the other, using the right hand on the right side of the face and then the left hand on the left side (Figure 15–1-13). Repeat eight to ten times.

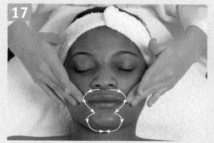

Draw the fingers from the center of the upper lip, around the mouth, under the lower lip, and under the chin. *(Figure P15–1-14)*

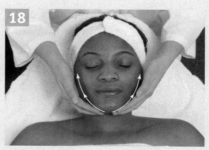

Begin a scissor movement from the center of the chin and then slide the fingers along the jawline to the earlobe. *(Figure P15–1-15)*

18 With the index finger above the chin and jawline (the middle, ring, and little fingers should be under the chin and jaw), start a scissor movement from the center of the chin and then slide the fingers along the jawline to the earlobe. Alternate one hand after the other, using the right hand on the right side of the face and the left hand on the left side of the face (Figure P15–1-15). Repeat eight to ten times on each side of the face.

17 With the middle finger of both hands, draw the fingers from the center of the upper lip, around the mouth, under the lower lip, and then continue a circle under the chin (Figure 15–1-14). Repeat six to eight times.

PROCEDURE 15–1, CONT.

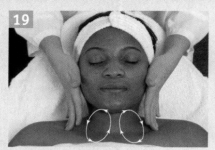

Apply light upward strokes over the front of the neck. *(Figure P15–1-16)*

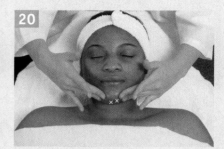

Tapping. *(Figure P15–1-17)*

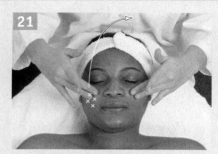

Tap and lift the cheek area. *(Figure P15–1-18)*

19 Apply light upward strokes over the front of the neck with both hands (Figure P15–1-16). Circle down and then back up, using firmer downward pressure on the outer sides of the neck. Repeat 10 times. Do not press down on the center of the neck.

20 With the middle and ring fingers of the right hand, give two quick taps under the chin, followed with one quick tap with the middle and ring fingers of the left hand. The taps should be done in a continuous movement, keeping a steady rhythm. The taps should be done with a light touch, but with enough pressure so that a soft tapping sound can be heard. Continue the tapping movement while moving the hands slightly to the right and then left, so as to cover the complete underside of the chin. Without stopping or breaking the rhythm of the tapping, move to the right cheek (Figure P15–1-17).

21 Continue the tapping on the right cheek in the same manner as under the chin, except the tapping with the left hand will have a lifting movement. The rhythm will be tap, tap, lift, tap, tap, lift, tap, tap, lift. Repeat this rhythmic movement 25 times. Without stopping the tapping movement, move the fingers back under the chin and over the left cheek, repeating the tapping and lifting movements. Move up and out on the area in a consistent pattern. Avoid tapping directly on the jawbone because this will feel unpleasant to the client (Figure P15–1-18).

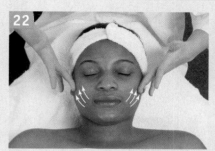

Begin a stroking movement at the mouth. *(Figure P15–1-19)*

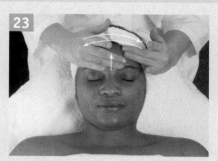

Move up to the outside corner of the left eye and across the forehead to the outside corner of the right eye. *(Figure P15–1-20)*

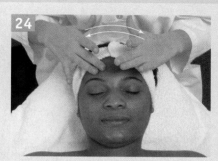

Let the movements grow slower, and feather off to end the massage. *(Figure P15–1-21)*

22 Without stopping the tapping movement, move back under the chin and over to the right corner of the mouth. Break into an upward, stroking movement with the first three fingers of each hand. One finger follows the other as each finger lifts the corner of the mouth. Repeat the movement 20 times. Continue the stroking movement as you quickly move under the chin to the left corner of the mouth (Figure P15–1-19). Repeat the stroking movement 20 times.

23 Without stopping the stroking movement, quickly move up to the outside corner of the left eye and continue the stroking, upward movement 20 times (Figure P15–1-20). Continue the stoking movement across the forehead to the outside corner of the right eye. Continue this stroking movement back and forth 20 times.

24 Continue the stroking movement back and forth across the forehead, gradually slowing the movement. Let the movements grow slower and slower as the touch becomes lighter and lighter. Taper the movement off until the fingers are gradually lifted from the forehead (Figure P15–1-21). This slowing down of movement is often called "feathering."

25 Finish the service, and complete your client consultation.

Clean-Up and Sanitation

Follow appropriate facial clean-up and sanitation steps.

FYI

Blood returning to the heart from the head, face, and neck flows down the jugular veins on each side of the neck. All massage movements on the side of the neck are done with a downward (never upward) motion. Always slide gently upward in the center of the neck and circle out and then down on the sides.

REVIEW QUESTIONS

1. Name at least five benefits of massage.

2. List the different types of classical massage movements, and describe each of the movements.

3. What is the Dr. Jacquet movement used for?

4. List the facial massage steps from memory.

5. What are some massage contraindications?

6. How do you find out what the licensing regulations for massage are in your area?

7. In what direction do you massage on the muscles?

CHAPTER GLOSSARY

Dr. Jacquet movement: beneficial for oily skin; it helps move sebum out of the follicles and up to the skin's surface by kneading.

effleurage: a soft, continuous stroking movement applied with the fingers and palms in a slow and rhythmic manner.

friction: a rubbing movement; pressure is maintained on the skin to create friction. Chucking, rolling, and wringing are variations of friction.

fulling: a form of petrissage in which the tissue is grasped, gently lifted, and spread out.

manual lymph drainage: stimulates lymph fluid to flow through the lymphatic vessels. This light massage technique helps to cleanse and detoxify the body.

massage: a manual or mechanical manipulation by rubbing, kneading, or other methods that stimulate metabolism and circulation.

petrissage: a kneading movement that stimulates the underlying tissues.

reflexology: treatment of the body through reflex points located on the bottom of the feet.

shiatsu: a form of acupressure.

tapotement: fast tapping, slapping, and hacking movements.

vibration: a rapid shaking movement in which the technician uses the body and shoulders, not just the fingertips, to create the movement.

CHAPTER OUTLINE

FACIAL MACHINES

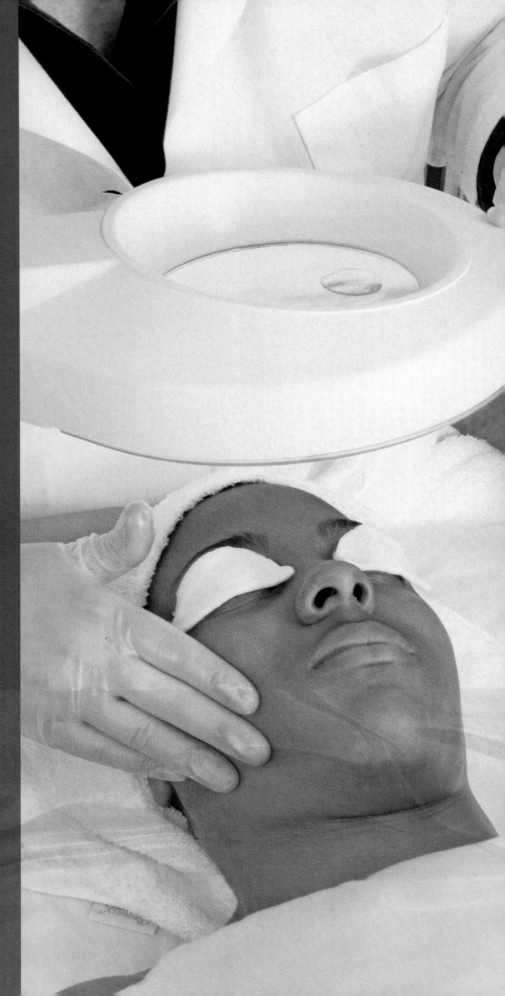

LEARNING OBJECTIVES

After completing this chapter, you will be able to:

- Explain electrotherapy.
- Identify the machines used in skin care treatments.
- Describe the mechanization used with each machine.
- Explain the benefits of each machine.
- Understand how to safely use each machine.
- Describe the contraindications for machines.

KEY TERMS

A variety of useful machines will enhance the esthetician's services. Each machine has a specific benefit for the skin and makes clients feel as though they are receiving a specialized service. In this chapter you will learn how these tools are integrated into the facial experience. Although facial treatments can be performed effectively without electrical devices, even better results can be achieved with electrical tools and electrotherapy.

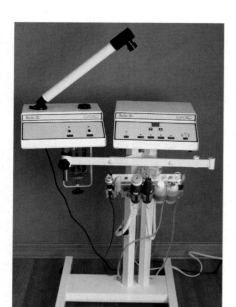

Figure 16–1 Multifunctional machines.

CAUTION!

To prevent physical harm, some machines should never be used on heart patients; clients with pacemakers or metal implants; pregnant clients; clients with epilepsy or seizure disorders; clients who are afraid of electric current; or those with open or broken skin.

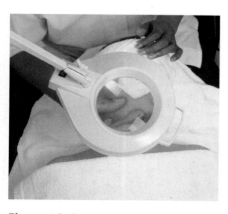

Figure 16–2 The magnifying lamp is used to analyze the skin.

Electrotherapy is the use of electrical devices for therapeutic benefits. It is important to be familiar with machines even if you choose not to work with them. Electrical devices enhance the facial by making it easier to give a skin analysis, achieve better product penetration (with galvanic current), or sanitize the skin (using high frequency). These tools are especially effective for more challenging skin conditions. Machines can be purchased separately or as multifunctional with many of the modalities (machines) all on one unit (Figure 16–1).

New machines and technology emerge each year. Estheticians must continue to be educated about the latest methods in skin care, while being cautious of expensive, trendy machines. Lasers, light therapy, and microcurrent are advanced topics discussed in Chapter 18. Clients today are well educated and have greater access to information, and they will expect you to be knowledgeable about such topics. To maintain professional credibility, it is important that you are aware of current technology.

Contraindications

There are several contraindications for electrotherapy. To prevent physical harm, some machines should never be used on heart patients, clients with pacemakers, metal implants, pregnant clients, clients with epilepsy or seizure disorders, clients who are afraid of electric current, or those with open or broken skin. Further, if you ever have any doubts about whether the client can have electrotherapy safely, request that the client get a note from her or his physician approving electrotherapy treatment.

Use all machines as directed by the manufacturer, because similar machines may have different mechanisms, and work differently. Most machines are used for approximately 5 to 10 minutes in a service.

MAGNIFYING LAMP (LOUPE)

The magnifying lamp (also referred to as a *loupe*; pronounced "loop") magnifies the face to help the esthetician treat and analyze the skin (Figure 16–2). The lamp uses a cool fluorescent light bulb. The magnifying lamp has various powers of magnification known as *diopters*. Most lamps in the industry come in values of 3, 5, or 10 diopters, which means 30 times the power magnification, 50 times the power magnification, or 100 times the power magnification. Five diopters is the most common magnification. A good-quality light should have a clear lens, free of distortion. Since you are using this light often, any distortion will add strain to your eyes and make it more difficult to see the skin.

Magnifying Lamp Procedure

The procedure for using a magnifying lamp is as follows:
1. Position the lamp where you want it during the room setup. Turn on the light, and carefully bring it back over the face. If necessary, move it away from the face and loosen the adjustment knob to change the light's angle so you can see through it comfortably.

2. Once the lamp is adjusted, bring it back over the face. Avoid startling the client by suddenly shining the light directly into the eyes, or by losing control of the lamp.

3. Eye pads can be used to protect the eyes from the bright light. Make sure your eye pads are not too large, or they may block the eye area you need to analyze or treat.

4. Gently move the client's head back and forth to examine the sides of the face.

It is important to loosen the adjustment knobs before moving the lamp arms up or down. If you force the lamp into positions without loosening the knobs first, you will wear out the light and then it will not stay in position at all. To avoid overreaching and hurting your back or wrists, you may need to stand up and adjust the lamp.

Magnifying Lamp Maintenance

To clean the lens, turn off the lamp and spray it with a disinfectant and wipe with a soft cloth. Avoid using paper products because paper towels or tissues will scratch the lens.

Sanitize the entire lamp and base with a high-level disinfectant. Magnifying lamps can last up to 10 years if they are well constructed and well-maintained. Conversely, if they are abused and roughly handled, their longevity is compromised. If problems do occur, they typically involve the adjustment arm. The spring on the arm can wear out and may break if not used with care. Some less expensive magnifying lights have hinges rather than knobs that adjust, but these may wear out faster. Periodically check the screws around the light to ensure that they are not loose. The arm and base may also need tightening.

WOOD'S LAMP

The **Wood's lamp,** developed by American physicist Robert Williams Wood, is a filtered black light that is used to illuminate fungi, bacterial disorders, pigmentation problems, and other skin problems (Figure 16–3). The Wood's lamp allows the esthetician to conduct a more in-depth skin analysis, illuminating skin problems that are ordinarily invisible to the naked eye. Under the lamp, different conditions show up in various shades of color. For instance, the thicker the skin, the whiter the fluorescence will be. Pigmentation that shows up under the Wood's lamp cannot be completely lightened with products or treatments, because the pigmentation is in the dermis.

Following are some examples of skin conditions and how they appear under the Wood's lamp:

* thick corneum layer—white fluorescence
* horny layer of dead skin cells—white spots
* normal, healthy skin—blue-white
* dehydrated skin—light violet
* oily areas of the face/comedones—yellow or sometimes pink
* pigmentation problems—brown

When using the Wood's lamp, the room must be totally dark. Put small eye pads on the client, making sure the area around the eye is still visible. Turn on

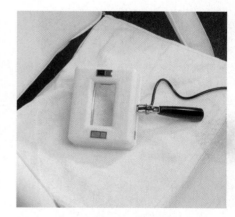

Figure 16–3 The Wood's lamp illuminates skin care problems that are ordinarily invisible to the naked eye.

FYI

Pigmentation that shows up under the Wood's lamp cannot be completely lightened with treatments, because it is in the dermis.

the light and hold it over the client's face. The bulbs can get hot, so be careful not to touch the skin or have the lamp turned on too long.

Treat the Wood's lamp carefully, as you would a magnifying lamp. Follow the manufacturer's directions for cleaning.

HOT TOWEL CABINET

Towel warmers, called *hot towel cabinets* or *hot cabbies,* are commonly used in the treatment room (Figure 16–4). Hot towels are used for both face and body treatments. Towels provide a warm, soothing, and softening benefit to the skin and are utilized for removing facial masks and softening the skin before doing extractions. Cotton pads and products can also be warmed in a cabbie or specialized product warmer. Some cabbies are equipped with ultraviolet lamps.

Hot Cabinet Maintenance

It is important to keep the hot towel cabinet clean and free from mold or mildew. After each client session, clean the inside of the cabinet with a topical disinfectant. Give cabbies a thorough cleansing at the end of the day. Leave the door open at night to allow the cabinet and rubber seals to dry thoroughly. Also empty and clean the water catchment tray underneath the cabbie daily.

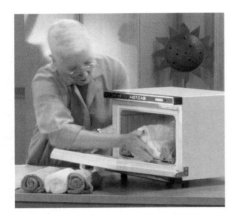

Figure 16–4 The towel warmer.

CAUTION!

Plastic melts in hot towel warmers—use heat-resistant dishes to warm products.

ROTARY BRUSH

The main purpose of the **rotary brush** is to lightly exfoliate the skin (Figure 16–5). The brush machine also assists in the cleansing process. The brush stimulates the skin and helps soften excess oil, dirt, and cell buildup. Do not use brushes on acne, couperose, or inflamed skin. Brushes come in smaller sizes for the face and larger sizes for body areas, such as the back. Brush machines vary. Typically they have two or three small brushes with different textures ranging from soft to firm. The brushes can be rotated at different speeds and directions. Moisten the brush before each use to soften the bristles. More sensitive skin requires a slow, steady rotation and soft brushes. Thicker, oily skin can tolerate a faster speed and firmer brushes.

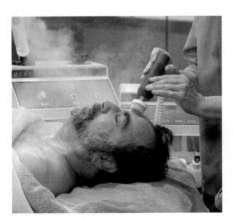

Figure 16–5 Using the brush machine.

MINI-PROCEDURE

THE BRUSH MACHINE

The following steps describe the safe and effective use of a rotary brush.

1. Before using the brush, lightly cleanse the client's skin.
2. Insert the appropriate size brush into the handheld device.
3. Apply more cleanser or water to the skin. Do not let water or cleanser drip down the face or into the eyes. Use a piece of cotton or a towel to catch any excess water.

MINI-PROCEDURE, CONT.

4. Dip the head of the brush into water, adjust the speed, and begin a horizontal pattern at the forehead. The brush should be damp, not drippy. Wipe excess water on a towel if necessary.
5. Continue the rotation down the cheeks, nose, upper lip, chin, jaw, and neck areas.
6. Do not apply pressure. Allow the rotating brush to do the work. The bristles of the brush should remain straight.
7. Use the brush approximately three times on each area, or for approximately 3 to 5 seconds, unless directed otherwise. Keep the brush moving across the face without stopping.
8. Lift the brush from the skin and turn off the machine.

Brush Maintenance

Rotary brush machines come with detachable brushes for cleaning. Here are some guidelines for maintaining the brushes.

- Remove the brushes after each use and wash them thoroughly with soap and water.
- After manual cleansing, immerse the brushes in a hospital-strength disinfectant for the time recommended in the manufacturer's instructions.
- It is important to clean, rinse, dry, and store the brushes so that they do not lose their shape when drying. If the bristles become bent or lose their shape, they will not rotate properly.
- Although they can be stored temporarily in a dry ultraviolet sanitizer, the brushes will break down if left in the sanitizer too long. When they are completely dry, transfer them to a closed container.

STEAMER

Many estheticians consider the steamer to be the most important machine used in esthetics. There are many benefits to steaming the skin (Figure 16–6). Steam helps to stimulate circulation. It also softens sebum and other debris. The warmth relaxes the skin and tissues, making it easier for the esthetician to extract comedones. Steam can be beneficial for the sinuses and congestion. Steamers with ozone (O_3) may have an antiseptic effect on the skin that is beneficial in treating acne and problematic skin. Do not use too much steam on couperose or inflamed skin, because it dilates the capillaries and follicles, causing more redness and irritation. Professional steamers come in various sizes and models. Use only distilled or filtered water in the steamer, because the mineral and calcium deposits in tap water can damage the machinery. The vapor is directed onto the skin's surface by a nozzle at the end of the arm. Steamers usually have a place for an aromatherapy ring on the inside of the nozzle head, and they may have a special feature for oils.

> ## Here's a Tip
>
> Using the brush machine while cleansing the skin saves time for both you and your client.

> ## CAUTION!
>
> To avoid damaging or further irritating the skin, do not use brushes or suction devices on acne, couperose, or inflamed skin.

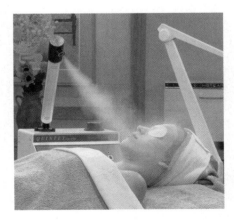

Figure 16–6 The steamer provides many benefits during the facial treatment.

CAUTION!

To avoid burning yourself, never touch the glass jar on the steamer when it is hot—it takes a long time to cool down. Ask your instructor for a demonstration on how to safely remove and replace the glass jar.

MINI-PROCEDURE

USING THE STEAMER

When using a steamer, or any equipment, always read and follow the manufacturer's directions. Steam treatments are timed according to the client's specific needs and the type of facial procedure. Ordinarily, treatment time is between 6 and 10 minutes.

1. Place distilled water into the designated container.
2. Before giving the facial, position the steamer where you want it. Adjust the height.
3. Preheat the steamer before the facial. Do not let water steam or boil for more than a minute. If the contents of the steamer evaporate, the glass may break.
4. Place a towel under the client's neck and over the shoulders to protect these areas from the steam or dripping water and keep the nozzle completely away from the body.
5. Turn the machine away from the client, and flip the power switch to on. Do not turn on the ozone (or vaporizer) switch until steam is visible.
6. When the water is boiling and steam is visible, flip on the ozone switch and slowly adjust the steamer arm close to the client. This will activate the generator inside the machine. You may hear the sound of a small motor. If the noise is too loud and the steam amount does not increase, turn the ozone switch back off because the steamer is not ready yet.
7. Keep the steam approximately 15 to 18 inches from the face. Place the steamer farther away, if necessary, so that it is warm but not too hot on the face. If placed too close, steam can cause overheating of the skin, possible irritation, or burning. Always check the client's comfort level.
8. When you are ready to discontinue the steam, move the steamer away from the client. Turn off the ozone/vaporizer switch first. Then turn off the power switch.
9. Do not spray the hot reservoir with disinfectant before it has cooled off, as this may cause it to shatter.

Steamer Maintenance

To ensure proper usage, always read and follow the manufacturer's directions for the steamer. Following these guidelines will keep your machine in peak working condition for years.

- After each use, wipe down the outside of the steamer with a high-level disinfectant.
- At night, empty the jar and let it dry. Make sure that the rubber seal along the rim of the jar is clean.
- Refill the steamer machine with fresh distilled water each morning. Turn it on to give it a chance to warm up. This will save valuable time when treating your first client of the day.

> # CAUTION!
>
> - Do not use too much steam on couperose or inflamed skin because it dilates the capillaries and follicles, causing more redness and irritation.
> - Do not leave the room while steaming the client in case the steamer starts spraying water—this may burn the client.
> - Do not overfill the steamer because the steamer may spray excess water and burn the client.
> - Clean the steamer regularly to avoid mineral buildup that causes water to spray and burn the client.
> - Do not let the water run low in the steamer—the glass may break.

- Water used inside the steamer should be as free of chemicals and minerals as possible. Therefore, it is always recommended that distilled, not tap, water be used. Most tap water contains chlorine, other chemicals, and mineral deposits.

- Do not leave water in the steamer overnight or on weekends. If the steamer is not emptied regularly, deposits can collect on the heater element. Empty the jar and lightly clean with vinegar and then with soap and water. Allow the coils to dry.

- Neglected steamers tend to spit hot water due to the buildup of mineral deposits that occur with daily use. Mineral deposits may appear as a white or yellow crusty film on the heating element. The hot water can land on the client's face and may cause a serious burn.

- Some steamer models have solid tanks, preventing you from seeing the element; therefore, they need to be cleaned at least two times a month. Use a cleaning solution of plain vinegar and water.

- Never put essential oils or herbs directly into the water. Essential oils are highly active. When dropped directly into a closed jar with boiling water, they can cause excessive spitting of water or, even worse, clog the steamer or cause the glass to break from pressure. Some steamers are equipped with a wick-type apparatus at the mouth of the nozzle. A couple of drops of essential oil can be placed here before the steamer is preheated. The steam picks up the aroma as it vaporizes out into the room.

- Other models make use of a special container for herbs. These specialized steamers are normally more expensive; however, they provide the esthetician with the added benefit of incorporating therapeutic herbs into the steaming process. You can also put a few drops of essential oil on your hands or a cotton pad or swab and hold it close to the steam for aromatherapy.

- Do not leave the room when preheating the steamer, or you may forget about it and run the water down too low and shatter the glass. Water levels must be kept above the safety line marked above the element on the glass jar. Not all steamers have automatic shutoffs.

? **Did You Know**

Ordinary oxygen in the atmosphere consists of two oxygen atoms (O_2). Ozone consists of three oxygen atoms (O_3). Ozone is created after a lightning storm. Ozone has antiseptic qualities. These molecules have the power to kill bacteria and other microorganisms. Ozone is also a strong oxidizer that creates free radicals.

Here's a Tip

You can place 1 to 2 drops of an essential oil onto two hot stones and place them beside the client's ears while steaming. First be sure to check for client allergies and preferences.

- Some machines may have automatic regulators that detect the water level. When it becomes too low or empty, a safety switch is triggered, turning off the machine. Some have timers that shut off after the set time. Timers are useful; but some may tick and then ding when the timer goes off, which can be a distracting noise. Try before you buy.

MINI-PROCEDURE

CLEANING THE STEAMER

The steamer should be trouble free if you follow these general cleaning guidelines.

1. Add two tablespoons of white vinegar, and fill jar to the top with water.
2. Turn on the steamer and let it heat to steaming. Do not turn on the ozone.
3. Let the machine steam for 20 minutes or until the water level is low, but make sure it stays above the low-level line.
4. Turn off the steamer and let the vinegar solution rest in the unit for 15 minutes. Because vinegar has a pungent smell, clean the steamer in your utility room or in an area away from the treatment rooms. Open a window, if possible, when performing maintenance to keep fumes from traveling to other areas of the salon.
5. After it cools, drain the steamer jar completely and then refill with water. Again let the steamer heat to steaming and operate for approximately 10 minutes. If there is still an odor, drain the unit and repeat the process.
   - Do not allow the caustic vinegar and water solution to sit on the heating coil without steaming immediately. If left overnight, it will corrode the copper coils.
   - Note that there is usually a reset button on steamers for additional safety in the event the steamer runs out of water. If the steamer is not running, check the reset button before you call for help. The reset button is ordinarily found on the back of the machine.

VACUUM MACHINE

The **vacuum (suction) machine** serves two main functions. One is to suction dirt and impurities from the skin. The other is to stimulate the dermal layer and blood circulation. This function is thought to help reduce the appearance of creases, such as laugh lines, and improve the overall appearance of the skin. (Figure 16–7). This machine can be used after desincrustation. It can also be used in place of massage. It should not be used on couperose skin with distended or dilated capillaries or on open lesions. Glass and metal suction cups come in different sizes and shapes, depending on their use.

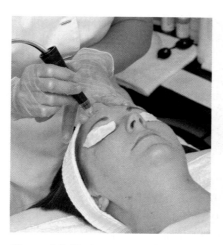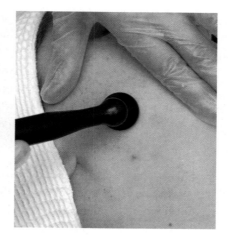

Figure 16–7 The vacuum apparatus.

MINI-PROCEDURE

THE VACUUM PROCEDURE

Use the vacuum to remove impurities according to these guidelines.

1. Attach the appropriate glass or metal tip to the hose after inserting a piece of cotton into the handpiece as a filter (without blocking the suction pressure).
2. Turn on the power and adjust the suction.
3. With the index finger, cover the finger hole on the handpiece when moving the suction across the skin.
4. Slowly move the device horizontally on moistened or damp skin. Be sure to include the vertical creases near the nose. Usually 3 to 5 passes on each area are enough.
5. Keep moving across the face without stopping. To avoid pulling on the skin, lift the finger off the hole before lifting the device off the face.

CAUTION!

To avoid harming the client's skin, do not use suction on inflamed, rosacea, or couperose skin. Never suction liquids or oils into the suction device. Avoid using strong suction because it may cause tissue damage or bruising.

Vacuum Machine Maintenance

To clean and maintain the vacuum machine, follow these guidelines.
- Clean all glass devices with soap and water and soak them in a hospital-strength disinfectant.
- Follow manufacturer's directions to clean the handpieces and hoses.
- Normally a filter is located at the end of the hose where the hose attaches to an orifice connected to the machine. The filter may have to be changed frequently, depending on use.

GALVANIC CURRENT

Galvanic current is used to create two significant reactions in esthetics: chemical (**desincrustation**; des-in-krus-TAY-shun) and ionic (**iontophoresis**; eye-ahn-toh-foh-REE-sus). See Figure 16–8.

The galvanic machine converts the alternating current received from an electrical outlet into a direct current. Electrons are then allowed to

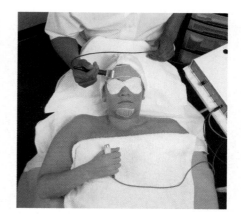

Figure 16–8 The galvanic machine is used to create two significant reactions in esthetics: chemical (desincrustation) and ionic (iontophoresis).

flow continuously in the same direction. This creates a relaxation response that can be regulated to target specific nerve endings in the epidermis. The machine can leave a metallic taste in the mouth, which is normal. To avoid harm to the skin, desincrustation should not be used on couperose skin, pustular acne, or inflamed areas. To avoid potential health complications, do not use galvanic current on clients who are pregnant or on those who have pacemakers, heart problems, high blood pressure, braces, or epilepsy.

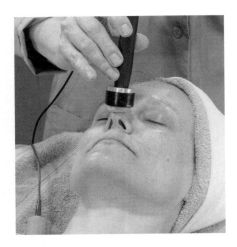

Figure 16–9 The desincrustation process.

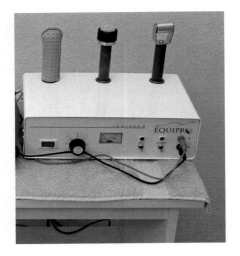

Figure 16–10 A selection of electrodes for the galvanic machine.

Desincrustation

Estheticians use desincrustation (**anaphoresis;** an-uh-for-EES-sus) to facilitate deep pore cleansing (Figure 16–9). During this process, galvanic current is used to create a chemical reaction that emulsifies or liquefies sebum and debris. This treatment is beneficial for oily or acne skin because it helps soften and relax the debris in the follicle before extractions.

To perform desincrustation, an alkaline-based electronegative solution is placed onto the skin's surface. This product helps soften sebum and follicles for deep pore cleansing. The solution is formulated to remain on the surface of the skin rather than being absorbed. When the esthetician is conducting desincrustation, the client holds the positive electrode, the positive polarity. The esthetician uses the negative electrode, set on negative polarity, on the face. This creates a chemical reaction that transforms the sebum of the skin into soap—a process known as **saponification** (sah-pahn-ih-fih-KAY-shun). Soap is made from fat and lye (sodium hydroxide). When the electrical current interacts with the salts (sodium chloride) in the skin, it creates the chemical known as sodium hydroxide—or lye. This soapy substance helps dissolve excess oil, clogged pores, comedones, and other debris on the skin, while softening it at the same time.

Various types of electrodes are available for the galvanic machine (Figure 16–10). The most common are the flat electrode and the roller. To make proper contact, each electrode must be covered with cotton, and the client must hold the electrode whose charge (either positive or negative) is the opposite of the electrode on the skin.

CAUTION!

To avoid health complications or harm to the skin, do not use galvanic current on clients who have the following conditions:

- metal implants or a pacemaker
- braces
- heart conditions
- epilepsy
- pregnancy
- high blood pressure, fever, or any infection
- diminished nerve sensibility due to diseases such as diabetes
- open or broken skin (wounds, new scars) or inflamed pustular acne
- couperose skin or rosacea
- chronic migraine headaches

MINI-PROCEDURE

DESINCRUSTATION

1. Gently cleanse the skin before treatment.
2. Instruct the client to remove any jewelry from the hand that will be used to hold the electrode. Cover the positive electrode to be held by the client with a moistened sponge, or place a piece of dampened 4" × 4" cotton gauze around the electrode. Give this to the client to hold. This electrode is connected to the red wire (the positive wire).
3. Prepare the handheld flat electrode by placing a small, dampened sponge or round cotton pad into the black ring. Slide the ring back onto the electrode.
4. Apply product and gauze to the face as directed. Dip the electrode into the desincrustation solution. Apply the electrode to the client's forehead. *Make sure the electrode is directly on the skin before turning on the galvanic current* (Figure 16–11).
5. Turn the switch to negative and set at the appropriate level for the client.
6. Beginning on the forehead, gently rotate the electrode while gliding it over the client's forehead. Do not lift the electrode or break contact once the machine is on the skin, or it will be uncomfortable to the client. Keep the electrode as flat as possible and parallel to the skin's surface at all times. Continue in the T-zone area down the nose and onto the chin area (or onto any area that is oily or needs desincrustation). Use desincrustation only in areas that need it, and avoid areas with dry skin conditions.
7. Keep the electrode constantly moving to avoid overstimulating an area. Keep the skin moist and the pads wet. Add water to the pad or face if it gets too dry to glide over the skin.
8. When you are finished, turn off the machine first and then remove the electrode. Rinse the skin thoroughly with warm 4" × 4" cotton pads. Discard the pads.
9. Proceed with extractions or the next step in the treatment.

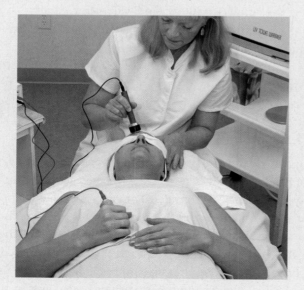

Figure 16–11 Do not let the galvanic electrode break contact with the skin.

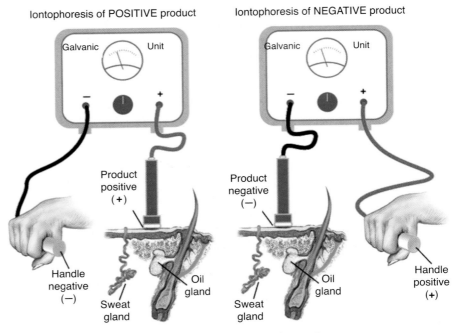

Iontophoresis of POSITIVE product   Iontophoresis of NEGATIVE product

Figure 16–12 A Iontophoresis of positive and negative products.

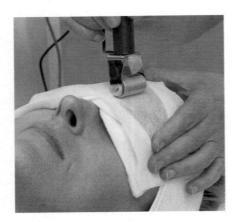

Figure 16–12 B Iontophoresis in use.

Iontophoresis

Iontophoresis is the process of using electric current to introduce water-soluble products into the skin. This process allows estheticians to transfer, or penetrate, ions of an applied solution into the deeper layers of the skin. **Ions** (EYE-ahns) are atoms or molecules that carry an electrical charge. Current flows through conductive solutions from the positive and negative polarities. This process is known as **ionization** (eye-ahn-ih-ZAY-shun)—the separating of a substance into ions.

Theoretically, iontophoresis is based on universal laws of attraction. For example, negative attracts positive, and vice versa. Similar to a magnetic response, iontophoresis creates an exchange of negative and positive ions or charges (Figure 16–12 A,B).

The process of ionic penetration takes two forms: **cataphoresis** (kat-uh-fuh-REE-sus), which refers to the infusion of a positive product; and **anaphoresis,** which refers to the infusion of a negative product.

Polarity of Solutions

It is important to identify the polarity of an ampoule (AM-pyool) or solution. Products that have a slightly acidic pH are considered positive. Products with an alkaline (or base) tendency are considered negative and are used for desincrustation. If the manufacturer indicates that the product is negative, the esthetician infuses the solution with the electrode set at negative; that is, the esthetician holds the negative electrode. The client holds the positive electrode.

If the product were positive, the client and esthetician would use the opposite electrodes. Some manufacturers may include ingredients in the same vial that are simultaneously positive and negative. In that case, the product should

Table 16-1

EFFECTS FROM THE GALVANIC CURRENT	
NEGATIVE POLE (CATHODE) ANAPHORESIS	**POSITIVE POLE (ANODE) CATAPHORESIS**
Negative Solutions: Desincrustation	*Positive Solutions: Iontophoresis*
causes an alkaline reaction	causes an acid reaction
softens and relaxes tissue	tightens the skin
stimulates nerve endings	calms or soothes nerve endings
increases blood circulation	decreases blood circulation

be ionized for 3 to 5 minutes on negative followed by 3 to 5 minutes on positive. If neither a negative nor positive polarity is indicated for an ampoule, as a general rule the esthetician should first use the negative and then the positive pole. This way you are stimulating and softening the skin first and preparing it for the treatment with anaphoresis, and then ending with the product penetration, skin tightening, and soothing with cataphoresis.

The molecular weight of a product is also a factor in permeability. Smaller molecules have greater penetration ability, while larger molecules cannot penetrate into the skin. Water-based products will also penetrate better than oil-based products. Several possible skin reactions can occur during ionization (Table 16-1).

MINI-PROCEDURE

IONTOPHORESIS

The steps in iontophoresis are the same as those used for the desincrustation procedure.

1. Set the switch on the machine to the appropriate setting while the client holds an electrode with the opposite charge. When the client holds the handheld electrode, all the water molecules in the skin become charged with the polarity of the electrode. For iontophoresis to occur, the client must hold the polarity opposite to that of the product, otherwise there will be no attraction or reaction.
2. To ensure proper connections, it is also important to moisten the electrodes. Have the client hold an electrode that is wrapped with a moistened cover or sponge. Place a sponge or piece of cotton that has been dipped into the solution onto the electrode before applying to the skin. No metallic electrode should ever be placed directly on the skin. Gels can be used with metallic electrodes as long as the skin is completely covered with the gel and gauze.
3. Apply the product as directed. You have the option of switching positive and negative poles when infusing solutions.

Galvanic Maintenance

Before attempting to clean the electrodes, always read and follow the manufacturer's directions for cleaning and disinfecting. Detach the electrode cord from the electrode. Remove any soiled sponge or cotton cover from the electrode and discard. Do not soak the electrode unless directed otherwise. Never place the metal electrode in an autoclave. The black plastic ring can be soaked in a germicidal solution for 10 minutes. In general, when cleaning rollers, detach the metal tip and soak it for 20 minutes in a disinfectant solution. Carefully spray and wipe the electrode attachment piece with a hospital-strength disinfectant.

Ionto Mask

The ionto mask works with galvanic current and can be used to facilitate either desincrustation (deep pore cleansing) or ionization (penetration of product). Depending on treatment goals, different solutions can be used to target specific skin conditions. The face is first covered with moistened gauze. This helps direct the current to the underlying tissue. The mask is then applied to the face and timed according to treatment parameters. Instead of the client holding an electrode, a wet pad is placed under the shoulder. The mask is then plugged into the source of the galvanic current.

HIGH-FREQUENCY MACHINE

The **high-frequency machine** is an apparatus that utilizes alternating, or **sinusoidal current** (sy-nuh-SOYD-ul KUR-unt). The oscillating circuit passes through a device that allows for the selection of a Tesla pulse current. This current can produce a frequency of 60,000 to 200,000 hertz, depending on how it is regulated. Remember that the frequency indicates the repetition of the current per second. Because high-frequency current is capable of changing polarity 1,000 times per second, it basically has no polarity and in effect does not produce chemical changes. This makes product penetration physically impossible. Product penetration is achieved by using galvanic current. The high frequency machine creates Ozone and this has a germicidal action on the skin.

The rapid oscillation created by the high-frequency machine vibrates water molecules in the skin. This can produce a mild to strong heat effect. It is important to note that esthetic high-frequency devices have a mild effect. An example of a stronger reaction is seen in **thermolysis** (thur-MAHL-uh-sus), which is used for electrolysis (ee-lek-TRAHL-ih-sis; permanent hair removal). High frequency should not be used on couperose skin, inflamed areas, or on clients who are pregnant, epileptic, or have pacemakers or high blood pressure.

The high-frequency machine is a useful and versatile esthetic tool (Figure 16–13 A,B). It may be applied after extractions or used over a product. It benefits the skin in the following ways:

- It has an antiseptic effect on the skin.
- It stimulates circulation.
- It helps oxygenate the skin.

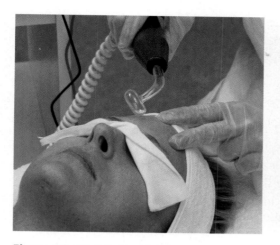 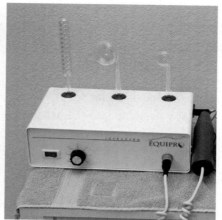

Figure 16–13 A,B The high-frequency machine produces a heat effect that stimulates circulation and has an antiseptic effect on the skin.

* It increases cell metabolism.
* It helps coagulate and heal any open lesion after extraction by sparking it with the mushroom electrode.
* It generates a warm feeling that has a relaxing effect on the skin.

Electrodes

During the manufacturing process, most of the air is removed from high-frequency electrodes, creating a vacuum in the tube. The air is replaced, mainly with neon gas. However, some electrodes may also contain argon gas. As electricity passes through these gases, they emit visible shades of light. Neon gas produces a pink, orange, or red light. Argon or rarified gas produces blue or violet light. Sometimes these lights are inaccurately called *ultraviolet* or *infrared* because of their colors. However, there are no infrared or ultraviolet rays in high frequency.

Several types of direct or indirect electrodes are available with high frequency. Each of these electrodes has unique benefits and features that produce specific physiological reactions in esthetic treatments. If you use the high-frequency machine, you will need to be trained in the procedure and on how to use the different electrodes (Table 16–2).

Maintenance

Follow these maintenance guidelines for the high-frequency machine.
* After each use, clean the glass electrode by wiping it with a solution of soap and water. Do not use alcohol on electrodes.
* Do not immerse the electrode directly in water. Place only the glass end (not the metal) into a sterilization solution for 20 minutes.
* Do not place electrodes in an ultraviolet machine or in an autoclave.
* Rinse electrodes with cool water. Do not get the metal end wet. Dry with a clean towel and store in a covered container.
* Unless they break or are damaged, most electrodes do not need replacing. However, electrodes are very fragile. Take extra care to wrap them in a soft material and then store them in a drawer where they will not be knocked

> **CAUTION!**
>
> High frequency should not be used on clients who have couperose skin or inflamed areas. Do not use high frequency on clients who are pregnant, have pacemakers, heart problems, high blood pressure, braces, or epilepsy. Be sure to know all the contraindications of using a machine before implementing it in treatments. To avoid being burned, the client should avoid contact with metal during electrical machine treatments. Clients should remove all jewelry prior to the treatment.

Table 16–2

HIGH-FREQUENCY PROCEDURES AND ELECTRODES	
ELECTRODE	**GENERAL APPLICATION**
Small mushroom The electrode is used to stimulate the skin during massage.	(Pink/orange light) for sensitive skin or (violet light) for normal to oily skin. 1. Place electrode into the handheld device. 2. Adjust the rheostat to the proper setting if the machine is not automatic. 3. Place an index finger on the glass electrode. 4. Apply the electrode directly onto dry skin beginning at the forehead. 5. Glide the electrode over the skin in circular movements (across the forehead area) and then to the nose, cheeks, and chin areas. Sometimes when skin is very clean, the electrode drags. In this case, place gauze between the skin and the electrode. 6. To remove from the skin, place an index finger over the glass and remove it. Turn the power switch off.
Large mushroom A large mushroom electrode in use on the face.	(Violet light) normal to oily or (pink/orange) sensitive. 1. The large mushroom is used in the same way as the small mushroom. 2. Another effective way to use this apparatus is to open a piece of cotton gauze and glide the mushroom electrode over the gauze. This produces a small spray of sparks onto the skin. This treatment is ideal for acne or problematic skin. 3. Facial finish: High frequency may be used at the end of a treatment over cream. Place cotton gauze between the cream and the electrode. Glide in circular motions over the entire area.
Indirect electrode (spiral)	Used indirectly to stimulate the skin during massage. This treatment is ideal for sallow and aging skin. 1. Apply cream to the client's face. 2. Give the wire glass electrode to the client who holds it with both hands. 3. The operator places the fingers of one hand to the forehead. 4. With the opposite hand, turn the high frequency on and move to a low setting. 5. Using both hands, perform a piano finger motion, gently tapping the skin. Move around in a systematic manner over the entire face. 6. To discontinue, remove one hand from the skin and turn the power switch off. 7. Do not lose contact with the skin during this procedure.
Sparking (glass tip)	A glass tip electrode is used to direct sparking to a specific area such as an acne lesion. It helps disinfect and heal the lesion. 1. Place the electrode into the handheld device. 2. Apply the index finger to the glass electrode and place it on the lesion area removing the finger so that the area is sparked. 3. Place the finger back on the electrode as you move from lesion to lesion releasing the finger in order to spark the skin. This is quick motion. 4. Remove the electrode from the skin by placing the finger once more on the glass. Turn the power switch off.
Comb electrode (rake)	Directly applied to the face. It may also be used in a scalp treatment. To apply, follow the directions for the mushroom electrode.

around or damaged. Some of the newer machines offer inserts for storing the electrodes right on the machine. Be sure to cover the electrodes so they remain clean.

- The high-frequency coil should be replaced after a few years of use if it is losing power. Check with the manufacturer for additional service requirements.

SPRAY MACHINE

Spray mists are beneficial in calming and hydrating the skin (Figure 16–14). The **spray machine** is part of the vacuum machine and is attached via a hose that is connected to a small plastic bottle with a spray nozzle. This bottle can be filled with a freshener solution or toner (1 part toner; 2 parts distilled water) to gently mist the client's face after cleansing or another treatment step, such as the massage.

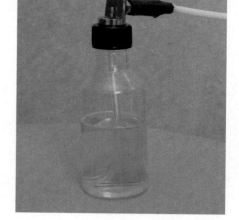

Figure 16–14 The spray machine.

MINI-PROCEDURE

THE SPRAY PROCEDURE

To mist the skin, use the following steps.

1. Place a towel under the client's chin to stop the mist from dripping down the neck. Remind the client to keep the eyes and mouth closed during the misting.
2. Turn on the power and adjust the velocity of the spray.
3. Hold the spray approximately 12 to 15 inches away from the face and mist for approximately 5 to 20 seconds. If necessary, pause and make sure the client can take a breath.
4. Turn off the power.
5. Gently pat or wipe off the product remaining on the skin.

Spray Machine Maintenance

Here are some general guidelines for spray machine maintenance.

- Follow the cleaning directions supplied by the manufacturer.
- Empty the bottle of fluid regularly to keep it fresh.
- Flush with distilled water regularly.
- Mineral buildup in the nozzle of the sprayer should be cleaned monthly or more often.

LUCAS SPRAYER

The **Lucas sprayer** (LOO-kus spray-ur) was invented by Dr. Lucas Championniere (sham-pee-awn-NARE) (1843–1913). It is the most unique of all atomizers and sprays. The Lucas sprayer is used to apply a very fine mist of plant extracts, herb teas, fresheners, or astringents (Figure 16–15). The mist is excellent for treating dehydrated, mature, and couperose skins. The mist can be used warm, to increase the blood flow to the skin's surface, or it can be used cool to calm couperose skin.

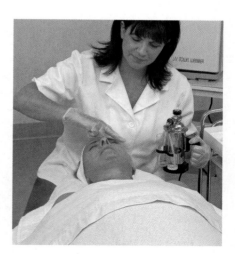

Figure 16–15 The Lucas sprayer.

MINI-PROCEDURE

USING THE LUCAS SPRAYER

1. Fill the Lucas sprayer 3/4 full with distilled water. A glass gauge on the side of the sprayer indicates the water level. Over-filling will cause the boiling water to spurt out. Add ingredients as directed.
2. Prepare the client by draping the body with a plastic cape. Place a towel around the neck to catch any dripping solution.
3. The spray should be flowing freely before directing it toward the client. The spray is held 14 to 16 inches from the client's face.
4. Circle the face with the spray, being careful not to spray directly at the client's nose or mouth.
5. Use cotton or a sponge to blot any solution that may drip down the client's face. Give the client some cotton to use if necessary.
6. The esthetician decides how long to use the spray. Usually the time does not exceed one minute.

Caution: Never let the water level drop from view on the water gauge. To do so could seriously damage the apparatus.

CAUTION!

To avoid burning the client's skin, never heat paraffin in anything other than an approved paraffin heater.

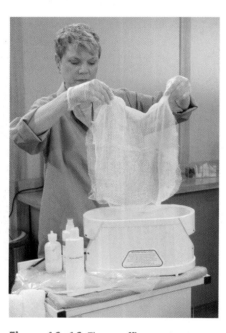

Figure 16–16 The paraffin wax treatment.

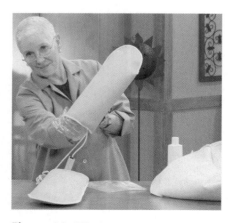

Figure 16–17 Electric mitts and boots.

PARAFFIN WAX HEATER

The paraffin wax heater is used to create a warm paraffin mask for hydrating dry skin (Figure 16–16). This device allows the esthetician to provide a treatment that offers quick results, but it lasts only for a limited period of time. Heated paraffin is applied to the face, creating an occlusive mask to hold in body heat and promote penetration of underlying products. The result is a hydrating and relaxing treatment that gives clients a glowing complexion. This is popular with women who want to look their best instantly, especially for special occasions. The paraffin mask procedure is in Chapter 14.

Paraffin wax heaters stay warm at a safe, low level of heat. They must be replenished as you discard the used wax. These heaters tend to take a long time to heat up in the morning. Always use a professional wax bath machine that emits low heat. A substitute heater, such as an electric cooking pot, regulates heat differently and is not recommended.

ELECTRIC MITTS AND BOOTS

Boots and mitts apply heat to the hands and feet to increase circulation and to promote overall relaxation (Figure 16–17). Often promoted as an add-on to a service, boots and mitts actually perform an important function. The heat helps lotion penetrate, and it soothes aching feet and hands. Paraffin wax is also used over lotion to warm and moisturize the skin.

To use these products, put lotion on the hands and/or feet and cover with plastic disposable liners before inserting into the warmers. Warm the mitts and/ or boots for approximately 10 minutes. Make sure the warmers do not get too hot. If the client feels sweaty, then the lotion cannot penetrate. To clean the electric mitts and boots, wipe them with a high-level disinfectant after each use.

THE ELECTRIC HEAT MASK

The electric heat mask produces heat at a comfortable temperature and is used to help soften the skin for better product penetration (Figure 16–18). The heat mask can be used on dry or oily skins, depending on the products being used with the mask. For dry skin, a moisturizer or deep penetration treatment cream is used. The heat and warmth of the mask will help the product to penetrate deeper into the skin. For oily, acne, or problem-blemished skin, the heat mask can be used with desincrustation solution to soften and liquefy grease deposits.

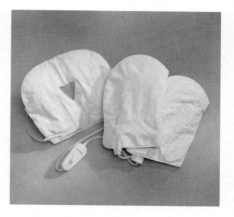

Figure 16–18 A heat mask and mitts.

The mask is not used on a face that has couperose or thin, sensitive skin. A fairly thick piece of moist cotton is placed over areas to protect it from the heating pad. The heat mask is also used for a combination skin that has an oily T-zone and areas that are dry. The desincrustation solution is applied to the oily areas of the skin with a wet cotton compress and the treatment cream for dry skin is applied to the dry area.

After application, the mask is left on the face for approximately 7 minutes. Should it be necessary for the esthetician to leave the facial area while the mask is in place, a timer should be set and the esthetician should take it with her so she can be aware of the time. This will let the client know that he or she is not being neglected. While the heat mask is on the face, most estheticians will take advantage of these few minutes and fill out the client's records.

To prevent the mask from burning out, turn it off immediately after use and disconnect it from the wall plug.

PURCHASING EQUIPMENT

Do your research before purchasing equipment. Regulations define what devices can be used within an esthetician's scope of practice. Another consideration is insurance coverage. Make sure the manufacturer claims are accurate and there is clinical evidence to support the claims. It is advisable to go slowly when considering purchasing expensive machines. Warranties and training provided from the manufacturer and distributor are two important considerations when purchasing equipment. Education and training are required for many high-tech machines.

Advances in science and technology have generated many new high-performance tools that enhance the esthetician's work. Estheticians must continue their education to keep abreast of the latest developments in therapeutic skin care. In this chapter, we have presented an overview of specialized tools and equipment designed to help the esthetician obtain the best results possible in skin care treatments.

Study and review the suggested guidelines for operating machinery, and practice your skills until you are comfortable working with equipment. Always be conscientious about safety issues and contraindications in using machines. Clients want instant results, so make sure you can deliver what you promise. Invest in high quality machines and your investment will increase your credibility and revenue as an esthetician. What machines would you like to incorporate into your services? High-tech equipment is the wave of the future.

Here's a Tip

It may be more affordable to purchase individual machines rather than the all-in-one machines that have the different modalities together on one unit. If anything needs to be repaired, you do not have to ship—or be left without—all of your machines.

REVIEW QUESTIONS

1. What skin conditions does a Wood's lamp reveal?

2. What is the purpose of a brush machine?

3. What are the benefits of the vacuum device?

4. List and define the two reactions of the galvanic current.

5. What are the contraindications for using a galvanic machine?

6. Define *anaphoresis*.

7. How does the negative pole of the galvanic current affect the skin?

8. Define *cataphoresis*.

9. How does the positive pole of the galvanic current affect the skin?

10. What is high frequency used for?

11. What are the benefits of the spray machine?

12. What are the benefits of electric mitts and boots?

CHAPTER GLOSSARY

anaphoresis: process of desincrustation or forcing negative liquids into the tissues from the negative toward the positive pole; an alkaline, stimulating reaction.

cataphoresis: process of forcing positive, acidic substances into deeper tissues using galvanic current from the positive toward the negative pole; tightens and calms the skin.

desincrustation: galvanic current is used to create an alkaline chemical reaction that emulsifies or liquefies sebum and debris.

electrotherapy: the use of electrical devices for therapeutic benefits.

galvanic current: a constant and direct current, it uses a positive and negative pole to produce chemical reactions, (desincrustation) and ionic reactions (iontophoresis).

high-frequency machine: apparatus that utilizes alternating or sinusoidal current to produce a mild to strong heat effect. High frequency is a *Tesla* current, sometimes called the *violet ray*.

ion: an atom or molecule that carries an electrical charge.

ionization: the separating of a substance into ions.

iontophoresis: process of introducing ions of water-soluble products into the skin by using an electric current such as the positive and negative poles of a galvanic machine.

Lucas sprayer: atomizer designed to apply plant extracts and other ingredients to the skin.

rotary brush: machine used to lightly exfoliate and stimulate the skin; also helps soften excess oil, dirt, and cell buildup.

saponification: chemical reaction during desincrustation where the current transforms the sebum into soap.

sinusoidal current: alternating current similar to faradic current; produces mechanical contractions and is used during scalp and facial manipulations.

spray machine: spray misting device.

thermolysis: a heat effect; used for permanent hair removal.

vacuum (suction) machine: device that vacuums/suctions the skin to remove impurities and stimulate circulation.

Wood's lamp: filtered black light that is used to illuminate skin disorders, fungi, bacterial disorders, and pigmentation.

CHAPTER 17

HAIR REMOVAL

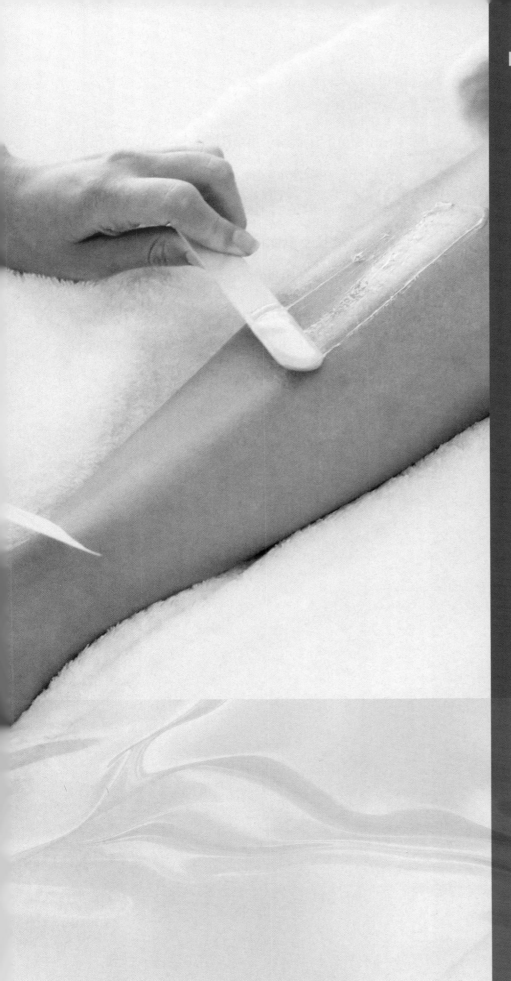

LEARNING OBJECTIVES

After completing this chapter, you will be able to:

- Explain the morphology of hair and its growth stages.

- Describe methods of temporary and permanent hair removal.

- Identify different hair removal equipment, tools, and accessories.

- Perform face and body waxing.

- Name the conditions that contraindicate hair removal.

- Provide a thorough client consultation before hair removal.

KEY TERMS

Throughout history, hair has been used for physical adornment and to enhance beauty. Different cultures have different views as to what is attractive; cultural norms also dictate if it is socially acceptable for women to have hair on their bodies. Hair removal for cosmetic reasons has become very popular. Consumers spend millions of dollars per year on hair removal products and services.

Unwanted hair has been removed throughout the ages by a variety of methods. Excavations of Egyptian tombs indicate that abrasive materials such as pumice stones were used to rub away hair. Ancient Greek and Roman women were known to remove their body hair by similar methods. Native Americans may have used sharpened stones and seashells to rub off and pluck out hair. The ancient Turks used a chemical method, a combination of yellow sulfide made of arsenic, quicklime, and rose water, as a crude hair removal agent.

Excessive or unwanted hair is a common problem that affects both men and women. Fortunately, a variety of hair removal methods are available, ranging from procedures such as shaving and tweezing to more advanced procedures that require special training. Face and body hair removal has become increasingly popular as evolving technology makes it easier to perform with more effective results.

Women comprise the vast majority of hair removal clients. Most often, they want hair removed from the eyebrows, upper lip, cheeks, chin, underarms, bikini line, and legs. Hair removal for men is also on the rise. Men may choose to have hair removed from their back and chest. If they compete in sports like bicycling and swimming, they may want hair removed from their legs and arms to facilitate faster competition times. Waxing is the most common method of hair removal in salons. Hair removal makes up a large part of a salon's business (Figure 17–1). In some cases, up to 50 percent of the services involve hair removal.

Understanding the techniques, the benefits and risks, and how to perform various techniques is key to an esthetician's success in this potentially profitable area. In this chapter, you will learn hair removal procedures, what tools are used, and what is involved in room preparation. Sanitation is an important part of hair removal procedures. Conducting services in a safe environment and taking measures to prevent the spread of infectious and contagious diseases are always primary concerns. Thorough client consultations and reviewing hair removal contraindications are necessary before providing any service.

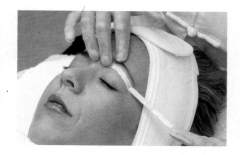

Figure 17–1 Hair removal is a large part of an esthetician's business.

MORPHOLOGY OF THE HAIR

Trichology (tri-KAHL-uh-jee) is the scientific study of hair and its diseases. *Trichos* is the Greek word for "hair." The main structures of the hair unit, or area below the skin's surface are the follicle, bulb, papilla, arrector pili muscle, and sebaceous glands. Hair is made from a hard protein called *keratin,* which is produced from the **hair follicle** (hair FAWL-ih-kul; Figure 17–2). A hair follicle is a mass of epidermal cells, extending down into the dermis and forming a small tube. Referred to as a *pilosebaceous follicle* (*pilus* [PY-lus] means hair; *pili* [PY-lie] is the plural), the unit contains both the sebaceous appendage and the **hair shaft.** How much hair you have is predetermined by genetics. Not all follicles contain a hair shaft. No hair grows on the palms of the hands, the soles of the feet, the lips, or the eyelids.

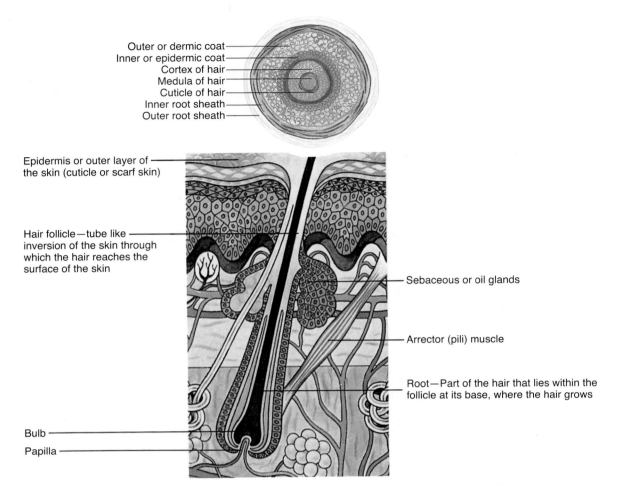

Outer or dermic coat
Inner or epidermic coat
Cortex of hair
Medula of hair
Cuticle of hair
Inner root sheath
Outer root sheath

Epidermis or outer layer of
the skin (cuticle or scarf skin)

Hair follicle—tube like
inversion of the skin through
which the hair reaches the
surface of the skin

Sebaceous or oil glands

Arrector (pili) muscle

Root—Part of the hair that lies within the
follicle at its base, where the hair grows

Bulb
Papilla

Figure 17–2 The hair follicle and appendages.

Hair follicles are slanted, sometimes growing in many different directions in one area (for example, under the arm). The main structures of the hair follicle are the root, bulb, and papilla. The arrector pili muscle and the sebaceous glands are attached to the follicles (Figure 17–3). The **hair bulb** is a thick, club-shaped structure that forms the lower part of the **hair root.** The lower part of the bulb fits over and covers the papilla. The **hair papilla,** a cone-shaped elevation at the base of the follicle, fits into the bulb. The papilla is filled with tissue that contains the blood vessels and cells necessary for hair growth and nourishment of the follicle.

Vitamins, minerals, and nutrients are needed for strong, healthy hair. The blood vessels bring nutrients to the base of the bulb, causing it to grow and form new hair. The **arrector pili muscle** (ur-REK-tohr PY-li) inserts into the base of the hair follicle. When the muscle contracts, the hair stands straight up, causing goose bumps. Oil ducts (sebaceous glands) attached to the follicle are responsible for lubricating the skin and hair. Moderate amounts of sebaceous oil are necessary for healthy skin and hair. The face contains approximately 3,200 follicles per square inch.

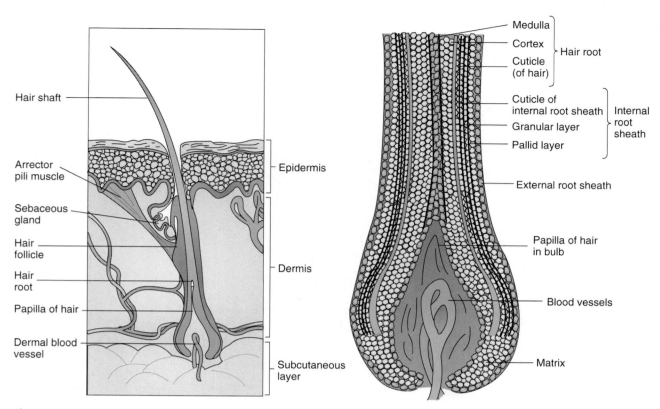

Figure 17–3 Hair morphology.

Hair formation actually begins before birth. The hair on a fetus is extremely soft and downy, known as **lanugo** (luh-NOO-goh). The lanugo hair is lost and then replaced with stronger, pigmented hair after birth. The shape, size, and normal function of the hair follicle are genetically determined, along with secretion activity and the depth of the hair shaft. Very fine, soft hair is referred to as **vellus hair** (VEL-lus). It is found in areas that are not covered by the larger, coarse hairs found on the head, brows, and pubic area. The cheeks are a good example. The terms *vellus* or *lanugo* are sometimes incorrectly used interchangeably to describe short, fine, and downy hair.

HAIR GROWTH CYCLE

Hair growth is a result of the activity of cells found in the basal layer. These cells are actually found within the hair bulb. Hair growth occurs in three stages: anagen, catagen, and telogen (Figure 17–4).

Anagen (AN-uh-jen) is the growth stage during which new hair is produced. New keratinized cells are manufactured in the hair follicle during the anagen stage. Activity is greater in the hair bulb, which pushes down into the dermis and swells with cell mitosis.

Catagen (KAT-uh-jen) is the transition stage of hair growth. In the catagen stage, the hair shaft grows upward and detaches itself from the bulb.

Telogen (TEL-uh-jen) is the final, or resting, stage of hair growth. During the telogen stage, the hair is at its full size and is erect in the follicle. It shows above the skin's surface. The hair bulb is not active, and the hair falls out. The

> **? Did You Know**
>
> The average hair growth on the scalp is one-half inch per month.

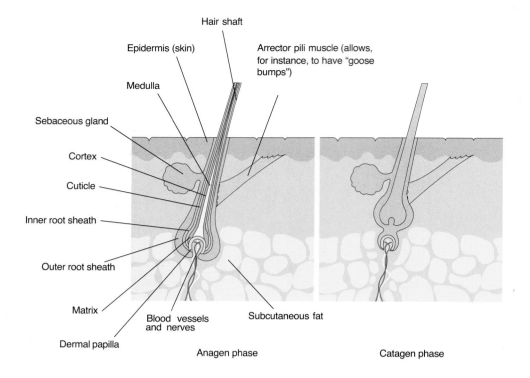

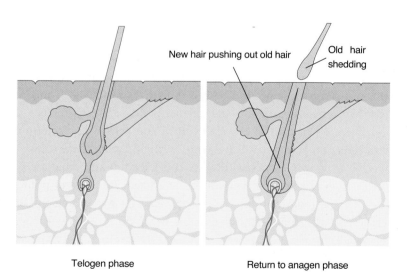

Figure 17–4 Hair growth encompasses three stages: anagen, catagen, and telogen.

bulb then moves upward into the dermis and begins to grow a new hair. The cycle then begins again. The follicle can be void of hair in the telogen stage until it cycles back into the anagen stage. If the hair does not fall out and the anagen stage begins again, two hairs can occupy the same follicle.

It is important to understand the three stages of hair growth. Two hairs can be growing next to each other and be at different stages of growth. It takes 4 to 13 weeks for the hair to grow from the papilla to the surface of the skin depending in part on the areas of the body. When offering services, the practitioner takes into consideration these stages and schedules appointments according to these cycles. Repeat visits are normally necessary. Remind clients that not all hair grows at the same rate and that hairs are at different growth stages in the follicle. Hairs removed in the anagen stage while the hair bulb is more "active" will be more effective for long-term hair reduction.

Indicator of Health

Hair and skin are good barometers of an individual's state of health. Dull, lifeless hair and sallow, listless skin tone may signal a health warning. Strong, healthy hair and good skin tone are signs of good health. Hair also responds to the outside elements. For instance, hair grows faster in a warm climate. Excessive cold can dry the hair and reduce its luster. The rate of oil secretions from the follicle determines whether the skin is oily or dry. Excessive heat or damaging products will dry the hair. Disease, drug use, and the aging process affect the hair's growth and overall appearance.

Excessive Hair Growth

Two medical terms are applied to excessive hair growth. The first is **hirsutism** (HUR-suh-tiz-um), which is excessive hair growth on the face, arms, and legs, especially in women (Figure 17–5). The second is **hypertrichosis** (hy-pur-trih-KOH-sis), or excessive growth of hair where hair does not normally grow. The amount of hair an individual has differs from person to person. Genetics accounts for how much hair you will normally have on the body. What would be normal hair growth in one person might be extreme in another. Excessive hair growth on a female body suggests an imbalance of hormones.

Hirsutism can be caused by various factors. A normal pregnancy increases adrenocortical activity, which may cause moderate hirsutism. Vitamin deficiency, certain diseases, particular drugs, and emotional shock or stress can result in glandular disturbances that stimulate excessive hair growth. Excessive hair growth on a female face or body may be attributed to hormonal imbalances. One of the more notable and prevalent causes being Polycystic Ovarian Syndrome (PCOS). Menopause may also cause excess facial hair. The "menopause mustache," as it is often called, is a sign of menopause. These changes may dissipate with time.

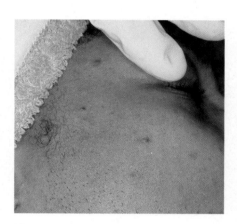

Figure 17–5 Hirsutism.

CHARACTERISTICS AND DIFFERENCES IN HAIR GROWTH

Hair protects the body from environmental elements and ultraviolet rays. It guards the nose, ears, and reproductive areas with fine hairs to filter out dust and other particles. Hair is a conduit of sensation for the skin and acts as a wick in the follicle, allowing for sebum to move up and out onto the skin's surface.

As cultures moved from region to region, individuals acquired mixed traits of hair color and thickness (Figure 17–6). In northern regions of the world, fine hair and lighter skin tones are common. Blond hair is finer and easy to remove. Red heads can have coarse hair that may be more difficult to remove. These individuals generally have fair skin that tends to be sensitive, a very important point to remember when performing hair removal.

In areas closer to the equator, the skin and hair are normally thicker and darker. These characteristics help protect the body from strong ultraviolet rays.

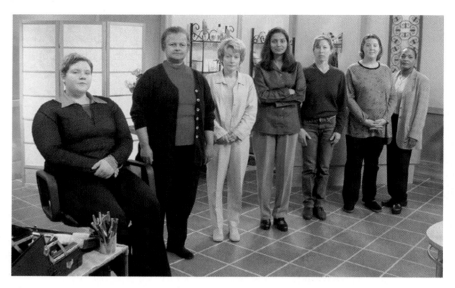

Figure 17–6 Genetic differences in growth and coloring.

Central and South American peoples, as well as those from Mediterranean regions and the Middle East, tend to have darker and more noticeable hair. Individuals with olive and darker skin tones can have pigmentation problems if epilation is not performed carefully. Individuals from Western Europe (France, Spain, and Portugal) generally have black hair, which is average in density. For those with thicker hair the root is quite deep in the follicle, thus very difficult to remove. With repeated removal, hair regrowth tends to become thinner and easier to remove.

Individuals originating from Africa and Australia tend to have black, coarse, curly hair, which has a tendency to become ingrown. The method of hair removal for these individuals needs to be chosen carefully. Native Americans and many Asians have thinner facial hair, but the roots tend to be deep.

Aging creates changes in the hair. Gray hair is a result of physiological changes, causing it to be coarse with a deep root system. Before hair grays, it is easier to remove. With the changes that take place during the aging process, the hair root system increases by almost 50 percent, making hair removal difficult. This explains the increase in coarse hairs on women's chins and lips.

METHODS OF HAIR REMOVAL

Methods of hair removal fall into two general categories: temporary and permanent. Temporary hair removal involves repeat treatments as hair grows. With permanent hair removal, the papilla is destroyed, making regrowth impossible. Salon techniques are generally limited to temporary methods such as waxing.

Electrolysis

Electrolysis (ee-lek-TRAHL-ih-sis), the process of removing hair by means of electricity, is considered the only true method of permanent hair removal (versus permanent hair reduction). Electrolysis should be performed by a certified and licensed (if the state requires it) electrologist. If the state does not license the profession, look for an electrologist who holds the designations "CPE" (certified professional electrologist) from the American Electrology Association (AEA). Talk with your instructor for additional information about classes and licensing.

There are three methods of electrolysis: *galvanic, thermolysis,* and *blend.*

Galvanic Electrolysis

This method uses direct current, which causes chemical decomposition of the hair follicle. The galvanic method decomposes the papilla, the source of nourishment for the hair. The needle is connected to the negative side of a direct current (DC) power source and is inserted into the follicle. The client holds the electrode connected to the positive side of the power source. When power is applied, the electrical charge begins transforming saline moisture inside the follicle into sodium hydroxide (lye) along with hydrogen and chlorine gas. Unstable sodium hydroxide destabilizes the follicle wall through a chemical action. It weakens the hold of the follicle wall on surrounding tissue. This allows the hair to be removed easily. In the case of galvanic electrolysis, the moisture content within the skin is important to conduct a proper current. This method is slower than thermolysis.

Thermolysis

This method utilizes a high-frequency current to produce heat, which coagulates and destroys the hair follicle. Electrocoagulation (**thermolysis**) destroys the hair by coagulating the papilla through heat. An alternating current (AC) passes through a needle, causing vibration in the water molecules surrounding the hair follicle. This action produces heat, which destroys the papilla.

Blend

This method combines both systems, sending a current through a fine needle or probe. The blend method combines the benefits of the galvanic and thermolysis methods by passing AC and DC current through the needle at the same time. Results are reported to be quicker than with the galvanic method alone.

Permanent Reduction and Semipermanent Hair Removal

Methods of "permanent" hair reduction include laser as well as photo light hair removal systems. Laser and photo light are normally performed in a medical setting. Food and Drug Administration (FDA) guidelines require that these procedures be defined as permanent hair reduction. While these methods are sometimes called "permanent," the hair bulb must be destroyed completely, or there may be some regrowth. This has led to the confusing, interchangeable terms of *permanent reduction* and *semipermanent removal* (these terms mean that hair removal is not permanent).

Laser and Pulse Light Technology

Photoepilation (FOH-toh-ep-uh-LAY-shun) uses intense light to destroy the growth cells of the hair bulb. Both *intense pulsed light (IPL)* and *laser hair removal* are used to reduce hair growth.

Laser hair removal technology has been around since the early 1980s. A variety of lasers are available, such as the diode, alexandrite, and Nd:YAG. The hair removal industry now has the ability to offer clients a choice of both treatments: epilation by traditional methods and photoepilation with intense pulse light and lasers. Clinical studies have shown that photoepilation can provide a 50 to 60 percent clearance of hair in 12 weeks.

Lasers. In **laser hair removal,** a laser beam is pulsed on the skin, impairing the hair follicles. It is most effective when used on follicles in the growth, or anagen, phase. As mentioned earlier, "permanent" laser hair reduction is defined as *semipermanent.* The laser will reduce the number of body hairs. It will not result, however, in the permanent removal of all hair. Nevertheless, laser hair removal is increasingly in demand by clients with excess hair problems.

The laser method was discovered by chance when it was noted that birthmarks treated with certain types of lasers became permanently devoid of hair. Lasers are not for everyone; some lasers work only if one's hair is darker than the surrounding skin. Coarse, dark hair responds best to laser treatments. For some clients, laser hair removal brings truly permanent results. The laser can also slow down hair regrowth.

Earlier-generation lasers restricted hair removal to Fitzpatrick skin types I, II, and III, and sometimes type IV. Darker skin ended up absorbing more energy, which often resulted in permanent pigmentation. Today, newer machines allow hair removal on darker Fitzpatrick skin types.

Intense Pulsed Light. Intense pulsed light (IPL) is different from a traditional laser. First-generation lasers were a solid beam of light. Pulsed light (or photo light) produces a quick "flash" of light. These short, powerful pulses shatter their target without allowing heat to build up and burn the surrounding skin. The flash destroys the targeted vein or hair bulb and reduces hair or spider veins. Improved since its introduction in the United States, it is widely used in the medical arena or in medi-spas. While there is always a risk of scarring with any laser procedure, this newer technology greatly reduces the risk of scarring, often to less than 1 percent.

All laser devices must have FDA approval. Many photoepilation hair removal machines must be used under the direct supervision of a physician. Each local regulatory agency regulates who can use these devices. Manufacturers of photoepilation equipment generally provide the specialized training for administering this procedure, but certification through an advanced training program is recommended and in some cases required. Training should be above and beyond manufacturers' training programs. Some advanced schools offer 60 hours of clinical training. This is an advanced treatment that is discussed more fully in Chapter 18.

TEMPORARY METHODS

Temporary methods of hair removal include depilation and epilation. **Depilation** (DEP-uh-lay-shun) is a process of removing hair at or near the level of the skin. Both shaving and chemical depilation are included in this category. Another temporary method of hair removal is **epilation** (ep-uh-LAY-shun), the

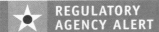

? Did You Know

The word *laser* is an acronym for "light amplification by stimulated emission of radiation." Lasers use intense pulses of electromagnetic radiation.

★ REGULATORY AGENCY ALERT

Laws regarding photoepilation services vary by region and province. Be sure to check with your regulatory agency for guidelines.

process of removing hair from the bottom of the follicle by breaking contact between the bulb and the papilla (Figure 17–7). The hair is pulled out of the follicle. Tweezing (manual), wax depilatories, and sugaring are all methods of epilation. Waxing, the most common epilation procedure estheticians perform, is the focus of this chapter.

Depilation

The main method of depilation is shaving. How long it takes for hair to grow back after removal depends on a person's hair growth pattern. After removal by any method, hair can take from days to weeks to reappear.

Shaving

Shaving is a daily ritual for most men. Many women shave the underarms, legs, and bikini area. As in any depilation method, the hair is removed down to the skin's surface. Shaving is a temporary method of hair removal that can also irritate the skin. Ingrown hairs are also a problem with shaving. **Barbae folliculitis** (BAR-bay fah-lik-yuh-LY-tis) is a term for infected follicles or ingrown hairs. This problem can be corrected by changing the direction of shaving. Contrary to popular belief, shaving does not cause hair to grow back thicker or stronger. It only seems that way because the razor blunts the hair ends and makes them feel stiff. *Pseudofolliculitis* are razor bumps or ingrown hairs without pus or infection.

Depilatories

A **depilatory** (dih-PIL-uh-tohr-ee) is a substance, usually a caustic alkali preparation, used for temporarily removing superfluous hair by dissolving it at the skin level. During the application time, the hair expands and the disulfide bonds break as a result of using such chemicals as sodium hydroxide, potassium hydroxide, thioglycolic acid, or calcium thioglycolate. Although depilatories are not commonly used in salons, you should be familiar with them in case your clients have used them.

Chemical depilatories are applied in a thin coating on the surface of the skin. Any chemical depilation cream should be patch tested first on the inside of the arm to make sure there are no allergic or sensitivity reactions. Normally, if there is no reaction—swelling, itching, or redness—within the first 10 minutes, the substance can then be applied to a larger area. A chemical depilatory is generally not recommended for use on the upper lip or other sensitive areas.

Methods of Epilation

Epilation methods and products continue to improve and become more effective.

Tweezing

The method of using tweezers to pull hair out by the root one at a time is called *tweezing*. Eyebrows can be shaped and contoured by tweezing (Figure 17–8). Tweezing is also used on remaining hairs after waxing. If clients are sensitive to waxing, tweezing is a slower, but effective alternative for removing the dark, coarse hair on the face.

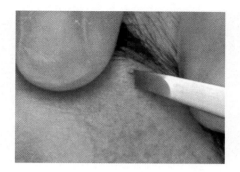

Figure 17–7 Epilation removes hairs from the follicles.

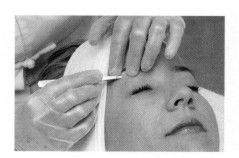

Figure 17–8 Tweezing hair from the eyebrows.

Electronic Tweezers

Another method for removal of superfluous hair used in salons and spas is the electronically charged tweezers. This method is supposed to transmit radio frequency energy down the hair shaft into the follicle area. The papilla is thus dehydrated and eventually destroyed. The tweezers are used to grasp a single strand of hair. Electronic tweezers are not a method of permanent hair removal. Furthermore, the process of clearing any area of hair by this method is slow.

Sugaring

Sugaring is an ancient method of hair removal, dating back to the Egyptians. It is an alternative for those who have sensitive skin or who react to waxes with bumps and redness. The sugaring solution is water soluble, meaning that it is easily removed with water. The original basic recipe is a mixture of sugar, lemon juice, and water. It is heated to form syrup, which is molded into a ball and pressed onto the skin and then quickly stripped away.

Sugaring is similar to waxing methods except that it uses a thick, sugar-based paste and is especially appropriate for more sensitive skin types. One advantage with sugar waxing is the hair can be removed even if it is only 1/8 inch long. It can be removed in the direction of the hair growth, which is less irritating.

Sugar mixtures are now manufactured in large quantities and sold in small containers ready to be placed in a heater. The sugar mixture melts at a very low temperature. A thin coat is applied and removed as recommended by the manufacturer. The sugar paste adheres only to the hair, making removal more comfortable.

Threading

Another ancient method of hair removal is *threading* (Figure 17–9), which is still practiced in many Eastern cultures today. It works by using cotton thread that is twisted and rolled along the surface of the skin, entwining the hair in the thread and lifting it out of the follicle. The skin usually reacts with a little redness and slight soreness. However, it is considered an effective hair removal method for clients unable to tolerate waxing due to the use of products like glycolic acid and Retin A®. Threading has become increasingly popular as an option to other methods and requires specialized training.

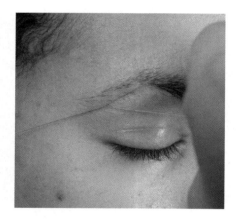

Figure 17–9 An example of threading.

Waxing

The primary hair removal method used by estheticians is waxing. Wax is a commonly used epilator, applied in either soft or hard form as recommended by the manufacturer. Both products are made primarily of resins and beeswax. Hard wax is thicker than soft wax and does not require fabric strips for removal. Wax is applied evenly over the hair and then removed. The benefit of waxing is that the hair takes longer to grow back and the skin feels smoother without the hair or stubble. The recommended time between waxing appointments is generally 4 to 6 weeks.

WAXING TECHNIQUES

Correct waxing techniques, appropriate materials, and proper wax temperatures are all factors in obtaining positive results from waxing services. Wax is designed to adhere to the hair as close to the skin as possible. When the wax is removed, it should adhere to the hair and remove the bulb from the follicle. If the wax is not applied correctly, is applied at the wrong temperature, or if the skin is not cleansed well, the hair will not be removed. If the wax is too hot, it can cause skin irritation and burns severe enough to cause blistering. During removal, the skin can be pulled off as well. The skin must be held as taut as possible to avoid skin damage. As with all esthetic methods, proper technique is the key to successful waxing. Understanding the "whys and hows" of proper waxing techniques and checking for contraindications that might cause injury is crucial to providing a satisfactory, safe, and comfortable hair removal service.

Types of Wax Products

There are two types of waxes: hard (no strip is used) and soft (a strip is used). Hard "stripless" waxes are applied directly to the skin in a thick, "wet" layer that hardens as it cools (Figure 17–10). The technician then uses the fingers to lift the wax off the skin. Soft "strip" waxes are applied in a thin layer and covered with a strip of pellon or muslin material, which removes the hair as it is pulled off quickly. All soft wax is applied in the same direction as the hair grows out of the follicle and is removed in the opposite direction of the hair growth. Hard wax is the only wax that may be removed differently, but additional training is needed to use this method.

Wax product consistencies vary, as do melting points. Waxes require a heater to liquefy them. Cold hard waxes are also available, primarily for home use. Formulas are derived from resins (some from pine trees), beeswax, paraffin, and other substances. Waxes may include additives to address the needs of different skin types. Azulene or chamomile may be used for sensitive skin. Tea tree oil may be added for its soothing and antiseptic benefits. Some waxes are water soluble and wipe off easily with water. Others, such as resins, are oil-soluble. Excess wax is removed with an oil-based solution if it is not soluble in water.

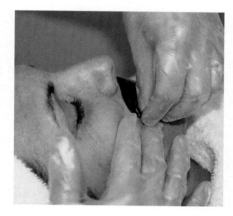

Figure 17–10 Hard wax application on the face.

Hard Wax

Hard waxes are available in blocks, disks, pellets, or beads (Figure 17–11). They are considered a no-strip wax. They must be liquefied before they can be used. Hard waxes are available at different melting points to address the needs of normal and sensitive skin. The harder the wax, the more heat it requires to melt it. Small, individual wax heaters are available and can be placed in each treatment room. The used wax is discarded after each use.

Some estheticians prefer hard waxes. They are gentle enough for the face area, yet strong enough to be used on hard-to-remove, coarse hairs. Some like to use it on the bikini and underarm area. Estheticians generally use soft wax in larger areas, such as the back and legs, and hard wax in smaller areas, such as the eyebrow.

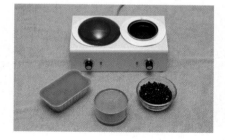

Figure 17–11 Hard waxes are available in blocks, disks, pellets, or beads.

Soft Wax

One of the most common methods of hair removal is soft, or strip, waxing. Soft waxes have a lower melting point. They come in tins or plastic containers and can be melted slightly in the microwave to make it easier to pour the wax into a wax heater or warming pot (Figure 17–12). With this method, a thin coat of wax is applied on the skin and removed immediately with a muslin, pellon, or cotton strip before it cools.

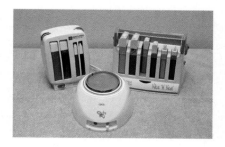

Figure 17–12 Soft wax products.

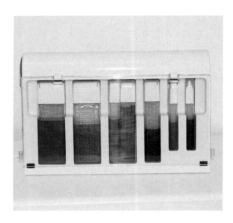

Figure 17–13 Roller-type waxes are convenient for various waxing applications.

Roll-On Wax

Another type of soft wax method uses roll-on applicators (Figure 17–13). The applicators contain wax and have roll-on heads. Applicators are warmed in a heating unit designed to fit the applicators. This method is very efficient and clean. Many estheticians prefer to use the roll-on waxer because it can be less messy and more efficient. Be sure to sanitize applicators and rollers properly.

ROOM PREPARATION

The waxing room should be clean and disinfected, with appropriate covers on the waxing table.

Furniture and Accessories

Some spas and salons have separate rooms for waxing. Others perform waxing services in the facial rooms. Waxing, especially on larger body areas such as the legs, is labor intensive. Furniture should be ergonomically designed so that both the technician and client are comfortable. Ideally, the waxing table should be adjustable to different heights. This allows each technician to adjust the table to the correct height that is comfortable for their back.

A multitiered, wheeled cart is useful for holding waxing pots and supplies (Figure 17–14). The cart can be moved near the client, keeping tools and supplies close at hand. A covered waste container is necessary for the proper disposal of all used supplies as you work. A stool should also be available to help the client safely get on and off of the table.

Tools and Supplies

Appropriate tools and supplies need to be replenished every day. Many items, such as applicators, are available as disposable items that are both convenient and sanitary. The trolley should be stocked with items such as the wax and

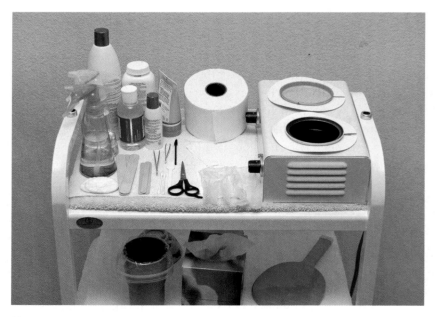

Figure 17–14 The wax cart setup.

warmer, cleansers, pre- and post-epilation solutions, tweezers, scissors, applicators, cotton supplies, and gloves. Follow the same sanitation procedures for all esthetic services.

Tweezers

Professional tweezers are available in different point sizes. Slant-tipped tweezers are best for general tweezing. A more pointed tip is ideal for ingrown hairs. Tweezers should be made of stainless steel so they will not corrode when disinfected in solution or in the autoclave. Always purchase the highest-quality tweezers and accessories you can afford. Tweezers are an important tool that will help make your work more precise and efficient. The result will be a more satisfied client.

Applicators

Disposable wax applicators are wooden, flat sticks, either large or small. (These are similar to popsicle sticks, cuticle pushers, and tongue depressors.) A stainless steel 5" spatula is ideal for spreading a thin coat on larger areas such as the legs; it must be disinfected after each use. All disposable applicators are used once and are not double-dipped. If they are, wax is exclusively used on each client, any leftovers are discarded, and the container must be disinfected.

Wax Strips

There are two popular types of wax strips: cotton muslin, which comes in rolls or precut packets, and pellon. Pellon® is a fiberlike material that does not shed or stretch. Strips can be used a few times on a client before disposal. When using a strip wax, prepare your strips ahead of time. Cut smaller strips for the eye and face areas. Trim a strip to the size of the area you are going to wax, plus an inch or two to hold onto. With correct strip sizes, less material is wasted and more accurate pulling is ensured.

Wax strip sizes: If strips are not precut, cutting the wax strip to the right size is important for client safety and proper technique. If the strips are too large, it interferes with your wax technique. It is not safe to wax too much surface area at one time. Your instructor will give you specific dimensions to use. The strips should be cut straight with no stray edges. The width for leg strips is the size of the wax roll, approximately 3" (Figure 17–15 A,B). Cut smaller sizes from the leg strips.

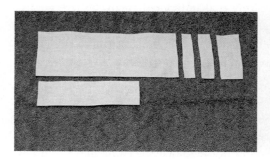 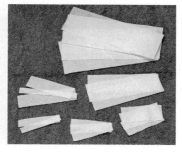

Figure 17–15 A,B Wax strips and sizes.

These are approximate sizes:

- Leg: 3" wide × 8" in length (cut 1/2 to 3/4 of the strip length for the knees)
- Brow/lip: 1/2", 3/4" to 1" wide × 3" in length
- Face (chin): 1-1/2" wide × 3" length
- Bikini/underarm: 1-1/2" to 2" wide × 5" to 6" length (half of the roll's width and 3/4 of the leg strip length). Or, you can use part of a small leg strip for larger areas.

Linens/Roll Paper

To keep the area clean, place a clean sheet or sheet of paper on the waxing table for each new client. Roll paper for waxing is normally ordered through esthetics or medical suppliers. You can also use bath towels or sheets. Keep these separate from nicer facial linens.

Pre- and Post-Epilation Products

Various products are available for treating the skin before and after waxing. A prep solution is applied to thoroughly clean the skin before waxing. Both pre- and post-waxing solutions may have antiseptic and calming ingredients such as witch hazel, arnica, chamomile, and calendula. Other desensitizing lotions ease discomfort. Powder and other pre-wax products protect the skin while waxing.

Post-waxing products contain antiseptic and soothing properties, such as azulene or aloe. Other post-waxing products are hair-growth inhibitors. Use caution when applying products to skin after waxing. Fragrances and other ingredients such as alcohol can be irritating to the skin. Irritation, reactions, and breakouts can occur. Aloe products are not always soothing—some contain irritating ingredients. Products to prevent ingrown hair are used after the skin has recovered from waxing and help keep the follicle open.

Sanitation

Waxing stations and supplies must be kept clean and sanitized. Wax drips on the side of a heater are unsightly. Waxing needs to be done carefully to avoid drips on the floor, linens, and furniture. Wipe excess wax off the spatulas before taking it from the pot, and move the spatulas carefully from the pot to the client. Do not double-dip the spatula unless you are disposing of the entire pot of wax after treating that individual client. Otherwise, use a new spatula each time to dip into the pot of wax. Place the waxing unit and all your accessories on a roll cart that can be pulled close to the client. Keep the clean disposable wooden applicators and cotton supplies in covered containers.

Always wear gloves. Use vinyl gloves rather than latex. Latex tends to get sticky and breaks down easily. Change your gloves if they become sticky during a waxing service. Hair removal often causes trauma to the follicle. When the hair is forcefully pulled out of the follicle, bleeding may occur and fluids may rise to the surface of the skin. All blood-stained gauze and materials should be discarded in a hazardous waste container and disposed of properly. When there is slight bleeding or even red bumps, place a small amount of antiseptic on a cotton 4" × 4" (or 2" × 2") pad and gently pat the area. This helps stop the bleeding and calms the area. A cold wet cotton compress is also soothing after waxing.

Sanitizers and Disinfectants

The wet sanitizer is normally a small, rectangular box with a lid. Tweezers should be thoroughly cleansed and placed into a wet sanitizer, depending on the manufacturer's instructions. Place the instruments into an approved, hospital-strength disinfectant solution that is designated to kill all microbes, including staphylococcus, tuberculosis, pseudomonas (a pathogen), fungus, and the HIV virus. These solutions are often listed in catalogs for the esthetics industry or are available at a medical supply house. Stainless steel instruments can also be sterilized in an autoclave.

CONTRAINDICATIONS FOR HAIR REMOVAL

The main reason for the client consultation is to determine the presence of any contraindications for hair removal (Table 17–1).

Table 17–1

CONTRAINDICATIONS FOR WAXING PROCEDURES

Leg waxing should not be performed on clients who have varicose veins, phlebitis, or diabetes.

Facial waxing should not be performed on clients who have any of the following contraindications:

- recent chemical peels using glycolic, salicylic, or other acid-based products
- recent microdermabrasion, injectables (Botox® or other dermal fillers)
- recent cosmetic or reconstructive surgery
- rosacea or very sensitive skin
- sunburn
- history of fever blisters or cold sores
- presence of pustules or papules on area to be waxed
- exfoliating topical medication including Retin-A®, Renova™, Tazorac®, Differin®, Azelex®, other peeling agents, or vitamin A topical products
- hydroquinone for skin lightening
- topical or oral cortisone medication
- Accutane® or other acne medications
- blood-thinning medications

CLIENT CONSULTATION ASSESSMENT FORM

Date _____

Name_____

Address _____

City _____ State _____ Zip _____

Have you been waxed before? Yes_____ No_____

1. Have you been seen by a dermatologist? Yes_____ No_____ If yes, for what reason?
   _____

2. Please list all medications that you take regularly. Include hormones and vitamins.
   _____

3. Are you taking Accutane or any other acne medications? Yes _____ No _____ If yes, for how long?
   _____

4. Do you use Retin-A, Renova, other topical vitamin A, or hydroquinone? Yes_____ No _____
   If yes, for how long?_____

5. Do you have any allergies? Are you allergic to any medications? Yes _____ No _____ If yes, please list allergies.
   _____

6. Are you pregnant or lactating? Yes _____ No _____

7. Have you had any of the following procedures?

   Laser resurfacing: Yes _____ Date _____ No _____

   Light chemical peel: Yes _____ Date _____ No _____

   Medium/heavy chemical peel: Yes _____ Date _____ No _____

8. Do you ever experience tightness or flaking of your skin? Yes _____ No _____

9. Do you tan or frequent tanning booths? Yes _____ No _____

10. Do you have a history of fever blisters or cold sores? Yes _____ No _____

Figure 17–16 A client assessment form.

CLIENT CONSULTATIONS

Before any hair removal service, a consultation is always necessary. A client assessment form (Figure 17–16) should be completed by each new client and kept in the client's file folder. Ask the client to complete a questionnaire that discloses all products and medications, both topical (applied to the skin) and oral (taken by mouth), along with any known skin disorders or allergies. Allergies or sensitivities must be noted and documented. Keep in mind that many changes can occur between client visits. Since the last time you saw them, clients may be taking new medications such as antidepressants, hormones, cortisone, medicine for blood pressure or diabetes, or such topical prescriptions as Retin-A, Renova, and hydroquinone. A client on any one of these prescriptions may not be a candidate for hair removal, because the client is more sensitive and the skin can actually be pulled off if waxed. See Table 17–1 for contraindications.

It is imperative that every client fills out a release form for the hair removal service you are going to provide. Have clients review their forms before every service because it reminds them to think about any topical or oral medication they may have started since the last visit (Figure 17–17).

RELEASE FORM FOR HAIR REMOVAL

I, _____, am _____ or am not _____ presently using:

____ Retin-A or any other topical vitamin A.

____ Accutane or any other acne medication.

____ any exfoliant or hydroxy-based products.

____ any medications such as cortisone, blood thinners, or diabetic medication.

____ any of the above are contraindicated for waxing and may result in skin irritation, peeling or hyperpigmentation.

____ I understand that if I begin using any of the above products and do not inform my esthetician/cosmetologist prior to hair removal, I am accepting full responsibility for any skin reactions. Minor redness and sensitivity is normal from waxing. Avoid sun, heat, and certain products as directed for at least 24–48 hours after waxing.

____ The hair-removal process has been thoroughly explained to me, and I have had an opportunity to ask questions and receive satisfactory answers.

Client Signature _____ Date _____

Technician Signature _____ Date _____

Figure 17–17 A sample release form.

Waxing Safety Precautions

Please note the following safety precautions for wax treatments:

- Before beginning a wax treatment, be sure to complete a client consultation card and have the client sign a release form.
- The hair should be at least ¼" (.6 cm) to ½" (1.25 cm) long for waxing to be effective. Trim before waxing if hair is longer than 3/4".
- Do not remove vellus hair; doing so may cause the hair to lose its softness.
- Wear disposable gloves to prevent contact with any possible bloodborne pathogens.
- Beeswax has a relatively high incidence of allergic reaction. Before every service, always do a small patch test of the product to be used.
- To prevent burns, always test the temperature of the heated wax before applying it to the client's skin.
- Use caution so that the wax does not come in contact with the eyes.
- Do not apply wax over warts, moles, abrasions, or irritated or inflamed skin. Do not remove hair protruding from a mole because the wax could cause trauma to the mole.
- The skin under the arms and other areas is very sensitive. If sensitive, use hard wax.
- Redness and swelling sometimes occur on sensitive skin. Apply aloe gel or cortisone cream to calm and soothe the skin after waxing.
- Give clients post-wax precautions: Avoid sun exposure, exfoliation, creams with fragrance or other ingredients that may be irritating, and excessive heat (hot tubs, saunas) for at least 24 to 48 hours after waxing.

CAUTION!

Never wax if you are in doubt about how a client's skin will react. Do a patch test on a tiny area if you are concerned about the results or reactions from a procedure or product.

GENERAL WAXING PROCEDURES

Here is an overview of waxing procedures to review before performing the hands-on procedure.

Client Preparation

Provide the client with a gown, disposable panties, or other item, depending on the service provided. Draping is important for client's modesty.

Prepare the skin per the instructor's or manufacturer's directions.

- *Brows/face.* The client's eyes should be closed. Completely remove any traces of makeup with a gentle cleanser. Follow with a preparation solution to remove any residue on the area. Allow the area to dry for a few moments. Some states require the use of client eyepads before some services, such as waxing or tweezing.

- *All areas.* Clean the skin thoroughly with pre-epilation solution such as witch hazel on a cotton pad. Powder is applied if a moist area needs to be dried (especially underarms). Powder can also protect the skin and make hairs more visible. However, it can interfere with waxing if too much powder is applied. Do not use talcum powder. Many talcs contain fragrances and other particles that can cause an allergic reaction. Cornstarch is a good alternative.

- *Excess body hair.* Trim any thicker or longer hair areas with scissors before applying wax. This allows the wax to adhere better with less trauma to the follicles and is more comfortable for the client. Trim hair to no shorter than 1/2".

Wax Application

Applications are either soft wax used with strips or hard wax without strips.

Soft wax. Dip the end of a small spatula into the warm wax. Following the direction of the hair growth, apply a very thin coat along the area to be waxed. Be careful not to drip wax on areas that are not being waxed.

Hard wax. Dip a spatula into the wax and apply it first in the opposite direction, then in the same direction of the hair growth in a smooth or figure-eight pattern over the area to be waxed. Apply to the thickness of a nickel. Apply a thicker area on the end to pull up with, lifting it up to make a tab that can be grasped between the thumb and index finger. Wait a few moments for the wax to set up. If hard wax becomes too dry or cool, it will be brittle and break off when you attempt to remove it.

Hard wax is a slower method, and the technician has to wait for the applied wax to set. With experience, one should be able to apply the second application to another part of the area, (although not immediately adjacent) while waiting for the first application to set. Remove the first application, then the second, otherwise it becomes slow (not cost efficient), laborious and uncomfortable for the client.

Wax Removal

The most important points in wax removal techniques are to hold the skin taut and to remove it quickly while pulling parallel to the skin.

Soft wax. Apply muslin or Pellon® evenly and with light pressure. Rub the strip firmly in the same direction as the wax application. Do not use too much pressure, or you could cause bruising. Leave approximately 1" of muslin or pellon free to grip for removing. Hold the skin tight next to the end you will be pulling, and remove the wax quickly with one continuous pull in the direction opposite the hair growth. If the end of the hair is pointing to the left, pull to the right. Because follicles do not grow vertically, but at an angle, the hair is "popped" out at an angle. The pulling method and direction are critical. When pulling, keep the strip parallel to the skin without lifting.

Follow through on the pull to avoid slowing down. Do not pull straight up, or you will remove skin or cause bruising or the hair to break off. Immediately after you remove the strip, place your other hand quickly over the area and apply pressure to block the nerves from sensing pain.

Hard wax. Follow the previous steps, only without the strips. Once the wax has set, grasp the thick edge between the thumb and index finger. Pull off the wax in the appropriate direction according to instructions.

Immediately put your other hand over the area to soothe nerve endings. Visually check the area with the magnifying light. All hair should have been removed in the pull. Remove any residual hair with tweezers. If there are ingrown hairs, pointed tweezers can be used to remove them.

Post-Wax Product Application

Remove residual wax with a wax remover made for the skin. Gently apply to the waxed area, removing any wax residue. Rub with a cotton pad to remove excess wax and product. Apply an after-wax soothing product (azulene or aloe) as directed. Some after-wax products have too much alcohol or other irritating ingredients and are not always soothing. Even some aloe vera products can be irritating. After waxing, open, irritated follicles are susceptible to more irritation. Keep epilated areas clean and free from any debris. If you are applying a hair growth inhibitor cream, follow the manufacturer's directions.

Post-Wax Clean-Up

Follow all sanitation procedures. Give the client post-wax instructions and precautions. Prepare the station for the next service.

Eyebrows

Correctly shaped eyebrows have a strong, positive impact on the overall attractiveness of the face (Figure 17–18). The natural arch of the eyebrow follows the top of the orbital bone, or the curved line above the eye socket. Most people have hair growth both above and below the natural line. These hairs can be removed to give a cleaner, more attractive appearance.

As with any procedure, always perform a client consultation before tweezing or waxing the eyebrows. Determine the client's wishes as to final eyebrow shape. If you remove too much hair, it will generally grow back, but the process takes a long time. You will also end up with an unhappy client who

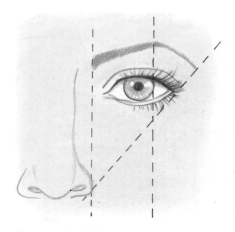

Figure 17–18 Brow shaping guidelines.

is not likely to return for your services. Conducting a thorough consultation beforehand will help you avoid such mistakes.

Brow Waxing Tips

Here are some guidelines to use when waxing the eyebrows.

* *Men's eyebrows.* Most men want the brows left natural with just cleaning up underneath and between the brows. Do not make an even line or tweeze to define unless the client requests it.
* *Sculpting.* Brows are arched according to the standard diagram.
* *Corrections.* If brows are uneven or too thin, leave the stray hairs to grow back in to match the shape the client wants. Recommend letting the hair grow back to achieve the desired shape. If hairs are removed, they may not always grow back. Hair density gets thinner with time, so in 10 or 20 years, there may be less hair in areas. Let clients know that overthinning now can affect the brow shape for years to come. Chapter 19 provides more information about corrective brow shaping.

Body Waxing Procedures

* Use the same equipment as for the eyebrow waxing procedure, with the addition of a larger metal or disposable wooden spatula. A metal spatula holds the heat longer, but it must not touch the client's skin as you apply the wax, and must not be used if prohibited by your regulatory agency. You may find disposable spatulas more convenient. Prepare the correct strip sizes.
* Drape the treatment bed with disposable paper, or use a bed sheet with paper over the top.
* Conduct the consultation and review the client release form and contraindications.
* Instruct the client on how to prepare, and be mindful of her or his modesty and comfort.
* If bikini waxing, offer the client disposable panties or a small sanitized towel.
* If waxing the underarms, have the female client put on a wrap. Offer a wrap when waxing the legs as well.
* Assist the client onto the treatment bed and drape the client with towels.

Here's a Tip

To remove hair with tweezers, first hold the skin tight around the area where you are removing the hair. Then place the tweezers at the base of a hair and gently but firmly pull the hair at a slight angle, matching the direction of the hair growth. Always check your work with the magnifying lamp. Some estheticians prefer to use their magnifying light while doing hair removal to allow for very detailed work. Some estheticians tweeze between the brows and above the brow line first, because the area under the brow line is much more sensitive; others start underneath.

PROCEDURE 17–1

EYEBROW TWEEZING

SUPPLIES
- towels
- tweezers
- cotton pads
- eyebrow brush
- emollient cream
- antiseptic lotion
- gentle eye makeup remover
- astringent
- disposable gloves
- station and sanitation supplies
- client release form and chart

Preparation

Set up the station and have the client sign the release form.

In preparing for the tweezing procedure, perform the following steps:

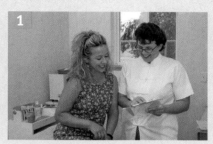
Discuss ideal eyebrow shape with client. *(Figure P17–1-1)*

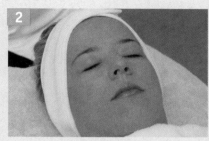
Seat and drape client. *(Figure P17–1-2)*

1. Discuss with the client the type of eyebrow arch suitable for his or her facial characteristics (Figure P17-1-1).

2. Seat the client in a facial chair in a reclining position, as for a facial massage. Or, if you prefer, seat the client in a half-upright position and work from the side (Figure P17-1-2).

3. Drape a towel over the client's clothing.

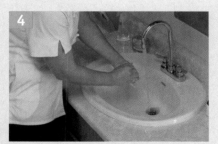
Wash hands. *(Figure P17–1-3)*

4. Wash and dry your hands, and put on disposable gloves. Washing your hands thoroughly with soap and warm water is critical before and after every client procedure you perform (Figure P17–1-3). The importance of proper sanitation in these procedures cannot be overemphasized.

PROCEDURE 17–1, CONT.

Procedure

The eyebrow tweezing procedure involves the following steps:

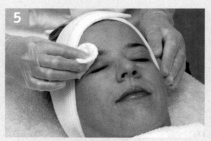

Apply a mild antiseptic before tweezing. *(Figure P17–1-4)*

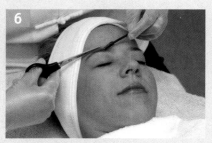

Trim long hairs outside the brow line. *(Figure P17–1-5)*

5 Use a mild antiseptic on a cotton pad before tweezing to clean and prepare the area (Figure P17-1-4).

6 Brush the eyebrows with a small brush. Carefully trim long hairs outside the brow line now or after tweezing (Figure P17-1-5). Brush the hair upward and into place to see the natural line of the brow.

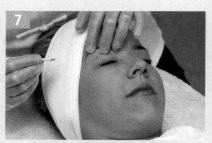

Stretch the skin taut with the index finger and thumb. *(Figure P17–1-6)*

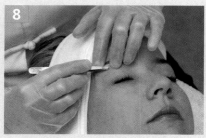

Remove hairs from below the brow line. Grasp each hair and pull with a quick, smooth motion. *(Figure P17–1-7)*

7 Stretch the skin taut with the index finger and thumb (or index and middle fingers) of your other hand (Figure P17-1-6).

8 Remove hairs from under the eyebrow line. Shape the lower section of one eyebrow; then shape the other. Grasp each hair individually with tweezers and pull with a quick, smooth motion in the direction of the hair growth (Figure P17-1-7). Grasp the hair at the base as close to the skin as possible without pinching the skin.

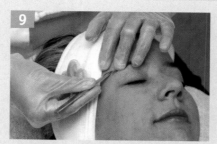

Remove stray hairs from above the brow line. *(Figure P17–1-8)*

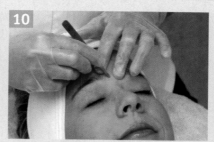

Remove hairs from between the eyebrows. *(Figure P17–1-9)*

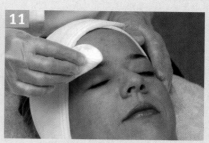

Apply an antiseptic lotion. *(Figure P17–1-10)*

9 Brush the hair downward. Remove hairs from above the eyebrow line (Figure P17–1-8). Shape the upper section of one eyebrow; then shape the other.

10 Remove hair from between the brows. (Figure P17–1-9).

11 Sponge the tweezed areas with a cotton pad, moistened with a nonirritating antiseptic lotion, to contract the skin and avoid infection (Figure P17-1-10).

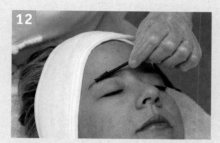

Brush eyebrow hair. *(Figure P17–1-11)*

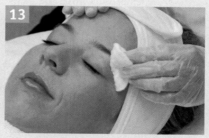

Apply soothing cream. *(Figure P17–1-12)*

12 Brush the eyebrow hair in its normal position (Figure P17-1-11).

13 *Optional:* Apply a soothing cream. Gently remove excess cream with a cotton pad (Figure P17-1-12).

14 Wash your hands with soap and warm water.

Clean-Up and Sanitation

15 Perform sanitation procedures. If eyebrow tweezing is part of a makeup or facial service, continue the procedure. If not, complete the next step.

16 Remove the towel from the client and place it in a closed hamper.

17 Accompany the client to the reception area and suggest rebooking. (The eyebrows should be tweezed about once a week.)

18 Discard disposable materials in a closed receptacle and disinfect the implements.

FYI

Always wash your hands before preparing and setting up for a service, after draping, and immediately after any service before walking the client out.

PROCEDURE 17–2

EYEBROW WAXING WITH SOFT WAX

SUPPLIES

- wax release form and chart
- facial chair
- high-level disinfectant
- roll of disposable paper or towels
- wax
- wax heater
- wax remover
- small disposable applicators or rollers
- fabric strips for hair removal and scissors
- hair cap or headband
- towels for draping
- disposable gloves
- plastic bag
- cotton pads and swabs
- powder
- surface cleaner (alcohol/oil)
- wax cleaning towel
- mild skin cleanser
- emollient or antiseptic lotion
- tweezers

This procedure for eyebrow waxing employs the use of a strip to remove soft wax. Adapt this procedure to all other body areas to be waxed.

Preparation

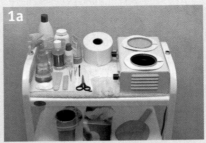
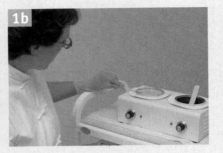

Prepare the wax. *(Figure P17–2-1 A,B)*

1 Melt the wax in the heater. The length of time it takes to melt the wax depends on how full the wax holder is; approximately 20 minutes if it is full; 10 minutes if it is a quarter to half full. Be sure the wax is not too hot (Figure P17-2-1).

2 Complete the client consultation, release form, contraindications, and determine what hair you need to remove.

3 Lay a clean towel over the top of the facial chair and then a layer of disposable paper.

4 Place a hair cap or headband over the client's hair.

5 Drape a towel over the client's clothing as necessary.

6 Wash and dry your hands, and put on disposable gloves.

Procedure

The soft pot wax procedure with strips includes the following steps:

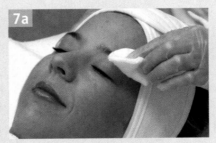
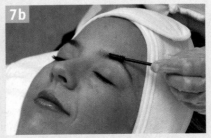

Cleanse the area thoroughly with a mild astringent cleanser, and dry. *(Figure P17-2-2)*

Brush the hair into place to see the brow line. *(Figure P17-2-3)*

7 Remove makeup. Cleanse the area thoroughly with a mild astringent cleanser, and dry (Figure P17-2-2). Apply a non-talc powder, if applicable. Brush the hair into place to see the brow line (Figure P17-2-3).

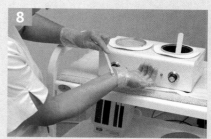

Test the temperature of the wax.
(Figure P17–2-4)

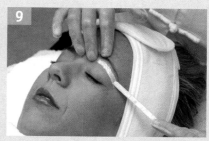

Spread a thin coat of wax evenly over
the area. *(Figure P17–2-5)*

8 Test the temperature and consistency of the heated wax by applying a small drop on the inside of your wrist. It should be warm but not hot, and it should run smoothly off the spatula (Figure P17–2-4).

9 Wipe off one side of the spatula on the inside edge of the pot, so it does not drip. Carefully take it from the pot to the brow area. If it is dripping off the spatula, there is too much wax, or it is too hot. Correct the problem to avoid drips or hurting the client.

10 With the spatula or applicator, spread a thin coat of the warm wax evenly over the area to be treated, following the direction of the hair growth (Figure P17–2-5). Be sure not to put the spatula in the wax more than once (do not double-dip). Be sure not to use an excessive amount of wax, because it will spread when the fabric is pressed and may cover hair you do not wish to remove. Hold the skin taut near the edge where the wax is first applied.

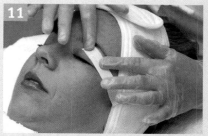

Apply a clean fabric strip over the area
to be waxed. *(Figure P17–2-6)*

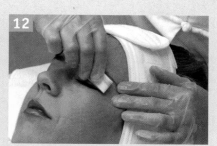

Hold the skin tight and remove the
strip. *(Figure P17–2-7)*

11 Apply a clean fabric strip over the area to be waxed. Start the edge of the strip at the edge of the wax where you first applied it. Do not cover the rest of the brow with the strip. This way you can see the exposed area that you do not want to wax. Press gently in the direction of hair growth, running your finger over the surface of the fabric three to five times (Figure P17–2-6).

12 Gently but firmly hold the skin taut, placing the middle and ring fingers of one hand on either side of the strip as close as possible to where you will start to pull. Hold the loose edge of the strip at the end and quickly remove the fabric strip by pulling in the direction opposite to the hair growth. Do not lift or pull straight up on the strip; doing so could damage or remove the skin (Figure P17–2-7).

PROCEDURE 17–2, CONT.

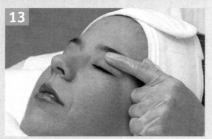

Apply pressure to the area after the wax strip is removed. *(Figure P17–2-8)*

13 Immediately apply pressure with your finger to the treated area. Hold it there for approximately five seconds to relieve the painful sensation (Figure P17–2-8).

14 Remove any excess wax residue from the skin with the cotton strip by gently lifting it sideways in the same direction as the hair growth. You can carefully remove excess wax without removing hairs this way.

15 Repeat the wax procedure on the area around the other eyebrow.

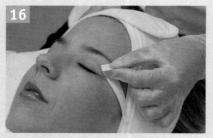

Remove excess wax residue. *(Figure P17–2-9)*

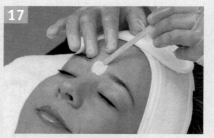

Wax between the brows. *(Figure P17–2-10)*

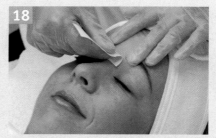

Pull the strip straight down. *(Figure P17–2-11)*

16 For the area between the brows, apply the wax (generally in an upward direction between the nose and the forehead). Line the bottom of the strip up to the bottom edge of the wax. Hold the skin tight on both sides of the strip above the brows with the middle and ring fingers. Hold the top of the strip and pull the strip straight down close to the nose without lifting. This can be done all in one section or in two halves—the right and the left (Figure P17–2-9).

17 Cleanse the skin with a mild wax remover, and apply a post-wax product or antiseptic lotion (Figure P17–2-10).

18 Tweeze the remaining stray hairs, and apply a cold compress if necessary. If it is too slippery or there is wax residue, apply the post-wax products after tweezing; or rinse the area with water and pat dry before tweezing.

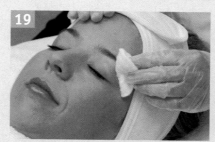

Cleanse the skin and apply an emollient or antiseptic lotion. *(Figure P17–2-12)*

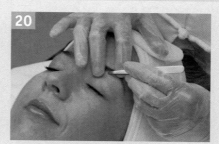

Tweeze stray hairs. *(Figure P17–2-13)*

CAUTION!

Never leave the wax heater on overnight, because it is a fire hazard and can affect the quality of the wax.

19 Finish all services with the client precautions and the post-consultation.

20 Follow all services with sanitation clean-up procedures.

Clean-Up and Sanitation for All Procedures

21 Remove the headband and towel drape from the client, and place them in a closed hamper.

22 Discard all used disposable materials in a closed waste container. Never reuse wax. Do not place the used spatula, muslin strips, wax, or any other materials used in waxing directly on the counter.

23 Wash your hands with soap and warm water.

24 Sanitize and disinfect the treatment area. This includes counter surfaces, the facial chair, the wax heater, the mag lamp, implements, containers, bottle caps/lids, and the floor.

Here's a Tip

Excess wax will get on the tweezers and interfere with tweezing. Remove all wax and post-products with a moist cotton pad before tweezing, and reapply soothing products after tweezing.

CAUTION!

If the wax strings and lands in an area you do not wish to treat, remove it with lotion designed to dissolve and remove wax. Do not apply the strip over any area that should not be waxed.

PROCEDURE 17–3

LIP WAXING PROCEDURE WITH HARD WAX

SUPPLIES
Use the same list of supplies as for the eyebrow waxing in Procedure 17–2.

Procedure

The lip waxing procedure with hard wax includes the following steps:

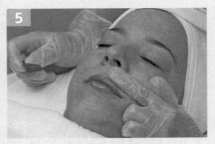
Test wax temperature. *(Figure P17–3-1)*

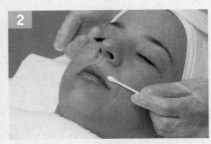
Prepare the skin. *(Figure P17–3-2)*

1. Prepare the client and test the temperature of the wax on your arm or wrist (Figure P17–3-1).

2. Prepare the skin (Figure P17–3-2). For lip waxing, have the client hold the lips tightly together to make waxing easier on the skin.

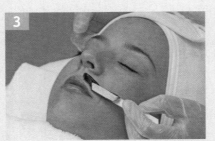
Apply wax to the upper lip, one side at a time, leaving a "tab or handle" to grasp. *(Figure P17–3-3)*

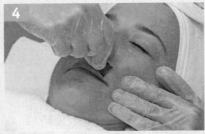
Pull off wax in the appropriate direction. *(Figure P17–3-4)*

3. Apply wax to one side of the upper lip outward from the center to the corner, leaving a "tab or handle" to grasp (Figure P17–3-3). (If using soft wax, apply the strip.)

4. Hold the skin tight, and quickly pull parallel to the skin without lifting up (Figure P17–3-4).

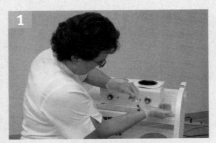

5. Immediately apply pressure to the waxed area to ease any discomfort (Figure P17–3-5).

Apply pressure. *(Figure P17–3-5)*

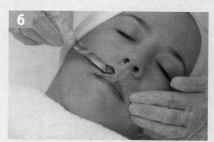

Repeat on other side. *(Figure P17–3-6)*

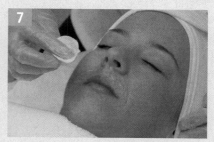

Apply soothing lotion. *(Figure P17–3-9)*

6 Repeat on the other side of the lip (Figure P17–3-6).

7 Apply after-wax soothing lotion (Figure P17–3-9).

8 Finish all services with the client precautions and the post-consultation.

9 Follow all services with sanitation clean-up procedures.

PROCEDURE 17-4

CHIN WAXING WITH SOFT WAX

SUPPLIES

Use the same list of supplies as for the eyebrow waxing in Procedure 17–2.

Procedure

1 Test the wax.

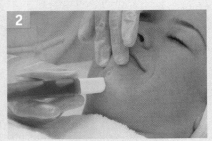
Apply the wax in small sections above the curve of the jawline. *(Figure P17–4-1)*

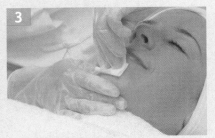
Hold the skin tight and pull opposite to the hair growth and parallel to the skin. *(Figure P17–4-2)*

2 Apply the wax in small sections above the curve of the jawline (Figure P17–4-1). Do not go over the curve. Wax above the jawline, then below it using separate pulls. Or you can wax below the jawline first, then above it.

3 Apply the strip, hold the skin tight, and pull opposite to the hair growth and parallel to the skin (Figure P17–4-2).

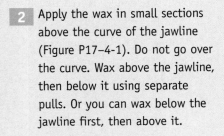
Apply the wax below the jawline. *(Figure P17–4-3)*

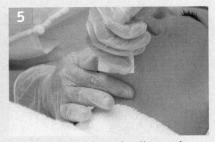
Hold the skin tight and pull opposite to the hair growth and parallel to the skin. *(Figure P17–4-4)*

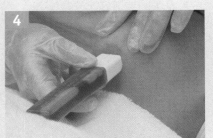

4 Apply the wax in small sections below the curve of the jawline (Figure P17–4-3).

5 Apply the strip, hold the skin tight, and pull opposite to the hair growth and parallel to the skin (Figure P17–4-4).

6 Apply pressure if necessary without pressing hard on the throat or neck.

8 Finish all services with the client precautions and the post-consultation.

7 Finish the procedure.

9 Follow all services with sanitation clean-up procedures.

★ REGULATORY AGENCY ALERT

Some states or provinces require estheticians to (1) sanitize the skin before tweezing or waxing and (2) apply an antiseptic at the end of the procedure. Always check with your regulatory agency to be sure you are complying with its requirements.

PROCEDURE 17–5	**LEG WAXING PROCEDURE WITH SOFT WAX**

SUPPLIES

Use the same list of supplies as for the eyebrow waxing in Procedure 17–2.

Procedure

Leg waxing can be started with either the front or the back of the legs. Visually divide the front of the legs in quarter sections (below the knees) and use a set pattern, starting removal at the bottom half of the lower legs. Make sure the skin is held tight, especially around the ankle, which is more sensitive.

1 Cleanse the area to be waxed with a mild astringent cleanser and dry. Apply a light dusting of powder if necessary.

2 Test the temperature and consistency of the heated wax.

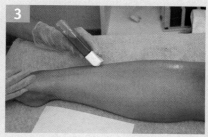

Apply the wax to the leg in a set pattern. *(Figure P17–5-1)*

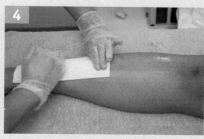

Apply the strip. *(Figure P17–5-2)*

3 Using a metal or disposable spatula or roller, spread a thin coat of warm wax evenly over the skin surface in the same direction as the hair growth (Figure P17–5-1).

4 Apply a fabric strip in the same direction as the hair growth. Press gently but firmly, running your hand over the surface of the fabric three to five times (Figure P17–5-2).

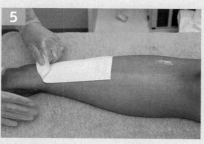

Hold the skin tight and remove the strip. *(Figure P17–5-3)*

5 Hold the skin taut with one hand close to where you will pull with the other hand, and quickly remove the wax in the opposite direction of the hair growth without lifting (Figure P17–5-3).

6 Quickly put your hand down to apply pressure to the treated area for approximately five seconds.

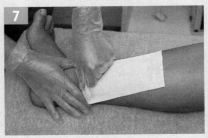

Repeat steps using fresh fabric strips.
(Figure P17-5-4)

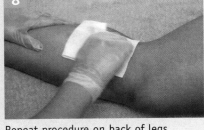

Repeat procedure on back of legs.
(Figure P17-5-5)

7 Repeat, taking a fresh fabric strip as each strip becomes too thick with wax (Figure P17–5-4).

8 Have the client turn over, and repeat the procedure on the backs of the legs (Figure P17–5-5).

9 Remove any remaining residue of wax from the skin, and apply an emollient or antiseptic lotion.

10 Finish all services with the client precautions and the post-consultation.

11 Follow all services with standard sanitation clean-up procedures.

Clean-Up and Sanitation

Follow these steps for leg waxing clean-up and sanitation:

12 Discard used disposable materials in a closed waste container.

13 Place linens and robe in a closed hamper.

14 Remove any wax from the metal spatula (if you used one) with wax removal solution. Disinfect the spatula and store it in a clean, covered container.

15 Disinfect the equipment, treatment bed, implements, waxer, and counters/surfaces.

16 Wash your hands.

Here's a Tip

If skin is too dry or cold, wax may stick and does not come off properly.

PROCEDURE 17–6

UNDERARM WAXING PROCEDURE WITH HARD WAX

SUPPLIES

Use the same list of supplies as for the eyebrow waxing in Procedure 17–2.

Procedure

Because the hair under the arms grows in several different directions, it is important to first determine the number of different growth patterns and then to wax in sections following those patterns. Cut strips to the appropriate size if using soft wax. Divide the underarm area into approximately three sections or as hair growth patterns allow.

1 Wearing gloves, cleanse and sanitize the underarm area.

2 Apply a small amount of powder to the area to dry the area and facilitate the adherence of wax.

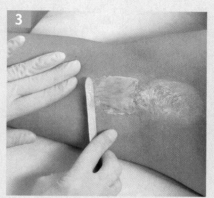

Apply wax to the first section of the underarm area. *(Figure P17–6-1)*

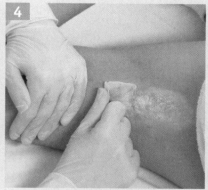

Grasp the wax edge or strip and pull against the hair growth. *(Figure P17–6-2)*

3 Apply wax to the first growth area, usually on the top or outer edge of the underarm. (Figure P17–6-1).

4 Grasp the wax "handle" or strip and quickly pull (Figure P17–6-2). Hold the skin tight when removing the wax.

5 Apply pressure immediately after wax removal to ease any pain.

6 Repeat the procedure on the next growth area—the bottom or inner edge of the underarm (Figure P17–6-3).

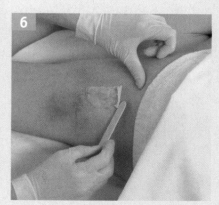

Repeat the procedure in the next area. *(Figure P17–6-3)*

PROCEDURE 17–6, CONT.

FOCUS ON . . .

THE CLIENT

Be mindful of your client's modesty. Try to make her as relaxed as possible, and do not expose the bikini area any more than she is comfortable with.

CAUTION!

When using hard wax, start with the lower sections of hair to apply the end section or "handle" of wax without hair underneath it. Each section then has a bare area at the bottom to form the next handle of the wax. Avoid pulling the hair underneath when first lifting the edge to grasp onto—it is very uncomfortable to lift the hair underneath with the wax stuck on it.

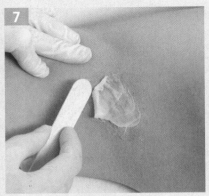

Repeat the procedure in the center of the underarm area. *(Figure P17-6-4)*

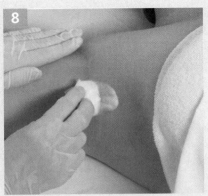

Apply a soothing after-wax lotion to calm any sensitivity. *(Figure P17–6-5)*

7   Repeat the procedure on the last growth area, or the center of the underarm (Figure P17–6-4). Remove any other stray hairs. Check in with the client to make sure she is comfortable and can handle any tweezing. It is a sensitive area, so the faster the procedure, the better.

8   Apply a soothing after-wax lotion; cold compresses are also nice to soothe the skin (Figure P17–6-5).

9   Finish with the client precautions and the post-consultation.

10 Perform sanitation clean-up procedures.

PROCEDURE 17–7

BIKINI WAXING PROCEDURE WITH HARD WAX

SUPPLIES

Use the same list of supplies as for the eyebrow waxing in Procedure 17–2.

Preparation

Prepare the station and the client. Always wear gloves.

Procedure

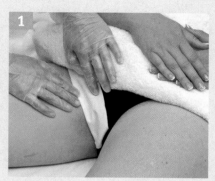

Drape the client. *(Figure P17–7-1)*

1 Tuck in a paper towel or wax strip along the edge of the client's bikini line. Cleanse and sanitize the area (Figure P17–7-1).

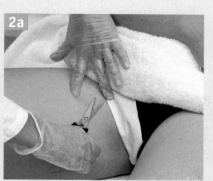

Trim the hair to 1/2 to 3/4 of an inch. *(Figure P17–7-2)*

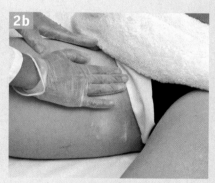

Apply powder. *(Figure P17–7-3)*

2 Trim the hair to 1/2" to 3/4" in length if necessary (Figure P17–7-2). Apply a small amount of powder (Figure P17–7-3).

3 Bend the client's knee with the leg facing out. This position assists in reaching the inner bikini area and stretches the skin tighter. Be confident in moving the client's body position around to reach the right angle for waxing, but make sure they are comfortable in the different positions.

PROCEDURE 17–7, CONT.

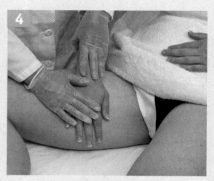

Show client where to place her hands. *(Figure P17–7-4)*

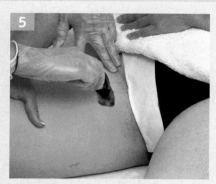

Apply wax above the curve. *(Figure P17–7-5)*

4 Have the client hold her skin tight next to the area being waxed. Show her where to place her hand and make sure that is not in the way of the parallel pull (Figure P17-7-4).

5 Apply wax to the first growth area, usually on the upper, outer edge of the bikini line (Figure P17-7-5).

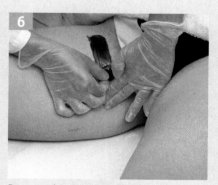

Remove the wax. *(Figure P17–7-6)*

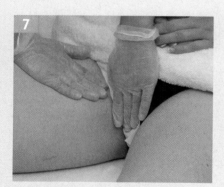

Apply pressure. *(Figure P17-7-7)*

6 Hold the skin tight, grasp the wax "handle," and quickly pull (Figure P17–7-6). Pull back parallel to the skin.

7 Apply pressure immediately to alleviate any discomfort (Figure P17-7-7).

Here's a Tip

When waxing sensitive areas such as underarms or bikini lines, trim the hair with scissors if it is more than 1/2" (1.25 cm) long.

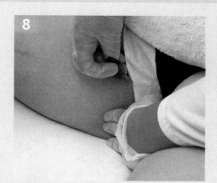

Work in sections. *(Figure P17–7-8)*

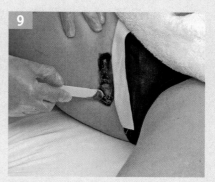

Apply wax below the curve. *(Figure P17–7-9)*

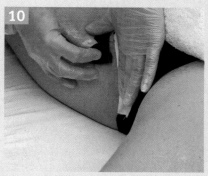

Remove the wax. *(Figure P17–7-10)*

8 Work in and down to the femoral ridge in sections. Do not wax over the curve of the femoral ridge (tendon). Wax the underside and the back side of the bikini area in separate sections (Figure P17–7-8).

9 To reach the back of the bikini area, have the client lift her leg toward her chest, grasping the ankle if possible. This also holds the skin tight (Figure P17–7-9).

10 Apply the wax and remove it without lifting (Figure P17–7-10).

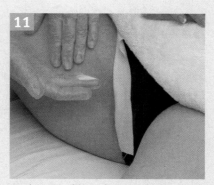

Apply a soothing after-wax lotion. *(Figure P17–7-11)*

11 Apply a soothing after-wax lotion (Figure P17–7-11). (Cold compresses are nice to soothe the skin.)

12 Finish all services with the client precautions and the post-consultation.

13 Perform sanitation clean-up procedures.

CAUTION!

Never go over the curve of the femoral ridge. Wax the top and bottom of the bikini area separately.

FYI

Brazilian waxing is an "extreme" bikini wax during which all of the hair is removed. Waxing procedures are the same; but hard wax must be used, and the skin must be held tight because the area is so sensitive. Get advanced training in this technique before attempting it on clients.

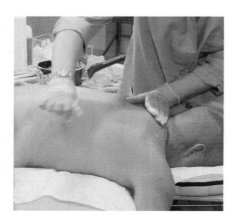

Figure 17–19 Waxing of the back and neck is common for many men.

WAXING FOR THE MALE CLIENT

The main areas men have waxed are the brow area and the nape of the neck (base of the back of the neck). Another common area that men have waxed is the back (Figure 17–9). Estheticians must proceed with caution in all cases. Men may be sensitive to waxing. The skin may become red and irritated. However, with subsequent services, your male clients typically get used to waxing. Men may grow wiry hair on the edges of their ears and on the inside of the nose. This growth tends to increase with age. It is not advisable to wax these sensitive areas. However, trimming the external hair is helpful.

PROCEDURE 17–8

MEN'S WAXING PROCEDURE WITH SOFT WAX

SUPPLIES
Use the same list of supplies as for the eyebrow waxing in Procedure 17–2.

Waxing of the back and neck is a common procedure for many men. First determine the number of different growth patterns, and then wax in sections following those patterns. Do not wax large areas at one time. Leg strip sections are generally too large. Cut the leg strips to 3/4 of the length. Save the leftover part of the strip for other body parts. Have the client lay face down and start at the lower back area working up to the shoulders. Then have them sit up for the top of the shoulder area if necessary. This procedure demonstrates a partial shoulder wax.

Procedure

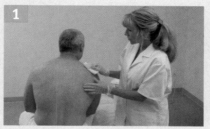

Sanitize the area. *(Figure P17–8-1)*

1 Cleanse and sanitize the area (Figure P17-8-1).

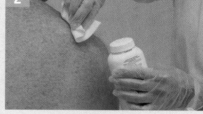

Apply powder. *(Figure P17–8-2)*

2 Apply a small amount of powder (Figure P17-8-2).

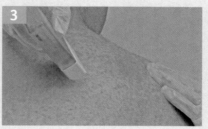

Apply the wax. *(Figure P17–8-3)*

3 Apply wax to the first growth area (Figure P17-8-3).

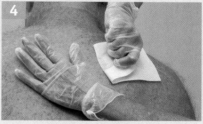

Remove the wax. *(Figure P17–8-4)*

4 Grasp the strip and quickly pull against the hair growth (Figure P17-8-4).

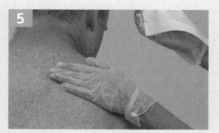

Apply pressure. *(Figure P17–8-5)*

5 Apply pressure immediately after wax removal to ease any pain (Figure P17-8-5).

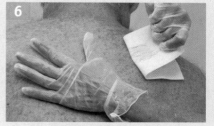

Repeat procedure. *(Figure P17–8-6)*

6 Repeat the procedure until all hair is removed (Figure P17-8-6).

PROCEDURE 17–8, CONT.

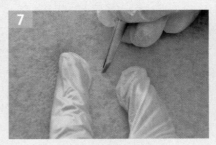

Remove stray hairs. *(Figure P17–8-7)*

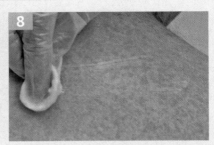

Apply soothing after-wax lotion. *(Figure P17–8-8)*

7 Remove any other stray hairs (Figure P17–8-7). Check in with the client to make sure he is comfortable. It is a sensitive area, so the faster the procedure, the better.

8 Apply a soothing after-wax lotion; cold compresses are also nice to soothe the skin (Figure P17–8-8).

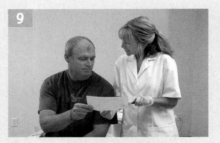

Client consultation. *(Figure P17–8-9)*

9 Clean-up and consultation: Remember to give your client post-wax precautions (Figure P17–8-9).

Here's a Tip

To wax a male client's shoulder and neck area, have him sit up and do the work from behind him.

REVIEW QUESTIONS

1. Explain the hair-growth cycle and stages.

2. What structures are found in the hair follicle?

3. Define the terms *hirsutism* and *hypertrichosis*.

4. Define *electrolysis*.

5. What is photoepilation?

6. What information should be entered in the client record during the consultation?

7. What conditions, treatments, and medications contraindicate hair removal in the salon?

8. What are the two major types of hair removal?

9. What is the difference between depilation and epilation?

10. What are temporary hair removal methods?

11. List safety precautions that must be followed for waxing.

12. Define *threading* and *sugaring*.

CHAPTER GLOSSARY

anagen: first stage of hair growth, during which new hair is produced.

arrector pili muscle: located in the hair follicle; when it contracts, the hair stands straight up, causing goose bumps.

barbae folliculitis: Infected inflammation of the hair follicle; ingrown hairs due to shaving. Pseudofolliculitis is inflammation of hair follicles without the infection.

catagen: second transition stage of hair growth; in the catagen stage, the hair shaft grows upward and detaches itself from the bulb.

depilation: the process on removing hair at skin level.

depilatory: substance, usually a caustic alkali preparation, used for temporarily removing superfluous hair by dissolving it at the skin level.

electrolysis: removal of hair by means of an electric current that destroys the hair root.

epilation: removes hairs from the follicles; waxing or tweezing.

hair bulb: the swelling at the base of the follicle that provides the hair with nourishment; it is a thick, club-shaped structure that forms the lower part of the hair root.

hair follicle: the tubular shield that surrounds the hair shaft; the "pore" where hairs grow.

hair papillae: cone-shaped elevations at the base of the follicle that fits into the bulb. The papillae are filled with tissue that contains the blood vessels and cells necessary for hair growth and follicle nourishment.

CHAPTER GLOSSARY

hair root: part of the hair that lies within the follicle at its base, where the hair grows.

hair shaft: portion of the hair that extends or projects beyond the skin, consisting of the outer layer (cuticle), inner layer (medulla), and middle layer (cortex). Color changes happen in the cortex.

hirsutism: growth of an unusual amount of hair on parts of the body normally bearing only downy hair, such as the face, arms, and legs of women or the backs of men.

hypertrichosis: excessive hair growth where hair does not normally grow.

intense pulsed light (IPL): A photoepilation hair-reduction method using flashes of light and different wavelengths; an intense pulse of electromagnetic radiation.

lanugo: the hair on a fetus; soft and downy hair covering most of the body.

laser hair removal: a photoepilation hair reduction treatment in which a laser beam is pulsed on the skin using one wavelength at a time, impairing hair growth; an intense pulse of electromagnetic radiation.

photoepilation: hair reduction methods using lasers and intense pulsed light (IPL).

sugaring: an ancient method of hair removal, dating back to the Egyptians. The original recipe is a mixture of sugar, lemon juice, and water that is heated to form syrup, molded into a ball and pressed onto the skin, and then quickly stripped away.

telogen: final hair-growth stage, the resting stage.

thermolysis: a heat effect; used for permanent hair removal.

trichology: the scientific study of hair and its diseases.

vellus hair: very fine, soft, downy hair covering most of the body.

CHAPTER OUTLINE

ADVANCED TOPICS AND TREATMENTS

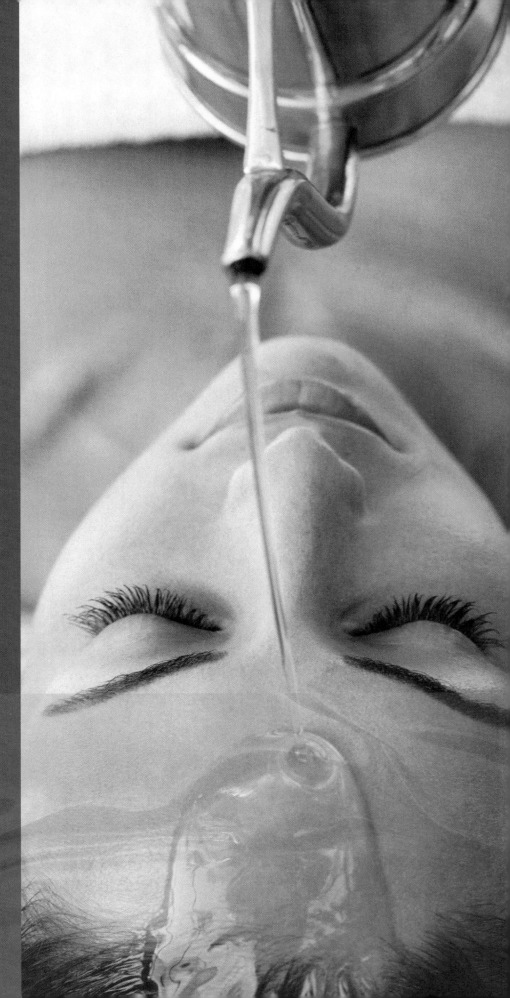

KEY TERMS

Advanced esthetics is an ever-expanding subject (Figure 18–1). There are many interesting topics to study and techniques to utilize. Advanced esthetics goes beyond the basics and is traditionally part of postgraduate studies. Chemical peels, microdermabrasion, light therapy, clinical skin care, and spa body treatments are just some of the specialized services offered in the world of esthetics. This chapter presents an overview of some of the advanced esthetic topics. Estheticians can incorporate many of these treatments into their service menus.

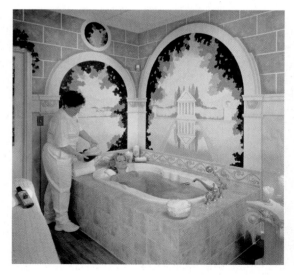

Figure 18–1 The world of advanced esthetics continues to grow.

The public's growing interest in maintaining the health of the body, coupled with tremendous scientific advances, has generated a trend toward integrating beauty, health, and therapeutic services. As a result, estheticians are required to be more knowledgeable about new tools and technology. Procedures such as microdermabrasion have expanded the esthetician's repertoire to include more results-driven services.

PEELS FOR SKIN CARE THERAPISTS

Offering peels in your skin care practice will be one of the most exciting and financially rewarding areas of your treatment "bag of tricks." In the field of skin care, we define the process of removing excess accumulations of dead cells from the corneum layers of the epidermis as *superficial peeling, exfoliation, keratolysis,* and *desquamation.* These are all interchangeable terms. This process can be accomplished mechanically (microdermabrasion), manually (scrubs), or chemically, by the use of specific products (glycolic acid) formulated to achieve these results.

Physicians use procedures designed to penetrate deeper into the skin (dermal layer) that are referred to as *medium* or *deep peels.* Skin care therapists, in contrast, use procedures designed to penetrate only the epidermis. These are referred to as *light peels.* These light peels are noninvasive and nonaggressive in nature and are designed to treat the epidermis—not the dermis, or living tissue.

Peel History

More than 5,000 years ago, the Egyptians used a form of chemical peeling. They understood the value of lactic acid from milk and the various fruit acids for skin conditioning. Thus, when Cleopatra relaxed in her milk bath, she was actually undergoing a chemical peel.

Physicians began using deeper peels in 1882, employing resorcinol, trichloroacetic acid (TCA), salicylic acid, and phenol. These procedures became very popular in the 1930s and 1940s, when Antoinette la Gasse brought the procedures from France to the United States. In the 1980s, the practice of superficially peeling clients by estheticians was just beginning. Alpha hydroxy acid (AHA) peels were the buzzword of the 1990s, and they are even more popular today.

The Cell Renewal Factor (CRF)

The **cell renewal factor (CRF),** or *cell turnover rate,* is the rate of cell mitosis and migration from the dermis to the top of the epidermis. This process slows down with age. The average rate of cell turnover for babies is 14 days; for teenagers, 21 to 28 days; for adults, 28 to 42 days; for those 50 and older, 42 to 84 days. Keeping the cell mitosis going is one of the goals for skin preservation.

Factors influencing CRF include genetics, the natural environment, and one's medical history, lifestyle, personal care, and exfoliation methods. The keratinized corneum layer is composed of approximately 15 to 20 layers and varies in thickness in different body areas. While peeling is great for the skin,

> ### CAUTION!
>
> Peels can result in burns that may require medical attention and they can scar a client. It is important to obtain as much training as possible in working with chemical peels. Make certain that you consult with the client before applying a peel, follow the manufacturer's instructions, and always patch (inside arm or behind ear) test 24 to 48 hours before giving a peel to watch for adverse reactions to the product.

a hydrolipidic balance must be maintained, especially for alipidic skins. Over-peeling is detrimental to the skin.

Deep Peels versus Light Peels

Deep peels are administered by physicians and make use of the following chemicals: resorcinol, phenol (carbolic acid, also called *Baker's peel*), tri-chloroacetic acid (TCA), glycolic acid (50 percent or more), and Jessner's peel (4 to 10 coats). **Jessner's peel** contains lactic acid, salicylic acid, and resorcinol in an ethanol solvent. It is very strong. TCA is a medium-depth peel that removes the epidermis down to the dermis. Phenol is a highly acidic deep peel that peels down into the dermis. Light peels are esthetician administered. These make use of glycolic acid (30 percent or less), lactic acid (30 percent or less), enzyme peels, and in some cases Jessner's solution (1 to 3 coats).

AHAs and BHAs

AHAs are mild acids. Glycolic acid is an alpha hydroxy acid derived from sugar cane that is used in different percentages and pH factors to dissolve the desmosomes between cells to keep skin cells exfoliated (Figure 18–2). Other AHAs promote superficial peeling as well. Beta hydroxy acids (BHAs), while milder, are also used to effectively exfoliate the skin.

AHAs are thought to penetrate the corneum via the intercellular cement and loosen the bonds between the cells. The intercellular cement between the skin cells consists of ceramides, lipids, glycoproteins, and active enzymes. AHAs also increase the production of intercellular lipids. Glycolic acid can penetrate into the epidermis more effectively because it has the smallest molecular size of the AHAs.

AHAs include glycolic acid derived from sugar cane; lactic acid derived from milk; tartaric acid derived from grapes; and malic acid derived from apples.

BHAs (salicylic and citric acid) also dissolve oil and are used for oily skin and acne. Salicylic acid, derived from sweet birch, willow bark, and winter-green—has antiseptic and anti-inflammatory properties. (Aspirin is derived from salicylates.)

Acid, Alkaline, and pH Relationships

The pH is an important consideration in peel products. Acids have a pH of 1 to 6, neutral is 7, and alkalies range from 8 to 14. The average pH of skin ranges from 4.5 to 5.5. Acids penetrate into the skin and can be a cause of irritation. A pH of less than 3 is not recommended for salon peels; most states do not allow using a lower pH. A 30 percent concentration of glycolic acid is usually formulated to have a pH of 3 if buffered properly. Buffering agents are ingredients added to products to help make them less irritating. Products with a higher percent of acid and a lower pH are more irritating. The acid needs to have a pH lower than the skin's pH to be effective (Figure 18–3). AHA product formulations contain from 2 percent to 15 percent of an acid. The most common products sold by salons range from 5 to 10 percent of an acid. Physicians carry products with higher percentages.

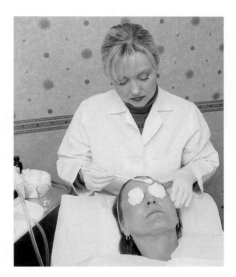

Figure 18–2 Glycolic peels.

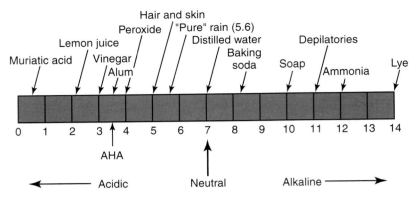

Figure 18–3 pH relationships.

Peel Benefits

Peels improve the texture of the skin and increase the CRF, hydration, and intercellular lipids. Peeling improves the barrier function, moisture retention, and elastin and collagen production. Peels also reduce fine lines, wrinkles, and surface pigmentation. After treatments, skin looks and feels smoother and softer. Peels are used to control skin conditions such as acne, hyperpigmentation, clogged pores, and dry skin.

Who Should Be Peeled?

Who are the best candidates for peels? When determining whether a series of peels is appropriate for a client, consider the following factors: skin type, sebaceous gland activity, skin conditions, the client's philosophy of sun exposure, her cosmetic and product use, and whether she is using Retin-A® or other acids/AHAs, Accutane®, or tetracycline.

CAUTION!

Peel contraindications include the following:
- recent cosmetic surgeries, laser resurfacing, chemical peels, or dermabrasion
- allergies or sensitivities to products or ingredients
- pregnancy
- herpes simplex
- hyperpigmentation tendencies
- use of Accutane, Retin-A, or other medications that exfoliate or thin the skin
- inflamed rosacea or acne
- infectious diseases
- open sores or suspicious lesions
- sunburn or irritated skin

Table 18–1

BENEFICIAL INGREDIENTS TO COMBINE WITH PEELS	
SKIN CONDITION	**BENEFICIAL INGREDIENTS**
mature and/or sensitive skin	glycolic acid, lactic acid, ceramides, hyaluronic acid; phospholipids, linoleic acid, aloe vera, allantoin, kojic acid, licorice root
hyperpigmentation	glycolic acid, kojic acid, licorice root, mulberry extract; bearberry extract, azelaic acid, ascorbic acid
acne	glycolic acid, lactic acid, salicylic acid, azelaic acid

Discuss the issues and contraindications listed in the Caution box (on the previous page) during the client consultation. Explain the procedures, the expected outcome, and realistic goals. In a diagnostic facial or skin analysis before scheduling peels, note the condition of the skin, dehydration, hyper-pigmentation, open lesions, and any other skin conditions on the client intake form. Also choose the type of peel based on the client's skin condition and the results desired. Additional ingredients added to peel formulas include pigment lighteners, acne ingredients, moisturizers or hydrators, and others (Table 18–1).

The Peel Procedure for AHAs

Your regulatory agency will determine the procedure guidelines regarding the strength of the peel. Peel selection will include the type of acid, the procedure time, strength, and the assisting ingredients. Protocols vary depending on the product line. Advanced training and certification are necessary to perform glycolic peels. The basic process consists of applying the peel and removing it within a few minutes. Exfoliation services are efficient and take less time than the more relaxing, in-depth facials.

Peels can be scheduled in a series of four to eight peels, one time per week for 4 to 8 weeks. More than eight weekly peels in a row is not recommended. A series of peels every 3 or 4 months is the typical recommendation. Peels can also be scheduled once a month or as needed. The optimum facial mainte-nance schedule is once a month, or every six weeks. The schedule will depend on the product strength and the client's tolerance to AHAs.

Post-Peel Home Care

Discussion of home care with clients includes issuing precautions and prod-uct advice. Peel clients should avoid the sun and additional exfoliation outside of the recommended home-care program. An example of a glycolic home-care product is a 5 percent cream in a moisturizer base. This product may be used approximately every other day. It is put on under sunscreen or at night on dry skin (not damp). Water or moisture on the skin can make the cream more active and cause it to sting. Peels do make the skin drier on the surface because the top layer is sloughed off, so keeping the skin hydrated is important. Make sure to communicate these points clearly to your clients.

It can take approximately six weeks to notice a difference in the skin, but sometimes improvements are visible after only one peel or one week of using the home-care products.

MICRODERMABRASION

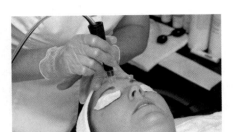

Figure 18–4 Microdermabrasion.

Microdermabrasion (my-kroh-der-mah-BRAY-shun), a form of mechanical machine exfoliation, originated in Europe. Some of the first machines entered the U.S. market around 1995. Today, many microdermabrasion models are available for both the esthetician's and physician's use. These machines are utilized in many skin care clinics, spas, and medical offices. The microdermabrasion machine is a powerful electronic vacuum. Microdermabrasion is achieved by spraying high-grade microcrystals, composed of corundum (kah-RUN-dum) powder or aluminum dioxide, across the skin's surface through a handpiece (Figure18–4). Crystals can also be used manually without the machine—this process is considered gentler on the skin. Other machines have hard applicators, such as the diamond tips, applied without crystals.

Microdermabrasion Benefits

Microdermabrasion can be used to diminish the following conditions: sun damage, pigmentation, open and closed comedones, fine lines and wrinkles, enlarged pores, and coarsely textured skin. The vacuum mechanism stimulates cell metabolism. Those who cannot tolerate acids may be candidates for microdermabrasion.

The difference between AHA peels and microdermabrasion is that peels are chemical and penetrate into the epidermis. The peel product and its penetration into the skin have many benefits. Microdermabrasion is a mechanical method of exfoliation. It exfoliates the epidermis more effectively than a 30 percent peel does, but the benefits of the chemical products are not produced. For example, acids penetrate into the skin and stimulate cell mitosis and the cell turnover rate more than microdermabrasion. The vacuum used in microdermabrasion does stimulate cell metabolism and circulation. Generally, you can think of microdermabrasion as a more effective tool for surface exfoliation and AHA peels as more effective below the surface.

Microdermabrasion Cautions

Technique plays a vital role in creating a positive outcome with the microdermabrasion machine. Proper use of the handpiece, rate of crystal flow, and vacuum setting all contribute to a successful treatment. Do not use microdermabrasion so aggressively that the client is uncomfortable. Once the skin shows erythema or redness, this is considered the stopping point for the procedure.

A series of treatments that incorporate complementary products, along with a complete home-care program, makes the difference in obtaining the best results. Vitamins and antioxidants are even more effective after exfoliation procedures. The esthetician's professional expertise in analyzing the skin and recommending the best program help make these procedures safe and effective.

Improper use of microdermabrasion can actually cause hypopigmentation and hyperpigmentation. It can also lead to sensitivity and other problems. Any strong exfoliation procedure requires sun abstinence and daily sunscreen. Microdermabrasion is not recommended for sensitive or couperous skin, rosacea, or for those with a predisposition to pigmentation problems.

Reading a manual does not provide instant experience in using this machine. Training and certification are absolutely mandatory. Microdermabrasion machines should be used by licensed, trained skin care professionals only.

Equipment Maintenance

Daily care and proper use prevents unnecessary machine repairs. Microdermabrasion machines consist of internal motors, hoses, filters, and handpieces.

Hoses and handpieces must be dry so that the crystals will flow properly. Use only the crystals recommended by the manufacturer. It is not necessary to overuse crystals to obtain good results. A constant, even flow of crystals will give a smooth and effective treatment. Crystals should flow onto the skin's surface only. Avoid breathing the crystals or getting them in the eyes or the nose.

Carefully clean up crystals while wearing rubber gloves and a mask. Machines that have separate crystal containers for both clean and used crystals are preferred. This way the used crystals stay contained and do not come into contact with the technician. These sealed containers are safer to dispose of properly. The treatment room and linens also need to be cleaned and checked for crystal residue and contamination.

LASER TECHNOLOGY

Lasers (LAY-zurs) are medical devices used for hair removal and skin treatments (Figure 18–5). Lasers are high-powered devices that use intense pulses of electromagnetic radiation and a single wavelength at one time. Different wavelengths affect different components of the skin. These different treatments can stimulate collagen production, reduce spider veins, reduce hair growth, or peel the skin. Some lasers target specific substances—such as melanin, dark hair, blood vessels, skin growths, and pigmentation—that absorb energy from the laser. Heating and damaging the dermal tissue stimulates fibroblasts to repair and rebuild tissue such as collagen. The laser is a precise tool used for surgical procedures. In laser skin resurfacing, pulsed lasers are so precise that they can be directed to "burn" off the surface of the skin without ever touching the lower dermis.

A laser produces colored light. Wavelengths are selected to treat a range of skin conditions. For instance, one laser is designed to produce yellow light. Yellow light will selectively absorb into the color red. Laser light passes harmlessly through the skin and targets only the hemoglobin of the red blood cell. The laser energy then heats and destroys the cell, leaving the normal skin cell completely intact.

Lasers are now more commonly used for noninvasive procedures. Lasers include the alexandrite, diode, and Nd:YAG lasers. Lasers combined with

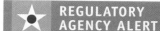

CAUTION!

To avoid eye damage or breathing in crystals during microdermabrasion, technicians should wear eye glasses and protective masks. Clients should keep eyes closed at all times. Avoid getting crystals in client's eyes, mouth, nose, or ears.

★ **REGULATORY AGENCY ALERT**

Check with your regulatory agency about advanced machine use such as microdermabrasion and light therapy laws.

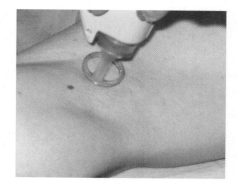

Figure 18–5 Lasers.

radio frequencies are considered to be even more effective. This combined energy technology targets and heats connective tissue to stimulate collagen production and produce a firming effect. It is also effective for hair removal and used for cellulite reduction.

Lasers and light therapy are advanced topics. It is not necessary at this stage to learn all of the details concerning these devices. They are mentioned to familiarize you with the technology, which continues to evolve.

LIGHT THERAPY

Light therapy is the application of light rays to the skin for the treatment of wrinkles, capillaries, pigmentation, or hair removal. Light therapy uses different types of devices: lasers, intense pulsed light (IPL), and LED light-emitting diode (LED) technologies. The power and effectiveness of the machines vary and depend on such factors as the wavelength, heat, and penetration power. Lasers and IPL are strong machines that are rated as Class IV medical devices by the Food and Drug Administration (FDA). LED is rated as a safer Class I or II device and is regulated less strictly.

The range of wavelengths used in light therapy are visible, infrared, and far infrared (Figure 18–6). Lasers such as Nd:YAG tighten skin and reduce wrinkles and spider veins. IPL devices use pulses of multiple wavelengths to reduce pigmentation, remove surface capillaries, and rejuvenate the skin. LED technology is nonthermal, meaning it does not use heat.

LED individual wavelengths are used at low intensity and are not as strong as the laser and IPL modalities. LED uses visible light such as blue, red or amber, and infrared (invisible). Blue light is considered effective in treating acne. Amber and red are used for muscles and healing. Infrared is used for rejuvenation. Infrared light is also used to detoxify the body and reduce pain. LED is likened to photosynthesis because it converts light to cellular energy that stimulates the body's collagen and metabolism.

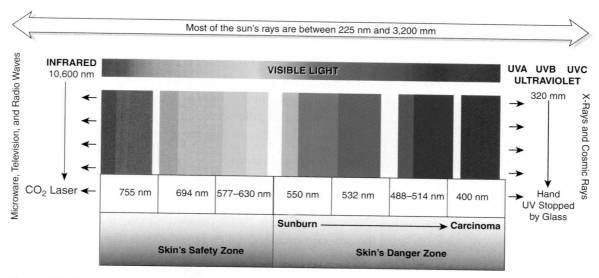

Most of the sun's rays are between 225 nm and 3,200 mm

Microware, Television, and Radio Waves

INFRARED
10,600 nm

VISIBLE LIGHT

UVA UVB UVC
ULTRAVIOLET

320 mm

X-Rays and Cosmic Rays

CO₂ Laser

| 755 nm | 694 nm | 577–630 nm | 550 nm | 532 nm | 488–514 nm | 400 nm |

Hand
UV Stopped
by Glass

Sunburn ⟶ Carcinoma

Skin's Safety Zone

Skin's Danger Zone

Figure 18–6 Wavelengths used in light therapy.

Photorejuvenation is a growing technology that utilizes light therapy to enhance the skin (Figure 18–7 A,B). Different light rays produce different effects on the skin. Light therapy has been used for years to treat physical conditions such as pain and to promote healing. LED has been shown to help the lymph system and increase ATP energy production in the cells. Therapeutic lamps are also used for light therapy. Different colors of light also have various psychological effects: red is considered stimulating, while green is calming. The use of machines, light therapy, and medical aesthetics continues to develop. Scientific discoveries and advances are changing the face of the antiaging industry.

> ## FYI
>
> Most high-tech devices require multiple sessions to achieve desired results.

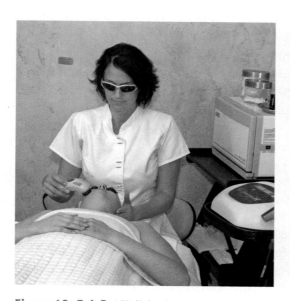
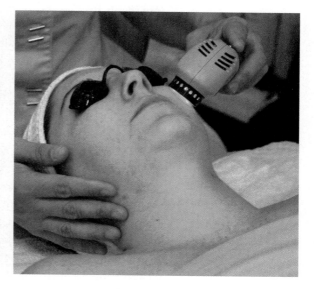

Figure 18–7 A,B LED light therapy.

MICROCURRENT MACHINES

Modern medicine utilizes microcurrent to treat many conditions, such as Bell's palsy and stroke paralysis. The growing uses of microampere electrical neuromuscular stimulation include healing muscles and wounds, controlling pain, and even fusing bones. There is even greater potential for this type of therapy. In the esthetics realm, microcurrent is used to tone the muscles by stimulating motor nerves and contracting the muscles.

Facial Benefits of Microcurrent

Microcurrent (MY-kroh-kur-runt), or wave therapy, devices mimic the way the brain relays messages to the muscles. In esthetics, microcurrent is used primarily to tone and stimulate facial muscles. Considered a passive form of exercise, this therapeutic technique helps stimulate motor nerves until a contraction of the muscles can be seen. Microcurrent has the ability to firm muscles and boost cellular activity. It can also assist with product absorption. In the past, faradic current has been used to stimulate motor nerves.

Many biological processes are associated with electrical impulses. Facial skin tone and muscles are all related to this system. As we age, impulses may slow down, causing the skin to sag. Muscles may not completely contract after use, such as in the case of sagging jowls (jaw muscles). The same effect can be seen on the rest of the body as well. That is why exercise and stretching are so important as one ages.

Microcurrent devices are designed to work in harmony with the natural bioelectrical currents found in the body. The technique utilizes two hand-held probes placed on facial muscle groups. A specific movement technique is used on facial points. A gel, such as a collagen ampoule, is placed on the skin before beginning the treatment. Current is regulated according to the skin's resistance.

Microcurrent is reported to aid in the healing and repairing of tissue and to influence metabolism and cellular activity. It works gently and helps speed up the natural regenerative processes of the body when the correct intensity of current and frequency are used. Treatment results are expected to show firmer and healthier skin. Microcurrent combined with light therapy can be even more effective. When using any electrical device, you should obtain a complete client health history and conduct a consultation before treatment. Contraindications are the same as those described for other electrical devices.

ULTRASOUND AND ULTRASONIC TECHNOLOGY

Ultrasound and *ultrasonic* are synonymous terms referring to a frequency that is above the range of sound audible to the human ear. This equipment uses noninvasive sound waves to create results-oriented treatments. Ultrasonic equipment is based on high-frequency mechanical oscillations produced by a metal spatula-like tool. The vibrations, created through a water medium, help cleanse and exfoliate the skin by removing dead skin cells. Contraindications include epilepsy, pregnancy, and cancerous lesions.

Ultrasound technology in esthetics is used for product penetration and for cellulite reduction. Ultrasound is deep penetrating. It stimulates tissue, increases blood flow, and promotes oxygenation. The lower the frequency, the greater the penetration. Conversely, the higher the frequency, the lower the penetration. Cellulite is affected through the heat manipulation of the tissue and lymphatic movements performed with the device. Heat is created, and the vibration in the cells stimulates circulation, metabolism, and lymph drainage. The heat damage from ultrasound and other modalities (such as lasers) is what stimulates collagen production.

Ultrasound also sends waves through the skin to assist in product penetration. This process is called sonophoresis (SAHN-oh-for-EE-sus), which is similar to iontophoresis (iontophoresis uses electrically charged ions, so an electrical charge is needed from electrodes). Esthetic ultrasound equipment is an FDA Class II device and may not be within an esthetician's scope of practice outside of a medical facility. Advanced training and technical research on equipment claims are necessary before using any advanced esthetic machine. Different frequencies of ultrasound are also used for medical imaging, physical therapy, and pain management. Lower-frequency ultrasonic devices are used for toothbrushes and jewelry cleaners.

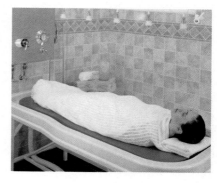

Figure 18–8 Body wrap.

SPA BODY TREATMENTS

Spa treatments provide a wonderful, relaxing experience. Body treatments have a therapeutic effect and treat the skin of the whole body. They include wraps, scrubs, and masks. Be mindful of contraindications and allergies to ingredients (seaweed) before working on clients.

- **Body wraps** are treatments where product is applied on the body and then covered or wrapped up. Wraps are used for various reasons and can either remineralize, hydrate, stimulate, detoxify, or promote relaxation. The product used will determine the effects and results. Aloe, gels, lotions, oils, seaweed, herbs, clay, or mud products can all be used for wraps. Linens or plastic can be used to wrap clients and to promote product penetration. Blankets or sheets are the cocoon of the "wraps." Inch-loss wraps, another type of wrap, are designed to flush toxins out of the body and promote inch loss. Inch-loss wraps have a diuretic effect and are controversial in their effectiveness. If done properly, detoxifying the body may aid in weight reduction (Figure 18–8).

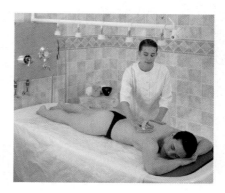

Figure 18–9 A salt glow.

- **Body scrubs** use friction to exfoliate and hydrate, increase circulation, and nourish skin using a combination of ingredients such as walnut husks, apricot kernels, cornmeal, jojoba beads, honey, salt, or sugar combined with oil or lotion. Exfoliation treatments are also called *polishes* and *glows* (Figure 18–9). Exfoliation prepares the skin to receive additional products or treatments.

- **Body masks** remineralize and detoxify the body using primarily clay, mud, or seaweed mixtures. Some body masks are used to treat cellulite. Clients are usually wrapped up after the mask application, and thus masks are similar to wraps. The ingredients and procedure used in the treatment determine whether the process is called a *mask* or a *wrap* (Figure 18–10).

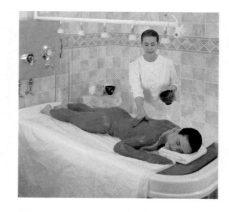

Figure 18–10 A body mask.

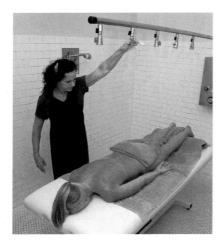

Figure 18–11 The Vichy shower.

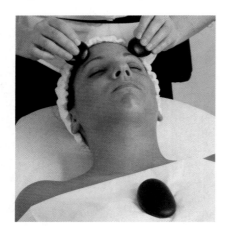

Figure 18–12 Stone therapy on the face.

- **Hydrotherapy** (hy-druh-THAIR-uh-pee) is another spa treatment that uses water in its three forms (ice, steam, and liquid). Hydrotherapy tubs, the Scotch hose, Vichy (VIH-shee) shower (Figure 18–11), Watsu® massage, hot tubs, steam rooms, saunas, the cold-plunge pool, foot soaks, and whirlpool baths are all different forms of hydrotherapy found in spas. All spa treatments, especially intensive hydrotherapy treatments, can be strong, so proper training is important before offering these services.

- **Balneotherapy** (bal-nee-oh-THAYR-uh-pee) is the treatment of physical ailments using therapeutic water baths. Mineral, mud or fango, dead sea salt, seaweed, enzymes, or peat are all used in baths (*balneum* is Latin for bath).

- **Stone massage** is the technique of using hot stones and cold stones in massage or other treatments (Figure 18–12).

- **Foot reflexology** (ree-flex-AHL-uh-jee) is the treatment of the body through reflex points located on the bottoms of the feet (Figure 18–13). It is balancing and relaxing for the entire body.

- **Ayurvedic** (eye-ur-VAY-dic) concepts are based on three *doshas*, or mind and body types. Treatments include Shirodhara (Figure 18–14), massage, and facials using ancient Indian concepts and ingredients suited to the three body/mind types: *pitta*, *kapha*, and *vatta*. Ayurveda originated over 5,000 years ago in India. It is a philosophy of medicine and balancing life and the body through various methods ranging from massage to eating habits. *Ayur* means "life, vital power"; *Veda* means "knowledge."

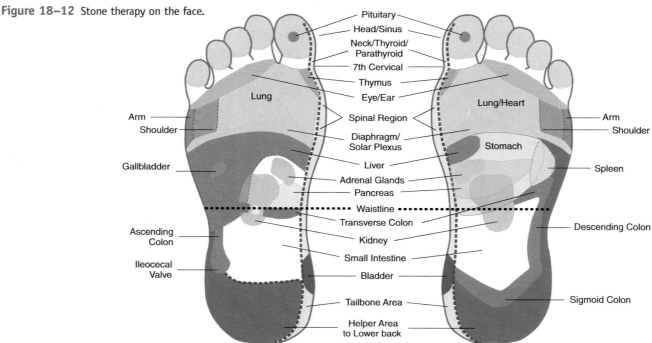

Figure 18–13 Foot reflexology chart.

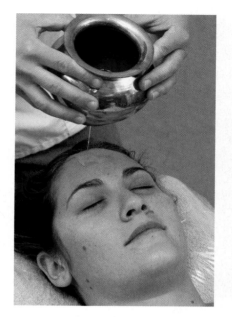

Figure 18–14 Shirodhara.

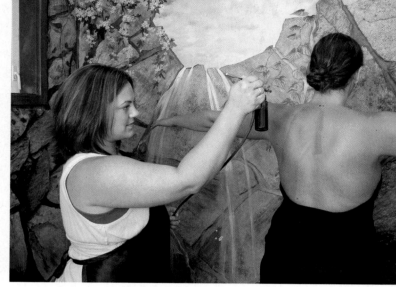

Figure 18–15 Sunless spray tanning.

- *Sunless tanning* product application is offered as an alternative to tanning. It is sprayed on (Figure 18–15) or applied manually.
- **Endermology** (en-dur-MAHL-uh-gee) is a treatment for cellulite. It helps stimulate the reduction of adipose tissue. Machines and other endermology methods are used in spas and in medical facilities.

Body Treatment Procedures

The following procedures briefly outline how the spa treatments are performed. Advanced training is needed to perform these treatments safely and efficiently. There are contraindications to be aware of and many variables in body treatments. Body services are wonderful treatments to offer clients.

MANUAL LYMPH DRAINAGE

Manual lymph drainage (MLD) (MAN-yoo-ul LIMF DRAY-nij) stimulates lymph fluid to flow through the lymphatic vessels. This technique helps to cleanse and detoxify the body. Congestion, water, and waste in the vessels create edema in the tissue. Moving this fluid out of the body with light massage movements will decrease the swelling from excess fluid (Figure 18–16). MLD is a great addition to a facial. It is also used both before and after surgery because it expedites healing and enhances cell metabolism. Advanced training courses are available for both estheticians and massage therapists.

Mechanical lymph drainage is an MLD service performed with machines.

> **CAUTION!**
>
> Instruct your clients to drink lots of water to flush the system and rehydrate the body after body treatments. If they do not replenish the water in the body, clients may feel sick. Detoxifying treatments are not as effective when the body is not flushed or rehydrated with water.

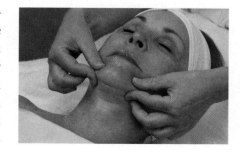

Figure 18–16 Manual lymph drainage.

ACTIVITY

To learn more about spa treatments, here is a research idea: Check out the spa menus and brochures in your area or on Internet sites. Professional trade journals and spa suppliers offer excellent information on treatment procedures. Many spa magazines are also good resources to gain insight into the industry.

MINI-PROCEDURE

THE BODY SCRUB

This procedure outline describes a basic body scrub. Follow the instructor's and manufacturer's directions for preparing the scrub.

1. Use a prepackaged body exfoliating product, or mix either salt or sugar with lotion or oil. Mix until the desired consistency is reached. Add two drops of aromatherapy oil if desired. A high-quality unrefined salt or sugar is recommended.

   Make sure the product is not too coarse or rough.

   Make sure your product rinses off easily because this treatment generally does not require a shower after the service.

   Prepare the bed with linens while the product and towels are warming in the hot cabby.

2. Use a set pattern to apply the warmed product, starting with the legs and using circular motions.

   Exfoliate the body using the hands, a brush, or a mitt (keep adding warm water if necessary).

   Most body products are applied first to the legs, followed by the arms, then the torso and back.

   To keep the client warm, cover each area with a sheet or body towel before proceeding to the next area.

3. Remove the scrub in the same order (legs, arms, torso) with warm, wet towels. Pat dry and cover each area before moving to the next.

4. *Optional:* Finish by spraying the treated areas with a skin freshener, and apply lotion if time permits.

   Note: A body wrap treatment can also follow the scrub.

MINI-PROCEDURE

THE BODY WRAP OR MASK

Use a body lotion, seaweed, or mud.

1. A dry brush or body scrub can be performed before the wrap or mask.
2. Apply the product with hands or a body "paint" brush.
3. Wrap the client for 20 to 30 minutes.
4. Add a facial or foot treatment, if desired, during the wrap.
5. Remove the product with warm towels if applicable, or have the client shower.

CELLULITE

Cellulite (SEL-yoo-lyt) is caused primarily by female hormones and genetics. Cellulite consists of fat cells. Dermal fat cells do swell, but that is not the only cause of cellulite. Cellulite is visible when dermal fat cells are closer to the surface of the skin. This occurs from damage to the dermis. If water is lost and the tissue is weakened, then dermal fat begins to push into the dermis. Additionally, if the epidermis is weakened or dehydrated, cellulite is more visible.

Keeping collagen and elastin healthy helps reduce cellulite. To repair cellulite, cells and connective tissue need to be strengthened and hydrated through nutrients and water intake. Drinking water is not enough—our cells have to be able to hold onto the water. Wasted water in the body builds up and leads to water retention and puffiness. Circulation of nutrients and blood flow through blood vessels up to the skin also affects cellulite. Repairing cell damage, connective tissue damage, and stratum corneum damage is important in treating cellulite.

The following recommended nutrients and ingredients may be beneficial for cellulite reduction:

- lecithin and lipids for cell walls
- glycosaminoglycans (GAGs) for moisturizing and firming
- glucosamine to build GAGs and connective tissue
- B vitamins to retain moisture and provide nutrients
- amino acids for building collagen and elastin
- essential fatty acids to attract water for connective tissue
- antioxidants
- anti-inflammatories
- aloe vera is anti-inflammatory, improves hydration, and contains enzymes and minerals
- AHAs
- alpha lipoic acid

The effectiveness of some endermology treatments is controversial. Detox diets, liposuction, and muscle-stimulating systems do not minimize cellulite. Some body wraps result in only a temporary water loss. Electronic devices with vacuums may reduce cellulite temporarily.

Manual lymph drainage, mesotherapy (microinjection to dermis to melt fat), dermal fillers, lasers, chemical peels, and microdermabrasion have all been tried to help reduce cellulite. Most of these techniques are considered temporary, and their effectiveness varies.

Increasing blood flow, stimulating collagen and elastin, attracting water to cells, and repairing cell membranes are recommended to reduce cellulite. Additionally, reducing wasted water, preventing free radical damage, and reducing inflammation is part of a healthy approach to treating cellulite and the skin.

Professional cellulite treatments must be performed consistently in continuous sessions. A common spa treatment consists of exfoliation with a scrub or dry brushing followed by a detoxifying mask and wrap. These stimulate the metabolism and circulation. To finish the service, a cellulite treatment cream is applied.

Exfoliation and skin brushing is also good for vessels and circulation. Another popular treatment is thalassotherapy (thuh-LA-soh-THAIR-uh-pee; *thalassa* is Greek for "sea"). Therapeutic benefits from sea and seawater products include minerals and nutrients. Massage can also help soften hardened cellulite. Cellulite is a common condition for most women, and improving the health of the skin is a continual process.

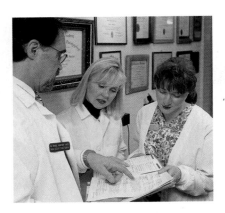

Figure 18–17 There are many opportunities for a medical aesthetician.

MEDICAL AESTHETICS

Medical aesthetics is a multibillion-dollar industry. The industry is constantly developing new products and services for our youth-oriented society. Plastic surgery, laser treatments, and injectables focus on maintaining a youthful appearance. Medical aesthetics integrates surgical and nonsurgical procedures with esthetic treatments. Estheticians perform services such as peels, microdermabrasion, and light therapy. Some assist in the medical procedures and monitor patient recovery. Additionally, recommending home-care products help patients heal faster and maintain their skin's health. Because medical aesthetics is evolving, the esthetician's role can be shaped to fit the facility's needs (Figure 18–17). Each setting varies, so it is important to define the responsibilities included in the esthetician's job description.

Medical aestheticians are well trained, experienced, and in some cases certified. However, not all estheticians must be certified to work in medical aesthetics. Most clinical procedures must be done in a medical office under a physician's supervision. Medi-spas are medical clinics and spas combined in one location and offer both esthetic and medical services.

The most popular medical spa services are peels, microdermabrasion, Botox®, fillers, laser hair removal, and photorejuvenation (FO-toh-rih-joo-vin-A-shun). Estheticians are not qualified to perform certain procedures, but it is important to be familiar with all of them because many clients will be asking questions and utilizing these procedures. Society is now flooded with information on medical aesthetics. It is part of modern society's continued quest for instant gratification and maintaining physical beauty. Medical spas are the fastest-growing segment in the beauty industry.

Pre- and Postoperative Care

Estheticians perform pre- and postoperative treatments and provide patient education before cosmetic surgery. These are important for faster patient recovery time. Estheticians also provide facials, light peels, extractions, and microdermabrasion. Camouflage makeup, retail sales, and patient home-care counseling are other responsibilities.

Preoperative care focuses on preparing the skin for the procedure. Getting the skin in its optimum state and as healthy as possible makes the surgery less traumatic on the tissue and shortens recovery time. Increasing the skin's metabolism and reducing cellular debris on the surface are part of conditioning the skin. Helping the patient stay calm is also a role the esthetician can fill. A plan and schedule for pre- and post-op care are outlined by the medical staff before a patient's surgery.

Post-op care includes providing skin care for rapid wound healing and the avoidance of infection. Decreasing inflammation, soothing and moisturizing, and providing for sun protection are the goals. Massage, hydration, protection, and camouflage makeup are all part of post-op care. Home-care instructions for long-term maintenance are also important. Permanent makeup, sometimes referred to as *micropigmentation,* is another technique utilized in clinical aesthetics.

Microdermabrasion and Peels

Glycolic peels (gly-KAHL-ik peels) can be performed to precondition the skin before laser resurfacing or surgery. These "lunchtime peels" can enhance the strength and barrier function of the epidermis. Microdermabrasion benefits to the epidermis are similar to those provided by peels, although the effects are more superficial.

Documentation

The patient charts are a record of what the patient conveys, what the esthetician observes, the assessment and analysis, and a plan of action to be taken. Protocols from standard clinical procedures are followed. Patient informed consent forms and treatment records are part of the standard charting procedure.

Other Clinical Procedures

Numerous opportunities for estheticians are found in specialized clinical settings. In laser and medical centers, hair reduction, spider vein removal, **nonablative** (non-uh-BLAY-tiv) wrinkle treatments, and other types of laser procedures are performed. Nonablative procedures do not remove tissue. Nonablative wrinkle treatments use intense pulsed light (IPL) to bypass the epidermis and stimulate collagen in the dermis to promote wrinkle reduction. Estheticians can assist physicians in these procedures if they are properly trained and certified.

Other common procedures performed by physicians include injectables of dermal fillers (DUR-mul fillers) and Botox (BOW-tocks).

Injectables

Botox® and dermal fillers are injectables that are a large part of the industry. Injectables have become the fastest-growing product in the medical spa industry. FDA-approved fillers are nontoxic, durable, biocompatible, and easy to use; these are the necessary attributes of a safe filler. **Injectable fillers** (in-JEK-tuh-buls) are substances used in nonsurgical procedures to fill in or plump up areas of the skin.

Botox. Botox® injection is the most popular nonsurgical clinical service performed. Botox (botulinum toxin) is derived from a botulism type A bacteria. Botox is injected into the muscles to cause paralysis or diminished movement by blocking neurotransmitters. This relaxes tissues and diminishes lines. The glabella (gluh-BEL-uh) is the area between the eyebrows where muscles cause creasing from squinting or frowning. The glabella has strong muscles and is the most common site for Botox injections (Figure 18–18). Over 3 million Botox injections are performed annually in the United States.

Dermal Fillers. Dermal fillers are used to fill lines, wrinkles, and other facial imperfections. As we age, dermal collagen, hyaluronic acid, and fat (lipotrophy) are lost and skin loses its shape. The first fillers were from animal sources, specifically bovine collagen. Collagen treatments use a filler, usually a bovine (cow) derivative, to fill in wrinkles or to make lips larger. Dermal fillers will last longer when used in conjunction with Botox.

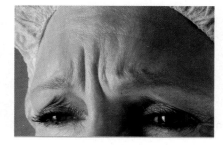

Figure 18–18 The glabella is the most common site for Botox injections.

Today's fillers are obtained from a variety of sources. Many are combined substances and materials. Collagen may be derived from human or animal sources. Synthetic sources are silicone and hyaluronic acids. The newest trend is to use nonanimal (Restylane®) and animal-based (Hylaform®) hyaluronic acid fillers. Hyaluronic acid is a polysaccharide found in the body and connective tissues. A component of the skin's natural moisturizing function, it holds up to 1,000 times its weight in water.

Another type of filler is aqueous calcium (Radiesse® FN), which is calcium-based. The newest injectable is not a filler, but a dermal stimulator called poly-L-lactic acid (PLLA). This product (marketed as Sculptra™) increases fibroblast activity and collagen production. New products are coming on the market regularly.

Surgical Procedures

There are two types of surgery: **reconstructive** and **cosmetic.**

- *Reconstructive* is defined as "restoring a bodily function." This type of surgery is necessary for accident survivors and those with congenital disfigurements or other diseases.
- *Cosmetic* (esthetic) surgery is elective surgery for improving and altering the appearance.

Cosmetic Surgical Procedures

Common plastic surgery procedures are face lifts, forehead lifts, eye lifts, nose reconstruction, laser resurfacing, and deep peels.

- A **rhytidectomy** (rit-ih-DEK-tuh-mee) is a face lift. This procedure removes excess fat at the jaw line; tightens loose, atrophic muscles; and removes sagging skin (Figures 18–19 and 18–20).
- A forehead lift, also called a *brow lift,* can be performed separately or in combination with an eye lift.

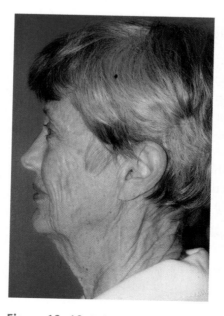

Figure 18–19 Before a face lift.

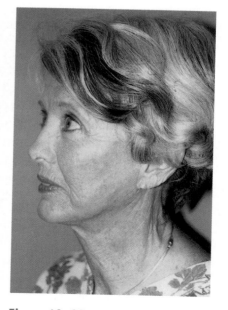

Figure 18–20 After a face lift.

- A **blepharoplasty** (BLEF-uh-roh-plas-tee) is an eye lift. It removes fat and skin from the upper and lower lids, making them less baggy and crinkled-looking (Figure 18–21). When sagging eyelids impede a patient's ability to see, it is a medical condition that may be covered by insurance.
- A **transconjunctival blepharoplasty** (trans-kon-junk-TIE-vul BLEF-uh-roh-plas-tee) is performed inside the lower eyelid to remove bulging fat pads, which are often congenital.
- **Rhinoplasty** (RY-noh-plas-tee) is nose surgery that makes a nose smaller or changes the appearance in some way. Sometimes rhinoplasty is necessary for health reasons and to improve the patient's breathing ability.
- **Laser resurfacing** (LAY-zur ree-SIR-fuh-sing) is used to smooth wrinkles or lighten acne scars. Collagen remodeling stimulates the growth of new collagen in the dermis (Figures 18–22 and 18–23). This type of laser treatment removes the epidermal layer and requires a recovery period.
- **Dermabrasion** (dur-muh-BRAY-zhun) is a strong exfoliation method that uses a mechanical brush to physically remove tissue down to the dermis. It is a very deep exfoliation used primarily on scars. Lasers are replacing the use of this medical procedure.

  Do not confuse dermabrasion with microdermabrasion. Microdermabrasion is a mild, superficial mechanical exfoliation method.
- **Trichloroacetic acid (TCA) peels** (TRY-klor-oh-uh-SEE-tik AH-sid peels) are used for sun damage and wrinkles.
- **Phenol** (FEE-nohl) peels are the strongest peels and can be toxic. They are still used and are less expensive, but they require a longer recovery period than TCA peels or laser resurfacing.

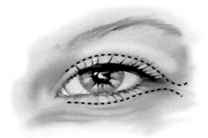

Figure 18–21 Blepharoplasty.

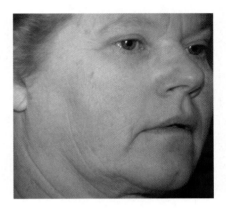

Figure 18–22 Before laser resurfacing.

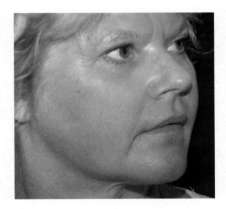

Figure 18–23 After laser resurfacing.

Body Procedures

Many individuals are having elective surgeries. It is therefore important to be familiar with these procedures, especially if you are offering body treatments.

- **Sclerotherapy** (sklair-oh-THAIR-uh-pee) minimizes varicose veins (dilated blood vessels) and other varicosities by injecting chemical agents into the affected areas. Lasers are a secondary method of vein therapy. Over 50 percent of women have varicose veins and smaller spider veins (telangiectasia) on their legs. Potential causes are heredity, race, gender, posture, hormones, and pregnancy. Trauma and injury causes inflammation to vessels. Phlebitis (fluh-BY-tus) is the inflammation of a vein. To take pressure off of veins, keep the legs elevated, wear compression stockings, avoid crossing the legs, exercise, and avoid being in stationary positions for long periods of time.
- **Mammoplasty** (MAM-oh-plas-tee) is breast surgery that enlarges the breasts or reconstructs them. This procedure is also referred to as breast augmentation, or implants. Breast reduction reduces or repositions the breasts. This is sometimes performed for health reasons.
- **Liposuction** (LY-puh-suck-shun) is the procedure that surgically removes pockets of fat.
- An **abdominoplasty** (ab-DOM-un-oh-plas-tee) removes excessive fat deposits and loose skin from the abdomen to tuck and tighten the area.

🌐 WEB RESOURCES

Here are some great Web sites for more information.

American Society of Plastic Surgeons:

http://plasticsurgery.org

eMedicine:

http://emedicine.com

Mayo Clinic:

http://mayoclinic.com

The medical journal for skin care professionals:

http://pcijournal.com

The Clinical Aesthetician

Working as a clinical aesthetician in medical aesthetics can be enriching. This specialty requires compassion and patience because you will work with people who are in pain or who are experiencing physical trauma. Many patients feel more comfortable with the esthetician than they do with a physician, who may not have time for more personal and empathetic discussions. Remember to stay focused on the treatment goals and maintain a professional role at all times. The role of an esthetician can be invaluable in a medical setting in providing pre- and postoperative care and other patient services and education.

A career in esthetics is always exciting and fascinating. Advanced areas of study range from medical aesthetics to exotic body treatments. Utilizing peels and light therapy for skin care are two of the most effective tools available today to estheticians. The opportunity for advanced training is limitless.

There are many services one can specialize in. As the industry continues to grow, keep up with new technology and changes, even if they are not on your service menu. After basic esthetic techniques are mastered, it is a natural progression to add advanced treatments to the services currently offered. This is the beauty of esthetics: the increased ability to improve the health of the skin as the industry evolves. Educated and skilled technicians will always be in demand.

REVIEW QUESTIONS

1. How do alpha hydroxy acids work?

2. What are the benefits of AHA peels?

3. What are the contraindications for AHA peels?

4. How does the microdermabrasion procedure work?

5. What effects does microdermabrasion have on the skin?

6. What types of laser services are offered?

7. What is light therapy?

8. What is light therapy used for?

9. What is LED?

10. What is microcurrent, and what does it do for the skin?

11. What is ultrasound used for in esthetics?

12. What are the benefits of body scrubs and wraps?

13. What services do medical aestheticians provide?

14. Give examples of pre- and post-op skin care treatments.

15. What is manual lymph drainage massage?

16. What is endermology?

17. What are injectables used for?

CHAPTER GLOSSARY

abdominoplasty: procedure that removes excessive fat deposits and loose skin from the abdomen to tuck and tighten the area.

ayurvedic: Indian philosophy of balancing life and the body through various methods ranging from massage to eating habits. It is based on three *doshas,* or mind and body types.

balneotherapy: body treatments that use mud or fango, dead sea salt, seaweed, enzymes, or peat baths.

blepharoplasty: an eye lift. It removes the fat and skin from the upper and lower lids.

body masks: remineralize and detoxify the body using clay, mud, gel, or seaweed mixtures.

body scrubs: use of friction to exfoliate, hydrate, increase circulation, and nourish the skin.

body wraps: remineralize, hydrate, stimulate, or promote relaxation by using aloe, gels, lotions, oils, seaweed, herbs, clay, or mud.

Botox: neuromuscular-blocking serum (botulinum toxin) that paralyzes nerve cells on the muscle when this serum is injected into it.

cell renewal factor (CRF): cell turnover rate.

cellulite: gel-like lumps of fat, water, and residues of toxic substances beneath the skin, usually around the hips and thighs of overweight people.

cosmetic (esthetic) surgery: elective surgery for improving and altering the appearance.

dermabrasion: a medical procedure; strong exfoliation method using a mechanical brush to physically remove tissue down to the dermis.

dermal fillers: products used to fill lines, wrinkles, and other facial imperfections.

endermology: a treatment for cellulite.

foot reflexology: treatment of the body through reflex points located on the bottom of the feet.

hydrotherapy: spa treatments that use water.

injectable fillers: substances used in nonsurgical procedures to fill in or plump up areas of the skin. Botox® and dermal fillers are injectables.

Jessner's peel: a light to medium peel of lactic acid, salicylic acid, and resorcinol in an ethanol solvent.

laser resurfacing: procedure used to smooth wrinkles or lighten acne scars. Collagen remodeling stimulates the growth of new collagen in the dermis.

lasers: acronym for "light amplification stimulation emission of radiation"; medical devices using electromagnetic radiation for hair removal and skin treatments.

light therapy: the application of light rays to the skin for the treatment of wrinkles, capillaries, pigmentation, or hair removal.

liposuction: procedure that surgically removes pockets of fat.

mammoplasty: breast surgery.

manual lymph drainage (MLD): stimulates lymph fluid to flow through the lymphatic vessels. This light massage technique helps to cleanse and detoxify the body.

CHAPTER GLOSSARY

microcurrent: a device that mimics the body's natural electrical energy to reeducate and tone facial muscles; improves circulation and increases collagen and elastin production.

microdermabrasion: a form of mechanical exfoliation.

nonablative: procedure that does not remove tissue; wrinkle treatments that bypass the epidermis to stimulate collagen in the dermis for wrinkle reduction are nonablative.

phenol: carbolic acid; a caustic poison; used for peels and to sanitize metallic implements.

reconstructive surgery: defined as "restoring a bodily function." It is necessary surgery for accident survivors and those with congenital disfigurements or other diseases.

rhinoplasty: nose surgery that makes a nose smaller or changes its appearance.

rhytidectomy: a face lift. This removes excess fat at the jawline, tightens loose, atrophic muscles, and removes sagging skin.

sclerotherapy: minimizes varicose veins (dilated blood vessels) and other varicosities by injecting chemical agents into the affected areas or by laser treatments.

stone massage: the use of hot stones and cold stones in massage or in other treatments.

transconjunctival blepharoplasty: procedure performed inside the lower eyelid to remove bulging fat pads, which are often congenital.

trichloroacetic acid (TCA) peels: a strong peel used to diminish sun damage and wrinkles.

CHAPTER OUTLINE

THE WORLD OF MAKEUP

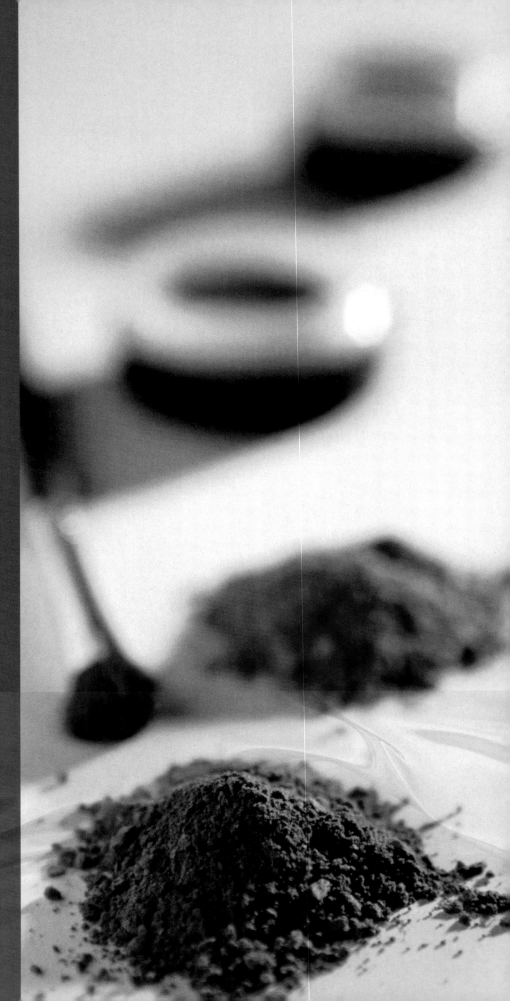

LEARNING OBJECTIVES

After completing this chapter, you will be able to:

- Describe the different types of cosmetics and their uses.

- Demonstrate an understanding of cosmetic color theory.

- Consult with clients to determine their needs and preferences.

- Identify different facial features and demonstrate procedures for basic corrective makeup.

- Perform a basic makeup procedure for any occasion.

- Demonstrate the application and removal of artificial lashes.

KEY TERMS

Makeup artistry is a fun, creative career choice. This is an area where one can be artistic and expressive. Different makeup looks can show off an individual's unique style. A wide range of makeup styles can be created, from basic daytime applications to makeup for dramatic photo shoots. It is both interesting and enjoyable to experiment with different colors and looks.

Makeup plays an important role in the fashion world and constantly changes with the seasons. Society has always taken great interest in the latest trends in fashion, hair, and clothing styles. Film and Hollywood continue to influence these trends. Makeup is also an important feature of weddings, proms, and other glamorous events. With ever-changing formulas and colors, every year brings increased sophistication to the art and science of makeup.

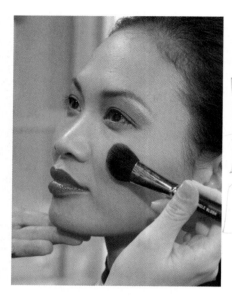

Figure 19–1 Makeup helps enhance a client's natural beauty.

The primary goal of makeup is to enhance the client's natural beauty by bringing out the most attractive features of the face, while minimizing those that are less attractive (Figure 19–1). Makeup is a tool that helps create a certain look. Every woman wants to look her best. Through the consultation, the client's individual needs can be determined. The natural skin tone, hair color, eye color, and face shape are taken into consideration. A person's lifestyle and preferences are also factors in determining the look. For most clients, makeup application should be subtle. The client's natural beauty can be enhanced by a blend of makeup artistry, hairstyle, and clothing choices.

This chapter covers all aspects of makeup artistry. Knowledge of color theory; analyzing facial features, including eyebrows; and corrective makeup techniques are all part of being a successful makeup artist. Client consultations, the makeup station, product descriptions, makeup application techniques, and lash procedures are all included in this comprehensive chapter. The key to creating beauty is in the details.

This is a large chapter, and you will not be expected to comprehend or memorize all of the information in one study session. The tables are included as guidelines that you can refer to again and again. The great thing about makeup is that it is not permanent—it washes off! After trying a few applications, you will find that the concepts will all come together.

PSYCHOLOGICAL ASPECTS OF MAKEUP

Many women are attached to their makeup kits and believe their attractiveness depends on their makeup. Others avoid makeup altogether. There are strong beliefs associated with makeup. What do you believe? Do you like makeup? Is it fun? Intimidating? Many women are not comfortable wearing makeup. Others play in front of the mirror every day, trying out different looks and colors. Adding color to our lives with cosmetics can be uplifting and give us a positive feeling.

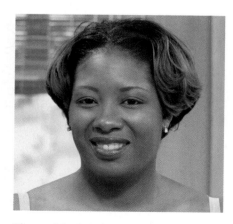

Figure 19–2 Makeup can influence our self-esteem.

Some women will not leave their home without "putting on their face." Unfortunately, they believe they need to wear makeup to look attractive enough to go out in public. This is a powerful mental disposition that is not healthy for an individual's self-esteem. However, makeup can give people a lift and make them feel more attractive, thereby enhancing their self-esteem (Figure 19–2). For those with disfigurements, makeup can be a wonderful tool that allows them to be more comfortable and live normal lives. For example, the American Cancer Society sponsors Look Good, Feel Better programs that help those with cancer by hosting hair and makeup clinics. Professionals volunteer their time, helping cancer patients look better and feel better by applying makeup and styling their hair or working with wigs.

Makeup artists have an opportunity to help clients feel better about themselves not just through makeup alone but also by boosting their self-confidence and focusing on their natural beauty. By finding out what clients believe about makeup, you can gain insight into what look will most satisfy them.

MAKEUP SERVICES OVERVIEW

The world of makeup offers a variety of opportunities. Makeup artists work in salons or spas offering makeup applications, makeovers, and lessons (Figure 19–3). Weddings are a big part of makeup services. Other opportunities include working with photographers, television stations, or video companies. Some artists become stylists on photo shoots or work in film and video production. Theaters also use makeup artists for theatrical makeup. Providing camouflage makeup applications for clinics or plastic surgeons is another avenue for makeup artistry.

MAKEUP PRODUCTS

Choosing a makeup product line is similar to choosing a skin care line. Makeup product choices range from private-label brands to exclusive spa lines. There are some good-quality, private-label cosmetics. Quality is important when choosing products and supplies. There is a difference between high-quality makeup and less expensive generic brands. The quality of the products and brushes makes a big difference in how makeup application will go for you, the artist, or for your client—smoothly or not so smoothly. Pigment quality, packaging, and applicators all vary. Advertising costs and overhead costs play a part in the cost of makeup. More advertising may mean more expensive products.

Explain to clients why they should buy quality makeup and brushes. Why are they better? Is quality going to make a difference on their skin? Will quality products glide on easier and not tug on the delicate eye tissue? Clients will be more satisfied with products that are easier to work with and will discover that quality is worth the extra money.

You will be better equipped to offer your professional expertise when you have learned about the products, supplies, and tools used in makeup application and services. The cosmetics industry offers a wide range of products designed to improve the skin's appearance as well as its condition (Figure 19–4). The cosmetics available today meet the needs of every skin type. Most products come in several forms: powders, creams, and liquids in an assortment of containers and packages. Makeup formulations are evolving and are now healthier for the skin. The product applications are introduced here before the hands-on procedures.

Foundation

Foundation evens out skin tone and color, conceals imperfections in the skin, and protects the skin from the outside elements of climate, dirt, and pollution.

Foundations that usually contain mineral oil or other oils are referred to as *oil based*. These products are a good choice for normal to dry skin.

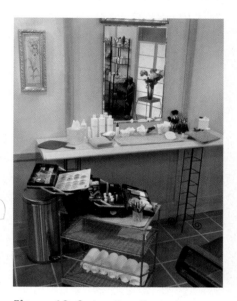

Figure 19–3 An attractive makeup station.

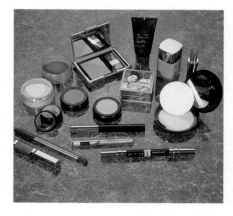

Figure 19–4 Makeup products and color choices are unlimited.

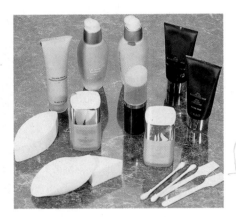

Figure 19–5 A wide selection of foundations.

Oil-free products are referred to as *water based*. Water-based foundations generally give a more matte (dull, not shiny) finish and help conceal minor blemishes and discolorations. These foundations are preferred for oily skin.

Foundation Chemistry

Foundations may contain water, mineral oil, stearic acid, cetyl alcohol, propylene glycol, lanolin derivatives, and insoluble pigments. Foundations may also contain surfactants (detergents, emulsifiers), humectants, perfume, and preservatives such as paraben.

Cream foundations are thicker and give medium to heavier coverage. These are generally suited for dry to normal skin. Liquid foundations are suspensions of organic and inorganic pigments in alcohol and water-based solutions. Bentonite is added to help keep the products blended. The formulation is generally suited for clients with oily to normal skin conditions who desire sheer to medium coverage. Pancake makeup is oil based and heavy.

Powder foundations, which consist of a powder base mixed with a coloring agent (pigment) and perfume, are good for oily skin. Cream-to-powder foundations are moist on application but dry to a powdery finish. Many foundations now contain barrier agents, such as sunscreen and silicone, to protect the complexion from environmental damage (Figure 19–5).

Mineral makeup is composed of micronized minerals and other ingredients and is designed to be healthy for the skin. A mineral-based foundation can be considered more noncomedogenic and natural than liquid foundations. It is not as heavy, and pigments are added to a range of products including eye shadows and blush. Mineral foundations give good coverage yet are lightweight. Many companies offer a mineral makeup line. Titanium dioxide is a physical sunscreen added to many mineral makeup products. If lightly applied, mineral makeup can refract light from lines and creases. Mineral makeup is popular to use as camouflage makeup after surgery.

Greasepaint (GREES-paint) is a heavy cream makeup used for theatrical purposes.

Cake (pancake) makeup is a heavy cream foundation. It is applied to the face with a moistened cosmetic sponge. It gives good coverage and is generally used to camouflage scars and pigmentation defects. It is also used for film and video applications.

Foundation Application

The success of makeup application depends on the correct color selection and begins with the application of the foundation. When correctly applied, foundation creates an even canvas for the rest of the makeup application. Skin tone determines the selection of foundation color. Skin tones are generally classified as warm, cool, or neutral. Warm tones are generally classified as yellow, orange, or red-orange. Cool tones are generally referred to as blue, blue-green (olive), or blue-red (pink). Neutral skin has equal amounts of warm and cool tones (see "Makeup Color Theory" later in this chapter).

Foundation should always be matched as closely as possible to actual skin tone. If the foundation color is too light, it will have a chalky or ghostly appearance and will "sit" on top of the skin. If the color is too dark, it will look dirty or artificial on the skin. The best way to determine the correct foundation color for your client is to apply a stripe of color near the jawline. Blend slightly and then try other colors if necessary. The color that "disappears" is the correct one. Avoid creating a contrast between the color of the face and the color of the neck. Makeup should blend smoothly with no visible line of demarcation. Two colors can be mixed together to custom-blend a color. Foundations are applied to the face with the fingertips or a makeup sponge. The sponge can be moist or dry.

Concealers

Concealers (kahn-SEEL-urs) are used to cover blemishes and discolorations and may be applied before or after foundation. They are available in pots, pencils, wands, or sticks in a range of colors to coordinate with or match natural skin tones. Concealers may contain moisturizers or control oil, depending on the formulation (Figure 19–6). The chemical composition of concealers is similar to that of cream foundation.

Concealer Application

Concealer is removed from the container with a spatula and may be applied with a concealer brush, fingertips, or a sponge. Place it sparingly over blemishes or areas of discoloration and blend. It is important to match concealer color to skin color as closely as possible. Concealer that is noticeably lighter than the skin can appear "raccoon-like" and can actually draw attention to a problem area such as dark circles. If covering a blemish, match skin tone closely to avoid highlighting the blemish. The principles that apply to choosing foundation colors also apply to concealer colors. Concealer may be worn alone, without foundation, if chosen and blended correctly. Be sure to use it sparingly and soften the edges so that the complexion looks natural.

Face Powders

Face powder is used to add a **matte,** or dull, finish to the face. It enhances the skin's natural color, helping to conceal minor blemishes and discolorations, and tones down excessive color and shine. Face powder is also used to set foundation (Figure 19–7).

> ### Here's a Tip
>
> For a smoother makeup application, remember to have clients exfoliate their skin.

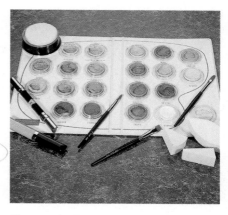

Figure 19–6 Concealers help to cover minor imperfections.

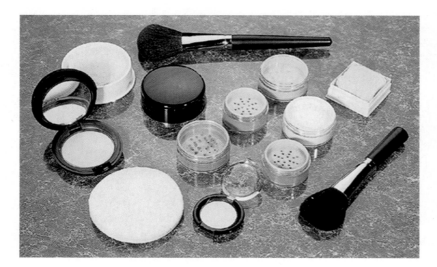

Figure 19–7 Powders come in two forms—loose and pressed.

Face Powder Chemistry

Two forms of face powder are widely used in the salon: loose powder and pressed powder. Both types have the same basic composition; pressed powders are compressed and held together with binders so they will not crumble. Coverage depends on the weight and formulation. Face powders consist of a powder base mixed with a coloring agent (pigment) and perfume. Ingredients in most powders include talc, zinc oxide, titanium dioxide, kaolin, chalk, zinc stearate, and magnesium stearate. Preservatives are also added to inhibit bacterial growth and preserve the product.

Face Powder Application

Face powders are available in a variety of tints and shades and in different weights. Face powder should match the natural skin tone and work well with the foundation. It should never appear caked or obvious. *Translucent* powder (colorless and sheer) blends with all foundations and will not change color when applied.

Apply face powder after foundation, using a brush or powder puff. Use a brush to blend and remove the excess. When suggesting products to a client, recommend both loose and pressed powders. Pressed powder is compact and easy to carry for quick touch-ups during the day. Loose powder is best used at home.

Blush

Cheek color is available in cream, liquid, dry (pressed), or loose powder form. It gives the face a natural-looking glow and helps create more attractive facial contours (Figure 19–8).

Blush Chemistry

Powder blush is the most common cheek color. Cream or gel cheek colors resemble cream foundation and are generally preferred for dry and

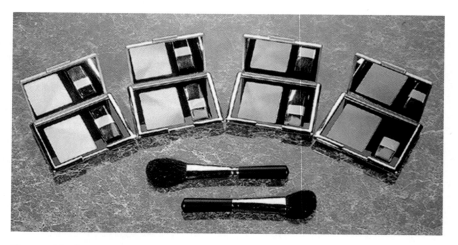

Figure 19–8 Blush contours cheekbones.

normal skin. Cream and liquid blush fall into two categories: oil-based and emulsions. Oil-based formulations are combinations of pigments in an oil or fat base. Blends of waxes (carnauba wax and ozokerite) and oily liquids (isopropyl myristate and hexadecyl stearate) create a water-resistant product. In addition, cream cheek colors contain water, thickeners, and a variety of surfactants or detergents that enable particles to penetrate the hair follicles and cracks in the skin. Because these ingredients can potentially clog the follicles, it is important to remind clients to remove their makeup each night.

Blush Application

Depending on the formulation, blush is usually applied with a brush or cotton puff. Creams are applied with fingers or sponges. Blend the color so that it fades softly into the foundation.

Eye Shadow

The eyes are the focal point in makeup design. Eye shadows accentuate and contour the eyes. They are available in almost every color of the rainbow—from warm to cool, neutral to bright, and light to dark. Some powder eye shadows are designed to be used either wet or dry. They also come in a variety of finishes, including matte, frost, or shimmer.

Eye Shadow Chemistry

Eye shadow is available in cream, pressed, and dry powder form (Figure 19–9). Stick and cream shadows are water based with oil, petrolatum, thickeners, wax, perfume, preservatives, and color added. Water-resistant shadows have a solvent base, such as mineral spirits. Pressed and dry powder eye shadow ingredients are similar to pressed face powder and powdered cheek color.

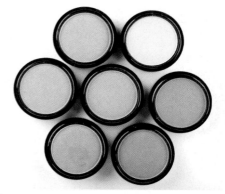

Figure 19–9 Eye shadows come in a variety of colors and forms.

Eye Shadow Application

Choose colors to bring out the eyes, even if the application is subtle. When applied to the lids, eye shadow makes the eyes appear brighter and more expressive. Matching eye shadow to eye color creates a flat field of color and should generally be avoided. Using color other than the eye color (that is, a contrasting or complementary color) can enhance the eyes. Using light and dark also brings attention to the eyes.

Generally, a darker shade of eye shadow makes the natural color of the iris appear lighter, while a lighter shade makes the iris appear deeper. However, the only set rules for selecting eye makeup colors are that they should enhance the client's eyes and color choices should be flattering. If desired, eye makeup color may match or coordinate with the client's clothing color. Look at the flecks in the iris of the eyes, and use colors to match or coordinate with these colors. Blending is the key, especially when using dark colors.

Eye shadow colors are generally referred to as highlighters, bases, and contour/dark colors.

- A *highlight* color is lighter than the client's skin tone and may have any finish. Popular choices include matte or iridescent (shiny). As the name suggests, these colors highlight a specific area, such as the brow bone. Remember that a lighter color such as white will make an area appear larger.
- A *base* color is generally a medium tone that is close to the client's skin tone. It is available in a variety of finishes. This color is generally used to even out the skin tone on the eye. It is often applied all over the lid and brow bone—from lash to brow, before other colors are applied—thus providing a smooth surface for the blending of other colors. If used this way, a matte finish is generally preferred.
- A *contour* color is deeper and darker than the client's skin tone. It is applied to minimize a specific area, to create contour in a crease, or to define the eyelash line.

To apply eye shadow, remove the product from its container with a spatula and then use a fresh applicator or clean brush. Unless you are doing corrective makeup, apply the base eye color close to the lashes on the eyelid, sweeping the color slightly upward and outward. Highlighters are used under the eyebrow. Darker colors are used in the crease. Blend to achieve the desired effect.

Eye makeup removers are either oil based or water based. Oil-based removers are generally mineral oil with a small amount of fragrance added. Water-based removers are a water solution to which acetone, boric acid, oils, lanolin or lanolin derivatives, and other solvents have been added.

Eyeliners

Eyeliner is used to outline and emphasize the eyes. It is available in pencil, liquid, and pressed (cake) forms. With eyeliner, you can create a line on the eyelid close to the lashes to make the eyes appear larger and the lashes fuller. Pencil is the most commonly used liner. Liquid eyeliners are more dramatic-looking. Powder liners or shadows can be applied wet or dry. Powder forms applied wet are more vivid and stay on longer.

Eyeliner Chemistry

Eyeliner pencils consist of a wax (paraffin) or hardened oil base (petrolatum) with a variety of additives to create color. They are available in both soft and hard form for use on the eyebrow as well as the eye. Liquid and cake eyeliners contain ingredients such as alkanolamine (a fatty alcohol), cellulose, ether, polyvinylpyrrolidone, methylparaben, antioxidants, perfumes, and titanium dioxide.

Eyeliner Application

Eyeliner can be applied before or after eye shadow. Most clients prefer eyeliner that is the same color as the lashes or mascara, for a more natural look. More intense colors may be preferred to match seasonal color trends.

? Did You Know

Any eye shadow can be used as either a brow color or an eyeliner.

Be extremely cautious when applying eyeliner. You must have a steady hand and be sure that your client remains still. Sharpen the eyeliner pencil and wipe with a clean tissue before and after each use. Also, remember to sanitize the sharpener after each use.

Apply to the desired area with short strokes and gentle pressure; the most common placement is close to the lash line. For powder shadow liner application, scrape a small amount onto a tissue or tray and apply to the eyes with a disposable applicator or clean brush. If desired, wet the brush before the application for more intense and lasting color.

Eye shadow may be applied as eyeliner with an eyeliner brush to create a softer lined effect. Whether you are using shadow or pencil liner, it may be helpful to gently pull the skin taut—from right below the eyebrow and upward—to ensure smooth application. Eye shadow can also be used for brow color.

Eyebrow Color

Eyebrows frame the eye. Eyebrow pencils or shadows are used to add color and shape to the eyebrows. They can be used to darken the eyebrows, correct their shape, or fill in sparse areas. For the best results, match the natural brow color or use a close shade of brown.

Eyebrow Color Chemistry

The chemistry of eyebrow products is similar to that of eyeliner pencils and eye shadows (Figure 19–10).

Eyebrow Color Application

Measure the brow shape and follow the shaping guidelines as closely as possible (Table 19–6). Avoid harsh contrasts between hair and eyebrow color, such as pale blonde or silver hair with black eyebrows. Taupe or grey are good color choices. Brown is usually a good choice, but reddish browns can be an unflattering tone.

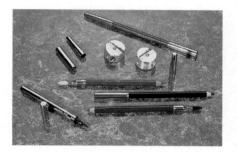

Figure 19–10 Pencils are used for the lips, eyes, and brows.

To color in the brows, follow the application instructions for eyeliner or eye shadows.

Mascara

Mascara darkens, defines, and thickens the eyelashes. It is available in liquid, cake, and cream form and in various shades and tints (Figure 19–11). The most popular mascara is a liquid in black or brown. These colors enhance the natural lashes, making them appear thicker and longer.

Mascara Chemistry

Mascaras are polymer products that contain water, wax, thickeners, film formers, and preservatives in their formulations. The pigments in mascara must be inert (unable to combine with other elements) and are made with carbon black, carmine, ultramarine, chromium oxide, and iron oxides. Some wand mascaras contain rayon or nylon fibers to lengthen and thicken the hair.

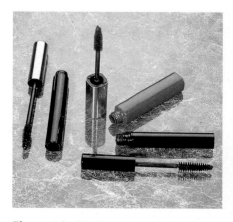

Figure 19–11 Mascara emphasizes the eyelashes.

Mascara Application

Dip a disposable wand into a clean tube of mascara, and apply from close to the base of the lashes out toward the tips, making sure your client is comfortable throughout the application. Dispose of the wand. Never double-dip the same wand back into the mascara that is used on different clients. Comb with a lash separator to avoid clumps.

If you are using an eyelash curler, you must curl the lashes before applying mascara. If lashes are curled after mascara, eyelashes may be broken or pulled out. Use extreme caution whenever you use an eyelash curler. It is easiest to learn how to use this tool by first observing its use. Ask your instructor to demonstrate before attempting to use an eyelash curler on someone else. Clients may prefer to curl their own lashes.

Apply mascara carefully. The most common injury with mascara application is poking the eye with the applicator. Practice applying mascara repeatedly until you feel confident enough to apply it on clients.

Lip Color

Most women have very definite ideas about their lip color. Lip color, lipstick, or gloss bring color to the face and finish a makeup design. Lip color worn alone enhances the face like no other product can. Some lip colors contain sunscreen to protect the lips from the harmful effects of the sun. Most contain moisturizers to keep lips from becoming dry or chapped.

Lip Color Chemistry

Lip color is available in several forms: creams, glosses, pencils, and sticks. All are formulas of oils, waxes, and dyes. Castor oil is a common ingredient in lipsticks; other oils used are olive, mineral, sesame, cocoa butter, petroleum, lecithin, and hydrogenated vegetable oils. Waxes commonly included in the ingredients are paraffin, beeswax, carnauba, and candelilla wax. Bromic acid, D & C Red No. 27, D & C Orange No. 17 Lake, and related tints are examples of common coloring agents. Iron oxides, mica, and annatto are natural colorants sometimes used in lip colors. Lip plumpers and stains are also popular.

Lip Color Application

Consider the client's preferences, eye color, skin tone, and lip shape before selecting and applying lip color. The current fashion trend may be lighter or darker lipstick colors, or a certain style, such as glossy, lightly stained, or matte (Figure 19–12).

Lip color must not be applied directly from the container unless it belongs to the client. Use a spatula to remove the lip color from the container and then take it from the spatula with a lip brush. Use the tip of the brush to line the lips. Connect the center peaks using rounded strokes, following the natural lip line. Aim for symmetry and balance. For long-lasting color, use a liner and then a lipstick with gloss over the lipstick.

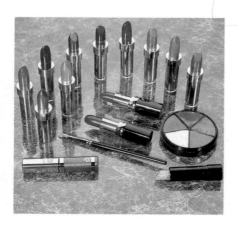

Figure 19–12 Lipsticks come in a variety of colors, textures, and forms.

Lip Liner

Lip liners are colored pencils used to outline and fill in the lips. Lining the lips also helps keep lip color on and keeps it from feathering. Lip liner is often used when doing corrective makeup. Lip liner comes in thin or thick pencil form. Some lip liners double as lipstick.

Lip Liner Application

To define and shape the lips, lip liner is usually applied before the lip color. Choose a lip liner that coordinates with the natural lip color or lipstick. The liner color should not be dramatically darker or brighter than the lip shade. If a darker liner is desired, fill in most of the lip with the liner and blend the lip color and lip liner to avoid harsh lines.

Sharpen the lip-liner pencil and wipe with a clean tissue before each use. Also remember to sanitize the sharpener before every use.

MAKEUP BRUSHES

Makeup brushes come in a variety of shapes and sizes (Figure 19–13). They may be made of synthetic or animal hair with wooden or metal handles. Commonly used makeup brushes and implements include the following items:

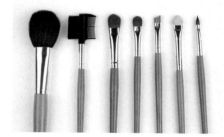

Figure 19–13 Quality brushes are important tools for the makeup artist.

- *Powder brush.* Large, soft brush used for blending and to apply powder or blush.
- *Blush brush.* Smaller, more tapered version of the powder brush used for applying powder blush.
- *Concealer brush.* Usually narrow and firm with a flat edge; used to apply concealer around the eyes or on blemishes.
- *Lip brush.* Similar to the concealer brush, but smaller and with a more tapered, rounded edge; also used to apply concealer.
- *Eye shadow brushes.* Available in a variety of sizes and ranging from soft to firm. The softer and larger the brush, the more blended the shadow will be. A firm brush is better for depositing dense color than for blending it. Small brushes are best for dark colors.
- *Eyeliner brush.* Fine, tapered, firm bristles; used to apply liner to the eyes.
- *Angle brush.* Firm, thin bristle; angled for use on the eyebrows or for eyeliner.
- *Lash and brow brush.* The comblike side is used to remove excess mascara on lashes, and the brush side is for brows.

Caring for Makeup Brushes

If you invest in high-quality makeup brushes, you will have them for years. Take good care of your brushes by cleaning them gently. A commercial sanitizer can be used for quick cleaning, although spray-on instant sanitizers contain a high level of alcohol and will dry brushes over time. A gentle shampoo or brush solvent should be used to thoroughly clean the brushes. These products will not hurt brushes and may actually help them last longer.

Brushes must be sanitized/disinfected properly after each client with liquid antibacterial soap and a disinfectant. Brush cleaners may not be enough to disinfect brushes for clients. The brush should always be put into running or still water with the *ferrule* (the metal ring that keeps bristles and handle together) pointing downward. If the brush is pointed up, the water may remove the glue that keeps the bristles in place. Rinse brushes thoroughly after cleansing. Do not pull on the brush fibers. Because they will dry in the shape they are left in, reshape the wet bristles and lay the brushes flat to dry. Cover brushes with a towel while drying and put in a closed container or drawer when dry.

MAKEUP COLOR THEORY

An understanding of how color works is vital to effective makeup application. Everyone sees color a little differently, and it may take a while to learn to see color shades naturally and easily. Primary, secondary, and tertiary colors, as well as warm, cool, and complementary colors are shown in the color wheels. Once you understand these basics of color theory, you can use your creative instincts to invent any color palette you desire (Figure 19–14).

- **Primary colors** are fundamental colors that cannot be obtained from a mixture. The primary colors are yellow, red, and blue (Figure 19–15).
- **Secondary colors** are obtained by mixing equal parts of two primary colors. Yellow mixed with red makes orange. Red mixed with blue makes violet. Yellow mixed with blue makes green (Figure 19–16).
- **Tertiary colors** (TUR-shee-ayr-ee KUL-urz) are formed by mixing equal amounts of a secondary color and its neighboring primary color on the color wheel. These colors are named by primary color first, secondary color second. For example, when we mix blue (a primary) with violet (a neighboring secondary), we call the resulting color blue-violet (Figure 19–17).

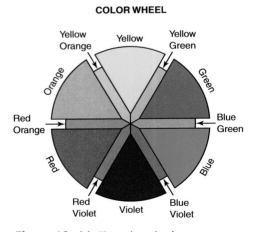

Figure 19–14 The color wheel.

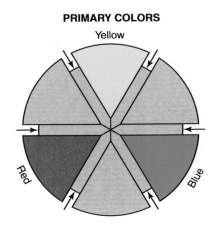

Figure 19–15 Primary colors.

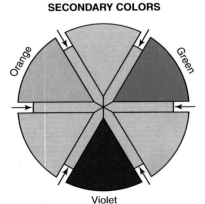

Figure 19–16 Secondary colors.

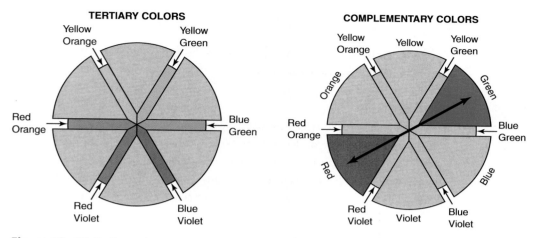

Figure 19–17 Tertiary colors.

Figure 19–18 Complementary colors.

- A primary and secondary color directly opposite each other on the color wheel are called **complementary colors.** When mixed, these colors cancel each other out to create a neutral brown or gray color. When complementary colors are placed next to each other, each color makes the other look brighter, resulting in greater contrast (Figure 19–18). For example, if you place blue next to orange, the blue seems bluer, the orange brighter. Try this with magic markers or colored paper to compare. The concept of complementary colors is useful when determining color choices. For example, the use of complementary colors will emphasize eye color, making the eyes appear brighter.

Warm and Cool Colors

Learning the difference between warm and cool colors is essential to your success as a makeup artist. This is the basis of all color selection, and understanding the difference will enable you to properly enhance your client's coloring (Figure 19–19).

- **Warm colors** have a yellow undertone and range from yellow and gold through the oranges, red-oranges, most reds, and even some yellow-greens.

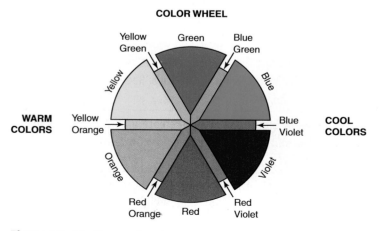

Figure 19–19 Warm and cool colors.

Warm colors have a yellow undertone (sunshine).

Cool colors have a **blue** undertone (water).

- **Cool colors** suggest coolness and are dominated by blues, greens, violets, and blue-reds.
- Reds can be both warm and cool. If the red is orange based, it is warm. If it is blue based, it is cool.
- Greens are similar: if a green contains more gold, it is warm; if it contains more blue, it is cool.

You may hear people refer to a color as having blue in it. For example: "This lipstick has a blue base/undertone" or "That is more of a cool blush than a warm one." This does not mean that the color is truly blue. Rather, it means that when the pigments were mixed to create that cosmetic, more blue color was added. Cool colors will be more pink or purple rather than peach or orange (Table 19–1).

Table 19–1

COLOR TEMPERATURES	
MAKEUP COLOR/ TEMPERATURE	**DESCRIPTION**
Pink—cool/warm	We think of pink as being a warm, rosy color, but a pastel (tint) is cool looking. When more red is added to white, the pink becomes warmer. Pink is flattering to skin tones unless the skin is ruddy. Pink combines well with other shades and tints of pink, blue, black, green, yellow, grey, purple, brown, beige, and white.
Blue—cool	Blue is complementary to most skin tones. Lighter blues enhance darker skin, while darker blue brings out color in lighter skin. Blue combines well with almost all other colors.
Purple—cool/warm	Mixed with pale tints of orchid and lavender, purple is cool. Darker shades (plum) with red undertones are warm. Purple is not kind to blemished or reddish skin tones and should be studied carefully against the skin. Purple combines well with pink, white, grey, and soft blue, beige, black, and pale yellow.
Green—cool/warm	Green is easy on the eyes and flattering to many skin tones. Bright green can intensify red in the skin. Blue greens are cool and generally attractive colors for both light and dark skin. Green combines well with other greens, blue, yellow, orange, beige, brown, white, and black.
Brown—warm	Brown can be kind to many complexion tones. Other reflecting or accent colors can be worn near the face if the skin is dark brown. Brown combines well with green, beige, blue, pink, yellow, orange, gold, white, and black.
Red—warm/cool	Red is a warm and exciting color, easy for most people to wear. Red with blue undertones is cool; with yellow undertones it is warm. Red of a specific tint or shade may not be kind to a ruddy complexion. Freckles will look darker when red is reflected onto the face. Red combines well with many other colors. Among them are black, white, beige, grey, blue, navy, green, and yellow.
Black—neutral	Black combines well with all other colors. A black costume can create a contrast for light skin and light or dark hair. When the skin and hair are dark, a color contrast near the face acts as a frame or highlight for the face.
White—cool/neutral	White is easy to wear, but be cautious of its undertones. Some materials reflect beige or yellow undertones (off-white), while others appear slightly blue. White combines well with all other colors.
Grey—neutral	A cool–neutral grey combines well with many other colors.

SELECTING MAKEUP COLORS

Now that we have determined warms and cools, it is time to learn a system that will help you feel more comfortable when choosing colors for your clients. Keep in mind this is simply one way of choosing colors. The art of makeup application allows for more than one way to achieve the result you desire. Once you learn the rules of a basic color selection system, you can then go on to expand them.

As you look at the color wheel, think of it as a tool for determining color choice. There are three main factors to consider when choosing colors for a client: skin color, eye color, and hair color. Assess the client's features during the consultation.

Determining Skin Color

When determining skin color, you must first decide if the skin is light, medium, or dark. Then determine whether the tone of the skin is warm or cool (use Table 19–2 as a guide). You may not see true skin colors in the beginning. Give yourself time and practice to develop your eye. Skin color also comes from the pigmentation in the skin and the blood showing through the skin.

A neutral skin tone contains equal elements of warm and cool, no matter how light or dark the skin is. Match the foundation color to the color of the skin, or use the corrective techniques discussed later in this chapter. Once you have determined if the skin is light, medium, or dark, you can choose eye, cheek, and lip colors to match the skin color level, or try contrasting colors for more impact. Most skin tones and levels (light to dark) can wear a surprisingly wide range of eye, cheek, and lip colors.

- If skin color is light, you can use light colors for a soft, natural look. Medium to dark colors will create a more dramatic look.
- If skin color is medium, medium tones will create an understated look. Light or dark tones will provide more contrast and will appear bolder.
- If skin color is dark, dark tones will be most subtle. Medium to medium-light or bright tones will be striking and vivid.

Table 19–2

SKIN TONES		
TONE	**UNDERTONES**	**ETHNICITY**
Ivory to fair	Fair, light skin with creamy or slightly pink undertones	Light Caucasians to light Asian, Hispanic
Beige or medium	Medium skin with pink or yellow	Medium Caucasians, medium Asian, Hispanic, black
Olive or warm	Olive skin with gold/yellow or orange/red	Tanned Caucasians, medium Asians, Hispanic, black
Deep or dark	Black skin with brown/yellow, brown/red, or brown/blue	Dark Hispanic to very black skin

Be cautious when choosing tones lighter than the skin. If the color is too light, it will turn grey or chalky on the skin. Look for translucent, shimmery colors if you are choosing these tones.

Complementary Colors for Eyes

As you begin recommending eye, cheek, and lip colors, neutrals will always be your safest choice. They contain elements of warm and cool and work well on any skin tone, eye color, or hair color. They come in variations of brown or grey. For instance, they may have a warm or cool base with brown tones. Or you might choose a plum-brown, which would be considered a cool neutral. An orange-brown would be considered a warm neutral. Charcoal grey is a cool neutral color, as is blue-grey.

Contrary to popular belief, matching eye color with shadow color is not the best way to enhance it; it only creates a flat region of color. By contrasting eye color with complementary colors, you emphasize the color most effectively. Matching the flecks of color in the eyes or clothing colors can also complement the color scheme.

The following are guidelines for selecting eye makeup colors. Refer to the color wheel for additional help in determining complementary colors.

- *Complementary colors for blue eyes.* Orange is the complementary color to blue. Because orange contains yellow and red, shadows with any of these colors in them will make your eyes look bluer. Common choices include gold, warm orange-browns like peach and copper, red-browns like mauves and plum, and neutrals like taupe or camel.
- *Complementary colors for green eyes.* Red is the complementary color to green. Because red shadows tend to make the eyes look tired or bloodshot, pure red tones are not recommended. Instead, use brown-based reds or other color options next to red on the color wheel. These include red-orange, red-violet, and violet. Popular choices are coppers, rusts, and purples.
- *Complementary colors for brown eyes.* Brown eyes are neutral and can wear any color. Recommended choices include such contrasting colors as greens or blues. Grey is not as flattering when combined with brown.

Cheek and Lip Color

After choosing the eye makeup, use the color wheel to determine whether your choices are warm or cool. Next, coordinate the cheek and lip makeup in the same color family as the eye makeup. For example, suppose your client has green eyes, and you recommended plums for her, which are cool. Now you should stay with cool colors for the cheeks and lips, so they will coordinate with the eye makeup. You could also choose neutrals because they contain both warm and cool elements and coordinate with any makeup colors.

It is not recommended to mix warms and cools on a face. They will compete with each other and create an "off" appearance. Staying within the color ranges you have chosen will ensure a balanced, beautiful look.

Here's a Tip

Be careful with orange or red tones in eye shadows because they can make the eyes look tired.

Hair Color

Hair color needs to be taken into account when determining makeup colors. For example, if a woman has blue eyes, your instinct might be to select orange-based eye makeup as the complementary choice. But if she has cool blue-black hair, the orange will not be flattering. In this case, you would choose cool colors to coordinate with the hair color. Red-violets (plums) would be a more flattering choice. Look at orange on the color wheel: it is warm. Go around the wheel toward the cool end. Red-violets are the closest to orange on the color wheel while still remaining cool. As mentioned earlier, there is a range of colors to choose from for any client.

Reviewing Color Selections

To review color selection, follow these steps:
1. Determine skin level: light, medium, or dark.
2. Determine skin undertone: warm, cool, or neutral.
3. Determine eye color: blue, green, brown, other.
4. Determine complementary colors.
5. Determine hair color: warm or cool.
6. Choose eye makeup colors based on complementary or contrasting colors.
7. Coordinate cheek and lip colors within the same color family: warm, cool, or neutral.
8. Apply makeup.

The best thing about choosing colors is the unlimited number of choices you have. Try one or all methods of choosing color. You can choose colors based only on skin tone, or you might find that working with complementary colors makes you feel more comfortable. Bring out hair color by matching or contrasting with it, or by blending all three areas as discussed here.

FACE SHAPES AND PROPORTIONS

Focusing on specific face shapes is not as popular as it used to be, because you mainly want to use light and dark to accentuate or diminish features. The rules are more relaxed with makeup; just about anything goes if you are not locked into rules about color or face shapes.

Analyzing Face Shapes

The basic rule of makeup application is to emphasize the client's attractive features while minimizing the less appealing features. Learning to see the face and its features as a whole and determining the best makeup for an individual takes practice. While the oval face with well-proportioned features has long been considered the ideal, other face shapes are just as attractive in their own way (Table 19–3). The goal of effective makeup application is to enhance the client's individuality, not to "remake" her image according to some ideal standard.

ACTIVITY

Apply makeup to a partner using color theory to choose and coordinate makeup colors. Have fun and experiment. Use the color selections and write down which colors enhance her appearance and coordinate with her wardrobe, and which ones do not. And remember, a haircut or hair color may represent a big commitment, but makeup does not. If you don't like it, just wash it off and try again!

Table 19–3

FACE SHAPES		
FACE SHAPE		**CHARACTERISTICS**
Oval		Widest at the temple and forehead, tapering down to a curved chin. This is considered the perfect or ideal facial shape because of its balance and overall look of symmetry. It is used as a standard for all face shapes.
Round		This face is widest at the cheekbone area, and is usually not much longer than it is wide, having a softly rounded jawline, short chin, and a rounded hairline over a rather full forehead.
Square		This face has a wide, angular jawline and forehead; the lines of this face are straight and angular.
Rectangle (Oblong)		This face shape is long and narrow; the cheeks are often hollowed under prominent cheekbones. Corrective makeup can be applied to create the illusion of width across the cheekbone line, making the face appear shorter and wider.
Triangle (pear-shaped)		Like a pyramid, this face is widest at its base or jawline, tapering up to slightly narrower cheeks, and reaching its apex at a narrow forehead. A jaw that is wider than the forehead characterizes the pear-shaped face. Corrective makeup can be applied to create width at the forehead, slenderize the jawline, and add length to the face.
Inverted triangle		This facial shape is wide at the temple and forehead area, forming a triangle that tapers down to a narrow chin.
Heart		Somewhat similar to the diamond shape, this face has a small, pointed chin and narrow jawline, but is wider at the forehead. It is usually soft rather than angular, and has some prominence in the cheekbone area.
Diamond		Widest at the cheekbones, this face has a narrow chin and forehead. It is angular in form, and the measurements of the jaw and hairline are approximately the same.

The Standard: An Oval-Shaped Face

The artistically ideal proportions and features of the oval face are the standard you will refer to when learning the techniques of corrective makeup application. The face is divided into three equal horizontal sections (Figure 19–20). The first third is measured from the hairline to the top of the eyebrows. The second third is measured from the top of the eyebrows to the end of the nose. The final third is measured from the end of the nose to the bottom of the chin. The ideal oval face is approximately three-fourths as wide as it is long. The distance between the eyes is the width of one eye (Figure 19–21).

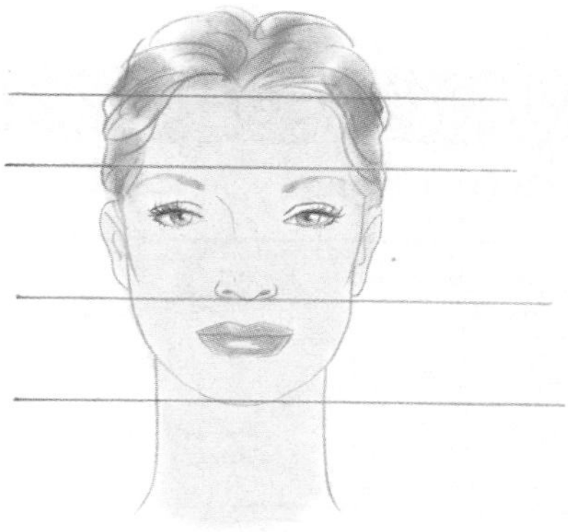

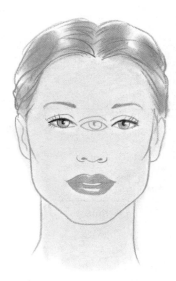

Figure 19–20 The oval face is divided into three equal horizontal sections.

CORRECTIVE MAKEUP

Corrective makeup mainly involves using light and dark colors to highlight and contour features. All faces are interesting in their own special ways, but none are perfect. When you analyze a client's face, you might see that the nose, cheeks, lips, or jawline are not the same on both sides; one eye might be larger than the other; or the eyebrows might not match. In fact, these tiny imperfections can make the face more interesting if treated artfully. In any case, facial makeup can create the illusion of better balance and proportion when so desired. Corrective makeup can be very effective if applied properly. However, a new makeup artist should proceed with caution because improper application, insufficient blending, or the wrong choice of colors can make the face look artificial.

Facial features can be accented with proper highlighting, subdued with correct shadowing and shading, and balanced with the proper hairstyle. A basic rule for makeup application is that highlighting emphasizes a feature, while shadowing minimizes it. A highlight is produced when a cosmetic, usually a concealer or pencil that is lighter than the original foundation, is used on a particular part of the face. Conversely, a shadow is formed when the product is darker than the skin color. The use of shadows (dark colors and shades) minimizes prominent features so that they are less noticeable.

Figure 19–21 The standard distance between the eyes is the width of one eye.

Before you undertake any kind of corrective makeup application, you should have a clear sense of how to contour and highlight the shape of the faces you will be working with (Table 19–4).

Jawline and Neck Area

When applying makeup, you can blend the foundation onto the neck so that the client's color is consistent from face to neck. Always set with a translucent powder to avoid transfer onto the client's clothing.

For a small face and a short, thick neck, use a slightly darker foundation on the side of the neck than the one used on the face. This will make the neck appear thinner.

Table 19–4

CORRECTIVE MAKEUP TECHNIQUES		
FACIAL FEATURE		**CORRECTIVE TECHNIQUES**
Round/square face		Use two foundations, light and dark, with the darker shade blended on the outer edges of the temples, cheekbones, and jawline, and the light one from the center of the forehead down the center of the face to the tip of the chin.
Triangular		Apply a darker foundation over the chin and neck and a lighter foundation through the cheeks and under the eyes to the temples and forehead, and then blend them together over the forehead for a smooth and natural finish.
Narrow face		Blend a light shade of foundation over the outer edges of the cheekbones to bring out the sides of the face.
Wide jaw		Apply a darker foundation from below the cheekbones, and along the jawline, and blend into the neck.
Double chin		To minimize a double chin, apply shading under the jawline and chin over the full area.
Long, heavy chin		To make a long or heavy chin appear less prominent, apply darker foundation over the area.
Receding chin		Highlight the chin by using a lighter foundation than the one used on the face.
Protruding forehead		Apply a darker shade of foundation over the area.

FACIAL FEATURE		CORRECTIVE TECHNIQUES
Narrow forehead		Apply a lighter foundation along the hairline and blend onto the forehead.
Wide nose		Apply foundation a shade lighter to the center of the nose. Apply darker foundation on both sides, and blend them together.
Short nose		A lighter shade of foundation is blended onto the tip of the nose and between the eyes.

Corrective Makeup for the Eyes

The eyes are very important when it comes to balancing facial features. Proper application of eye colors and shadow can create the illusion of the eyes being larger or smaller and will enhance the overall attractiveness of the face (Table 19–5).

- Round eyes can be lengthened by extending the shadow beyond the outer corner of the eyes.
- Close-set eyes are closer together than the length of one eye. For eyes that are too close together, lightly apply darker shadow on the outer edge of the eyes and light on the inside near the nose.
- Protruding eyes can be minimized by blending a dark shadow carefully over the prominent part of the eyelid, carrying it lightly toward the eyebrow. Use a medium to deep shadow color.
- For heavy-lidded eyes, shadow evenly and lightly across the lid from the edge of the eyelash line to the small crease in the eye socket.
- To make small eyes appear larger, extend the shadow slightly beyond the side of the eyes.
- To correct wide-set eyes, apply the shadow to the inner side of the eyelid toward the nose, and blend carefully.
- For deep-set eyes, use bright, light, reflective colors. Use the lightest color in the crease, and a light to medium color sparingly on the lid and brow bone.
- To diminish dark circles under the eyes, apply concealer over the dark area, blending and smoothing it into the surrounding area. Set lightly with translucent powder.

Table 19–5

EYE SHAPES	
EYE SHAPES	**CORRECTIVE TECHNIQUES**
Hidden lids	1. With a darker color, create a crease in the middle of the upper lid. Avoid strong colors. 2. Highlight the brow bone. 3. Softly line upper and lower lashes. 4. Apply light (brown) mascara.
Small eyes	1. Place a lighter shadow over the lid, blending it out toward the temple and up to the eyebrow. 2. Apply a darker shadow to the crease and outer corners of the lower lids. 3. Blend eyeliner softly from the center to the outer corners of both eyes along the eyelashes. 4. Apply mascara, brushing the lashes carefully.
Round eyes	1. Apply a medium shade of shadow, blending it over the eyelid toward the eyebrow. 2. Apply dark shadow onto the crease and blend it out toward the temple. 3. Line the eye with an eyeliner pencil. 4. Extend and blend the colors applied in steps 1 and 3 toward the outer corner of the eye. 5. Apply mascara to the lashes heavier at the outer corners of the eyes.
Protruding eyes	1. Apply a medium color on the entire eyelid, and blend it toward the eyebrow. 2. Line the eye using a brown or grey eyeliner pencil. 3. Apply mascara.
Deep-set eyes	1. Apply a light eye shadow along the crease of the lid. 2. Blend in a medium color next to the outer corners of the eyelids. 3. Use a soft color to accentuate the eyes. 4. Clearly outline the eyes along the lashes. 5. Choose a dark shade of mascara.
Close-set eyes	1. Apply a paler shade to the lid and a darker shade to the outer corner. 2. Line the eye from the middle to the corner, and blend the shadow outward. 3. Apply mascara in an upward and outward motion.
Wide-set eyes	1. Extend a darker shadow to the inner corner of the eye toward the nose. 2. Blend a lighter shadow from the middle toward the outer corner. 3. Apply mascara with an inward motion toward the nose.

EYE SHAPES	CORRECTIVE TECHNIQUES
Drooping eyes	To offset the droop of the eye, which is often accompanied by a low bone structure or low lid fold, it is necessary to give the appearance of a lift to the entire eye area. **1.** Tweeze the under area of the outer portion of the brow to allow a better arch. **2.** Apply shading shadow in a band across the fold and smudge it outward. **3.** Apply highlighter directly under the arch of the brow. **4.** Apply eyeliner (if used) in a very thin line, and thicken it very slightly at the outside in a wedgelike point to give a lift to the eye.

Eyebrows

Reshaping and defining eyebrows can be an art unto itself. Well-groomed eyebrows are part of a complete makeup application. The eyebrow is the frame for the eye. Over-tweezed eyebrows can make the face look puffy or protruding, or they may give the eyes a surprised look. Subtle changes in the shape of the brows can make a big difference in the overall look (Table 19–6).

When a client wants to correct her eyebrow shape, begin by removing all unnecessary hairs and then demonstrate how to use the eyebrow pencil or shadow to fill in until the natural hairs have grown in again. When there are spaces in the eyebrow hair, they can be filled in with hairlike strokes of an eyebrow pencil or shadow applied with an angled brush. Use an eyebrow brush or finger to soften the pencil or shadow marks.

The Ideal Eyebrow Shape

The ideal eyebrow shape can be measured by using three lines (Figure 19–22). The first line is vertical, measuring from the side of the nose and inner corner of the eye upward. This is where the eyebrow should begin. The second line is from the outer corner of the nose to the outer corner of the eye. This is where the eyebrow should end. The third line is vertical, from the outer circle of the iris of the eye upward. The client should be looking straight ahead as you determine this line. This is where the highest part of the brow arch would ideally be. Of course, not everyone's eyebrows fit exactly within these measurements, so use them only as guidelines.

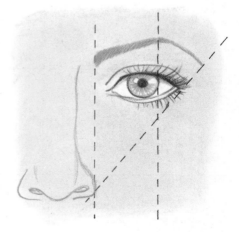

Figure 19–22 The ideal eyebrow shape.

The Lips

Lips are usually proportioned so that the curves or peaks of the upper lip fall directly in line with the nostrils. In some cases, one side of the lips may differ from the other. Lips can be very full, very thin, or uneven (Table 19–7). Various lip colors can be used to create the illusion of better proportions. It is best to follow the natural lip line as closely as possible.

Table 19–6

BROW SHAPES	
BROW SHAPES	**CORRECTIVE TECHNIQUES**
High arch	When the arch is too high, remove the superfluous hair from the top of the brow and fill in the lower part with eyebrow pencil or shadow. Build up the shape by layering color lightly until the desired effect is achieved. Adjustments to eyebrow shape can also be used to enhance other facial features.
Low forehead	A low arch gives more height to a very low forehead.
Wide-set eyes	The eyes can be made to appear closer together by extending the eyebrow line closer together past the inside corners of the eyes. However, care must be taken to avoid giving the client a frowning look.
Close-set eyes	To make the eyes appear farther apart, widen the distance between the eyebrows and extend them slightly outward.
Round face	Arch the brows high to make the face appear narrower.
Long face	Making the eyebrows almost straight can create the illusion of a shorter face. Do not extend the eyebrow lines farther than the outside corners of the eyes.
Square face	The face will appear more oval if there is a higher brow arch.

Table 19–7

LIP SHAPES	
LIP SHAPE	**CORRECTIVE TECHNIQUES**
Thin lower lip	Line the lower lip to make it appear fuller. Fill in with lip color to create balance between the lower and upper lips.
Thin upper lip	Use a lip-lining pencil to outline the upper lip and then fill in with lip color to balance with the lower lip.
Thin upper and lower lips	Use a lip-lining pencil to outline the upper and lower lips slightly fuller, but do not try to draw far over the natural lip line. Use a lighter color to make lips appear larger.
Cupid bow or pointed upper lip	To soften the peaks of the upper lip, use a medium lip-lining pencil to draw a softer curve. Extend the line to the desired shape. Fill in with a light to medium lip color.
Large, full lips	Draw a thin line just inside the natural lip line with a lining pencil. Use soft, flat lipstick colors that will attract less attention than frosty or glossy lip colors.
Small mouth and lips	Use a lip-lining pencil to outline both the upper and lower lips. Fill in lips with soft or frosted colors.
Drooping corners	Line the lips to build the corners of the mouth. This will minimize the drooping appearance. Fill in lips with a soft, flattering color.

continues on next page

Table 19–7 *(continued)*

LIP SHAPE	CORRECTIVE TECHNIQUES
Uneven lips	Outline the upper and lower lips with a soft color to create the illusion of matching proportions.
Straight upper lip	Use a lip-lining pencil to create a slight dip in the center of the upper lip, directly beneath the nostrils. Fill in with a flattering color.
Fine lines around the lips	Outline the lips with a noncreamy lip pencil, and then fill in with a product formulated to keep lip color from running into fine lines. Lighter colors work better and do not show the lines as much as dark or red colors do.

Skin Tones

For various reasons, some clients may wish to alter their skin tone. In terms of corrective makeup, you will be dealing with two basic skin tones.

- For ruddy skin (skin that is red, windburned, or affected by rosacea), apply a yellow or green-tinted foundation to affected areas, blending carefully. You can then apply a light layer of foundation with a yellow base over the entire complexion. Set it with translucent or yellow-based powder. Avoid using red or pink blushes. The skin color should still be natural-looking.
- For sallow skin (skin that has a yellowish hue), apply a pink-based foundation on the affected areas and blend carefully into the jaw and neck. Set with translucent powder. Avoid using yellow-based colors for eyes, cheeks, and lips.

CLIENT CONSULTATIONS

The first step in the makeup process, as with all services that take place in the salon, is the client consultation. A service should always begin with a warm introduction to your client. Visually assess the client to understand her personal style. This will give you cues as you continue your consultation (Figure 19–23). Ask the client questions that will elicit her preferences and concerns. Have the client fill out a questionnaire to get insight into her makeup needs (Table 19–8). Listen closely, and try not to impose your own opinions. Record the client's needs, and make recommendations based on the general application guidelines. If the client chooses not to act on your recommendations, do not take it personally. In time, perhaps she will.

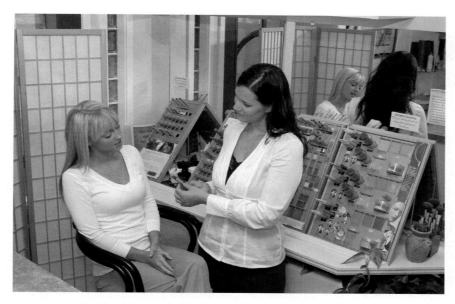

Figure 19–23 The makeup consultation.

Gather information on the client's skin condition, how much or how little makeup she wears, the amount of time spent applying makeup, colors she likes or dislikes, and any makeup problem areas. Record this information on a client consultation card. Also write down the colors you use and your recommendations on the client chart (Table 19–9) so that you can refer to them at the end of the makeup application. Reviewing and restating your written advice with the client at the end of the service will also help you recommend the retail products that would be beneficial for her.

After the service, escort your client to the retail or reception area, where you can assist her in choosing the products you have recommended. Ask if the client has any other questions. If possible, set up a time for the next appointment. Present a business card with your name on it and thank the client as you say good-bye, or bring the client to the receptionist, who will check her out.

The Makeup Station and Consultation Area

The area that you use for services and consultations must be clean and organized (Figure 19–24). No one wants to see a messy makeup unit or dirty brushes lying about. Clean your brushes after each use, and organize your makeup area daily. Also keep a portfolio in the consultation area that includes photographs of your own work or pictures from magazines. The client can go through your portfolio to find styles and colors that appeal to her. Try to have the makeup station in a visible yet semiprivate area of the salon for client privacy.

Lighting

Adequate and flattering lighting is essential for the application. Natural light is the best choice, but if it is necessary to use artificial light, it should be a combination of incandescent light (warm bulb light) and fluorescent light (cool industrial tube light). If you must choose between the two, incandescent light is warmer and will be more flattering.

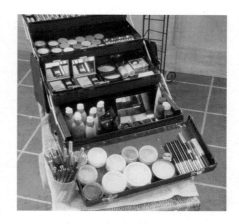

Figure 19–24 A professional makeup kit.

Table 19–8

THE CLIENT QUESTIONNAIRE

Confidential Makeup Questionnaire

PLEASE PRINT   Today's Date_____

First Name _____ Last Name _____ Date of Birth _____ / _____

Street _____ Apt# _____ City _____ State _____ Zip _____

Phone—Home ( ) _____ Work ( ) _____ Cell ( ) _____
_____ Phone ( ) _____

Your Occupation _____

Referred by ☐ Friend ☐ Mailer ☐ Walk-by ☐ Yellow Pages ☐ Gift Certificate ☐ Other
_____

1. Have you ever had a professional makeover? ☐ Yes ☐ No
2. If yes, what did you like (dislike) about the session? _____
3. If no, how did you learn to apply makeup? _____
4. What are some of your goals today? _____
5. What special areas of concern do you have? _____
6. Do you wear contact lenses? ☐ Yes ☐ No   If yes, are they ☐ Hard ☐ Soft
7. Do you take any medications that cause your eyes to be dry or itch?
   ☐ Yes ☐ No If yes, what? _____
8. Are you currently taking Accutane® or have you taken it in the past? ☐ Yes ☐ No
   If yes, describe the course of treatment and how long. _____
9. Do you have any health condition that may cause sensitivity in your skin or eye area?
   ☐ Yes ☐ No If yes, what? _____
10. Do you have any allergies? ☐ Yes ☐ No   If yes, please indicate. _____
11. Do you have any allergies to skin care products? ☐ Yes ☐ No   If yes, What? _____
12. Do you smoke? ☐ Yes ☐ No
13. What are your favorite colors: _____
14. Describe an ideal look for your makeup. _____

I understand that the services offered are for educational purposes only. I fully acknowledge that I do not have any known allergies to makeup products. I authorize the makeup artist to apply products to my face.

Salon Policies
1. We require a 24-hour cancellation notice.
2. Please arrive on time for appointments.
3. There is a $25 charge for a no-show appointment.
4. Health regulations do not allow us to accept returned products unless they are unopened and in their original packaging.
5. Returns are given salon credit only. No cash refunds.

I fully understand and agree to the above salon policies.

_____   _____
Client's Signature   Date

Table 19–9

THE CLIENT CHART

Name_____ Date_____

Skin Care _____

Makeup remover _____

Cleanser _____

Freshener _____

Moisturizer _____

Makeup

Foundation ☐ Liquid ☐ Wet/dry

Color _____

Concealer _____

Powder _____

Brow pencil _____

Eye shadows _____

Orbital area _____

Crease _____

Lid _____

Other _____

Eyeliner pencil _____

Mascara _____

Lip pencil _____

Lipstick _____

Special Instructions

_____

_____

_____

Next Appointment

_____

Day   Month

Make sure that the light always shines directly and evenly on the face. Check the makeup on both sides of the face for evenness, and take the client over to a window if necessary to check the final look in natural light. Clients who can see the finished look in natural light are more comfortable with purchasing the products you recommend. Makeup changes with the lighting, so it is important to use the appropriate lighting to match the lighting that the makeup is being applied for, such as an outdoor wedding.

Sanitation

For all products:

- Do not touch product containers to hands or previously used applicators. Distribute onto clean pallets, brushes, or sponges.
- Scrape powders with clean brushes or spatulas onto a tissue or clean tray.
- Scrape off powders and other products before and after use if contaminated.
- Do not apply lipstick or gloss directly to the lips from the container or tube. Use a spatula to remove the product, and then apply with a clean brush.
- If the product is accidentally contaminated, follow your supervisor's directions either to throw away the product or give it to your client. Do not put it back with your clean products to reuse.

For applicators, pencils, testers, and so forth, follow these sanitation guidelines:

- *Applicators.* Use sanitary applicators, brushes, and spatulas to distribute products. Disinfect after each use. Do not double-dip dirty spatulas, wands, or brushes back into products.
- *Pencils.* Sharpen pencils, spray to disinfect, and wipe with tissue—if they cannot be sharpened, they cannot be sanitary.
- *Testers.* Keep testers clean and sanitary. To avoid contamination, assist clients who are using testers.
- *Pallets and supplies.* Wash and disinfect artist trays, brushes, sharpeners and mixing cups after each use.

PRODUCTS, TOOLS, AND SUPPLIES

Supplies and Accessories

Numerous supplies and accessories are useful for makeup applications (Figure 19–25; Table 19–10). These supplies include the following:

- *Sponges* are good for blending foundation, concealer, and powder. Wedge shapes are the most versatile. Use the large, thicker end of the sponge for foundation to get more coverage and control. Use the smaller sides to blend around the eyes.
- *Brushes* to blend powder, blush, and eye shadows work better than sponge tips or fingers. Brushes allow for better control and better blending. They also feel nicer to the skin and are more professional. Make sure you sanitize brushes between clients. Be prepared and have enough brushes on hand for multiple uses throughout the day. Buy good-quality brushes. Art stores or brush wholesalers are good places to buy brushes.
- For straight lashes, a lash *curler* can be used before applying mascara.
- Use a sanitary disposable *wand* to dip into the mascara. Do not double-dip. Roll the wand around in a circle rather than pumping it in and out because this dries out the mascara.
- A lash *comb* separates lashes so lashes look finished and are not clumpy or messy looking. Metal combs work the best. Do not point combs or brushes toward the eyes or poke the skin. Point the prongs down or up away from the eye. Rest the hand on the face to steady the application. If the client moves too much, let her apply the mascara.

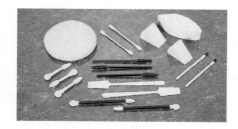

Figure 19–25 Disposable applicators are necessary for sanitation.

Table 19–10

MAKEUP SUPPLIES CHECKLIST		
SKIN CARE	**MAKEUP**	**SUPPLIES/ACCESSORIES**
cleanser	concealer	cape
toner	highlighter	disinfectant/sanitation supplies
moisturizer	contour color	tweezers
	foundation	hair clip/headband
	powder	brushes
	eye shadow	pencil sharpener
	eyeliner	mirror
	mascara	lash comb
	blush	lash curler
	lip gloss	disposables (spatulas, cotton swabs, mascara wands, mixing cups, sponges, tissues, applicators)
	lip liners	
	lipsticks	

- Use hair *clips* or a headband to hold the hair away from the face. Remove these items and fix the client's hair before showing her the finished look.
- Use a *cape* or towel around the client's neck to protect her clothes. Have her lean toward you to protect clothing from powder application. Put a tissue or disposable *neck strip* under the collar and around the neck to keep the cape clean for other clients, or wash the cape each time.
- Use sanitizing agent to clean hands, surfaces, and tools.
- Use *tissue* for blotting lipstick or powder. Hold it under the eye when applying dark shadow so it does not flake onto the skin.
- Use *spatulas* to remove products such as concealer or lipstick from jars and containers. Do not put fingers into products. Use a clean spatula each time. Do not double-dip.
- *Cotton* swabs are great for fixing mistakes. They are useful for blending under the eyes and especially when fixing mascara messes. Put a little foundation on the cotton swab, place it on your fingertip, and roll off the excess before using.
- Mixing *cups* can be used for blending foundation colors together or mixing foundation and moisturizer for a lighter tinted foundation. Artist's *palettes* are also great for holding products.

Here's a Tip

Use an artist's palette to distribute your makeup products into once you narrow your color choices. This keeps the original product sanitary and it is easy to work with. A palette is especially helpful when using loose mineral makeup. Remember the colors you used, so you can recommend and record them on your client charts.

Products

Common products for makeup application include the following:

- *Cleanser*
- *Toner (freshener or astringent)*
- *Moisturizer*
- *Lip conditioner*
- *Concealer* is usually one to two shades lighter than foundation. You can apply this under or over the foundation beneath the eyes. It can also be used as a highlighter because it is lighter than the skin color, accentuating and bringing out features. A darker shade can be used as a contour. Light brings out the features, and dark causes them to recede.
- *Foundation* covers the skin to even out the skin tone and mask imperfections. Dark circles, blemishes, pigmentation, redness, and other facial features can be toned down with foundation. Face makeup comes in different forms—mainly cream, liquid, and powder. Mineral makeup is in vogue right now. Most skin tones have a yellow undertone. Most people need different makeup colors in the summer (darker) and winter (lighter).
- *Highlighters* are lighter than the skin color, and they accentuate and bring out features such as the brow bone under the eyebrow, the temples, the chin, and the cheekbones. Highlighters are used more extensively in photography than in everyday use.
- *Contouring* colors are darker shades used to define the cheekbones and make features appear smaller. Dark colors recede or diminish features.
- *Powder* sets the foundation and finishes the makeup blending. This is usually applied after the foundation and before the blush. It is also applied again after the blush to help blend and set the blush.
- Eye *shadow* can be applied as one color or a blend of colors. Powders or creams are packaged in palettes or big pencils, and they come in mattes, frosts, cools, and warms.
- *Eyeliner* accentuates the eyes. Liners are usually pencils. Eye shadow used with a thin brush dipped in water works as a wet liner. Dry shadow applied with a thin, firm brush also works well. Liner can be applied to the top and bottom edge of the eye on the outside of the lashes, not the inner part of the eye (unhealthy for the eye and can lead to infections).
- *Brow pencils* are typically light brown shades of pencil. They also come in cake form.
- *Mascara* enhances the eyes and lashes and finishes the makeup.
- *Blush* gives color to the face and accentuates cheekbones. Apply blush just below the cheekbones, blending on top of the bones toward the top of the cheeks (Figure 19–26).
- Lip *gloss* can give a shiny, moisturized look to the lips. Put on a gloss or lip moisturizer when starting the makeup application, so it can soak in and moisturize before starting to apply the liner. If the lips have too much gloss, the liner will not stick.

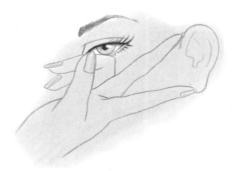

Figure 19–26 Measuring blush placement.

- Lip *liner* helps define the lips and keeps lipstick on longer.
- *Lipstick:* Light colors make lips appear larger; dark colors make lips look smaller. However, brighter colors show up more. Lip color can be tricky. Clients can be very selective about their lip color. Give them two or three shades to choose from.

MAKEUP APPLICATION TIPS AND GUIDELINES

The following guidelines should be considered in applying makeup:

- Fingernails should be short with smooth edges. Be especially cautious when working around the client's eyes!
- Blending and evenness are the most important factors in a good makeup application.
- Apply creams or liquids before powders, not afterward. Creams over powders do not blend, and you might end up with a big mess.
- Avoid tugging on the skin or rubbing too hard. If the client's head is moving or you have to hold it to keep it steady, your touch is too heavy.
- Do not hold the client's head or lift the eye skin unless it is absolutely necessary. Holding the head can feel too rough to the client. Lifting the skin will change the look when you let go of the skin around the eyes.
- To avoid getting products in the client's eyes, be sure they are closed when applying powder or eye shadow.
- Makeup is one area in esthetics where you have to apply downward, with the hairs on the face, when applying foundation and powder for better blending.
- If nothing else, mascara and lipstick are the two items that can enhance and give color to the face and eyes.

Table 19–11

MAKEUP APPLICATION CHECKLIST
1. Cleanse, tone, moisturize
2. Lip conditioner
3. Concealer
4. Foundation
5. Highlight
6. Contour
7. Powder
8. Eyebrows
9. Eye shadow
10. Eyeliner
11. Mascara
12. Blush
13. Lip gloss/moisturizer
14. Lip liner, lipstick

PROCEDURE 19–1

PROFESSIONAL MAKEUP APPLICATION

SKIN CARE PRODUCTS
- cleanser
- toner
- moisturizer

MAKEUP
- concealer
- highlighter
- contour color
- foundation
- powder
- eye shadow
- eyeliner
- mascara
- blush
- lip gloss
- lip liner
- lipstick

SUPPLIES
- cape
- disinfectant
- tweezers
- hair clip/headband
- brushes
- pencil sharpener
- mirror
- lash comb
- lash curler

DISPOSABLES
- spatulas
- cotton swabs
- mascara wands
- sponges
- tissues
- applicators

Your instructor may prefer a different method that may be equally correct. Completing a makeup application includes the consultation, setup, application, and clean-up procedures (Tables 19–10 and 19–11). Some artists like to apply the makeup working from the top to the bottom of the face—eyes, cheeks, and then lips. There are pros and cons to every method. You will likely come up with your own application procedure when working as a makeup artist.

Preparation

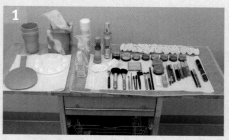

Set up products and colors. *(Figure P19–1-1)*

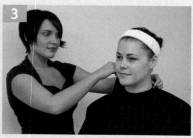

Drape the client. *(Figure P19–1-2)*

1 Determine the client's needs, and choose products and colors accordingly (Figure P19–1-1). Focus on your client's features and preferences. Discussing skin care or waxing is appropriate with a makeup client. Ask the following questions:
- Do you wear contacts or have allergies?
- What look do you want?
- What makeup products do you normally wear?
- What are your typical clothing colors?
- What is the special occasion or event?

2 Wash your hands.

3 Drape the client and use a headband or hair clip to keep her hair out of her face (Figure P19–1-2).

Procedure

Basic Makeup Applications

Preparing the face is like preparing a painting canvas for the palette of colors. The skin needs to be exfoliated and hydrated for the makeup to be applied successfully.

4 *Cleanser.* After washing your hands, cleanse the face if the client is wearing makeup or if the skin is oily.

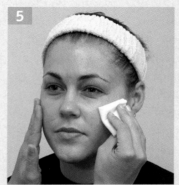

Apply toner or witch hazel. *(Figure P19–1-3)*

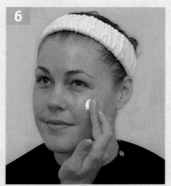

Apply moisturizer. *(Figure P19–1-4)*

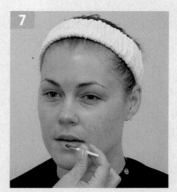

Lip conditioner. *(Figure P19–1-5)*

5 *Toner.* Use a cotton pad to apply the toner or witch hazel to cleanse the skin (Figure P19–1-3).

6 *Moisturizer.* Apply a moisturizer to prepare the skin for makeup (Figure P19–1-4).

7 *Lip conditioner.* Use a spatula to get the product out of the container. Apply with a brush (Figure P19–1-5). To give it more time to soak in and moisturize, put on the lip conditioner when starting the makeup application.

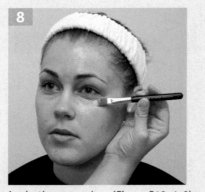

Apply the concealer. *(Figure P19–1-6)*

8 *Concealer.* Use a spatula to get the product out of the container. Choose a color one to two shades lighter than the foundation. You can apply this under or over the foundation beneath the eyes with a brush, sponge, or finger (Figure P19–1-6). It can also be used as the highlighter.

Note: Always use creams and liquids before applying powders, or they will not blend. If you are using a powder concealer or contour powder, apply these after the foundation.

PROCEDURE 19–1, CONT.

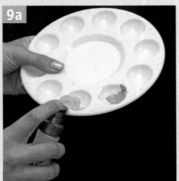

Choose the foundation. *(Figure P19–1-7)*

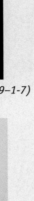

9 *Foundation.* Choose two colors to match the right shade. Use a spatula to get the product out of the container, or put some on a clean sponge or in a small container (Figure P19–1-7a,b). Apply to the jawline to match the skin color (Figure P19–1-8). Cover the skin to even out the skin tone and cover imperfections without over-rubbing the skin. Blend along the jaw and edges of the face (Figure P19–1-9). Blend downward to blend with facial hair and up around the hairline so the product does not stick in the hairline.

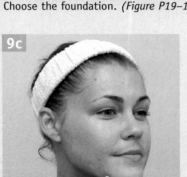

Apply to the jawline. *(Figure P19–1-8)*

Blend the foundation. *(Figure P19–1-9)*

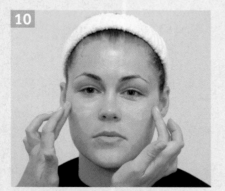

Apply highlighter to bring out features. *(Figure P19–1-10)*

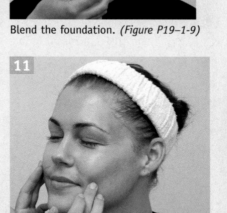

Apply contour for shading and minimizing features. *(Figure P19–1-11)*

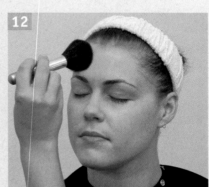

Lightly apply powder. *(Figure P19–1-12)*

10 *Highlighter.* Use a spatula to get the product out of the container. Apply a white or light color to accentuate and bring out features along the brow bone, the temples, chin, or above the cheek bones. Blend with your brush, a sponge, or your finger (Figure P19–1-10).

11 *Contouring.* Use a spatula to get the product out of the container. Apply a darker shade under the cheekbones and to other features you want to appear smaller (Figure P19–1-11).

12 *Powder.* Pour a little powder on a tissue to avoid cross-contamination. Apply to the brush and tap off excess powder onto the tissue. Use a powder brush or puff, and sweep downward all over the face to set the foundation (Figure P19–1-12).

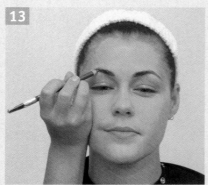

Color the brows using a pencil or brow powder. *(Figure P19–1-13)*

13 *Eyebrows.* Use a shade that is close to the hair color, or a shade the client likes. Apply color by using a pencil or cake eye shadow with a brush (Figure P19–1-13). Smudge with your finger, going in the opposite direction of the hair growth to blend. Then smooth back into place with a brow brush.

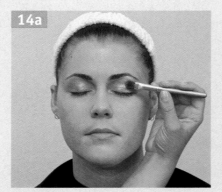

Apply the eye shadow base or light color all over the eye area. *(Figure P19–1-14)*

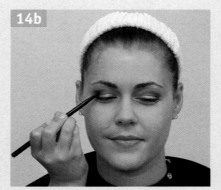

Apply a small amount of the darker eye shadow. *(Figure P19–1-15)*

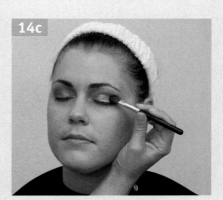

Blend the dark shadow. *(Figure P19–1-16)*

14 *Eye shadow.* Choose a light base color and apply all over the eyelid, from the lash line up to the brow. Stop color at the outside corner of the eye up to the outside corner of the brow (Figure P19–1-14).

Apply a darker shade to the crease: partially on top of the crease and partially underneath the crease. First tap the excess powder off the brush. Apply the color from the outside corner of

the eye to the area above the inside of the iris (Figure P19–1-15). Blend the color (Figure P19–1-16). *Optional:* Apply the eyeliner before applying the dark shadow color.

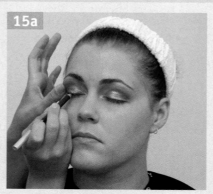

Line the eyes. *(Figure P19–1-17)*

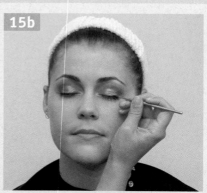

Blend and set the liner. *(Figure P19–1-18)*

15 *Eyeliner.* Sharpen the liner before and after use. Wet liner can also be used with a disposable or sanitized brush. Eye shadow can be applied as liner with a thin brush dipped in water; dry shadow can also be applied with a thin, firm brush for a more natural look. Make sure the liner is not too rough or so dry that it drags on the eye.

Have the client shut her eyes when you apply the liner on top of the eyelids. Then have her look up and away as you apply the lower liner under the eyes (Figure P19–1-17).

Apply to the top and bottom edge of the eye on the outside of the lashes. Bring the liner three-fourths of the way to the center of the eye, ending softly at the inside of the iris. Blend so that the color tapers off. Bringing the liner closer to the nose can make the eyes appear closer together. Lining only the outside corner makes the eyes appear farther apart. Blend the liner with a firm, small liner brush (Figure P19–1-18).

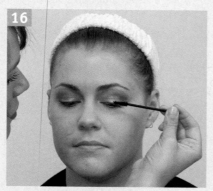

Carefully apply the mascara. *(Figure P19–1-19)*

16 *Mascara.* Dip a disposable brush into the mascara. Wipe off the excess. Have the client look down and focus on a fixed point to apply mascara to the top of the lashes (Figure P19-1-19). Comb with a lash comb before the product dries. Then have the client put her chin down while looking up at the ceiling to apply mascara to the bottom lashes. Comb before the client looks down to avoid smudging under the eye.

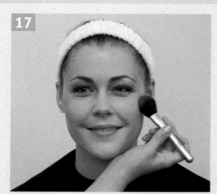

Apply the blush on the cheekbones. *(Figure P19–1-20)*

17 *Blush.* The blush color will depend on whether you choose a warm or cool color scheme. Tap off the excess powder on the brush. Apply blush just below the cheekbones, blending on top of the bones toward the top of the cheeks. The color should stop below the temple and not be

closer than two fingers away from the nose. It should not go lower than the nose, because this can "drag down the face." Blush should blend to the hairline, but not into it. Do not apply too much blush on the apple of the cheek; this makes the face look fatter. A horizontal line makes the face appear wider, whereas a vertical line makes it look thinner. Following the cheekbones usually works best (Figure P19–1-20).

18 ***Optional:*** *Lip conditioner/lip gloss.* This step applies if you did not already apply lip moisturizer in step 4. Use a spatula to get the product out of the container. Use a brush to apply. Put on a gloss or lip moisturizer when starting the makeup application,

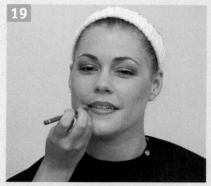

Line the lips. *(Figure P19–1-21)*

so it can soak in and moisturize before you start applying the liner. If the lips have too much gloss, the liner will not stick.

19 *Lip liner.* Sharpen the liner. Have the client smile and stretch her lips. With the lips pulled tight, the liner and lipstick brush glide on more smoothly. Line the outer edges of the lips first; then fill in and use the liner as a lipstick (Figure P19–1-21). This keeps the lipstick and color on longer.

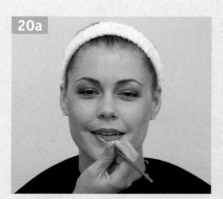

Apply and blend lipstick. *(Figure P19–1-22)*

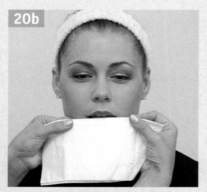

Blot lipstick. *(Figure P19–1-23)*

20 *Lipstick.* Use a spatula to get the product out of the container. Have the client select a color from among two or three choices. Apply the lipstick evenly with a lip brush. Rest your ring finger on the client's chin to steady your hand. Ask the client to relax her lips and

part them slightly. Brush on the lip color. Then ask the client to smile slightly so that you can smooth the lip color into any small crevices (Figure P19–1-22). Blot the lips with tissue to remove excess product and set the lip color (Figure P19–1-23).

21

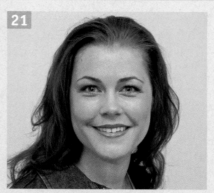

The finished look. *(Figure P19–1-24)*

21 Show the client the finished application (Figure P19–1-24).

Clean-Up and Sanitation

After the service is completed (and before the clean-up), fill out the client chart and make retail product suggestions and sales.

22 Wash your hands.

23 Discard all disposable items, such as sponges and applicators.

24 Disinfect implements such as eyelash curlers and tweezers.

25 Clean and disinfect brushes.

26 Place washable items in the laundry.

27 Disinfect product containers, used supplies, and the workstation.

FYI

Blending is the key to a professional makeup application.

SPECIAL-OCCASION MAKEUP

When a client asks for makeup for a special occasion, it is an opportunity to use your creativity. Special occasions often come with special conditions to consider, such as the lighting. For instance, many of these events take place in the evening, when lighting is subdued. That means more definition is required for the eyes, cheeks, and lips. You may also add drama by applying false lashes and using shimmery colors on the eyes, lips, cheeks, or complexion. If the special occasion is a wedding, however, where photography is an issue, matte colors are recommended because shimmer may reflect light too much. Follow the basic makeup procedure above, but consider the following pointers.

It is not recommended that you intensify every feature, because this will result in an overdone and harsh look. For example, you can intensify the eyes and lips, but not the eyes, cheeks, and lips (Figure 19–27).

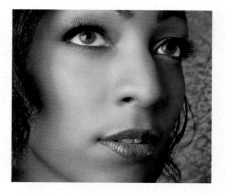
Figure 19–27 Bold eyes and lips.

Special-Occasion Makeup for Eyes

Evening Makeup

Follow these techniques for more glamorous eyes (Figure 19–28):
1. Apply the base color from the lashes to the brow with a shadow brush or applicator.
2. Apply a colorful medium tone on the lid, blending from lash line to crease with the shadow brush or applicator.
3. Apply medium to deep color in the crease, blending up toward the eyebrow but ending below it. Take the color further—just outside of the eye.
4. Apply a shimmery highlight shadow under the brow bone with the shadow brush or applicator.
5. Apply eyeliner (liquid or dry) on the upper lash line from the outside corner in, tapering as you reach the inner corner. Blend with the small brush or applicator.
6. Apply shadow in the same color as the liner, directly over the liner. This will give longevity and intensity to the liner. Repeat on the bottom lash line, if desired.
7. Apply two coats of mascara with a disposable wand.

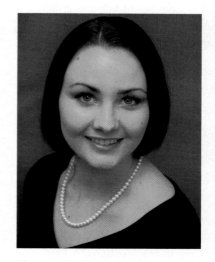
Figure 19–28 Glamorous eyes!

Dramatic Smoky Eyes

The techniques for dramatic smoky eyes (Figure 19–29) include the following:
1. Encircle the eye with dark grey, dark brown, or black eyeliner.
2. Smudge with a small shadow brush or disposable applicator.
3. Apply dark shadow from the upper lash line to the crease, softening and blending as you approach the crease. The shadow should be dark from the outer to inner corner. You can choose either shimmery or matte finish eye shadows.
4. Repeat on the lower lash line, carefully blending any hard edges.
5. If desired, add a highlight color in a shimmering or matte finish to the upper brow area with the shadow brush or applicator.
6. Apply heavier mascara with a disposable wand.
7. Add individual or band lashes if desired.

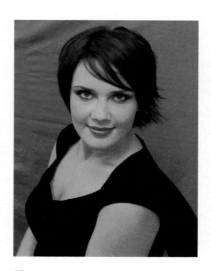
Figure 19–29 Dramatic smoky eyes.

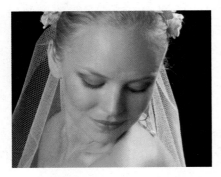

Figure 19–30 Bridal makeup is one example of a specialty makeup service.

Special-Occasion Makeup for Lips

Most clients prefer brighter or darker colors for special occasions. You can use shimmer colors or matte colors, if the client desires.

1. Apply the liner, and then fill in the entire lip area with the pencil and blot.
2. Add a similar color in lipstick over the entire mouth with a lip brush or applicator.
3. Apply gloss or a shimmery product to the center of the lips.

Makeup Application for the Camera

Makeup for photography, film/video, or weddings essentially uses the same basic application techniques, but with additional special features (Figure 19–30).

Bridal makeup is an important part of the bride's wedding. A classic, timeless look is best. Try to have a practice makeup session before the wedding day. Have the bride bring in examples of the looks she wants. The makeup should be applied after the hair and is the last thing to do before she puts on her dress. Put a scarf carefully over the hair and face to protect the dress or clothing while it is put on over the head. Makeup should be finished as close to the time of the wedding as possible, especially the lipstick. During the wedding, it is helpful for the main attendant to carry the bride's touch-up kit that includes lipstick and powder.

More product, color, and powder are generally used for photography for print work such as newspaper or magazine ads. For photos or film/video, the main difference is the powder and depth of color. Lighting will also influence the look. The amount of makeup applied does not show up in photos and videos, so a heavier application is needed for these occasions. Theatrical and fantasy makeup must be seen throughout the theater far away from the stage, and it is the most exaggerated type of makeup application (Figure 19–31).

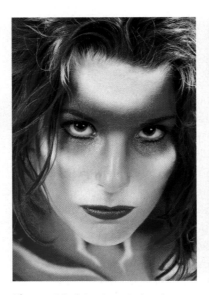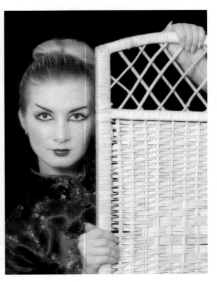

Figure 19–31 Theatrical makeup.

Airbrush makeup is a spray-on technique popular for video and photography (Figure 19–32).

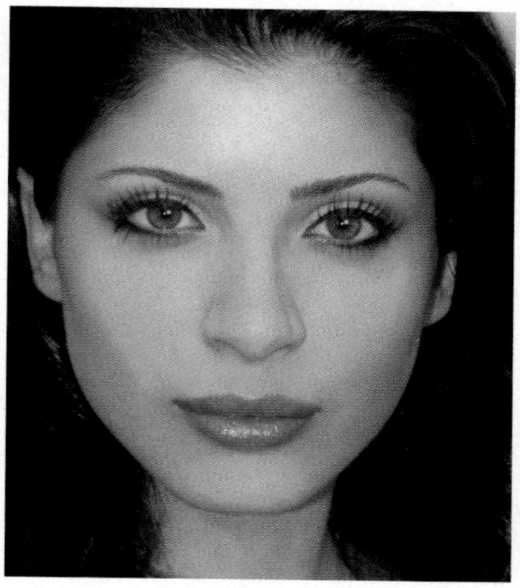

Makeup Lessons

Lessons are services that are offered to teach application techniques to clients and introduce new colors to them. This helps clients expand their confidence in applying their own makeup. Lessons are a step beyond *makeovers*, which focus on giving clients a new look. In a lesson, clients are shown how to apply makeup. These services are more time-consuming and expensive because you are sharing your knowledge. Lessons are a good opportunity to retail products, so that clients can reproduce the look you have created for them at home.

CAMOUFLAGE MAKEUP

Camouflage makeup is another area where makeup artists can utilize their skills (Figure 19–33). Post-surgery patients often need camouflage makeup to conceal their healing facial scars. Working with patients in medical offices after surgery is important to help clients look better and thus feel better about themselves. Individuals with permanent scars or disfigurements can benefit greatly from camouflage makeup (Figure 19–34). Teaching clients how to apply their own makeup is important. Camouflage makeup is challenging, and advanced training is recommended.

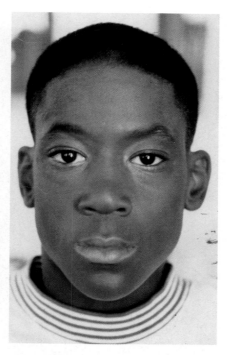

Figure 19–32 Airbrush makeup.

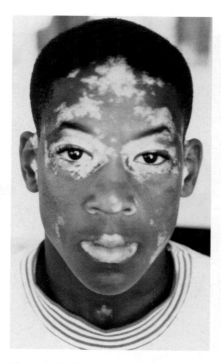

Figure 19–33 Camouflage makeup—before.

Figure 19–34 Camouflage makeup—after.

RETAILING

Retailing cosmetics is a significant part of the business. It is also an effective way to increase your income. Most salons will pay you 5 to 10 percent of every product you retail. If you focus on retailing to every client, this amount will add up quickly. You will be helping your client by giving her professional advice, and it is convenient to shop for makeup while receiving salon services. One of the biggest challenges women face when purchasing cosmetics is finding the correct colors and finishes.

When you start to use specific and "colorful" language, you will see a great improvement in your selling technique. Consider persuasive phrases such as these:

- "This cocoa shadow will make your green eyes look even more beautiful."
- "You have a great smile. This new peach lipstick will really show it off."
- "What a great dress! This silver eyeliner would look beautiful with it."

While retailing is important, always keep a person's best interests in mind. Never sell anything that you honestly feel will not benefit clients. Genuine advice is the best advice, and clients know the difference. If they trust you, they will return as well as recommend you to their friends, which is the best advertisement.

Makeup displays should be attractively presented and should stimulate interest in retail products (Figure 19–35).

The price of services and products will vary depending on the geographical location of the salon and client demographics. Generally the cost of a makeup application service ranges from an average of $25 up to $50. Lessons, makeovers, and special-occasion applications cost more.

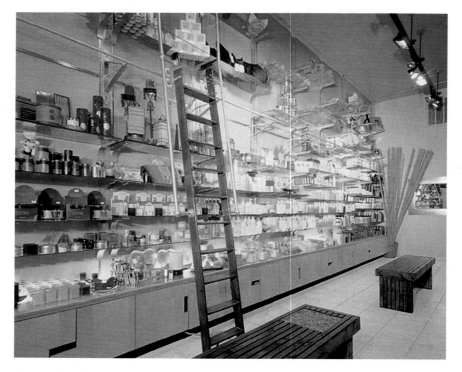

Figure 19–35 Displays should stimulate interest in products.

ARTIFICIAL EYELASHES

Artificial eyelashes are still popular makeup and fashion accessories. Clients with sparse lashes and clients who want to enhance their eyes for special occasions are most likely to request this service. Unless they want a dramatic look, the objective is to make the client's own lashes look fuller, longer, and more attractive without appearing unnatural.

Two types of artificial eyelashes are commonly used. **Band lashes** (also called *strip lashes*) are eyelash hairs on a strip that are applied with adhesive to the natural lash line (Figure 19–36).

Individual lashes are separate artificial eyelashes that are applied on top of the lashes one at a time. These are more natural-looking than band lashes (Figure 19–37). Individual eyelashes are synthetic and attach directly to a client's own lashes at the base. This process is sometimes referred to as **eye tabbing.**

Eyelash adhesive is used to make artificial eyelashes adhere, or stick, to the natural lash line. Some clients may be allergic to adhesive. When in doubt, give the client an allergy test before applying the lashes. This test may be done in one of two ways:

1. Put a drop of the adhesive behind one ear.

2. Attach a single individual eyelash to an eyelid.

In either case, if there is no reaction within 24 hours, it is probably safe to proceed with the application.

Artificial lashes are available in a variety of sizes and colors. They can be made from human hair, animal hair, or synthetic fibers. Synthetic fiber eyelashes are made with a permanent curl and do not react to changes in weather conditions. Artificial eyelashes are available in natural colors, ranging from light to dark brown and black or auburn, as well as in bright, trendy colors. Black and dark brown are the most popular choices.

Removing Artificial Eyelashes

To remove artificial eyelashes, use pads saturated with special lotions. The lash base may also be softened by applying a facecloth or cotton pad saturated with warm water and a gentle facial cleanser. Hold the cloth over the eyes for a few seconds to soften the adhesive. Starting from the outer corner, remove the lashes carefully to avoid pulling out the client's own lashes. Pull band lashes off parallel to the skin, not straight out. Use wet cotton pads or swabs to remove any makeup and adhesive remaining on the eyelid.

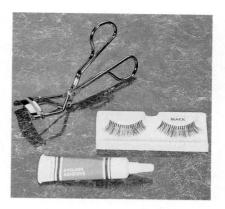

Figure 19–36 False eyelash kit.

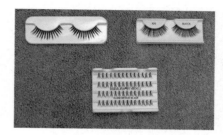

Figure 19–37 Individual and band lashes.

PROCEDURE 19–2

APPLYING ARTIFICIAL LASHES

SUPPLIES
- headband or hair clip
- tweezers
- eyelash comb/brush
- eyelash curler
- hand mirror
- small (manicure) scissors
- adjustable light
- adhesive tray or foil to put adhesive on
- makeup cape
- trays of artificial eyelashes

PRODUCTS
- eyelid and eyelash cleanser
- lash adhesive
- eyelash adhesive remover
- eye makeup remover
- hand sanitizer

DISPOSABLES
- cotton swabs
- cotton pads
- toothpick or hairpin
- mascara wand

Preparation

The following steps should be performed in preparation for applying artificial eyelashes.

1 Discuss with the client the desired length of the lashes and the effect she hopes to achieve.

2 Wash your hands.

3 Place the client in the makeup chair with her head at a comfortable working height. The client's face should be well and evenly lit; avoid shining the light directly into the eyes. Work from behind or to the side of the client. Avoid working directly in front of the client whenever possible.

4 Prepare for the makeup procedure, if applicable.

5 If the client wears contact lenses, she must remove them before starting the procedure.

6 If the client is only having artificial lashes applied and you have not already done so, remove mascara so that the lash adhesive will adhere properly. Work carefully and gently. Follow the manufacturer's instructions carefully.

Note: If the artificial lash application is in conjunction with a makeup application, complete the makeup without applying mascara to the lashes, and then finish with the false lashes.

Procedure

7 Brush the client's eyelashes to make sure they are clean and free of foreign matter, such as mascara particles (unless this is part of a makeup application). If the client's lashes are straight, they can be curled with an eyelash curler before you apply the artificial lashes.

8 Carefully remove the eyelash band from the package.

9 Start with the upper lash. If it is too long to fit the curve of the upper eyelid, trim the outside edge. Use your fingers to bend the lash into a horseshoe shape to make it more flexible so it fits the contour of the eyelid.

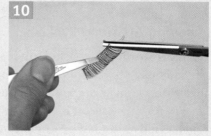

Feather the lashes with scissors. *(Figure P19–2-1)*

10 Feather band lashes to make uneven lengths on the end ("w" shapes) by nipping into it with the points of your scissors. This creates a more natural look (Figure P19-2-1).

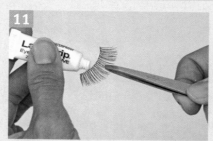

Apply adhesive to false lashes. *(Figure P19–2-2)*

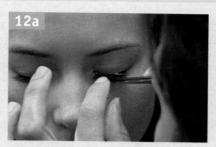

Apply lashes to the base of the natural lash line. *(Figure P19–2-3)*

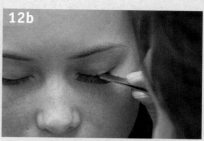

Press the lash on with an implement. *(Figure P19–2-4)*

11 Apply a thin strip of lash adhesive to the base of the false lashes with a toothpick or hairpin and allow a few seconds for it to set (Figure P19–2-2).

12 Apply the lashes by holding the ends with the fingers or tweezers.

For band lashes: Start with the shorter part of the lash and place it on the inner corner of the eye, toward the nose (Figure P19-2-3). Position the rest of the artificial lash as close to the client's own lash as possible.

For individual lashes: Apply five or six lashes, evenly spacing each one across the lash line. Use longer lashes on the outer edges of the eye, medium in the middle, and small on the inside by the nose.

Use the rounded end of a lash liner brush, a hairpin, or tweezers to press the lash on (Figure P19-2-4). Be very careful and gentle when applying the lashes. If eyeliner is to be used, the line is usually drawn on the eyelid before the lash is applied and retouched when the artificial lash is in place.

13 Apply the lower lash, if desired. Lower lash application is optional; it tends to look more unnatural. Trim the lash as necessary, and apply adhesive in the same way you did for the upper lash. Place the lash on top or beneath the client's lower lash. Place the shorter lash toward the center of the eye and the longer lash toward the outer part.

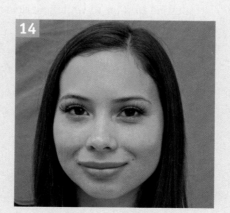

The finished look. *(Figure P19–2-5)*

14 Check the finished application and make sure the client is comfortable with the lashes (Figure P19-2-5). Remind the client to take special care with artificial lashes when swimming, bathing, or cleansing the face. Water, oil, or cleansing products will loosen artificial lashes. Band lash application lasts one day and are meant to be removed nightly. Individual lashes may last longer.

PROCEDURE 19–2, CONT.

Clean-Up and Sanitation

15 Discard all disposable items.

16 Disinfect implements, such as the eyelash curler.

17 Clean and sanitize brushes using a commercial brush sanitizer.

18 Place all towels, linens, and the makeup cape in a laundry hamper.

19 Disinfect product containers, supplies, and the workstation.

20 Wash your hands with soap and warm water.

ACTIVITY

Examine industry journals or women's magazines:

- Find five pictures of makeup looks that you like and five that you dislike.
- Find one of each: natural, business, evening, and dramatic looks.
- Find a brow look you like and one you dislike.
- What is in style right now for makeup? Present an example in class.
- Find two professional articles about applying makeup.
- Make index cards with the list of supplies and the makeup application outline to refer to while practicing.

LASH AND BROW TINTING

Lash and brow tinting is used to darken lashes and brows. It is nice for clients with light hair to have some color that lasts a few weeks, rather than penciling in brows or having light eyelashes without mascara. Tint is effective for those who have enough hair to darken. If the hair is sparse, tinting may not show up enough to be effective. Tinting is a quick procedure and can be a great add-on service to facials or waxing. It is very important to keep the tint off of the skin unless requested, especially for the brow area. The application must be precisely placed inside the brow shape. Color takes very quickly, so any excess on the skin must be removed within seconds. Lashes or brows can be tinted—clients do not always want both areas tinted.

PROCEDURE 19–3

LASH AND BROW TINTING PROCEDURE

SUPPLIES
- headband
- hand towels
- plastic mixing cup
- distilled water
- small bowl of water
- timer
- brow comb or mascara wand
- eyeliner brush
- disinfectant

PRODUCTS
- cleanser or eye makeup remover
- witch hazel
- petroleum jelly/occlusive cream
- lash tint kits: black for lashes and brown for brows unless client requests otherwise

DISPOSABLES
- cotton swabs (10 to 12)
- round cotton pads (6 to 8)
- paper sheets (1 under each eye)
- baggie

> ### CAUTION!
> Do not use tints with aniline derivatives. These are not FDA approved and can cause blindness. Some tints are illegal in the United States, but they may still be available from retailers for use. Do not use them if they are not legal in your region. You may be fined and lose your license. Vegetable dyes are allowed in some regions. Check your local laws to be sure.

Preparation

1 Wash hands.

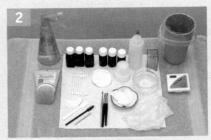

Gather supplies. *(Figure P19–3-1)*

2 Gather and set out supplies (Figure P19–3-1).

3 Wet 5 cotton pads and 5 to 6 cotton swabs. Cut supply amounts in half if doing only one procedure on either the brows or lashes.

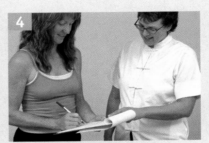

Conduct client consultation. *(Figure P19–3-2)*

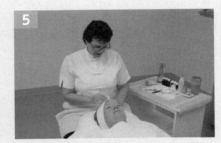

Drape client. *(Figure P19–3-3)*

4 Conduct the client consultation, and have the client sign the release form (Figure P19–3-2).

5 Drape the client with a headband and towel around the neck (Figure P19–3-3).

Procedure

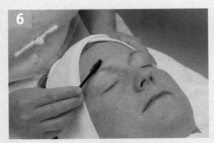

Brush brows in place. *(Figure P19–3-4)*

6 Cleanse the brow and/or lash area. All makeup must be removed and the area clean and dry before applying tint. Brush brows into place (Figure P19–3-4).

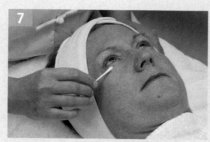

Apply protective cream around area.
(Figure P19–3-5)

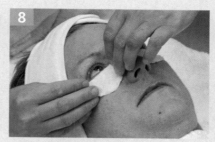

Apply pads. *(Figure P19–3-6)*

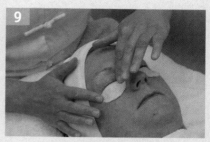

Adjust the pads. *(Figure P19–3-7)*

7 Apply protective cream with a cotton swab directly next to the area where you are tinting to protect the skin, covering the area where you do not want the tint. Do not touch the hairs with cream, because this interferes with the color. Apply cream around the brow area. Apply under the eyelashes on the skin below the eye and above the lashes just next to the lash line (Figure P19-3-5).

8 *For lash tinting:* Apply pads under the eyes and over the cream to keep tint from bleeding onto the skin. Use the paper sheaths in the tint kit, or you can make thin cotton pads from cotton rounds. Wet the pads and squeeze out excess water, tearing them so they are half as thick. Then fold in half to make half-moon-shaped pads. You may have to cut or adjust pad shapes to fit under the eyes. Pads should be under the lashes as close to the eye as possible without hiding or interfering with the lower lashes (Figure P19-3-6).

9 Have the client close her eyes, and adjust the pad so it sits next to the eye—not bunched up too close to the eye (Figure P19-3-7). If the pad is too close or too wet, tint may wick into the eye.

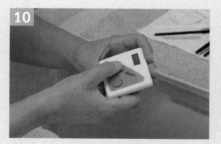

Set timer. *(Figure P19–3-8)*

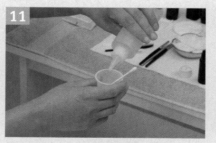

Optional for brows: Dilute tint with water. *(Figure P19–3-9)*

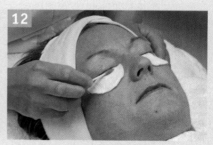

Apply tint. *(Figure P19–3-10)*

10 Set timer according to manufacturer's directions, and have wet pads and cotton swabs ready to use for rinsing (Figure P19-3-8).

11 For brows, the tint can be diluted with water in a 1:1 ratio in a mixing cup to lighten the color (Figure P19-3-9).

12 *Apply tint:* Dip cotton swab or brush applicator into tint (bottle 1), blot excess, apply and carefully saturate the area (Figure P19-3-10).

PROCEDURE 19–3, CONT.

13 Leave on for three minutes or as directed. Some tint kits have only one bottle and combine the tint and developer into one application. Alter the procedure accordingly. Do not double-dip—use a new applicator each time.

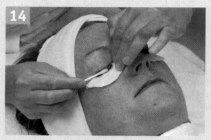

Apply developer. *(Figure P19–3-11)*

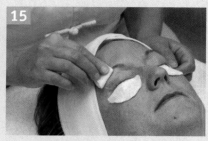

Rinse well. *(Figure P19–3-12)*

14 With a new applicator, apply the developer (bottle 2) for one minute (Figure 19–3-11).

15 Rinse each area with water at least three times with wet cotton swabs and cotton pads without dripping into eyes (Figure 19–3-12). *Tip:* Before rinsing, you can replace the under-eye shields if necessary (if color is bleeding through to skin).

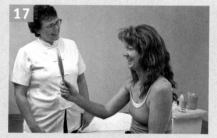

The finished look. *(Figure P19–3-13)*

16 Ask the client if her eyes feel all right, and have her flush them with water at the sink if necessary. It is common for the eyes to feel a little grainy after tinting, so rinsing is a good idea.

17 Show the application to the client. (Figure P19–3-13).

Clean-Up and Sanitation

After the service is completed (and before the clean-up), fill out the client chart, and make retail product suggestions and sales.

18 Wash your hands.

19 Discard all disposable items.

20 Disinfect implements.

21 Clean and disinfect brushes.

22 Place linens in the laundry.

23 Disinfect product containers, supplies, and the workstation.

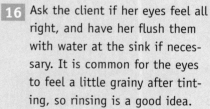

CAUTION!

To avoid eye damage, do not let tint or water drip into the client's eyes. Have the client keep her eyes closed the whole time.

OTHER EYELASH SERVICES

Lash Extensions

Lash extensions are single synthetic or natural hairs that are applied one-by-one to the client's natural lashes with a special adhesive. Fine-tipped forceps or tweezers are used to apply the lash extensions, and it can take up to two hours to apply a set. Partial applications and touch-ups take less time. Clusters or groups of hairs should not be applied as extensions, because doing so can damage the natural hairs. The bond will last for the life cycle of the natural lash—approximately two months. Fills, or touch-ups, are necessary as the hair grows and the extension needs to be replaced. For extensions to last, makeup application and cleansing should be gentle around the lash area. Research on the adhesive quality and safety is recommended. Advanced training and practice are necessary before performing this intricate procedure on clients.

Lash Perming

Lash perming is the process of curling the lashes. Research on the quality and safety of the perm solution is recommended. Advanced training and practice are necessary before performing this delicate procedure on clients. Always check with your regulatory agency about the legalities of performing lash services.

PERMANENT COSMETIC MAKEUP

Permanent cosmetic makeup is cosmetic tattooing. The specialized techniques used for permanent cosmetics are often referred to as *micropigmentation, micropigment implantation,* or *dermagraphics*. The cosmetic implantation technique deposits colored pigment into the upper reticular layer of the dermis. Eyeliner and eyebrow tattooing are the most popular services (Figure 19–38). Scar camouflage and body art are also offered as permanent cosmetic services.

Permanent cosmetics procedures are performed using various methods, including the traditional tattoo machines, the pen or rotary machine, and the hand method. The process includes an initial consultation, then application of pigment, and at least one or more follow-up visits for adjusting the shape and color or density of the pigment.

Technically, permanent cosmetics procedures are considered permanent because the color is implanted into the upper reticular part of the dermal layer of the skin and cannot be washed off. However, as with any tattoo, fading can and often does occur, requiring periodic maintenance and touch-ups.

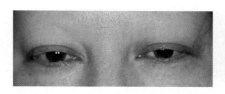 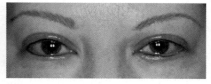

Figure 19–38 Permanent "tattoo" makeup.

WEB RESOURCES

For more information on permanent makeup, contact the Society of Permanent Cosmetic Professionals:

http://www.spcp.org.

Estheticians, tattoo artists, and medical technicians perform these services. Licensing and training requirements vary from state to state. A thorough training program and hands-on experience are necessary to perform these technical services. It is recommended that clients choose a technician carefully by considering their training and experience and by looking at their portfolio. It is important to remember that the shape and proper placement of the procedure is as important as the right color. It is permanent and there is no room for error.

The initial procedure will generally take approximately 1 to 2 ½ hours to perform. Touch-up procedures do not usually require as much time. Most clients experience some discomfort. This varies according to an individual s pain threshold as well as the skills of the technician performing the service. Generally, there is some swelling of the treated area. While eyebrows may show little aftereffect, eyeliner and lips may show more, and the edema may last from 2 to 72 hours. During the procedure, there may be some bleeding and or bruising. There is usually some tenderness for a few days. The color is much darker for the first 6 to 10 days.

AIRBRUSH MAKEUP

Airbrush makeup is sprayed on and techniques include both freehand and stencil. Airbrushing has the following benefits:

- hygienic, long-lasting, rub- and water-resistant, yet simple to remove
- more efficient and faster to apply than traditional makeup
- lightweight, natural, and a flawless look

Airbrush makeup is used for the following applications:

- face and body art, washable tattoos, and tropical tans (lasting 4 to 5 days)
- makeup application: foundations, shading and highlighting, use of stencils
- hair and nail art application: hair adornments, coloration, and scalp covering
- popular for photography, film, theater, fantasy, and bridal makeup

A CAREER AS A MAKEUP ARTIST

Makeup artists play an important role in the esthetics field. Many opportunities are available for makeup artists in clinical offices, film/video, theater, and fashion. These art forms give individuals a chance to be creative. A natural part of the full-service menu for spas and salons, makeup services are complementary to other services offered by estheticians. To thrive in this business, it is important to keep up with current styles, sell yourself, and present yourself well. The key to building up a loyal client base is staying professional. Be punctual and prepared. Makeup artistry is a great addition to your repertoire of services.

Makeup services are another opportunity to work with facial and waxing clients and assist them with their makeup needs in a professional, sanitary environment. Clients benefit from the personalized service offered during a professional makeover. Each client is different, and that keeps the job interesting and challenging—because what may look good on one person does not look good on another. Enhancing our appearance through makeup is also an easy way to boost our self-image. The satisfying part of working as an artist is client satisfaction—the look on their faces when they see how much they can improve how they look. This gives them encouragement and helps them feel better about themselves. Makeup is not simply a trend or fashion statement. It has evolved over the years into a natural finishing touch to healthy skin.

REVIEW QUESTIONS

1. What is the main objective of makeup application?
2. List eight different types of cosmetics/makeup products.
3. List the primary and secondary colors.
4. Give six examples of warm and cool colors (three each).
5. What are complementary colors?
6. What does contouring do?
7. Where do you use highlighter?
8. What color tones down red?
9. What are the color selections or guidelines used to choose makeup colors?
10. How do you measure the ideal eyebrow shape?
11. List the cosmetics and supplies used in a basic makeup procedure.
12. List the steps of makeup application in the order they are performed.
13. What questions do you ask the client in a makeup consultation?
14. Name and describe the two types of artificial eyelashes.
15. List at least five safety and sanitation measures that should be followed when applying makeup.

CHAPTER GLOSSARY

band lashes: eyelash hairs on a strip that are applied with adhesive to the natural lash line.

cake (pancake) makeup: shaped, solid mass; heavy coverage.

complementary colors: primary and secondary colors opposite one another on the color wheel.

concealers: cosmetics used to cover blemishes and discolorations; may be applied before or after foundation.

cool colors: colors with a blue undertone that suggest coolness and are dominated by blues, greens, violets, and blue-reds.

eye tabbing: procedure in which individual synthetic eyelashes are attached directly to a client's own lashes at their base.

greasepaint: heavy makeup used for theatrical purposes.

individual lashes: separate artificial eyelashes that are applied on top of the lashes one at a time.

matte: dull; not shiny.

primary colors: yellow, red, and blue; fundamental colors that cannot be obtained from a mixture.

secondary colors: colors obtained by mixing equal parts of two primary colors.

tertiary colors: colors formed by mixing equal amounts of secondary color and its neighboring primary color.

warm colors: the range of colors with yellow undertones; from yellow and gold through oranges, red-oranges, most reds, and even some yellow-greens.

BUSINESS SKILLS

CAREER PLANNING

mage whatsoever res

formation.

ile in Your Employ___

urity Number ___

mployment ___

on ___

APPLICATION

PERSONAL INFOR

NAME (LAST NAME FIRST)

PRESENT ADDRESS

PERMANENT AD

OU 18

LEARNING OBJECTIVES

After completing this chapter, you will be able to:

- Describe those qualities that are needed to be successful in a service profession.

- Explain the steps involved in preparing for and passing the licensing exam.

- Discuss the essentials of becoming test-wise.

- Demonstrate effective techniques for writing a good resume.

- Discuss methods for exploring the job market and researching potential employers.

- List and describe the various types of esthetics practices and determine your employment options.

- Be prepared to complete a successful job interview.

- List the habits of a good salon team player.

- Recognize the importance of a job description.

- Describe the different methods of compensation that are utilized in esthetics.

- Explain the importance of meeting financial responsibilities and managing money well.

- List several ways you can benefit from good role models.

- Understand the importance of continuing your education.

KEY TERMS

A desire to help people is often at the top of the list of reasons why individuals choose a career in esthetics. Esthetics is a caring, nurturing profession that helps others to feel positive about their appearance. However, there are many facets of esthetics to consider in planning your career.

Whether this is your first job or you are making the transition from another occupation, defining your reasons for entering the field of esthetics is an important first step in developing long-term goals and short-term objectives.

As you embark on your newly chosen career path, take some time to think about your personal goals. Begin by naming at least three reasons why esthetics appealed to you. Then list three services that you especially like to perform. What other aspects of being an esthetician do you enjoy? For example, do you like to consult with clients or recommend products, track your sales progress, or make follow-up phone calls to see how clients are doing with a new skin care program? Name at least two tasks that are not hands-on that you find rewarding. Next, state what you would like to be doing five years from now. Perhaps this involves moving on to another aspect of skin care, such as education, running your own salon, or becoming a sales representative. Developing a better understanding of your long-term goals and short-term objectives will help you to make the best choices as you plan your esthetics career.

PREPARING FOR LICENSURE

The preparation period before you enter the workforce is an exciting time. But before you can actually apply for a job, you must first fulfill the required number of hours for esthetics training and pass your state licensing exam (Figure 20–1).

Hopefully, you have developed good study habits and practice skills during the course of your esthetics program. These will come in handy as you prepare for the exam. Your school may offer additional assistance for test preparation. If so, you should take advantage of these options. However, there is no substitute for a solid understanding of the material. Mastery of the course content is essential to passing the exam.

Preparing for the Test

Test anxiety can be a real issue for many students. If you are subject to pre-test jitters, there are several simple strategies that can help to alleviate much of the stress involved. A **test-wise** student begins to prepare for taking a test by practicing the good study habits and time management skills that are such an important part of effective studying. The following are some tips that will help you to gain control of the test situation.

- Read content carefully and become an active studier.
- Take effective notes during class.
- Organize your notebook and class handouts for easy review.
- Separate vocabulary lists and study these carefully.
- Scan your text and review end-of-chapter questions.
- Listen carefully in class for any cues and clues about what questions could be expected on the test.
- Use any study guides that are available from the state board of examination or in conjunction with your text.
- Review tests or quizzes taken as part of your course work.
- Plan your study schedule so that you are not cramming the night before the test.
- Pay attention to any tips offered by your instructors.

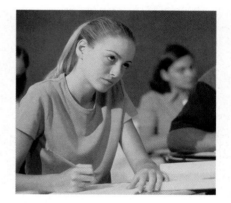

Figure 20–1 Developing good study habits and practice skills now will help you prepare for the state licensing exam.

In addition to good study habits, there are other, more holistic test-wise habits to keep in mind as you prepare to take the test.

- Take good care of yourself in the weeks before your exam; eat right, exercise, and get plenty of rest.
- Maintain a positive attitude that supports passing the test as a necessary and useful step in the process of achieving your goal of becoming a licensed esthetician.
- Anticipate feeling some anxiety (but note that a certain amount of anxiety may actually help you to do better).

Taking the Test

Many techniques can be useful in preparation for testing. For instance, it may help you to practice relaxation methods or to arrive early to become familiar with the surroundings. But the most important thing to keep in mind is that you must have knowledge of the test material. If you are unsure of certain information, take time to review the material beforehand.

Deductive Reasoning

One of the best techniques that students should learn to use for better results is called **deductive reasoning.** Deductive reasoning is the process of reaching logical conclusions by employing logical reasoning.

Some strategies associated with deductive reasoning follow.

Eliminate options known to be incorrect. The more answers you can eliminate as incorrect, the better your chances of identifying the correct one.

Watch for key words or terms. Look for any qualifying conditions or statements. Keep an eye out for such words as *usually, commonly, in most instances, never, always,* and the like.

Study the stem. The stem is the basic question or problem. It often provides a clue to the answer. Look for a match between the stem and one of the choices.

Watch for grammatical clues. For instance, if the last word in a stem is *an,* the answer must begin with a vowel rather than a consonant.

Look at similar or related questions. They may provide clues.

In answering essay questions, watch for words such as *compare, contrast, discuss, evaluate, analyze, define,* or *describe* and develop your answer accordingly.

In tests that contain long paragraphs of reading followed by several questions, read the questions first. This will help you identify the important elements in the paragraph.

Test Formats

Tests are developed using numerous styles and formats. These commonly include *true or false, multiple choice, matching,* and *essay* questions. We present some points to consider when answering each of these kinds of questions.

True or False

True or false questions offer only two choices. Sometimes the question can be presented so that it seems there is an element of truth in each answer. But it is important to remember that for an answer to be true, the entire sentence must be true. In general, long statements are more likely to be true than short statements are because it takes more detail to provide truthful, factual information. When in doubt, look for qualifying words such as *all, some, no, none, always, usually, sometimes, never, little, equal, less, good,* or *bad.* For the most part, questions that use absolutes such as *all, none, always,* or *never* are generally not true.

Multiple Choice

Multiple-choice questions typically offer the tester a selection of four to six responses (Figure 20–2). However, in some cases more than one choice may be true, so it is always important to look for the best answer. A process of elimination can be helpful in determining the right choice. Note that when

1. You are most likely to see the word "aesthetician" used in which environment?
    a) medical setting
    c) small independent salon
    B) large chain salon
    d) beauty school

2. An important part of good personal hygiene is:
    a) washing your hands as often as possible throughout the day
    b) selecting a strong perfume that will mask any potential body odor
    c) avoiding the use of floss when caring for your teeth
    d) following a regular skin care regimen

3. Which of these must be signed by the client before you administer an aggressive treatment?
    a) health insurance form
    c) intake form
    b) consultation card
    d) consent form

4. Skin types include:
    a) dry skin
    c) normal skin
    b) oily skin
    d) all of the above

5. It is important to inform clients that exposure to the sun can contribute to:
    a) weight gain
    c) collagen growth
    b) elastin growth
    d) hyperpigmentation

6. Which of these would you find on an MSDS?
    a) product disposal guidelines
    b) instructions for using a product
    c) product warranty information
    d) all of the above

7. Which kind of disinfectant is used in salons and spas?
    a) hospital disinfectant
    b) tuberculocidal disinfectant
    c) neither hospital nor tuberculocidal disinfectant
    d) both hospital and tuberculocidal disinfectant

8. Which type of bacteria are shaped like short rods?
    a) spirilla
    c) diplicocci
    b) bacilli
    d) staphylococci

Figure 20–2 Sample of a multiple-choice test.

two choices are close or similar, one is probably right; when two choices are identical, both must be wrong; when two choices are opposites, one is probably right and one is probably wrong. (However, this also depends on the other choices.) Often, but not always, if one of the choices states "all of the above," it is the correct answer. If you are unsure, it is helpful to pay attention to qualifying words such as *not, except,* and *but.* It is also possible to find the answer to one question in the stem of another. If after exhausting all of these methods you are completely unsure of an answer, it does not hurt to guess on multiple-choice questions, provided there is no penalty for doing so. As you work through the answer it can be helpful to cross out wrong answers, provided you are allowed to write on the text exam booklet.

Matching Questions

Matching questions to answers is a relatively straightforward method of testing, because the right answer is always available. However, these questions assume that you have knowledge of the material. Sometimes matching responses to questions can be similar or confusing. It may be helpful to check off items from the response list as you use them to eliminate the number of choices as you go along.

Essay Questions

Essay questions are open-ended and allow the test taker some leeway in how she or he can present an answer. Before putting pen to paper, always take a few moments to organize your thoughts. Frequently, the question itself will suggest a method for organizing your response. Look for cue words in the question to help you, and begin by creating an outline to structure your response. When you have completed your answer, always review what you have written. Be sure you have addressed the question asked completely and accurately and that you have provided the information in an organized and clear manner.

On Test Day

When you are taking written exams, it is also wise to do the following:
- Listen carefully to all verbal directions given by the examiner.
- Do not hesitate to ask the examiner questions if something is not clear.
- Enter identifying information, such as your name, before you begin answering questions.
- Read all written directions carefully before you begin.
- Scan the entire test before you start.
- Wear a watch to monitor your time.
- Read each question carefully before answering.
- Answer those questions you are sure about first.
- Save difficult questions or ones you are unsure of for last.
- Mark any questions you skip, so that you can find them easily later.
- Answer as many questions as possible.
- If you have time at the end of the exam, review your answers. If you feel compelled to change an answer, make sure there is sufficient reason to do so.
- Check that you have entered all pertinent information correctly.

The Practical Examination

Although requirements vary, in most states you must also be prepared for a test of your practical or hands-on skills. If your state requires a practical examination, you will probably receive some notice of the materials that you will be required to bring to perform this portion of the test, including whether it is necessary to bring a model. Always take time to review any notices, materials, or pamphlets you receive. This information will give you a good idea of what to anticipate. Your instructors can also be useful resources in helping you to prepare for this part of the test. If a trial run is available, take advantage of any opportunities to participate. If you do not, it is a good idea to perform your own trials, paying close attention to timing, sanitation, and safety procedures. Finally, make sure you are familiar with the location of the test site and the amount of time it will take you to get there on time. Arriving late will only increase your anxiety level and may even prevent you from taking the exam.

PREPARING FOR EMPLOYMENT

When you chose a career in esthetics, your primary goal was to get a good job. To fulfill that goal, you will need to showcase your best qualities to prospective employers. To define these qualities, you will need to answer two very important questions:

1. What are my strongest practical skills?

2. What personal qualities do I possess that will make me a good hire?

The inventory of personal characteristics and technical skills (Figure 20–3) will help you to answer these questions. After you have completed this inventory and identified the areas that need further attention, you can then determine where to focus the remainder of your training,

Surveying Your Options

Deciding on the type of esthetics practice that is right for you is an important part of the job search. Traditionally, the field of skin care grew out of the beauty salon business, where the main focus was on hair and nail services. Since acquiring separate licensing, the field of esthetics has expanded to include several new business opportunities. While there are many variations of skin care practices, the following general categories highlight those that are referenced frequently.

- *The independent skin care clinic or day spa* offers a variety of skin care treatments and may include facial and body treatments, makeup artistry, nail care, massage therapy, and other holistic health practices.

- The *full service salon* provides a total beauty experience including hair services and nail and skin care; it also may offer a combination of other holistic health practices similar to those available at the skin care clinic or day spa.

- The *wellness center* or *spa* is focused on maintaining optimal health and may combine several holistic, complementary, or alternative health care practices with more traditional medical practices, exercise and nutrition counseling, medical esthetic procedures, beauty treatments, skin care, and spa services to promote an inclusive wellness program. The wellness center or spa may exist as an independent operation or can be incorporated within a health, fitness, or destination-type spa facility.

INVENTORY OF PERSONAL CHARACTERISTICS

PERSONAL CHARACTERISTIC	Exc.	Good	Avg.	Poor	Plan for Improvement
Posture, Deportment, Poise					
Grooming, Personal Hygiene					
Manners, Courtesy					
Communications Skills					
Attitude					
Self-Motivation					
Personal Habits					
Responsibility					
Self-esteem, Self Confidence					
Honesty, Integrity					
Dependability					

INVENTORY OF TECHNICAL SKILLS

TECHNICAL SKILLS	Exc.	Good	Avg.	Poor	Plan for Improvement
Skin Analysis					
Skin Conditions					
Fitzpatrick Scale					
Basic Facials					
Advanced Skin Care					
Body Treatments					
Use of Equipment					
Waxing					
Make-up					
Retail Sales					
Other					

After analyzing the above responses, would you hire yourself as an employee in your firm? Why or why not?

State your short-term goals that you hope to accomplish in 6 to 12 months:

State your long-term goals that you hope to accomplish in 1 to 5 years:

Figure 20–3 Inventory of personal characteristics and technical skills.

- The *medical spa* integrates a variety of medical esthetic and surgical procedures with esthetic skin care treatments and spa services. The *medi-spa*, as it is often referred to, may exist in a hospital setting, laser center, or independent medical practice, such as a cosmetic surgery or dermatology office. The medical esthetic practice employs a diverse, well-trained staff that can include physicians, nurses, estheticians, and other professionals such as massage therapists and electrologists. Treatments in the medical spa are mainly focused on clinical procedures, such as dermal filler injection therapy, chemical peels, laser treatments, and dermatological and cosmetic surgery procedures that require pre- and postoperative skin care (Figure 20–4).
- The *destination spa* is an all-inclusive spa retreat that offers patrons a wide range of health, beauty, and wellness programs such as fitness, nutrition, massage, skin care, beauty treatments, educational classes, and more. This environment, as the name implies, involves travel to a specific location and includes hotel accommodations.
- The *resort or hotel spa* is an amenity spa that provides guests with a variety of spa services that may include skin care, massage, and hair and nail services. The amenity spa may also be available to local patrons and residents who wish to receive services on a regular basis.
- *Booth rental* establishments, or the practice of leasing a room to provide services independently, is an option in some states. This is possibly the least expensive way of owning your own business. Booth rentals may be available in a variety of skin care salon and spa businesses.

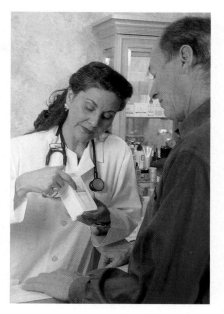

Figure 20–4 The medical spa integrates medical esthetic and surgical procedures with skin care and spa services.

PREPARING YOUR RESUME

The **resume** (REH-zuh-may) is your ticket to employment. It provides employers with a summary of your education and work experience and highlights relevant accomplishments and achievements. Before you begin the task of writing your resume, you should consider that, on average, a potential employer spends about 20 seconds scanning your resume to decide whether to grant an interview.

To create a positive reaction, it is a good idea to know as much as possible about the culture you are targeting and tailor your resume accordingly. For example, if you are interested in working in a medical esthetics practice, you should use terminology that is commonly accepted in the medical profession and highlight any experience you have that is relevant to this setting. You may also want to take a more conservative approach in your presentation style. However, if you are interested in working for a chic day spa, you might want to take a more stylish approach that demonstrates your knowledge of the latest trend setting spa techniques.

Formatting Your Resume

There are many styles of resumes. Finding the format that works best for you will require a bit of research. Fortunately, there are numerous resources available to help you. Some esthetic training programs provide vocational guidance counseling or include resume development as part of the curriculum. If your program does not, many resources can be easily accessed at your local library, located online, or purchased from a bookstore.

Once you have determined the resume style and format that is right for your needs, you can begin to address more functional requirements. To be effective, your resume should be neat, concise, easy to read, grammatically correct, and error free. Ideally, it should fit on one page and be presented on good-quality white, buff, or grey bond paper. The content of your resume should incorporate several important areas, including practical knowledge, interpersonal skills, administrative and management skills, and sales abilities. In general, this information is integrated using a structure that includes the following information:

- name, street address, telephone number, and e-mail address
- career goals and objectives
- a summary of professional qualifications
- a history of employment or experience
- any awards or achievements that highlight your credentials

Rather than providing a detailed account of your duties and responsibilities, it is often a good idea to focus on presenting your accomplishments (Figure 20–5). The goal is to get the reader's attention in a way that demonstrates your broad-based skills. Notice the difference in impact in the following statements:

- Performed facials on individuals with varying skin types and conditions.
- Developed and retained a personal client base of over 75 individuals of all ages, both male and female, with various skin types and conditions.

If you are applying for your first position as an esthetician, you may be concerned that your qualifications are inadequate compared to those of more seasoned estheticians. Do not let this discourage you; many employers are looking for eager self-starters. Highlighting student achievements such as attendance, academic awards, clinic performance, or volunteer work can also stimulate the interest you need to obtain an interview.

The Resume Checklist

A well-written resume is an excellent marketing tool. As you tackle putting the right words on paper, the following checklist will help you avoid problems and make the most of your individual skills.

- Use clear, concise language and avoid elaborate or cliché phrases.
- Think about writing separate resumes to target different markets if you are applying for positions that have distinct requirements, such as a medical spa.
- Consider your audience, and use specific words they can relate to.
- Highlight your accomplishments and the methods you used to achieve them. For example, were you selected student of the month for your academic performance or for exemplary attendance?

MARY SMITH
143 Fern Circle
Anytown, USA 12345
(123) 555-1234

An esthetician with honors in attendance and practical skills who is creative, artistic, and works well with people of all ages.

ACCOMPLISHMENTS/ABILITIES

Academics Achieved an "A" average in theoretical requirements and excellent ratings in practical requirements. Exceeded the number of practical skills required for graduation.

Sales Named "Student of the Month" for best attendance, best attitude, highest retail sales, and most clients served. Increased add-on services to 30 percent of my clinic volume by graduation. Achieved a client ticket average comparable to $33.00 in the area salon market.

Increased retail sales of cosmetic products by over 18 percent during part-time employment at local department store.

Client Retention Developed and retained a personal client base of over 75 individuals of all ages, both male and female.

Image Consulting Certified as an Image Consultant who aids in providing full salon services to all clientele.

Administration Supervised a student "salon team" which developed a business plan for opening a full-service salon; project earned an "A" and was recognized for thoroughness, accuracy, and creativity.

As President of the Student Council, organized fundraising activities including car washes, bake sales, and yard sales which generated enough funds to send 19 students to a skin care show in El Paso.

Externship Trained one day weekly at the salon for ten weeks under the state-approved student externship program.

Special Projects Reorganized school facial room for more efficiency and client comfort.

Organized the school dispensary, which increased inventory control and streamlined operations within the clinic.

Catalogued the school's library of texts, books, videos, and other periodicals by category and updated the library inventory list.

EXPERIENCE

Salon Etc. Spring 2006
Student Extern in Esthetics

Dilberts Summer 2006
Retail Sales, Cosmetics

Food Emporium 2003–2005
Cashier

EDUCATION

Graduate, New Alamo High School, 2005

Graduate, Milady Career Institute of Cosmetology, August 2007

Licensed as Esthetician, September 2007

Figure 20–5 A sample resume.

- Present your career goals in a nonthreatening manner that encourages trust in your willingness to work cooperatively in the position that is available.
- Emphasize any **transferable skills,** such as sales training or administrative abilities, that you have mastered at other jobs and can apply to a new position.
- Choose your words carefully, using action or power words such as *established, accomplished, increased, managed, developed,* or *coordinated* for emphasis.
- Avoid making any reference to salary levels or requirements.
- State only professional references, and include the person's title, phone number, and business name on a separate page.
- Be honest in the way that you present yourself, stating only those experiences and achievements that are valid.
- Avoid including personal commentary and hobbies that are not directly related to business.

Writing Your Resume

Many people find it difficult to start the actual resume writing process. But with a little organization and the right materials, writing your resume can be a lot easier than you might imagine. A computer or word processor is an ideal tool if you are creating your own materials. However, if you are not computer literate or do not have access to a computer, other resources are available. Try searching your local community directory for print shops or individuals that specialize in formatting resumes. Libraries are also a good resource and typically have several computers available for public use if you are without one.

A good way to start organizing the content of your resume is to compile all of the documents in your possession relating to your education or work experience. These can include diplomas, continuing education or training certificates, copies of previous job applications, achievement awards or letters of recommendation, and memberships in professional organizations. Using this information, you can begin to create an outline listing pertinent information under each of the headings discussed previously. For example, make a list of your accomplishments and achievements, professional qualifications, and career objectives. Condensing this information into small bulleted phrases is a good way to begin developing sentences. Next, you can focus on choosing the best words to define your experience. A dictionary and thesaurus can be useful tools in performing this task.

When you have completed a rough draft, have someone with knowledge about resume writing review it for you. An objective opinion can lend valuable insight, pointing out areas that you may have overlooked. You should also double-check your spelling and grammar for errors. In this technological age, resumes are often delivered electronically via the internet. If you are mailing a hard copy of your resume, the right stationery and envelopes are also important in creating a positive impression. Remember to keep your target market in mind when selecting paper, and be sure to buy enough for a coordinating cover letter.

Your Name
Your Address
Your Phone Number

Ms. (or Mr.)_____
Salon Name
Salon Address

Dear Ms. (or Mr.)_____,
We met in August when you allowed me to observe your salon and staff while I was still in skin care training. Since that time, I have graduated and have received my license, which allows me to practice esthetics. I have enclosed my resume for your review and consideration.

I would very much appreciate the opportunity to meet with you and discuss either current or future career opportunities at your salon. I was extremely impressed with your staff and business, and I would like to discuss with you how my skills and training might add to your salon's success.

I will call you next week to discuss a time that is convenient for us to meet. I look forward to meeting with you again soon.

Sincerely,
(your name)

Figure 20–6 A sample resume cover letter.

The Cover Letter

Your cover letter completes the presentation of your professional qualifications and should be written using a professional letter format (Figure 20–6). Begin your letter with a statement that identifies the position you are interested in, and include the reason you are interested in working for that particular salon or spa. Briefly define the qualifications you will bring to the position, and include a statement explaining your philosophy of teamwork and the ways in which your contribution will benefit the spa or salon. It is also a good idea to offer some input on why you chose a career in esthetics. Both your cover letter and resume should be typed. Never handwrite these important presentation pieces. However, it is appropriate to send a handwritten thank-you note after you have interviewed for a position.

In addition to your written resume, you may also have a portfolio of your work that includes before and after photos relating to skin care or makeup artistry, award certificates, or letters of recognition for community service or volunteer work. Materials of this nature should not be included with your resume; however, they make an excellent presentation when interviewing. If you intend to use such materials, arrange them in a neat portfolio so the interviewer can review them easily.

THE JOB SEARCH

With a completed resume in hand, you are now ready to present yourself to prospective employers. The job search is an exciting process that will open up many new doors. To make the most of your efforts, it is a good idea to be clear about any personal prerequisites you may have and to gather as much information as possible before calling on employers.

Finding the Salon or Spa That Is Right for You

Finding the right work environment takes careful planning and preparation. With loans to repay and living expenses to meet, of course you are eager to earn real wages. But money does not necessarily guarantee satisfaction. Before you accept the first job opportunity that comes along, take time to find out as much as possible about a salon's history and philosophy. This will help you to make critical choices about whether you will be happy working there.

When searching for a good job fit, ask yourself the following important questions (Figure 20–7).

SALON VISIT CHECKLIST

When you visit a salon, observe the following areas and rate them from 1 to 5, with 5 considered being the best.

_____ **SALON IMAGE:** Is the salon's image pleasing to you and appropriate for your interests? Is it neat and clean? Is the decor warm and inviting? Is the physical layout user-friendly? If you are not comfortable, or if you find it unattractive, it is likely that clients will also.

_____ **PROFESSIONALISM:** Do the employees present the appropriate professional appearance and behavior? Do they give their clients the appropriate levels of attention and personal service or do they act as if work is their time to socialize?

_____ **MANAGEMENT:** Does the salon show signs of being well managed? Is the phone answered promptly with professional telephone skills? Is the mood of the salon positive? Does everyone appear to work as a team?

_____ **CLIENT SERVICE:** Are clients greeted promptly and warmly when they enter the salon? Are they kept informed of the status of their appointment? Are they offered a magazine or beverage while they wait? Is there a comfortable reception area? Are there changing rooms, attractive smocks?

_____ **PRICES:** Compare price for value. Are clients getting their money's worth? Do they pay the same price in one salon but get better service and attention in another? If possible, take home salon brochures and price lists.

_____ **RETAIL:** Is there a well-stocked retail display offering clients a variety of product lines and a range of prices? Do the estheticians and receptionist (if applicable) promote retail sales?

_____ **IN-SALON MARKETING:** Are there posters or promotions throughout the salon? If so, are they professionally designed and relevant to contemporary skin care treatments?

_____ **SERVICES:** Make a list of all services offered by each salon and the product lines they carry. This will help you decide what earning potential estheticians have in each salon.

SALON NAME: _____

SALON MANAGER: _____

Figure 20–7 Salon visit checklist.

- *What is the most important consideration for me in terms of work conditions?* Each individual will have his or her own agenda; however, things to think about might include flexibility in scheduling, salary, benefits, opportunity for advancement, safety, or ethical considerations.

- *Am I in agreement with the salon or spa's philosophy?* Learning that you are opposed to meeting a sales quota, performing a particular treatment, or using certain products after you have accepted a position makes it hard to exit gracefully. By taking a look at all aspects of a company's philosophy or policies, you can decide what you are comfortable with beforehand.

- *Do I have any other obligations that may interfere with the demands of this particular situation?* It is always best to be honest. Trying to work around other duties or responsibilities may become a burden that will compromise your ability to do a good job and jeopardize your position. If you are unavailable at certain times or days of the month, make sure your employer is informed and willing to consent to your schedule.

- *What support will I need to ensure my success?* The salon or spa industry has become increasingly competitive. To maintain credibility, you must continue to keep abreast of new treatments and techniques. Finding the support you need to do your job well can become a critical issue after you have graduated. Mentors may not be readily available, and workshops and seminars could become prohibitively expensive. It is always best to find out what options are available to continue your education before you start a job. Learning that your employer is not invested in providing you with opportunities to enhance your performance may ultimately become a lesson in frustration.

- *Are there any causes that you feel passionate about?* Some people have ethical or moral issues that are compelling enough to make them take a stand. These may be related to personal, cultural, or political differences. For example, you may have strong feelings about working on Sundays or using products that are tested on animals. If you hold certain opinions or views that you feel strongly about, be sure these are a good fit and can be tolerated within the environment where you will be working. Becoming a crusader for certain rights or privileges may or may not make you employee of the month.

Qualifying Your Options

Many people enter the field of esthetics with the dream of working in a particular setting. Some might want to work at a chic urban day spa or a health and wellness center, while others will crave a more intimate atmosphere. Understanding more about the qualitative differences in salon and spa environments will help you to narrow your search and find the best fit for your personality and style.

There are many variations of the general categories stated previously. Skin care salons and spas range from basic to glamorous, and prices vary according to location and clientele. These options can exist in urban, suburban, or rural settings. Salons or spas may be franchised, independent, or corporately owned. They can be full service, specialized, or health oriented, and they may be categorized as skin care clinics, salons, and day, destination, or medical spas. A **franchised salon or spa** (FRAN-chyzed suh-LAHN or SPAH) is owned by individuals who pay a certain fee to use the company name, and it is part of a larger organization or chain of salons. The franchise operates according to a specified business plan and set protocols and is able to offer certain advantages associated with more corporate environments, such as national marketing campaigns and employee benefits packages. Important decisions such as the size, location, décor, and menu of services are dictated by the parent company.

Small *independently owned skin care clinics* and *day spas* afford the owner greater freedom and control in decision making, which in turn can allow them to be more flexible in their dealings with employees. Benefits may be fewer; however, this does not necessarily mean that income is inadequate. Practitioners who prefer a more intimate setting and like to work closely with a smaller group of practitioners may find this experience very rewarding. Many also associate the small salon or spa with a greater opportunity to build long-lasting relationships with clientele.

The *full-service salon* or *day spa* can be a fast-paced hub of activity appealing to those who appreciate the full spectrum of beauty and the opportunity to become part of a larger team or network. Chic, high-end image salons or day spas may appeal to more cosmopolitan personalities who like to be on the cutting edge of beauty and fashion.

The *resort* or *destination spa* is associated with a hotel facility and can be just the right fit for the esthetician who likes to work with a constantly changing clientele. This climate may also afford more corporate style benefits and educational opportunities.

Finally, the *medical spa* or *wellness center* may be an ideal situation for those estheticians who are more focused on the health benefits or age-management aspect of skin care.

Before you decide on the setting that is best for you, take time to visit and research a variety of operations. If you do not find the type of spa or salon you are looking for in your locale, there are many trade publications, consumer magazines, and Web sites that can provide you with more in-depth information to help you make your decision.

The Salon Visit or Information Interview

One of the best ways to learn about a salon or spa is to request an **information interview.** Whether in person or over the telephone, having a chat with the owner, employees, or clients who frequent a salon you are interested in is a good place to start. Asking questions without the added pressure of being a job candidate may also be a less stressful approach to getting the answers you want. Just be sure to be diplomatic and prepared; remember those granting an information interview have taken valuable time to help you. In turn you should be prompt, courteous, and respectful of any boundaries they may impose.

Visiting salons before you graduate is also a good way to network. Many salon owners or managers are eager to meet students looking for employment. At the same time, this will give you the opportunity to compare different types of esthetic salons, service menus, pricing, and styles of management. When requesting an information interview, always use professional telephone etiquette. Begin the conversation by identifying yourself as a student interested in learning more about salon operations. Ask to speak to the owner or manager, and politely request a few moments of his or her time. Remember that an information interview is not the same as a request for a job interview, although managers frequently will consider enthusiastic students for positions that become available.

If your request for an information interview is turned down or limited, do not be offended. Some salon owners may have time for only a brief telephone conversation or may be unwilling to disclose what they consider privileged information. Others may generously offer you an opportunity to visit the salon and meet them in person. If you are lucky enough to be granted an interview, it is a good idea to prepare very specific questions, limiting topics to key areas that will give you a general idea of how the salon or spa operates. Possible subjects might include:

- the duties and responsibilities required of estheticians on staff.
- how management makes important decisions related to product selection, new techniques, pricing, and other policies.
- what customer service policies the manager believes are critical to operating a successful salon or spa.
- how the salon attracts new customers or markets its services.
- who is responsible for retail sales, and if there are any sales quotas that estheticians must meet.
- whether there are specific policies or procedural guides for employees.

If you would like to solicit additional information directly from employees or clients afterward, always ask permission from the salon owner first. After your visit, it is considered proper professional etiquette to send a handwritten thank-you note (Figure 20–8).

Those who are uncomfortable with conducting an information interview with the owner or manager may choose to gather information anonymously, frequenting different salons and spas as a client. Interacting with estheticians and other patrons will give you the opportunity to ask questions indirectly in a relaxed and nonthreatening fashion. In such situations, remember that you should always practice professionalism, tact, and diplomacy.

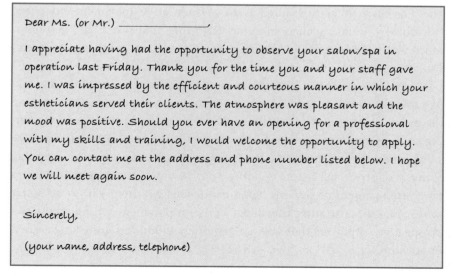

Dear Ms. (or Mr.) _____,

I appreciate having had the opportunity to observe your salon/spa in operation last Friday. Thank you for the time you and your staff gave me. I was impressed by the efficient and courteous manner in which your estheticians served their clients. The atmosphere was pleasant and the mood was positive. Should you ever have an opening for a professional with my skills and training, I would welcome the opportunity to apply. You can contact me at the address and phone number listed below. I hope we will meet again soon.

Sincerely,

(your name, address, telephone)

Figure 20–8 A sample thank-you note for the salon visit or information interview.

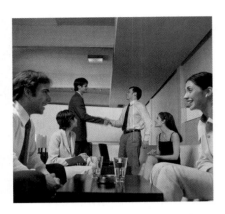

Figure 20–9 Networking is a good way to increase contacts that can enhance your career.

Networking

Establishing contacts that eventually lead to employment opportunities is another important part of the job search. There are many ways to network or build relationships to further your career; finding the one you are most comfortable with is part of the process (Figure 20–9).

Networking is a subtle approach to increasing the breadth and scope of your contacts. It is far less intimidating than a direct request for a job interview and is a useful exercise in developing important communication skills. Students can begin to develop networking skills in many ways. The following list of suggestions will help you to get started.

- Join professional organizations. Most offer student discounts and encourage membership.
- Attend industry trade shows and educational seminars. Talk to presenters and participants.
- Create a list of ideal affiliations, for example, dermatologists, massage therapists, and nutritionists. Develop a "script" for introducing yourself.
- Find out who's who in the area of skin care, and request a 10-minute information interview. This can be conducted over the phone or by e-mail.
- Subscribe to trade publications and get in the habit of checking into calendars of events.
- Ask your instructors about local, regional, and national happenings.
- Participate in field trips sponsored by your school.
- Keep a list of guest speakers who have visited your school, for future reference.
- Become involved in a charity project.
- Be open-minded and attend business functions or health seminars that will provide positive learning experiences, even if they are not completely focused on skin care.

The Employment Interview

The first step in getting hired is to arrange an employment interview. Hopefully, you have spent some time narrowing your search and getting in touch with your personal job requirements. Now you are ready to focus exclusively on finding a job.

Many students have a list of spas and salons where ideally they would like to work, but it is always a good idea to begin your search by scouting the many advertised positions that are available. The first step toward gaining an interview is to send your resume, prefaced by a cover letter, to those salons and spas you are interested in. Even if you have general knowledge about a salon or spa before sending your resume, it is wise to request a brochure or menu of services beforehand. This will help you to be better informed. Demonstrating knowledge of the employment setting also shows prospective employers that you are genuinely interested in making a good impression.

Here's a Tip

To help you stay organized during the employment search, create a chart that lists the name of the salon or spa, the contact person responsible for hiring, the date you sent your resume or called to inquire about a job, a planned time to follow up, and a brief summary of your results (Figure 20–10).

Salon	Position available	Website	Brochure	Contact date	Follow-up date	Resume sent
Salon #1	☐	☐	☐	☐	☐	☐
Salon #2	☐	☐	☐	☐	☐	☐
Salon #3	☐	☐	☐	☐	☐	☐
Salon #4	☐	☐	☐	☐	☐	☐

Figure 20–10 Interview checklist.

You may need to send several resumes and make many phone calls before you are actually granted an interview. Do not get discouraged; you may not begin your career in your dream job, but the right job will come along. Just speaking with someone responsible for hiring over the phone is a move in the right direction. Often, salon managers will not have an immediate position available but may be interested in having a copy of your resume or meeting you in case an opening becomes available later. Do not consider this effort a waste of your time. Each interview is a valuable learning experience that will help you build confidence in your interpersonal skills and become familiar with what to expect. Interviews can also be an excellent occasion to network. Whatever the outcome, always be polite and thank those in charge for their time and consideration. If you are granted an interview, following it up with a handwritten thank-you note is standard protocol. This should include a positive statement about why you want the job, if in fact you do want it.

Preparing for the Interview

Does the thought of being interviewed make you anxious? If so, you are not alone. It is common to feel a bit nervous when preparing for a job interview.

There are many ways to alleviate the pressure of being interviewed. Being organized and prepared with the appropriate documents will put you at ease and help you make a positive first impression. Even if you have already mailed your resume, be sure to have an additional copy in case the interviewer has misplaced it. You should also have some form of identification, such as your driver's license and your social security card. Other important documents include a copy of your esthetics license, any other pertinent licenses you may hold, training certificates or awards, professional memberships, references or letters of recommendation from former employers, and any photos of your work that may enhance your status. Presenting these in a covered binder or portfolio is a good way to appear efficient and organized (Figure 20–11).

We have already discussed the importance of personal appearance in the esthetics industry. This is especially important when presenting for a job interview. Employers will expect you to reflect healthy skin care practices.

PREPARING FOR THE INTERVIEW CHECKLIST

RESUME COMPOSITION

1. Does it present your abilities and what you have accomplished in your jobs and training?
2. Does it make the reader want to ask, "How did you accomplish that?"
3. Does it highlight accomplishments rather than detailing duties and responsibilities?
4. Is it easy to read, short, and does it stress past accomplishments and skills?
5. Does it focus on information that's relevant to your own career goals?
6. Is it complete and professionally prepared?

PORTFOLIO CHECKLIST

_____ Diploma, secondary and post-secondary

_____ Awards and achievements while in school

_____ Current resume focusing on accomplishments

_____ Letters of reference from former employers

_____ List of, or certificates from, trade shows attended while in training

_____ Statement of professional affiliations (memberships in esthetics organizations, etc.)

_____ Statement of civic affiliations and/or activities

_____ Before and after photographs of technical skills services you have performed

_____ Any other relevant information

Ask: Does my portfolio portray me and my career skills in the manner that I wish to be perceived? If not, what needs to be changed?

GENERAL INFORMATION

Describe specific methods or procedures you will employ in the salon/spa to build your clientele.

Describe how you feel about retail sales in the salon/spa and give specific methods you would use in the salon/spa to generate sales.

State why you feel consumer protection and safety is so important in the field of esthetics.

After careful thought, explain what you love about you new career. Describe your passion for esthetics.

Figure 20–11 Interview preparation checklist.

Keep perfume subtle and your makeup simple, with the focus on a natural glow. Nails should be clean, short, and manicured. If you wear polish, choose a neutral shade. Your jewelry and hairstyle should be unpretentious and conform to the practice of esthetics. If you have long hair, it is a good idea to style it neatly away from your face, particularly if you will be performing a facial. Wear a flattering neutral-colored suit that is cleaned and pressed, and make sure your shoes are polished and in good condition (Figure 20–12). To complete your professional appearance, carry a briefcase or portfolio to store your documents. If you do not have a briefcase, a simple handbag and a folder for your materials are appropriate.

There is always an element of surprise when it comes to the interview. However, there are certain commonly asked questions. For example, expect to answer questions related to the following issues:

* your previous job experience or academic performance
* your attendance record
* what you liked best about your esthetics training program
* your individual strengths and weaknesses
* ways that your skills will contribute to the success of the salon or spa
* your ability to be a team player
* your method for handling common problems or conflicts
* how flexible you are willing to be in terms of scheduling
* your philosophy of skin care
* your approach to customer service
* your methods for increasing client retention
* how you feel about promoting retail sales
* your long-term career goals and objectives

Many prospective employers will also ask you to perform a facial. This situation can be stressful for some. However, others may find the opportunity to demonstrate practical skills a plus. Whichever category you fall into, it is ultimately in your best interest to cooperate. If by chance you do falter, do your best not to bring attention to your mistake.

The Interview

Finally, the moment you have been waiting for has arrived: you have been granted an interview (Figure 20–13). Many books are available that offer lengthy discussions on the do's and don'ts of interviewing. You may want to spend some additional time browsing through a few of them. Here are a few basic survival tips.

* Dress professionally.
* Be on time; or better yet, arrive 10 to 15 minutes early.
* Use good manners. Be polite and courteous at all times.
* Do your best to appear relaxed and confident.
* Project a warm, friendly smile.
* Never smoke or chew gum, even if one or the other is offered to you.
* Do not come to an interview with a cup of coffee, a soft drink, snacks, or anything else to eat or drink.
* Do not bring children, friends, or significant others with you.

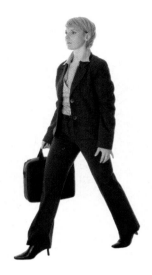

Figure 20–12 A professional appearance is important when presenting yourself for a job interview.

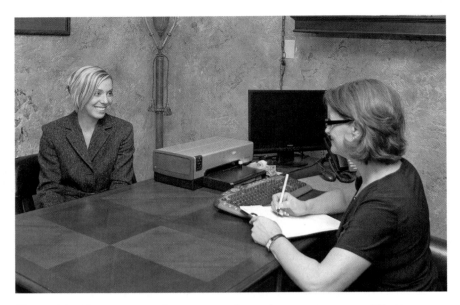

Figure 20–13 An interview is an opportunity to demonstrate your qualifications.

- Never lean on or touch the interviewer's desk. Some people do not like their personal space invaded without an invitation.
- Listen respectfully without interrupting.
- Answer questions thoughtfully, but do not elaborate for more than two minutes at a time.
- Be honest with your answers.
- Speak clearly, and use good language.
- Do not make critical remarks about previous employers or instructors.
- Always thank the interviewer for the opportunity to present your skills.

Another crucial part of the interview comes when you are invited to ask the interviewer questions of your own. You should think about those questions ahead of time and bring a list if necessary. Doing so will show that you are organized and prepared. Some questions to consider include the following:

- Is there a job description? May I review it?
- Is there a salon manual?
- How frequently does the salon advertise?
- How long do practitioners typically work here?
- Are employees encouraged to grow in skills and responsibility? How so?
- Does the salon offer continuing education opportunities?
- Is there room for advancement? If so, what are the requirements for promotion?
- What benefits does the salon offer, such as paid vacations, personal days, and medical insurance?
- What is the form of compensation?
- When will the position be filled?
- Should I follow up on your decision, or will you contact me?

Do not feel you have to ask every question on your list. The point is to create as much dialogue as possible. Be aware of the interviewer's reactions, and stop

WEB RESOURCES

Many women find it difficult to afford the two or three outfits necessary to project a confident and professional image when going out into the workplace for a job interview. Fortunately, several nonprofit organizations have been formed to address this need. These organizations receive donations of clean, beautiful clothes in good repair from individuals and manufacturers. These are then passed along to women who need them. For more information, visit Wardrobe for Opportunity at http://www.wardrobe.org and Dress for Success at http://www.dressforsuccess.org.

when you think you have asked enough questions. By obtaining answers to at least some of your questions, you can compare the information you have gathered about other salons and then choose the one that offers the best package of income and career development.

Legal Aspects of the Interview

While the opportunity to be interviewed can elicit a response to tell all, you should know that many questions are considered inappropriate or illegal. As a job applicant, you have certain rights as established by the *Equal Employment Opportunity Commission* and federal and state laws. It is important to be aware of those questions that cannot be asked either on an application form or during an interview. These include questions about your age or date of birth, race, religion, national origin, marital status, disabilities, medical conditions or health problems, and citizenship status. Employers are permitted to inquire about drug use or smoking habits and may also obtain an applicant's consent to conform to the company's drug and smoking policies or to submit to drug testing.

Sometimes interviewers are unaware when they are crossing a boundary that is illegal. You can always choose not to answer inappropriate questions. However, it is in your best interest to be tactful and diplomatic whether or not you want the job.

The Employment Application

Even if you have submitted a resume, you should also expect to fill out an employment application (Figure 20–14). Forms can vary; however, most request the same basic information—such as name, address, telephone and Social Security number, education and employment history, the position you are applying for, languages you speak, references, and emergency contacts. Your resume and portfolio will help you to answer the employment application form quickly and efficiently. To ensure credibility, be sure that the information you supply is the same on all documents. For practice, you may want to fill out the sample form in Figure 20–14.

Application for Employment

Applicant Information (please print)   Date _____

Name (Last, First, Middle) _____

Address _____

Home Phone _____ Cell Phone _____

Email Address _____

Position Desired _____ Date Available _____

Shift (day/night/rotating) _____

How did you hear about this opening?

_____

If you are under 18 years of age, do you have a permit to work?   ☐ Yes   ☐ No

Are you legally authorized to work for any employer in the United States?   ☐ Yes   ☐ No

_____

Position/Availability:

Position Applied For

_____

Days/Hours Available

Monday _____
Tuesday _____
Wednesday _____
Thursday _____
Friday _____
Saturday _____
Sunday _____

Hours Available: from_____ to _____

What date are you available to start work?

_____

Figure 20–14 A typical job application form.

2

Education

	Name and Location	Course of Study/Major	Highest Grade/Degree Completed	Diploma/Degree Received
High School or GED Equivalent				☐ Yes ☐ No
College or University				☐ Yes ☐ No
Technical/ Vocational				☐ Yes ☐ No
Other (including military training)				☐ Yes ☐ No

Please list any other professional licenses or certifications you may have:

_____

Employment History

Please list your previous employers in the past 10 years starting with your most recent. Please account for all periods of time, including military service and any periods of unemployment. You may include as part of your employment history any work performed on a volunteer basis.

Last or Present Employer
Organization Name _____
Address _____
Job Title _____
Primary Responsibilities _____
Dates of Employment _____ to _____
Salary (Starting / Leaving) _____ / _____
Supervisor (Name and Phone) _____
Reason for Leaving _____

_____
_____

Figure 20–14 *Cont.*

3

Previous Position:

Employer: _____

Address: _____

Supervisor: _____

P _____

E-mail: _____

Position Title: _____

From: _____ To: _____

Responsibilities: _____

_____

Salary: _____

Reason for Leaving: _____

May We Contact Your Present Employer?

Yes _____ No _____

References:

Name/Title/Address/Phone

_____

_____

_____

I hereby certify that all of the information provided by me in this application (or any other accompanying or required documents) is correct, accurate and complete to the best of my knowledge. I understand that the falsification, misrepresentation or omission of any facts in said documents will be cause for denial of employment or immediate termination of employment regardless of the timing or circumstances of discovery.

Acknowledgement (applicant signature): _____

Printed Name _____

Date _____

Figure 20–14 *Cont.*

ON THE JOB

Congratulations! You have worked hard to finish your esthetics training program, pass your licensing exam, and gain employment—your career as an esthetician is about to begin. This is your opportunity to put your learning to the test.

To make the transition from school to work successfully, you will need to establish and prioritize your goals. Now more than ever, you will need to practice putting your best self forward. Learning to discipline and conduct yourself in a positive and professional manner will help you develop a standard of behavior that will last throughout your career (Figure 20–15).

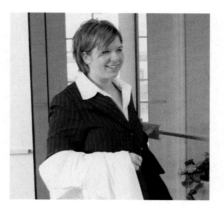

Figure 20–15 Getting off to a good start.

Moving from School to Work

Entering the workforce is an exciting time. However, earning a salary commands a new level of responsibility.

As a student, chances are you were given many opportunities to perfect your skills by performing a procedure several times before you got it right. Having instructors to guide you and peers to support you no doubt gave you a good deal of security as you learned the trade. School may also have afforded you a more flexible schedule that allowed you to juggle personal or work commitments to complete your training program. When you become an employee of a salon or spa, you will be expected to conform to a new set of rules.

Thriving in a Service Profession

The most important thing to remember as you embark on a career in esthetics is that your work revolves around serving clients. Although some people consider the idea of serving the public demeaning in some way, many find this type of work extremely rewarding.

As you continue on your journey to provide quality customer service, the following key points are emphasized to help guide you in providing client-focused service.

- *A professional appearance.* Maintain a clean, neat work environment and a polished personal appearance. These are important considerations in building client confidence.
- *Courteous behavior.* Use good manners when interacting with clients. Practicing proper etiquette is an important part of conducting yourself professionally.
- *Prompt service.* Remember that no one wants to wait. Punctuality shows clients that you value and respect their time.
- *Personal consideration.* Give each client your undivided attention. Respectful listening demonstrates a genuine interest in the client's concerns.
- *Honesty.* False claims damage the client's trust. Be sure to tell the truth when it comes to the products and services you provide.
- *Competence.* Clients need to know they can rely on your expertise. Make sure you are knowledgeable about the treatments you are practicing and the products you use. When in doubt, seek support from supervisors, manufacturers, or other educational sources.
- *Positive attitude.* A pleasant and helpful attitude makes clients feel welcome and cared for. If you cannot provide a particular service or certain information, make an effort to find out how the client can obtain it.

Joining a Successful Business

Joining a successful team is an incredible opportunity to use the training and skills that you have worked so hard to obtain.

Estheticians should always remember that the main goal of a salon or spa is to promote business. Maintaining work habits that foster this goal, such as keeping a schedule that benefits the salon's clients, will become a top priority. You will also be responsible for producing good work and following set standards. Learning to put the needs of the salon and its clients ahead of your personal concerns and performing whatever services and functions your job requires, regardless of personal circumstances, is an ordinary part of the working world.

Being a Team Player

Most spas employ several individuals and are dependent upon their working cooperatively to achieve success. In today's fast-paced and competitive business environment, salon and spa owners simply cannot tolerate individual agendas that would undermine their prosperity. Skin care services are expensive, and customers are demanding. There are bills to pay and quotas to meet to earn a profit. To increase productivity and keep customers satisfied, smart managers realize that all employees must be equally invested in achieving a common goal (Figure 20–16).

Unless you intend to be a one-person operation, it is important to understand how to get along with others and work productively. While it is the responsibility of management to create a climate that promotes each person's success, and to build a solid team effort in the most stress-free and supportive atmosphere possible, each individual should be aware of the traits that support these efforts. The following behavioral characteristics are crucial to becoming a good team player.

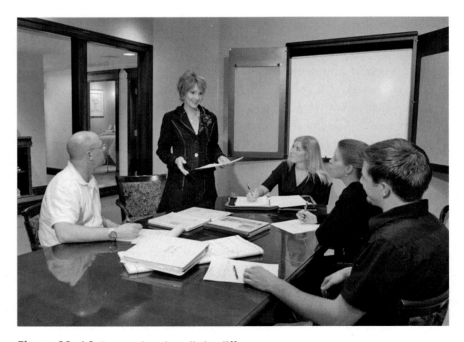

Figure 20–16 Teamwork makes all the difference.

Be Dependable

It is important for all team members to have a sense of being able to depend upon one another. Be punctual, keep your word, and be willing to help out whenever a colleague needs your assistance.

Be Cooperative

Understand what your boss expects of you, and work hard to meet those objectives. If you have finished your own work, be willing to pitch in and help others to meet team goals. Sharing the workload in a cooperative and pleasant manner benefits everyone.

Be Supportive

If you are knowledgeable in a particular area, be willing to share that information with others. Offering support in a humble and genuine fashion is a good way to earn the respect of coworkers and receive positive recognition from your employer.

Be Responsible

For a salon to be successful, each employee must be successful. Be ready, willing, and able to pull your own weight and accept additional responsibilities whenever necessary.

Be Caring

Show an interest in others. At times your coworkers may be stressed or overwhelmed with their duties and responsibilities. When you encourage and support your teammates to do their best, particularly through difficult times, everyone wins.

Be Respectful

Each of us has unique talents and methods of doing things. At times you may disagree with another's approach. However, it is important to be patient and work to solve problems in a kind and productive way. As you learn to value differences in others, you will no doubt find new ways to approach tasks and increase your ability to express yourself positively (Figure 20–17).

> **? Did You Know**
>
> In some cases, those working for someone else may be held liable for errors in professional judgment. It is always best to understand the limits of your employer's liability protection and seek additional insurance coverage when applicable.

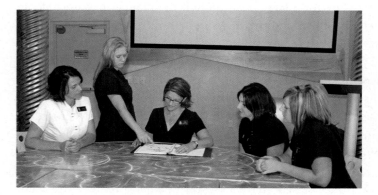

Figure 20–17 Staff meetings are essential for building high-functioning teams.

Recognizing the Value of Policies and Procedures

Knowing what the rules are is an important part of functioning in the work world. Rules and regulations help us navigate many situations. For example, rules and guidelines help us maintain a healthy and productive existence by telling us how fast we can drive on the highway, what forms of payment are acceptable when purchasing goods and services, or what our rights are when applying for health insurance, credit cards, or loans.

Successful businesses also recognize the need for clear directives and work hard to see that all employees are aware of expectations. To keep personnel informed and maintain quality control, most well-run businesses will provide a written statement of their policies and procedures. These may come in the form of an employee handbook or company manual. Rules and regulations are instrumental in keeping operations running smoothly; they also help to guarantee customer satisfaction. It is every employee's responsibility to be aware of company policy; ignorance is no excuse for not following the rules.

Chances are you will receive some explanation of how your employer expects you to behave when you are hired. Whether this comes in the form of a verbal discussion or written statement, you will want to be clear about what your duties and responsibilities are. The following list targets critical issues every employee should know about.

- correct protocol for calling in sick or late
- number of sick days allowed
- length of vacation time and number of days that can be accrued over time
- paid and unpaid holidays
- dress code
- a detailed job description highlighting specific duties and responsibilities
- insurance plan and payment procedure
- person responsible for human resource issues
- person responsible for your direct supervision

Many salons incorporate a mission statement or philosophy in their company manual. This may explain their vision for the future as well as their position on various issues, such as what products they believe in or how they feel about supporting employee education. This statement can help you determine whether your own goals and objectives will be a good fit.

If you are working for a large organization, the manual may include an organization chart. Understanding who is in authority and how you fit into the company's "big picture" is important in terms of diplomacy. Knowing who's who may save you from an embarrassing moment or give you the motivation you need if you are looking to advance within the company.

Some salons may also insist on performing treatments in a certain way. Do not be surprised if the salon you work for dictates exactly how a procedure should be performed. Because estheticians work closely with the public, it is imperative in today's litigation-oriented society for businesses to provide specific guidelines on such topics as sanitation, sterilization, and standard precautions. It also makes sense to have a set way of administering a treatment or task to ensure that each customer receives the same quality of treatment and is ultimately satisfied with whoever performs the service.

Liability Issues

Liability is a topic that deserves a good deal of attention. The skin care business has become increasingly sophisticated, incorporating treatments that are far more aggressive and complex than they were 10 years ago. And while no one looks for problems, accidents do happen. Reactions or sensitivities to cosmetic products are commonplace. Clients may not fully disclose information, or they may suddenly develop an allergic reaction to a substance they have been using without a problem for some time. Therefore, it is in everyone's best interest, employers and employees alike, to take a cautious approach.

Ideally, the esthetician should have the opportunity to practice using a new product or treatment several times under direct supervision before administering it to a paying customer. This helps businesses to avoid more costly errors. However, smaller salons and spas may not be able to afford such practices—the cost of products may be high, and management may be limited in their capacity to bring in professional consultants. To ensure the safety of your clients and to protect yourself and your employer from liability issues, take time to consider these recommendations.

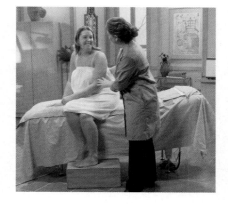

Figure 20–18 Always exercise care and caution to ensure the safety of your clients.

- Before beginning any new procedure, be sure to take a complete client history, noting any contraindications, allergies, or sensitivities (Figure 20–18).
- Administer patch tests before allowing a client to undergo the complete treatment process.
- As a general rule, when in doubt, don't! Whenever you have a question, seek supervision from someone more knowledgeable than you.
- Always have the client sign a consent form that explains the procedure and what to expect, as well as the benefits and possible side effects or risks.
- Review the consent form, and go over any special instructions with clients before beginning the procedure.
- Be sure to have clients sign a consent form each time they undergo a procedure, updating information as necessary.
- Should a problem arise, inform your supervisor immediately and document the incident carefully, noting specific side effects and client concerns in the client's profile.

As a professional working for someone else, it is your duty to practice with care and caution. Although you should expect to be covered against any claims that may arise, you should know that, in some cases, even those working for someone else could be held liable for errors in professional judgment. To be safe, it is always best to ask your employer for documentation of the business's professional liability insurance and the limits of protection. Regardless of coverage, it is also a good idea to make inquiries about the cost of obtaining an additional individual professional liability insurance policy. Professional organizations, training schools, and small business associations can be helpful in referring you to appropriate resources.

THE JOB DESCRIPTION

The **job description** is an important tool that helps employees understand exactly what is expected of them.

Once you are hired as an employee, you will be expected to conduct yourself professionally and perform those services required of you as an esthetician in compliance with salon or spa policy. To carry out your responsibilities to the best of your ability, you should be given a job description. If the salon or spa you are working for does not provide one, it is a good idea to write down those duties that were discussed during your interview or training and review them with your employer or manager. This way you will both have a clear understanding of the requirements. If you do have any questions or some areas seem vague, this would be a good time to clarify them with your boss.

Job descriptions are as varied as the types of salons that exist, and they are typically based on the needs of the salon or spa. Expect that the small clinic or day spa will have a different set of demands than a large resort spa or medical esthetics practice. The number of employees may also determine which tasks you are required to perform. However, in general, estheticians are expected to perform some variation of the following duties and responsibilities.

- Analyze skin types and conditions.
- Perform facials and other specialized skin care treatments.
- Develop therapeutic skin care programs to treat certain skin conditions.
- Explain treatment protocols and review possible side effects with clients.
- Apply facial masks.
- Apply basic and corrective makeup.
- Conduct hair removal services.
- Conduct spa services such as body wraps and polishes.
- Recommend skin care products.
- Educate clients on new treatment programs.
- Advise clients on home-care programs.
- Make follow-up phone calls.
- Investigate new products and techniques.
- Advise management on new methods, products, and services.
- Educate staff on products and services.
- Encourage salon clients to try new services.
- Promote retail sales.
- Participate in sales events or promotional activities.
- Refer clients to colleagues for additional services or other professionals whenever appropriate.
- Create retail displays and perform merchandising tasks.
- Clean and sanitize the treatment room and utensils.

Estheticians may also be asked to perform other administrative duties such as the following.

- Answer the telephone.
- Schedule appointments.
- Confirm appointments.
- Initiate and update the client profile or intake questionnaire.
- Record client information and treatment results.
- File client data.

- Review consent forms with clients.
- Maintain product inventory.
- Supervise new employees.

Some salons and spas may incorporate other objectives in their job descriptions. These can specify the attitudes that are expected and the opportunities for growth that are available to employees (Figure 20–19).

Job Description: Entry Level Esthetician

Every Entry Level Estheticians must have an esthetics license as well as the determination to learn and grow on the job. All estheticians are expected to follow specified skin care protocols, and must attend all training seminars and workshops proposed by management for their job level. In addition, Entry Level Estheticians must report weekly to an assigned Senior Level Esthetician for a period of six weeks to review skin care protocols and raise any questions they may have regarding salon operations or procedures. This helps the Salon to maintain quality control, a significant factor in client satisfaction and repeat business. As an Esthetician, you must be willing to cooperate with coworkers in a team environment, which is most conducive to learning and to good morale among all employees. You must display a friendly yet professional attitude toward coworkers and clients alike.

Excellent time management is essential to the operation of a successful salon. All estheticians must perform services in accordance with set time allowances for each treatment. This helps to keep all service providers on schedule. Estheticians should be aware of clients who arrive early or late and should also keep track of other scheduled service providers who may be running ahead or behind in their schedule. In those situations the esthetician should be willing to make the appropriate adjustments to their schedule if needed. Be prepared to stay at work up to an hour late when necessary. Keep in mind always that everyone needs to work together to get the job done.

The Responsibilities of an Entry Level Esthetician include the following:
1. Analyze skin types and conditions.
2. Perform facials and other entry level specialized skin care treatments.
3. Develop therapeutic skin care programs in accordance with set salon protocols for specific skin types and conditions.
4. Explain treatment protocols and review possible side effects with clients.
5. Apply facial masks.
6. Apply basic and corrective makeup.
7. Conduct hair removal services.
8. Recommend skin care products.
9. Educate clients on new treatment programs.
10. Advise clients on home-care programs.
11. Encourage salon clients to try new services.
12. Promote retail sales in accordance with specified sales goals for your job level.
13. Participate in sales events or promotional activities.
14. Refer clients to colleagues for additional services or other professionals whenever appropriate.
15. Clean and sanitize the treatment room and utensils after each use.
16. Supervise the client intake questionnaire.

Figure 20–19 A sample job description.

17. Review the appropriate consent forms with clients as necessary.
18. Record client information and treatment results.
19. Maintain inventory control in treatment room at regularly scheduled daily and weekly intervals set by management.
20. Inform management of any equipment malfunctions, treatment room or building maintenance problems that would impact the safety of clients and/or service providers.

Continuing Education

Your position as an Entry Level Esthetician is the first step toward becoming a successful member of the salon's skin care team. In the beginning, your training will focus on set protocols and procedures. Once you have mastered those, your training will focus on the sales skills you will need to promote proper client home care. As part of your continuing education in this salon, you will be required to:

• Attend all salon classes as required for your job level.
• Attend our special Sunday sales seminars four times a year.
• Meet the established retail sales goals set for all Entry Level Estheticians.

Advancement

Upon successful completion of all required classes and seminars and your demonstration of the necessary skills and attitudes, you will have the opportunity to advance to the position of a Level II Esthetician. This advancement will always depend upon your successful performance as an Entry Level Esthetician as well as the approval of management. Remember: How quickly you achieve your goals in this salon is up to you!

Figure 20–19 *Cont.*

EMPLOYEE EVALUATION

Developing a productive process for measuring an employee's progress is critical to setting employee and business standards. The esthetician's evaluation is likely to begin with a reference to her or his job description. The job description provides an excellent standard for evaluating the functional aspects of employee performance, that is, how well you perform the practical tasks that are expected of you. Keep in mind that attitude is a critical factor in evaluating employee performance and may be specified in your job description. Maintaining a running checklist of your job requirements will help to ensure that you are meeting these important obligations.

Most salons today also use computerized information systems to analyze retail and service sales. This generally includes a detailed account of each employee's productivity levels. Be prepared to review the results of your individual sales performance with your supervisor in an open-ended manner. When queried, try not to respond to questions with a simple yes or no. This approach may not supply you with the feedback you will need to move forward in the best way possible. Whenever you have the opportunity, it can also be helpful to ask your employer for suggestions that will help you to do your job better. This demonstrates that you are willing to grow and learn and are mature enough to handle constructive criticism.

Although the evaluation process may take some getting used to, it should ultimately supply employees with incentive for performing their duties in a way that also helps management to meet their goals, creating a win–win situation for both. In general, estheticians starting out should expect to be evaluated 90 days or 3 months after they are hired, and on a yearly basis thereafter. In the meantime, developing a method for critical self-analysis and soliciting important feedback from management can help you to become comfortable with the process.

Employers generally appreciate personnel who are proactive in assuming responsibility for their own success and may automatically supply monthly sales and service reports to help individuals evaluate their progress. If your employer does not, consider requesting such information or keep track on your own. You may also want to ask a trusted colleague to critique your sales technique, or you can ask clients for suggestions about how to provide better service. Understanding your productivity and client satisfaction levels can validate those things that you are doing right and provide additional incentive for making necessary changes. Learning to use this information wisely will help you fulfill job requirements and develop solid career management skills.

COMPENSATION

Just as the bottom line for salons is making money, getting paid is the primary incentive for estheticians. You undoubtedly enjoy what you do, but it is not likely that you would go to work if you did not receive a paycheck at the end of each week. In today's competitive market, *how much* an esthetician is paid varies, and compensation can be a determining factor in whether he or she accepts a position.

Historically, esthetics grew out of the salon industry, which used a percentage-based or commission-based wage structure. As a result, many skin care salons and day spas adopted this method of compensation. Since acquiring separate licensing, estheticians have gained entry to many other professional arenas. This has opened the door to new ways of thinking about how to pay estheticians.

Methods of Compensation

Skin care salons, day spas, and other businesses that employ estheticians differ in how they compensate employees. Pay structures may be based on **salary, commission,** or on some combination of both.

Salary

Salaries can be based on either a *flat* or *hourly* rate. If you are compensated using a flat rate, you can expect to be paid a certain amount that has been agreed upon per week. Salary levels for estheticians vary, and in some cases are negotiable, but remember: If you are offered a set salary each week, instead of an hourly rate, it must be equal to at least minimum wage; and you are entitled to overtime pay if you work more than 40 hours per week. The only exception would be if you were in an official salon management position.

The hourly rate is a popular method of payment for estheticians and is generally based on company standards. For example, a senior-level esthetician may earn a higher rate of pay than does an entry-level esthetician. Those compensated using this method can expect to be paid only for those hours they work. For example, if you worked 35 hours at the rate of $10 per hour, you would be paid $350. If you worked more hours you would earn more money; and, conversely, you would earn less money for working fewer hours.

Commission

Commission-based wages are directly related to your performance, which means that you earn a certain percentage of whatever services you perform. In the salon industry straight commission rates typically fluctuate and can range anywhere from 25 to 60 percent depending on the length of your employment, your performance level, and the benefits that are part of your employment package. This means that if you take in $1,000 in services for the week and your commission is 25 percent, your gross earnings (before taxes) would be $250. If your commission rate were 50 percent, your gross earnings would be $500. At 60 percent, your gross earnings would be $600. In addition to a commission on services, a percentage of retail sales, generally between 10 and 15 percent, is also calculated.

This compensation method continues to appeal to a number of salon owners. However, as newer methods of compensation become more readily accepted, and salon owners recognize inherent differences in the role of individual service providers and the costs of services, many of those using this system of payment to pay estheticians are establishing lower commission rates and implementing tiered schedules to motivate staff to increase their income. This means the service provider must meet a certain volume of sales and services dollars to earn higher commission rates. Others are implementing a fixed percentage or flat rate for each service. If you are comfortable with this method of payment, be aware that the commission-based model varies according to the employer and may or may not include additional benefits or other bonuses. In addition, some salons may apply surcharges to cover the cost of products used to perform services. This policy can make earning a living difficult for the esthetician who is starting out and has yet to develop a clientele.

Hybrid Pay Structures

Many salons are now using a combination of salary and commission-based structures. Generally speaking, these incorporate a base salary plus a certain commission on services and/or products. Again, the salary-plus-commission model varies and is dependent on the philosophy of the individual salon owner. Typically, this model offers a salary that is established by an hourly or flat rate, plus anywhere between 10 and 20 percent

ACTIVITY

Go through the budget worksheet and fill in the amounts that apply to your current living and financial situation. If you are unsure of the amount of an expense, put in the amount you have averaged over the past three months or give it your best guess. For your income, you may need to have three or four months of employment history in order to answer, but fill in what you can.

- How do your expenses compare to your income?
- What is your balance after all your expenses are paid?
- Were there any surprises for you in this exercise?
- Do you think that keeping a budget is a good way to manage money?
- Do you know of any other methods people use to manage money?

FOCUS ON . . .

THE GOAL

Always put the team first. While each individual may be concerned with getting ahead and being successful, a good teammate knows that no one can do it alone.

commission on products and/or services. Some salons also incorporate bonuses or other incentives that are fixed according to performance **quotas.** In some cases these quotas will be based on team rather than individual performance.

Other Factors Affecting Wages

Estheticians can also expect wages to vary according to several criteria, such as an individual's level of training and experience. Other business factors, for example, the type of salon (that is, full service, day or resort spa, skin care clinic, or medical practice), geographic location (urban or suburban), and pricing (moderately priced or high end) will come into play.

Today, many opportunities are available to estheticians in a variety of work environments. Each will have its own basis for establishing wages. Although pay scales and methods continue to vary, there appears to be a growing movement toward establishing more professional salary levels and benefits. As you make important decisions about employment, it is a good idea to analyze all aspects of compensation, such as salary, health benefits, vacation pay and allowances for sick days, and any retirement benefits that might be included.

Gratuities

Similar to other service oriented industries such as the hair, hotel, and restaurant business, in the esthetics world, tips or gratuities, have become a customary way of expressing appreciation for satisfactory service. However, not all salons and spas allow tipping. Most salons and spas today make their policy on gratuities clear to clients before they purchase a service by posting a sign at the front desk or checkout area or by incorporating their position in a brochure or menu of services.

Estheticians can expect the amount a client tips to vary, with most gratuities ranging between 15 and 20 percent of the total service ticket. For example, if a client spends $120 on a facial treatment, and tips 15 percent, then the tip to the service provider would be about $18. The most important thing for estheticians to remember about tips is that the Internal Revenue Service (IRS) considers tips additional income. As such, tips must be tracked and reported on your income tax return. While this may seem like a nuisance, it can actually prove beneficial in some situations, for example when applying for a loan or mortgage, where you want your income to appear stronger than it might be otherwise.

MANAGING MONEY

Once you are earning a salary, you will want to keep careful track of what you are spending. Understanding the value of a dollar that you have earned is a valuable lesson in economics and long-term financial success. Particularly if this is your first job, you will need to learn to plan and budget your money according to your needs.

Meeting Financial Responsibilities

Perhaps you took out a loan to pay for your esthetics education or you need to purchase a car to get to work. How will you pay for these expenses? Creating a personal budget is an important task that will help you to meet your financial obligations responsibly.

Money management is a complex issue that often generates a great deal of anxiety for people. But with careful planning and thoughtful deliberation, learning to manage your money can actually be fun. Many businesses provide automatic mechanisms for taking care of important basics such as depositing an employee's salary into his or her personal checking account, managing savings, planning for retirement, and paying health and dental insurance. Unfortunately, smaller salons and spas may not be able to afford these types of employee benefits. If you work for such an organization, you will need to learn to manage most of these things for yourself.

Keeping track of where your money goes is the first step in financial planning. To get started, write down all of your expenses and then weigh these against your total income (Figure 20–20). Once you understand the amount of money you have coming in and going out, you can make critical choices about your spending habits. Cutting down on certain unnecessary expenses can help you obtain other, more desirable items. Perhaps you would like to save for a special trip or purchase your own home. Learning to manage your money well can make these dreams a reality.

Maintaining important obligations such as car loans, mortgage payments, and other bills will also help you establish good credit. Although some may take a nonchalant attitude toward meeting financial responsibilities, it is ultimately in everyone's best interest to be mature and responsible about handling money. Defaulting on loans or claiming bankruptcy can have serious consequences for your personal and professional credit rating—an important consideration for those planning to own or operate their own business someday.

Personal Budget Worksheet

A. Expenses

1. My monthly rent (or share of the rent) is $ _____
2. My monthly car payment is   _____
3. My monthly car insurance payment is   _____
4. My monthly auto fuel/upkeep expenses are   _____
5. My monthly electric bill is   _____
6. My monthly gas bill is   _____
7. My monthly health insurance payment is   _____
8. My monthly entertainment expense is   _____
9. My monthly bank fees are   _____
10. My monthly grocery expense is   _____
11. My monthly dry cleaning expense is   _____
12. My monthly personal grooming expense is   _____
13. My monthly prescription/medical expense is   _____
14. My monthly telephone is   _____
15. My monthly student loan payment is   _____
16. My IRA payment is   _____
17. My savings account deposit is   _____
18. Other expenses: _____

TOTAL EXPENSES $ _____

B. Income

1. My monthly take-home pay is   _____
2. My monthly income from tips is   _____
3. Other income: _____

TOTAL INCOME $ _____

C. Balance

Total Income (B)   _____
Minus Total Expenses (A)   _____

BALANCE $ _____

Figure 20–20 A personal budget worksheet.

Seek Professional Advice

Finally, if you have difficulty managing money or feel unsure about how to handle certain areas of finance, such as putting money away for retirement, it may be helpful to seek professional advice. Your local bank may offer such services or be able to refer you to other resources. There are many qualified financial advisors who can offer sound advice on such topics as investing, retirement planning, and credit card debt. If you decide such a service could be helpful to you, it is always best to be cautious. Take time to investigate the person's credentials, and do not feel obligated to act on anything that you are uncomfortable with.

FINDING THE RIGHT ROLE MODELS

As a student, you are given the opportunity to practice techniques and perfect skills under the umbrella of a supportive environment that includes teachers and fellow students. However, once you are in a work environment, at times you may feel isolated or insecure about your ability to handle certain situations. Seeking the advice of someone more experienced than you can be a good way to alleviate concerns and gain the support you need.

Take a look around you. Is there anyone whose career status impresses you? Finding role models who inspire and invigorate you is an important part of career development. A **role model** is a person whose behavior and success you would like to emulate. People often think of role models only as those who have acquired significant fame or status within their industry. But the truth is, you may not have to look very far to find people with skills and habits worth imitating.

Perhaps there is a more experienced coworker or boss you admire. Take note of how she handles situations with clients and colleagues. Are there any special techniques she uses to enhance her job performance? What character traits does she possess that keep clients coming back? Does she read certain publications or attend trade shows to keep herself informed? Paying attention to the habits that have made those successful in your immediate environment is a good place to begin your search. But do not limit yourself: the world is full of positive role models unaffiliated with the field of esthetics whose work habits or character traits are worth modeling. Consider them as well when you focus on how you can apply success strategies to your personal goals.

If you are lucky enough to find a role model who is willing to share her knowledge, use the time wisely. Be thoughtful in the way you present your questions and listen attentively without interrupting, even if you take issue with what the individual is saying. Remember: you asked for this person's advice.

CONTINUING YOUR EDUCATION

Upon graduation, you will have a solid base of knowledge to use in building your success. Where you go from there depends largely on your willingness to grow and develop new skills. Esthetics is a dynamic industry that has made great strides over the past several decades. Advances in equipment and product technology have introduced sophisticated new skin care methods that have changed the way estheticians work and heightened media attention. Greater awareness of treatment options has resulted in a more educated consumer who expects estheticians to have answers to more complex questions about skin care treatments and techniques. In today's continually evolving esthetics market, there is every reason to expect that this trend will continue.

To keep up with consumer demands and job requirements, estheticians must find other sources of advanced education once they have graduated. Fortunately, there are many opportunities available to those interested in increasing their knowledge. Alumnae and trade associations are a good place to start and are often good resources for accessing other information. Manufacturers and distributors are another viable source of education about

---

FOCUS ON . . .

THE GOAL

Always remember that success does not just come to you. You make it happen. How? By being a team player, having a positive attitude, and keeping a real sense of commitment to your work foremost in your mind.

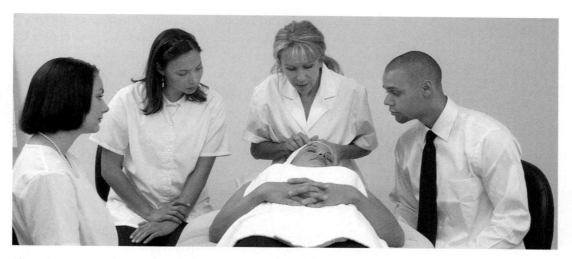

Figure 20–21 Make continued education part of your long-term planning.

new products and techniques, although you should be aware of vested interests and take care to substantiate all scientific data using unbiased methods. Subscribing to trade publications and professional newsletters will help you to keep up with important news and trends on a regular basis. You can also benefit from attending workshops and seminars sponsored by allied health professionals (Figure 20–21). This will not only increase your knowledge of associated therapies, but it can also be an excellent opportunity to network.

If you are interested in learning more about management or operating your own salon or spa, you might also consider enrolling in other business-related courses such as those offered at local adult education centers and community colleges. Becoming Internet savvy is another way to broaden your information base, although it is a good idea to follow through with additional research, particularly if topics are promotion or advertising based. Many books and videos are available that can be purchased or borrowed for independent reading and study. Of course, all of these options involve a certain expenditure of time, effort, and money. However, those committed to success understand that taking responsibility for advancing their education is ultimately worth the investment.

PLANNING YOUR SUCCESS

Many factors contribute to a successful career. We have already discussed several of them, including having a clear vision of the type of environment that best suits you, meeting the demands of your job description, and being committed to advancing your education. However, an important area that should not be overlooked is character or personality development.

We already know that efficient time management and a strong work ethic are important ingredients for success. But there are other qualitative factors to consider. Take a closer look at those who have made it. Successful people are *motivated* or driven to achieve their goals. This requires discipline and, at times, a great deal of flexibility. Success is not something that happens overnight. It requires hard work and dedication. There will be times when you hit roadblocks and need to rethink your plan. When this happens, it is important not to give up. Learn to use your setbacks as opportunities for growth, and stay focused on your goals. As you find your own way, it is also important to maintain a code of conduct that you can be proud of. Be clear about what you stand for, and remain ethical in your dealings with others. This will establish you as a person of integrity and credibility. Finally, it is important to remember to be true to yourself—there is no stopping success if you believe in yourself.

REVIEW QUESTIONS

1. Name several ways you can begin to investigate job opportunities as a student.

2. Discuss the best methods for preparing for your state licensing exam.

3. List several techniques that can be utilized to improve your results when taking written exams.

4. What is the best way to approach your response to multiple-choice questions on a test? True and false questions?

5. List the topics that should be covered in a resume, and identify the general categories they apply to.

6. Name at least five things that should not be included in your resume.

7. List the components of a good cover letter. Practice writing a cover letter that includes these criteria.

8. What should you look for in determining whether a salon or spa is right for you?

9. What is the purpose of an information interview?

10. Describe four types of salon or spa environments. Comment on the one that suits you best, and state the reasons for your decision.

11. Create a list of possible questions that you might ask during an information interview based on your target environment.

12. Name eight possible ways to network.

13. Discuss several practical steps you can take to prepare for a job interview.

14. What questions are not allowed during a professional interview?

15. What is the purpose of a job description?

16. Name and describe two ways in which the esthetician is compensated for his or her work. Which method do you consider the most advantageous? State your reasons.

17. Name several possible candidates for role models, and discuss the best way to approach these individuals for an information interview. List at least three questions that you would like to ask these people.

CHAPTER GLOSSARY

commission: a method of compensation that is percentage-based and is directly related to the employee's performance; for example, the employee earns a certain percentage of whatever services he or she performs and/or a certain percentage of the amount of product he or she sells.

deductive reasoning: the process of reaching logical conclusions by employing logical reasoning.

franchised salon or spa: a salon or spa owned by an individual(s) who pays a certain fee to use the company name and is part of a larger organization or chain of salons. The franchise operates according to a specified business plan and set protocols.

information interview: a scheduled meeting or conversation whose sole purpose is to gather information.

job description: specified list of duties and responsibilities that are required of an employee in the performance of his or her job.

networking: a method of increasing contacts and building relationships to further one's career.

quota: a method for gauging the amount of sales and targeting production levels.

resume: a summary of education and work experience that highlights relevant accomplishments and achievements.

role model: a person whose behavior and success are worthy of emulation.

salary: a method of compensation that specifies a certain amount of pay based on either a flat or hourly rate.

test-wise: refers to a student who begins to prepare for taking a test by practicing good study habits and time management as part of an effective study program.

transferable skills: those abilities, such as sales training or administrative skills, that were mastered at other jobs and can be applied to a new position.

THE SKIN CARE BUSINESS

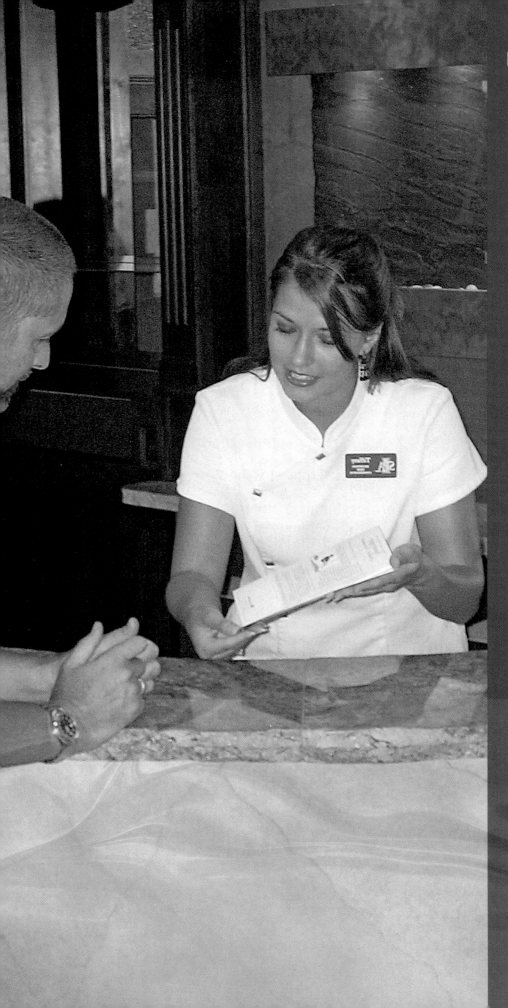

After completing this chapter, you will be able to:

- Describe the qualities necessary to be successful in a service profession.

- Evaluate options for going into business for yourself.

- List the most important factors to consider when opening a salon.

- Name and describe the types of ownership under which a skin care salon or spa may operate.

- Explain why it is necessary to keep accurate business records.

- Discuss the importance of the front desk and receptionist to a salon's success.

- Demonstrate the best practices for telephone use.

KEY TERMS

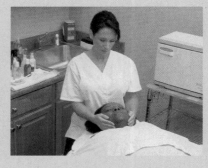

Figure 21–1 Professional skin care has become a significant part of the health, beauty, and wellness movement.

Over the past several decades, the beauty business has grown tremendously, becoming a multibillion-dollar industry that has moved beyond traditional hair and nail care to include total body services. This more holistic approach to beauty has given birth to a new era that has broadened treatment options and created a much stronger connection between beauty, health, and wellness, expanding the role of the salon and spa. From this new perspective, professional skin care has emerged from what traditionally has been a minor role in the U.S. beauty market to become the focus of many new business opportunities (Figure 21–1).

GOING INTO BUSINESS FOR YOURSELF

Perhaps you are thinking about starting your own business. Many service providers enter the field of skin care with the thought of owning their own salon or spa one day. If you are focused, disciplined, and driven to achieve your goals, this may be a viable option for you. However, motivation and commitment are only the beginning. To be successful, you will need to have lots of energy, a clear vision of what you would like to accomplish, and solid business skills. You should also have some real, practical experience in the business.

Operating your own business is a big responsibility, and it will involve many hours of careful planning and preparation. You will need to become familiar with several basic business principles, such as accounting, finance, business and tax laws, insurance, sales, and employee and customer relations. Managing day-to-day operations requires the ability to solve problems on a regular basis. Be prepared to address any number of issues, such as scheduling employees, booking appointments, tracking inventory, and ordering supplies.

Booth Rentals

For many, renting a booth or space within an established salon is a good way to gain the experience of operating a business on a much smaller scale. **Booth rentals,** as they are commonly called, have become popular in various settings including beauty salons, skin care clinics, and day spas. They offer the practitioner an opportunity to be his or her own boss within a certain set of parameters. In a booth-rental arrangement, the esthetician is required to pay the owner a set rental fee, along with payment of utilities as agreed upon, to operate in a specific space within the owner's establishment. The renter is responsible for conducting all necessary business functions, such as managing her own clientele, supplies, and records. However, renting space does not necessarily mean that you have complete control over your situation.

Before you agree to a booth-rental arrangement, take time to investigate the many legal and business aspects of conducting business as a booth renter. The first thing you will want to determine is whether it is lawful to operate as a booth renter in your state. Some states require a separate license for booth rentals. Other states may not recognize this business structure at all. So it is important to check with all of the state regulating agencies that apply, including your esthetic licensing board, before adopting this model. Note that some state boards require an apprenticeship before an esthetician can be self-employed. Renting a space from a qualified practitioner may or may not meet the criteria, so be sure to learn whether your current esthetician license is sufficient to operate on your own. Other state business and licensing requirements for operating a separate business may also apply to you. It is also imperative that you have a complete understanding of Internal Revenue Service (IRS) laws governing this form of business ownership. As a booth renter, you are responsible for paying all taxes associated with being self-employed, including higher Social Security taxes (double that of an employee; (Figure 21–2).

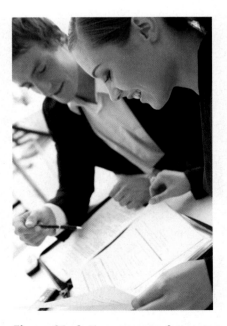

Figure 21–2 There are many factors to consider when opening your own salon.

Once you are clear about the legalities, weigh the pros and cons of this business structure carefully. There are several advantages to booth rentals. For example, booth rentals offer the individual practitioner an opportunity to establish his or her own business with minimal investment, generally require lower maintenance fees, and give the practitioner the flexibility of creating his or her own schedule. In some situations, the booth renter may be allowed to engage in joint advertising efforts, sharing costs at a lower rate. Additionally, there may be an opportunity to access clients from the owner's existing clientele. These benefits can be appealing, but it is wise to learn as much as you can about the business and owner before signing any contracts. Take a close look at the owner's track record. How many years has the establishment been in business? What is its turnover rate for booth renters and/or employees? Do you agree with the accepted practices of the salon owner? Sharing similar philosophies goes a long way in resolving any problems that may arise.

There are other practical matters to consider. For some, the idea of keeping records for legal and tax purposes can be a challenge. Being the sole person responsible for all day-to-day operations such as scheduling appointments, managing clients, purchasing products, and maintaining inventory is a huge undertaking when there is no partner or team to support you. If you do not enjoy working alone, this arrangement may not suit you. Keep in mind that you will be required to retain separate malpractice and health insurance, and you will not have the luxury of additional benefits that are typically supplied by employers, such as paid vacation time and sick days. In addition, you may be limited to certain hours during which you can conduct business, and you will be responsible for marketing and developing your own clientele.

Weigh all of these pros and cons cautiously, and be sure to obtain the appropriate legal advice before signing any documents or contracts. Carefully researching all matters before you act can help to avoid problems.

Developing a Plan of Action

Everyone has a different vision of the type of esthetics practice he or she would enjoy. For some, results are most important; for others, health and wellness are the top priority. Deciding which treatments you would like to offer will help you determine the type of facility, products, and equipment that will be most effective in accomplishing your goals.

Once you are clear about your overall concept, you will be ready to develop a strategic business plan. Many factors go into operating a successful business and are far beyond the scope of this chapter. It is a good idea to read and research your ideas extensively before making any final decisions. A review of the following basics will help you to get started.

Location

"Location, location, location!" How often have you heard that phrase? Although it may seem obvious, deciding where to conduct business is an important consideration that requires careful deliberation. The right location can significantly affect your success.

In searching for various places to open your salon or spa, it is important to keep your target market in mind. If you want to attract a high-end clientele, explore high-income areas. If you are interested in attracting a variety of

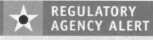

REGULATORY AGENCY ALERT

Some state boards require a special license for booth rentals. Before entering a booth-rental arrangement, always check with local and state board officials to determine rules and regulations as they apply to your individual situation.

clients with moderate incomes, search for a high-volume area that is conveniently located and offers easy access to public transportation. While many people starting small businesses like the convenience of being close to home, understand that you may have to travel a bit to reach the market your spa or salon hopes to attract.

After defining your target market, you can begin to address other factors. Two of the most important are *visibility* and *accessibility*. Ideally, a good location is easy to get to and highly visible. Most people are juggling busy schedules, and being close to other thriving businesses such as supermarkets, restaurants, department stores, or specialty shops offers clients the added convenience of "one-stop" shopping that is so crucial. High-traffic areas also provide access to a larger number of potential clients. More remote locations generally require a good deal of advertising to attract business, and this can be costly for the new small business owner (Figure 21–3).

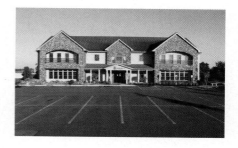

Figure 21–3 Visibility and accessibility are two of the most important factors to consider when searching for a business location.

Parking Facilities

One of the most crucial elements in attracting business is parking. Frequently, clients may be pleased with your services but become frustrated over the inability to find convenient or affordable parking. Particularly in these uncertain times, safety and convenience are important marketing features. As spa and salon hours become increasingly flexible, it is only natural for clients to want to feel safe walking in an area, especially at night or in bad weather. Well-lit, ample, and affordable parking is a good way to alleviate these concerns.

Demographics

How do you know if an area meets the criteria of your target market? One of the best ways to find out is to study the *demographics*. The term **demographics** (DEM-uh-GRAF-iks) refers to particular identifying characteristics of an area or population, such as the specific size, age, sex, or ethnicity of its residents; average income; and buying habits. This important information is available from various sources including town census bureaus, the government, local chamber of commerce and real estate agents, and special marketing agencies. Information may be obtained in a variety of formats including electronic media such as CD-ROM or print publications that distribute "cluster snapshots" or demographic synopses.

From a more subjective perspective, you can also gain valuable information by speaking with other business owners in the area or by attending local meetings and events. Learning more about who lives in a particular area, what they like to do, how they spend their money, and what they value, need, or want will help you to decide if the type of salon or spa you would like to open is a good fit.

Competition

The skin care and spa industry has grown tremendously in recent years, creating a far more competitive marketplace than the one existing even a decade ago. While it is important to investigate the services being offered at other salons in your area, do not let your findings intimidate you. The mainstay of business in the United States is competition, and in many cases it has played a positive and motivating role in driving successful businesses.

Here's a Tip

A building that is highly visible is not necessarily easy to access. Be sure the facility you are renting has a convenient way to enter and leave during the salon's regular business hours. Learning that the building's main entry or exit opens or closes before or after your salon may make it difficult for you to conduct business and can require extra security measures. Be sure to consider these factors when negotiating the terms of a lease.

Nevertheless, it is usually in your best interest to look for an area that has a limited number of salons or spas. It is also wise to develop a unique menu of services that will attract your specific target market. There is always room for a different approach that does not directly compete with those of existing businesses. In fact, similar businesses often exist side by side quite successfully simply because they are targeting different markets.

However, before you sign a lease, it still makes good sense to conduct a thorough investigation of what others are offering and the prices they are charging. You may also want to visit other reputable and established salons that are not in your general vicinity. It never hurts to find out what other successful businesses are doing right. As you conduct your research, keep a journal of those practices that make a positive impression. You also might want to create a list of ways to improve upon those ideas.

The Business Plan: Costs, Revenue, and Profits

How will you get to your destination if you do not know where you are going? The **business plan** gives the practitioner a strategy for understanding key elements in developing business. It serves as a sort of map or blueprint to help guide you in making informed decisions.

Many resources are available, including computer software that provide several methods for developing a business plan. Alternatively, hiring a professional consultant may ultimately be the most cost-effective way to approach this task. If you are unsure about how to locate a professional in this area, consider asking other small business owners for referrals or call the professional organizations to which you belong. Your local chamber of commerce or small business association is usually a good place to start.

Your plan should include a general description of your business and the services you will provide, a detailed explanation of how you will finance and manage your operation, and a discussion of area demographics, the competition, and the personnel you intend to hire. Be prepared to identify all costs related to operations, including a price structure for products and services, employee salaries, the cost of any additional benefits, and other ordinary expenses such as the cost of equipment, supplies, rent, utilities, insurance, taxes, and marketing and advertising.

Learning to think in terms of *costs, revenues,* and *profits* can help you gain a more global perspective of business functions as you develop your plan. Expenses related to operating your salon can be broken down into *fixed* and *variable costs*. **Fixed costs** are operating costs that are constant, for example, rent and loan payments. **Variable costs** are expenses that can fluctuate, such as utilities, supplies, and advertising. To a certain extent, you will have some control over variable costs. **Revenue** is the income generated from selling services and products; that is, money coming in. **Profit** is the amount of money available after all expenses are subtracted from all revenues.

As you become familiar with the specific costs related to running your business and the number of services or products you must sell to meet costs and earn a profit, you will be able to forecast or make projections about your business. Of course, to make viable projections, you will need to consider many variables on a weekly, monthly, or yearly basis. The smart businessperson also factors in changing circumstances such as economic trends and down periods. An in-depth analysis of the actual business you do over a certain time period versus forecasting will give you a more accurate idea of your situation and also help you make good business decisions (Table 21–1).

Table 21–1

AN INCOME STATEMENT				
	1ST QTR	**2ND QTR**	**3RD QTR**	**4TH QTR**
Net Sales or Revenues:				
Less the Cost of Goods Sold	————	————	————	————
Gross Profit:	————	————	————	————
Operating Expenses				
Salaries, Wages, & Commissions	————	————	————	————
Operating Supplies	————	————	————	————
Repairs & Maintenance	————	————	————	————
Laundry	————	————	————	————
Advertising & Promotion	————	————	————	————
Loan Interest	————	————	————	————
Rent	————	————	————	————
Utilities	————	————	————	————
Telephone	————	————	————	————
Insurance	————	————	————	————
Payroll Taxes	————	————	————	————
Benefit Costs	————	————	————	————
Administrative Costs	————	————	————	————
Legal Fees	————	————	————	————
Licenses	————	————	————	————
Training & Development	————	————	————	————
Depreciation	————	————	————	————
Total Operating Expenses:	————	————	————	————
Profit [or Loss] before Taxes:	————	————	————	————
Taxes:	————	————	————	————
Net Profit [or Loss] after Taxes:	————	————	————	————

Regulations, Business Laws, and Insurance

Understanding the law is critical to operating a successful business. Before opening the doors to your salon, be sure you are in compliance with all local, state, and federal regulations. You should be aware that laws vary from state to state. It is your responsibility to check into the specific laws that govern business owners in the state you are working in, particularly as they apply to your licensing or ability to establish your own business. In some states, there are levels of licensure that may require a practitioner to work under another experienced and licensed professional for a certain period of time before being allowed to operate independently.

After confirming your ability to own and operate a salon, you must contact local authorities to investigate other necessary business licenses and regulations. Ordinarily, local officials supervise building renovations and business codes. You should seek information regarding sales tax, licenses, and employee compensation laws from state administration. The federal government oversees laws regarding Social Security, unemployment compensation or insurance, cosmetics, and luxury taxes. Although some people may be annoyed by the idea of complying with so many rules and regulations, keep in mind that regulations and laws exist to protect the consumer and enforce fair and reasonable standards for best business practices. Prospective business owners should also be aware that failure to comply with state and federal regulations and tax obligations can result in serious legal consequences. If you do not understand your obligations as a business owner, seek the advice of a qualified business attorney and certified public accountant (CPA).

Insurance is another primary concern for business owners. You will need it to guard your business against such unforeseen events as malpractice, liability, disability, fire, burglary, theft, and business interruption. Before purchasing insurance, it is always best to seek professional advice to determine the right amount and type of coverage for your particular business needs. It is also a good idea to contact the department of insurance in your state to learn more about laws regulating insurance. You will need to comply with certain insurance obligations that are required by law, such as workers' compensation.

Although insurance may give the business owner some peace of mind, it should not be considered protection against inappropriate conduct. If you decide to become a business owner, it will be your job to ensure that everyone in your salon practices within the boundaries of their license. Always review the limitations of your insurance policy carefully, and take time to establish appropriate guidelines for your employees.

Salon owners must also be aware of state and federal guidelines for regulating sanitation and occupational safety. The Occupational Safety and Health Administration (OSHA) is a government agency responsible for overseeing safety in the workplace. Those working in the skin care industry should be familiar with OSHA guidelines, particularly as they apply to the correct procedure for handling bloodborne materials, instruments, and equipment. For more information on this topic or other issues more specific to skin care, visit one of OSHA's numerous Web sites on the Internet or contact the Department of Public Health in your state.

Ownership Options

Various options are available to those interested in becoming a salon owner. To choose the one that is right for you, it is important to understand the specific parameters associated with each. Hiring an attorney who specializes in such matters can be invaluable in helping you reach a decision. However, before you seek legal advice, it is a good idea to conduct your own research. This will help you formulate the right questions, thus saving time and money. A salon can be owned and operated by an individual, a partnership, or a corporation. The following are brief descriptions of each type of ownership.

Sole Proprietorship

Under individual ownership or **sole proprietorship,** the proprietor acts as sole owner and manager. A *sole proprietor* is responsible for determining all policies and making all of the necessary decisions associated with running a business. In turn, a sole proprietor is also accountable for all expenses, receives all profits, and bears all losses. If you are an independent, self-motivated individual who likes to be in charge and does not mind assuming all of the duties and obligations associated with operating a business, this may be the best arrangement for you.

Partnership

In a **partnership,** two or more people share ownership, although this does not necessarily mean an equal arrangement (Figure 21–4). There are several benefits to a partnership, including increased **capital** for investment, a greater pool of skills and talent to draw from, and the added advantage of shared responsibilities and decision making. However, when it comes to sharing, partners also divide profits. In a partnership each partner also assumes the other's unlimited liability for debt.

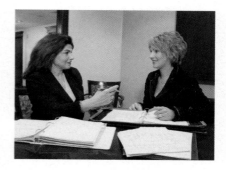

Figure 21–4 A partnership can be a mutually satisfying experience.

If you like the security of working jointly with others and you are willing to assume the risk of liability, a partnership may be ideal for you. A partnership can be a mutually satisfying experience for the right partners. It can also be a lesson in frustration if you find yourself affiliated with the wrong partner. To avoid any long-term repercussions, seek qualified legal counsel. Also, before entering any binding agreement, learn as much as possible about your prospective partner's ethics and philosophies.

Corporation

Incorporating is one of the best ways that a business owner can protect his or her assets. Most people choose to incorporate for solely this reason, but this form of ownership has other advantages. For example, the corporate business structure saves you money in taxes, provides greater business flexibility, and makes raising capital easier. It also limits your personal financial liability if your business accrues unmanageable financial debts or otherwise runs into financial trouble.

A **corporation** raises capital by issuing stock certificates or shares. Stockholders (people or companies that purchase shares) have an ownership interest in the company. The more stock they own, the larger their interest becomes. You can be the sole stockholder (or shareholder) or have many stockholders. In a corporation, income tax is limited to the salary that you draw, not the real profits of the business. However, a stockholder in a corporation is required to pay unemployment insurance, whereas a sole proprietor or partner is not.

Corporations are managed by a board of directors who determine policies and make decisions according to the corporation's charter and bylaws. Corporate formalities such as director or stockholder meetings are required to maintain a corporate status. The corporation also costs more to set up and run than a sole proprietorship or partnership does. For example, there are the initial information fees, filing fees, and annual state fees. However, many people believe the advantages of incorporating outweigh any necessary legal and accounting obligations. Should you decide that a corporation is right for you, many resources—including computer software—are available to guide you through the process of incorporating. Additionally, you will require the services of a competent lawyer and tax accountant to be sure your business complies with more complex state rules and regulations. Nevertheless, corporations can offer excellent benefits and opportunities, particularly for businesses with a larger number of employees.

Other corporate models and business entities, such as the S corporation and the limited liability company (LLC), may be better suited to your needs. A competent business attorney familiar with the laws in your state is the best resource for answering more specific questions about these models.

Purchasing an Established Salon

Buying an existing salon or spa is often advantageous. For example, you will have the opportunity to begin working right away and will not have to worry about buying furnishings or fixtures. Before you buy, however, thoroughly investigate what you are buying. Most buyers are concerned about the initial return on their investment and the possibility of increasing future sales. Many become disappointed when an existing clientele fails to frequent the salon under new ownership or when equipment does not operate as expected. This does not mean that buying an established business is out of the question. You should simply understand that some risk is involved, and take preventive measures wherever possible. For example, you may be able to obtain an extended warranty for equipment that is several years old, or you could negotiate the owner's staying on for a certain time period to ease the transition. Another important consideration is finding out whether current employees will continue to work for you. If that is your desire, it is wise to develop a protocol that keeps staff informed during the process.

If you decide to purchase an established salon, always seek the professional advice of an accountant and business lawyer (Figure 21–5). You may also want to consider a broker who specializes in the transfer of business ownership. In general, any agreement to buy an established salon should include the following parts:

* a formal written and legal purchase and sale agreement that dictates the terms of your agreement, noting any specific arrangements in detail
* a complete and signed statement of inventory that includes all products, equipment, fixtures, furnishings, and so forth and indicates the value of each article

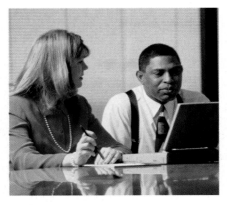

Figure 21–5 It is best to seek the appropriate legal advice when making important business decisions.

- information that clearly establishes the owner's identity
- free and unencumbered use of the salon's name and reputation for a defined period of time
- complete disclosure of all information, records, and files regarding the salon's clientele, purchasing, and service habits
- a non-compete clause stating that the seller will not compete directly with the new owner, work in, or establish a new salon within a specified distance of the present salon location

Finally, whenever there is a transfer of a note, lease, mortgage, or bill of sale, the buyer should always conduct a thorough investigation to be sure there has not been any default in payments.

Leases

Owning your own business does not necessarily mean that you own the building where your salon or spa is located. Many businesses rent or lease space in buildings owned by others. When renting or leasing space, be prepared to negotiate the terms of your agreement with your landlord. The final agreement should be clearly written and should specify who owns what and who is responsible for which repairs and expenses. If this is your first time renting commercial space, it may be helpful to seek guidance from a commercial real estate broker. It is also wise to have an attorney who specializes in real estate review the contract for you. Here are some points to consider as you negotiate your lease.

- Allow an exemption for fixtures or appliances that might be attached to the salon so that they can be removed without violating the lease.
- Specify how any necessary renovations and repairs—such as painting, plumbing, fixtures, and electrical installation—will be handled, clearly stating who is responsible for what.
- Include an option that allows you to assign the lease to another person. In this way, the obligations for the payment of rent are kept separate from the responsibilities of operating the business should you need to bring in another person or owner.

Protecting Your Business against Fire, Theft, and Lawsuits

Once your salon is up and running, you will want to do everything possible to protect it from any unfortunate mishaps or incidents. To avoid more costly dilemmas, consider taking the following precautions:

- Install adequate locks, a fire alarm, and a burglar alarm system. It can also be helpful to create a security checklist, so that those responsible for closing or opening the salon are aware of all the necessary measures required to lock and secure the premises.
- Maintain adequate amounts of liability, fire, malpractice, and burglary insurance. Note the expiration dates of your policy, and take special care not to allow a lapse in coverage during the course of business.
- Make certain that all personnel practice within the boundaries of their professional license, performing only those services they are properly trained for. Licensed professionals must never offer advice or make recommendations outside of their area of expertise. Never violate the

medical practice laws of your state by attempting to diagnose, treat, or cure a disease or illness. Always refer clients to a physician for diagnosis and treatment.

- Ignorance of the law is no excuse for violating it. Make sure you are familiar with and adhere to all laws governing the practice of esthetics in your state, including any sanitary codes that may apply in the city or state where you are operating. If you are an esthetician operating a full-service salon or spa that employs other licensed professionals such as cosmetologists or massage therapists, be aware of all laws and any limitations pertaining to their supervision or practice. If you have any questions about a law or regulation, always check with the appropriate regulatory agency.

- As an employer, it is your duty to keep accurate records of the number of people you employ as well as their salaries, length of employment, and Social Security numbers. You must also be aware of and comply with various state and federal regulations as required by law to monitor the welfare of workers.

Business Operations

To operate a successful salon, you will need a variety of business and management skills. Owning your own skin care business can be extremely demanding. There are employees to manage, customers to please, appointments to schedule, services to perform, and business issues to address. For many, the list of tasks can seem endless, leaving even the most motivated individual feeling overwhelmed occasionally. Be patient: it takes time, discipline, and focus to become a good business manager.

As you develop a clear understanding of your business objectives, you can begin to address more practical requirements. Start by making a list of all the functions necessary to operate your salon successfully. Follow this with a critical self-analysis. If you find yourself lacking in certain areas, decide how you will address these issues. The smart businessperson recognizes that she or he cannot be all things. Perhaps you will enroll in a course to learn more about a subject, or you might decide to outsource certain responsibilities. For example, you could hire an accountant to manage your bookkeeping or a marketing consultant to handle advertising and promotions.

To keep your business running smoothly, consider the following successful business strategies.

Manage Finances Well

Working from your business plan, carefully determine how much capital or money you will need to operate your salon for at least two years. Understanding the amount of money that will be required to meet your expenses before you open your salon will help you develop a strategic plan for financing your operation and managing your money. We discussed costs, revenues, and profits earlier. Tracking these on a regular basis is vital to an established business. A reliable accounting system will help you to access this information and plan the allocation of your funds to maintain good business practices.

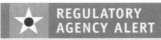

Develop Solid Business Management Skills

When starting out, you often will need to know more than you do. Running a successful business will require you to make thoughtful decisions. This means carefully researching your options and/or consulting with other professionals who can give you the information or support you need. When in doubt, do not be afraid to ask for help. As you become more informed, you will be able to make better choices and develop an effective management program.

Create Pricing Based on Value

Before you can determine a price for goods and services, you need to understand their value. Proper pricing begins with exact knowledge of what it costs to provide each service and retail product. Keeping in mind the old adage, "You get what you pay for," set your prices according to the level and quality of the service or goods you are providing. In general, the type of salon and the clientele it serves determine the cost of goods and services. For example, you must understand what your clients need, want, and value as well as the price they are willing to pay for these products or services. It also makes good business sense to explore the competition, compare pricing, and regularly make appropriate adjustments to remain competitive.

Work Cooperatively with Employees

To stay in business and accomplish your goals, you must learn to work cooperatively with your staff. This requires effective management and communication skills. To develop harmonious working relationships, you must set clear boundaries and objectives, communicate respectfully, and resolve conflicts quickly and diplomatically. A good manager sets an appropriate example and encourages employees to achieve individual and salon goals that will keep clients coming back. To attract quality and experienced help, you must also be willing to offer competitive salaries and benefits, such as continuing education.

Develop Positive Customer Relations

Working with people in a service-oriented business such as skin care requires a variety of interpersonal skills. Clients come to you for a professional service. They should expect to receive quality care in a confidential, respectful, and courteous manner. Good communication is essential to reassuring clients and building a reputation for exemplary business practices. The well-run salon offers clear, concise policies and makes them highly visible—for example, by displaying them in the reception area. Many salons also state their policies directly in their brochure or menu of services (Figure 21–6). Although misunderstandings and conflicts are still bound to occur, if handled well they can be an opportunity for you to develop a reputation for tact and diplomacy. To ensure client satisfaction and a positive outcome, be prepared to address common problems such as cancellations, no-shows, late arrivals, and product returns before they happen.

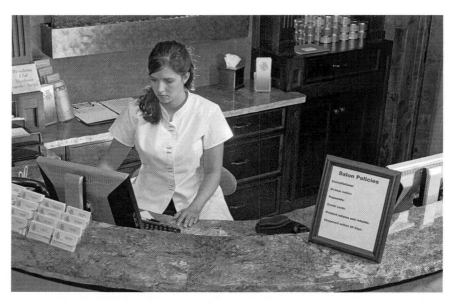

Figure 21–6 Salon policies should be displayed in a highly visible area.

THE IMPORTANCE OF KEEPING GOOD RECORDS

Keeping track of daily, weekly, and monthly records pertaining to your business may seem like one of the more mundane tasks associated with owning your own salon. However, this information is invaluable to you in understanding how well your business is functioning. Accurate records will help you determine income, expenses, profits, and loss. This information is also useful in assessing the net worth of your business and in arranging financing. Maintaining proper business records is also necessary for meeting the requirements of local, state, and federal laws regarding taxes and employees.

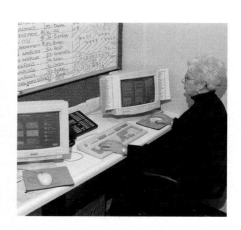

Figure 21–7 Accurate records are crucial to understanding how well your business is functioning.

Many useful computer programs can simplify the task of keeping good records (Figure 21–7). However, it is recommended that you hire a professional accountant and skilled bookkeeper to assist you. (A bookkeeper is someone who is trained in financial record-keeping and follows proper bookkeeping standards.) To ensure that information is accurately applied, it should always be recorded clearly, correctly, concisely, and completely. Income is generally recorded as receipts from sales and service. Expenses include but are not limited to rent, utilities, salaries, insurance, advertising, equipment, supplies, and repairs. Be sure to retain all receipts, cancelled checks, check stubs, and invoices associated with your income and expenses. You will need these to manage your accounts efficiently and correctly.

Daily Records

A day-to-day accounting allows the business owner to measure various important functions. Most importantly, accurate daily records supply key information regarding gross income and the cost of operations. Whether you choose a computerized program or manual method, you will need to keep track of all sales on a daily basis. A review of your daily sales slips and appointment book will allow you to determine the number of products and services sold at your salon each day and the amount of income generated from these products and services. You will also want to note expenses that have been paid out. These should be registered in the appropriate accounting system and checkbook. Do not forget to document any miscellaneous or cash expenses for tax reporting purposes. This information may be kept in a cash journal or "petty cash" notebook. Your accountant can instruct you on the best way to handle daily slips and receipts. In general, cancelled checks, payroll, and monthly and yearly records are held for at least seven years.

Weekly and Monthly Records

Certain financial records are easier to assess on a weekly or monthly basis. These reports may be used to compare the salon's performance to previous years, gauge promotional efforts, or check the demand for a service or product. Understanding the amount and types of services that are being performed in your salon can also serve as a check-and-balance system for utilizing products and staff more efficiently, controlling expenses, and eliminating waste.

Purchase and Inventory Control

Tracking inventory and supplies is an important part of conducting business. Inventory and purchase records will help you to prevent shortages, avoid overstocking, and alert you to any signs of pilfering. They are also important factors in measuring the net worth of your business at the end of the year.

Inventory can be broken down into two categories: *consumption* and *retail supplies*. **Consumption supplies** are items used to conduct business operations on a daily basis. Items available for sale to clients are referred to as **retail supplies.** Accurate records can help you determine which items are used or sold most frequently. This information will help you to reorder supplies in a timely and cost-effective way. (Figure 21–8).

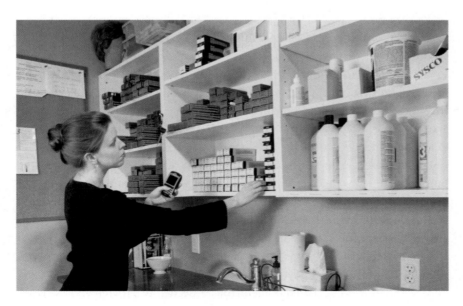

Figure 21–8 Tracking inventory and supplies helps owners prevent shortages and avoid overstocking.

Client Service Records

Maintaining accurate client records serves several business objectives, including customer service and performance analysis. Building relationships is an important factor in the service industry. To ensure client satisfaction, all service records should include key facts such as a client's name, the date and type of each treatment or product purchased, the amount charged, and the results obtained. It is also wise to note a client's particular preferences. In today's impersonal world, the simplest of details can significantly affect how the client perceives your efforts.

Client records are also instrumental in measuring the overall performance of a salon or individual practitioner. Analyzing sales and service can provide useful information for tracking customer trends and performing marketing tasks. Understanding what services and products clients need or want and when they are most likely to purchase them will ultimately increase sales and improve client satisfaction.

OPERATING A SUCCESSFUL SKIN CARE BUSINESS

Ask anyone operating a successful business what the key to his or her success is, and he or she will probably mention several things: the quality of services and staff, an efficient and pleasant workspace, eagerness to learn more about new treatments and techniques, or consistent marketing efforts. However, one thing all owners most likely have in common is the willingness to work hard. Certainly an element of luck is involved, you might be thinking—and indeed, in some cases, luck may be a factor. We have all had someone tell us, "I was just in the right place at the right time." Given the possibility that fate plays a role, we must still consider that without a great deal of planning, dedication, and continued hard work, most businesses would ultimately fail.

Planning the Physical Layout

Creating an efficient and user-friendly workspace requires careful planning. To obtain the best results, you will need to work closely with other experts such as architects, contractors, electricians, plumbers, and product and equipment vendors. You will also need to establish a positive working relationship with local planning board officials and state licensing agents. This can be an exciting time. However, it can also be a stressful time when you must think quickly and act decisively.

Your business plan will serve as a useful tool throughout the planning process. You will want to have this plan readily available and refer to it often during the various stages of construction. It will help you to stay on task and within budget as you make all the necessary decisions and purchases associated with operating your salon on a day-to-day basis.

Before construction begins, think carefully about the primary services you will offer as well as the ambiance you would like to create. Follow up by carefully researching all of the equipment that is needed to provide your services. Certain apparatus and design features may require special handling or modifications. You will want to be aware of any hidden costs, such as special power sources, that will be needed to operate mechanical or technological devices. Naturally, the safety and comfort of both clients and practitioners should always be a top priority as you make these important decisions (Figure 21–9).

As you plan your spa or salon (Figures 21–10 and 21–11), the following checklist may be helpful.

* Does the layout provide maximum efficiency and a safe and comfortable environment for practitioners and clients?
* Does the style of the salon evoke a professional ambiance that instills client confidence?
* Is the color scheme inviting to a broad spectrum of clients (men and women, older and younger clients)?
* Are amenities such as refreshments, music, and reading materials conducive to a friendly, relaxed, and professional ambiance?
* Does the reception area give clients a warm and welcoming first impression?
* Do services flow easily from the reception area to each treatment room?
* Is aisle space adequate for safety and efficiency?
* Is there enough space to allow for each piece of equipment that will be used in the treatment room?
* Have you chosen furniture, equipment, and fixtures on the basis of cost, durability, safety, utility, and appearance?
* Have you purchased the appropriate warranties or insurance necessary to protect your initial investments?
* Does your dispensary supply adequate storage space and ease of mobility?

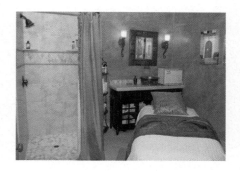

Figure 21–9 The safety and comfort of both clients and practitioners should be a primary concern when planning the treatment room.

ACTIVITY

Create a physical plan for your own salon, designating the equipment that you will need to conduct facial and body services. Then estimate the cost of equipment. Be sure to include the cost of any special design or construction considerations.

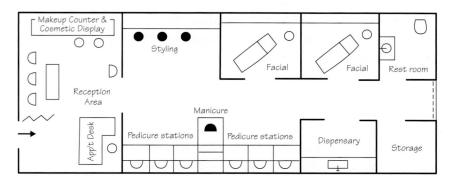

Figure 21–10 A full-service salon.

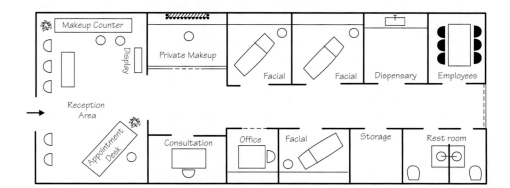

Figure 21–11 A facial and makeup salon.

- Are plumbing, lighting, and utilities adequate for the services that you intend to provide?
- Do air conditioning and heating systems supply adequate ventilation and comfort?
- Are restrooms clean and easily accessible?

Personnel

Skilled workers are an invaluable asset to any salon. How do you hire and keep good workers? The answer to that question is a multifaceted one that deserves special attention. How many times have you heard a business owner say, "It is not easy to find good help these days"? Although the phrase may seem overworked, it certainly highlights the frustration many salon owners feel when looking for new employees.

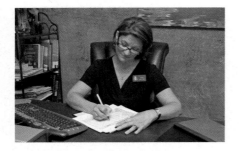

Figure 21–12 Hiring good employees requires careful thought.

Searching for good employees is expensive. Advertising can be costly, and the process of reading resumes and interviewing takes a good deal of time, effort, and energy. To maximize your efforts, develop a list of questions and criteria for evaluating prospective employees beforehand. You will want to consider such factors as experience, skill level, overall attitude, communication skills, personal presentation, and philosophy of skin care as it relates to your practice. If you are interested in a candidate, you will want to follow up by requesting references from previous employers or supervisors. When dealing with more inexperienced candidates, you may wish to ask for recommendations from the school they attended and a demonstration of the required skills (Figure 21–12).

For some salons, the opportunity to increase clientele is an important prerequisite for employment. If that is a priority for hiring in your salon, you will want to learn more about a prospective employee's clients and the possible number of clients that will follow him or her to your spa or salon. However, bear in mind that for various reasons, clients may be unwilling to follow an esthetician to a new establishment.

After determining that a candidate is a good fit for your salon and completing the hiring process, you will need to teach the new employee the way you would like things done. Training new staff takes time and patience. To get the best return on your investment, you will want to establish sensible rules and direction.

Efficiently run salons provide employees with clear expectations. These generally come in the form of job descriptions and employee manuals on policies and procedures. As we learned in Chapter 20, **job descriptions** are extremely useful in helping employees understand exactly what is expected of them. They can also provide a reasonable standard for evaluating an employee's performance. But it is important to remember that job descriptions vary from salon to salon. Larger salons or spas may hire a greater number of employees to perform very specific functions, while smaller salons may employ fewer **personnel** and require them to perform a greater number of services. For example, depending upon licensing regulations, an esthetician may be hired to perform facials as well as hair removal, body treatments, and makeup services.

Employee manuals have very distinct purposes. The **employee manual** or handbook may cover general information about salon operations: the number of sick days or amount of vacation time allowed, holiday closings, the procedure for calling in late or sick, the appropriate dress code for estheticians, the policy on purchasing goods or services from the salon, and how the company's health insurance plan works. A **procedural guide** is designed to standardize operations and may include specific protocols for conducting individual services, such as the expected method for performing a glycolic or microdermabrasion treatment. Although some may find this approach restrictive, keep in mind that guidelines are generally put in place to maintain a certain quality or standard of care. They may also address specific safety concerns such as sanitation, sterilization, or universal precautions that are intended to protect the consumer as well as the practitioner.

Hopefully, your relationship with employees will be long and fruitful, satisfying the needs of both parties (Figure 21–13). However, mutually beneficial relationships require work. To encourage lasting and profitable relationships, you must develop fair and ethical employee practices. Expect that it will take time to build trust, cooperation, genuine caring, and respect. The following guidelines are suggested to encourage good employee relations:

- *Treat employees with dignity and respect.* Acknowledge good work, and reward exemplary behavior whenever possible. This may come in the form of verbal praise or a tangible bonus.
- *Practice positive communication skills and take time to guide workers through difficulties.* Learn to actively listen, and provide positive feedback whenever the opportunity arises.
- *Let employees know you appreciate them.* If the company does well, share as much of the wealth as possible by offering profit sharing or year-end bonuses.
- *Meet payroll obligations on time.* Remember that employees have bills to pay and personal obligations to meet. Make the payroll a top priority.
- *Offer as many benefits as possible, and cover as much of the cost as possible.* If you are a small business and cannot afford certain benefits such as health insurance, at least consider the option of making it available.
- *Set clear goals and objectives, and be consistent.* Knowing what the expectations and consequences are encourages trust. To be recognized as a person of your word, be sure to create salon policies that you can stick to. *Set standards for how you will pay employees.* Everyone wants

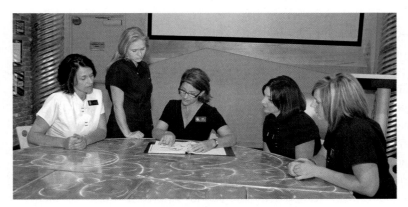

Figure 21–13 Sharing pertinent information with employees promotes understanding and strengthens relations.

to be acknowledged for his or her contribution. Let employees know what your standard of measurement is. For example, is salary based on knowledge, ability, experience, or training? Also, if you intend to incorporate commissions for specific sales or services put this information in writing and provide a copy for each employee.

- *Evaluate productivity, and furnish pay increases fairly.* Establishing set criteria for pay increases sets the tone for a fair and equitable system.
- *Learn to motivate your employees.* Create incentives for employees by offering bonuses—money, prizes, or tickets to educational conferences or trade shows.

Managing Personnel

Managing your staff can be a difficult but rewarding job. Motivating others to do their job well may be a challenge at first. However, if you are patient and dedicated to building a team, you will succeed. To become a good manager, you will need a variety of interpersonal and communication skills. Not all of these skills will come naturally, and they may require additional education on your part. Management skills can be learned from various sources, including other salon managers or owners. Do not be afraid to seek support from others more seasoned than you are. Joining managerial support groups or enrolling in courses designed specifically for new managers can be excellent opportunities for personal growth and development. As you acquire new methods for managing your team, think about the character traits that are most important to you in becoming a quality manager. The following suggestions may be helpful.

- *Honesty is always the best policy.* You will frequently have to share difficult information with employees, such as letting them know that their performance is not up to par. Learn to provide truthful, constructive feedback.
- *Act decisively.* Do not let situations linger. When issues and differences arise, address them as quickly and diplomatically as possible.
- *Learn to expect the best.* Before jumping to a negative conclusion, give your employees the benefit of the doubt and listen to all the facts. Good intentions may not always result in a positive outcome.
- *Show leadership.* Your employees will view you as the leader of the team. It is your job as the manager of your salon to support, guide, motivate, and mentor your staff.
- *Share information.* Show your employees that they are valuable members of your team by keeping them aware of important salon decisions. This does not mean you should tell all; some matters may cause employees to become overly concerned or worried. Share only pertinent and appropriate information on a need-to-know basis.
- *Follow the rules.* Rules are important to a well-run organization. To enforce them you must set a positive example. Be sure to follow your own rules: employees will have greater respect for them if you provide a good example.
- *Be reliable.* Keeping your word builds credibility and trust. Employees need to know they can depend and rely on you. To promote confidence, do not make promises you cannot keep.

• *Teach them well.* Learn to share your methods and reasoning for performing tasks or making certain judgments. This will help employees to understand that business decisions are determined in a thoughtful and rational way. It is also a good idea to provide a forum for employee input. Showing your employees you also value their opinion promotes mutual respect and strengthens relationships.

The Front Desk

We have already mentioned the importance of developing positive customer relations in the esthetics industry. Establishing a caring, nurturing, and trusting relationship with clients is a key factor in building any skin care practice. However, it is important to recognize that client relations are not limited to interactions with the esthetician. A good salon owner or manager understands that a salon must consistently provide quality treatments and products to achieve success. More importantly, he or she knows that how well the front desk is managed has just as much to do with client satisfaction as the practitioner's performance does.

The Reception Area

In the reception area, your clients get that all-important first impression of your salon. Take extra care to make a positive impression by keeping the area attractive, neat, clean, and comfortable. Clients need to feel confident when they walk through your doors. To assure them, you must create a sense of calm, order, and organization. The front desk should be easily accessible and clutter free, allowing clients to check in and out with a minimum amount of effort and confusion. While waiting for service, clients should be kept as comfortable as possible. Offer refreshments and reading materials for their pleasure. These should reflect the ambiance of your salon; for example, you will want to have educational materials that encourage good skin care habits (Figure 21–14).

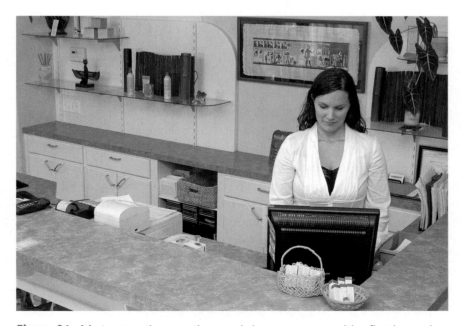

Figure 21–14 An attractive reception area helps to create a positive first impression.

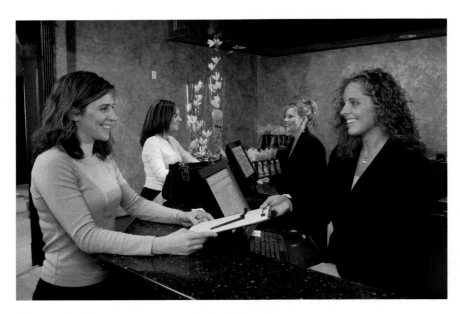

Figure 21–15 The reception area is the hub of salon operations.

But the reception area offers more than a polished image. It is the hub of salon operations, where the receptionist does his or her job, appointments are made, retail merchandise is displayed and sold, and communication systems are located. To manage all these functions effectively, the reception area should be stocked with ample resources for accomplishing tasks quickly and efficiently. Essential items such as business and appointment cards, brochures, gift certificates, product guides, and price lists should be readily accessible at all times. The reception area is also the ideal place to display your menu of services, pricing information, spa policies, and promotional materials (Figure 21–15).

The Receptionist

The receptionist is instrumental in managing a well-run salon. He or she should be a valued member of your team and a resource for all products and services. It is imperative that you hire the right person for the job and train him or her well. This should include a complimentary sampling of all salon services. Having firsthand experience with all treatments will help the receptionist do a better job of selling them to clients.

The receptionist performs a variety of tasks that are critical to maintaining the flow of business. These include greeting clients, answering the telephone, booking appointments, keeping staff informed and on schedule, recommending services and products, and informing customers about policies and procedures. In many salons, the receptionist also performs other business functions. For example, he or she might maintain inventory, generate sales reports, perform marketing-related tasks, conduct follow-up or reminder phone calls, and prepare staff schedules.

It is the receptionist's job to promote goodwill, instill client confidence, and ensure customer satisfaction. To do the job well, he or she should enjoy working with people and have excellent interpersonal communication and public relations skills. The receptionist's work can be demanding and stressful, requiring the ability to juggle tasks simultaneously. The phone may be ringing, colleagues may have questions, and several clients may be standing in front of the desk waiting for service. Nevertheless, the receptionist must remain calm, courteous, and pleasant. He or she should also be conscious of personal presentation. As the first person clients come in contact with, the receptionist should reflect the image of the salon. A friendly smile and neat, clean appearance help create that all-important positive first impression.

Scheduling Appointments

To generate business, you must book appointments. To do the job well, you should be aware of all scheduling parameters and time constraints. Managing time well is the key to successful business operations, particularly in the esthetics industry. In this fast-paced world, clients simply do not want to wait. To keep customers satisfied, those responsible for scheduling appointments should be aware of several crucial factors.

In most salons the receptionist is the primary person responsible for booking appointments. Whether appointments are made over the telephone or in person, the receptionist must be able to communicate clearly and effectively. Clients often have several questions when making decisions about appointments. The receptionist should be prepared to provide concise, direct, and courteous answers to such frequently asked questions as the cost of a service and how long it takes to perform that service. There may be additional information that goes along with scheduling a treatment; for example, a client may need to be prepared to arrive early or dress in a certain way. This means the receptionist must be knowledgeable about all treatments and procedures and know how long it takes each practitioner to provide the requested service (Figure 21–16).

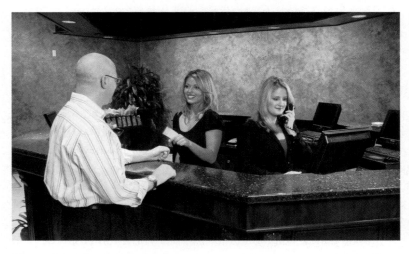

Figure 21–16 Scheduling repeat appointments is an important aspect of generating business.

Appointments may be written in an actual book that is kept at the reception desk. However, most contemporary salons use computerized programs to schedule appointments. In many busy or larger salons, appointment information is networked to other areas of the facility to help staff stay on schedule. Whichever method is used, the receptionist must take care to enter information precisely. It is critical to obtain the clients' first and last names, phone number, and the service they have requested.

To keep business flowing smoothly, most salons have specific policies for confirming and cancelling appointments as well as for handling late arrivals. There may also be general guidelines for assigning services. In larger facilities, requesting a particular practitioner may not be an option. Smaller salons may honor such requests; however, it is sometimes difficult to fulfill a client's desire for a certain time or practitioner. In such cases the receptionist should always give the client other options that may include suggesting another practitioner, offering to reschedule at another time, or putting the client on a waiting list for cancellations. Some clients may insist on being "squeezed in" for a special occasion or event. The receptionist must be careful not to overbook services, stating policies in an assertive but diplomatic way. Staying on schedule is critical to the ease and flow of operations and ultimately promotes customer satisfaction. The receptionist must also consider how each practitioner works. In turn, practitioners must do their part to stay on schedule and work cooperatively with the receptionist. If schedules change or rotate monthly or weekly, the receptionist should be informed and display this information in a prominent place as a general reminder to others who may require it.

Scheduling appointments is generally the receptionist's main job. However, at times others may be required to answer the phone. It is important for management to instruct all staff members responsible for answering the phone in all aspects of booking appointments. Presenting the wrong information or keeping clients waiting for answers does not instill confidence.

As a final note, those scheduling appointments should remember that repeat business is essential to maintaining a full appointment book. It should be standard practice to remind clients to book their next appointment. Some salons offer incentives for rebooking, such as special discounts or frequent-buyer programs. A good receptionist will make clients aware of any valuable savings when making appointments.

Telephone Skills

Although many businesses are becoming comfortable with e-commerce, using the Internet effectively to schedule appointments and make purchases online, the telephone is still considered the lifeline of business operations, offering direct personal service to clients. Therefore, proper training in the correct procedure for handling calls is essential.

For quality control purposes, it is often helpful to identify the specific language that should be used when answering calls and to supply examples of the best way to handle common problems. Many well-run businesses will print this information and store it in a strategic location near the telephone along with other important administrative manuals. Planning ahead in this way can prevent the necessity of urgently training a substitute for the receptionist. It also provides easy access to the correct protocols should employees who answer the telephone occasionally need a quick reminder.

The telephone is an important part of the salon's business. It is regularly used to do the following:

- answer questions and provide friendly service
- make, change, or confirm appointments
- receive messages
- promote client services
- handle complaints
- follow up with clients
- order equipment and supplies from vendors
- seek new business opportunities

Here are some suggested guidelines for making the most effective use of the telephone.

- Assign a specific person to answer the phone.
- Answer calls promptly, and return messages directly.
- Locate the telephone in a convenient and quiet area.
- Keep the necessary tools near the phone: pens, pencils, and a pad of paper for taking notes; directories; a list of important numbers; client records; and the salon's appointment book (or computer displaying the salon's appointment screen).
- Make business calls at a quiet time.
- Use a pleasant, natural tone of voice, speak clearly at a moderate pace, and use correct professional language. Do not use slang.
- Be polite, respectful, courteous, and attentive.
- Handle price objections or complaints with patience and tact. Do not say anything that might be construed as irritating or annoying.
- Practice appropriate greetings and answers to frequently asked questions.
- Plan and practice a "script" for marketing and business calls. This helps project an image of confidence and efficiency.
- Take notes so you will remember the main points of a conversation and be able to respond intelligently.

Incoming Calls

Salons spend a good percentage of their earnings on marketing. Getting the phone to ring is critical to stimulating business. Once your phone is ringing, you will want to make every effort to show how important that call is to you. Although voice mail and answering machines have become standard practice and are used in many smaller salons that may not be able to afford a full-time receptionist to answer the phone, proper etiquette still applies.

The following general guidelines are suggested as professional telephone etiquette:

- *Answer your phone within three rings.* No one likes to wait. Show clients you care by answering calls promptly.
- *If you must place a caller on hold, be polite.* Always ask permission before placing a caller on hold, allowing enough time for a response.
- *Program your voice-mail system to be user friendly.* Your message should be brief, but provide enough information for clients to identify the salon.

Use simple, easily understood instructions that encourage clients to leave their name, telephone number, and reason for calling.

- *Return calls promptly.* Check your messages often, and respond as quickly as possible. If you will be away from the telephone for any length of time, let clients know how long and specify when you will return calls. Waiting longer than 24 hours to respond to a call is inappropriate.

- *Project a positive attitude.* Let clients know you are eager to serve them by greeting them in a sincere, welcoming tone of voice. Remember: a first-time caller is your first opportunity to make a good first impression.

- *Be courteous and attentive.* Use polite words and phrases such as "Please," "Thank you," and "Excuse me." Never chew gum or eat while engaged in a conversation. This is extremely unprofessional.

- *Listen respectfully.* Give the caller your undivided attention; carrying on a conversation with someone else while the caller is on the line is impolite. If you need to obtain additional information for a client, ask to place him or her on hold or take his or her number to return the call.

- *Confirm appointments 24 to 48 hours in advance.* Reminder calls show customers you value their business. Whether speaking directly to a client or leaving a message, be sure to state the details of the appointment, including the exact time, date, day of the week, and service scheduled.

- *When leaving messages, always address the client properly by name.* Clearly identify yourself and the salon. Keep your message simple and to the point, providing exact information in a polite voice.

PUBLIC RELATIONS

Developing a reputation for quality service and fair business practices will increase your standing not only with employees and clients but also in the community where you work. Public relations is a significant factor in building business. Although we hear the term *public relations* often, many are not clear about its meaning. **Public relations—or PR,** as it is commonly referred to—is all about planning and developing relationships to achieve a certain desired behavior. When making important decisions about your business, it is wise to weigh factors based on the overall image you would like to project. What are your goals, and how would you like to be perceived by others? These are questions that require thoughtful deliberation and ongoing assessment.

In operating your own skin care business, you will have many opportunities to interact with a wide variety of people including clients, employees, vendors, colleagues, business leaders, and local officials. To maintain productive relations and positive outcomes, you will need to work on developing effective communication and management skills. Your customer and employee policies will guide you in this process. When reviewing these materials, think earnestly about how comfortable you are with enforcing your "rules." If there are certain issues that you regularly dismiss, decide whether you can continue to stand behind them. You may decide to make changes to your commitments and philosophies over time. As you think about the many topics discussed in this chapter, take stock of how you handle difficult situations and treat others. Ongoing and critical self-evaluation is instrumental to growth and positive public relations.

REVIEW QUESTIONS

1. List the advantages and disadvantages of a booth-rental arrangement.

2. What should you look for when considering a location to open your own skin care salon?

3. Why are demographics important to the prospective salon owner?

4. How can a business plan help you to make good business decisions?

5. List the types of ownership under which a skin care salon may operate. Define each.

6. How do local, state, and federal government regulations affect the small business owner?

7. Why is it important for the small business owner to keep accurate records?

8. List several factors to consider when planning the physical layout of your salon.

9. Discuss the importance of insurance to the salon owner.

10. List several ways that you can safeguard your business.

11. Name several things you should look for when hiring employees.

12. Describe the qualities of a good manager.

13. List the qualifications that are important in a good receptionist.

14. Develop a script for receiving incoming calls, and discuss the best way to place clients on hold.

15. What important information should you provide when leaving a telephone message on a machine or service?

16. How can employee manuals and procedural guides help you manage personnel?

17. How might public relations affect the way you operate your own skin care salon?

CHAPTER GLOSSARY

booth rental: an arrangement in which the esthetician is required to pay the owner a set rental fee, along with payment of utilities as agreed upon, to operate in a specific space within the owner's establishment.

business plan: a strategy for understanding key elements in developing business; also serves as a guide to making informed business decisions.

capital: the money needed to start a business.

consumption supplies: items used to conduct daily business operations.

corporation: form of business ownership whereby one or more stockholders share ownership; the corporation is considered an independent legal entity separate and distinct from its owners with its own rights, privileges, and liabilities.

demographics: the particular identifying characteristics of an area or population, such as the specific size, age, sex, or ethnicity of its residents; average income; and buying habits.

employee manual: a handbook or guide for employees; contains important general information about salon operations, such as the number of sick days or vacation time allowed, holiday closings, how to call in late or sick, and the appropriate dress code for estheticians.

fixed costs: those operating costs that are constant, for example, rent and loan payments.

job descriptions: specified list of duties and responsibilities that are required of an employee in the performance of his or her job.

partnership: form of business ownership in which two or more people share ownership, although this does not necessarily mean an equal arrangement. In a partnership, each partner assumes the other's unlimited liability for debt. Profits are shared among partners.

personnel: employees; staff.

procedural guide: manual or set of instructions designed to standardize operations; supplies specific protocols for conducting individual services, such as the expected method for performing a glycolic or microdermabrasion treatment.

profit: amount of money available after all expenses are subtracted from all revenues.

public relations (PR): the planning and developing of relationships to achieve a certain desired behavior.

retail supplies: items available for sale to clients.

revenue: income generated from selling services and products, or money taken in.

sole proprietorship: form of business ownership in which an individual acts as sole owner and manager and is responsible for determining all policies and making all of the necessary decisions associated with running a business.

variable costs: business expenses that fluctuate, such as utilities, supplies, and advertising.

CHAPTER OUTLINE

SELLING PRODUCTS AND SERVICES

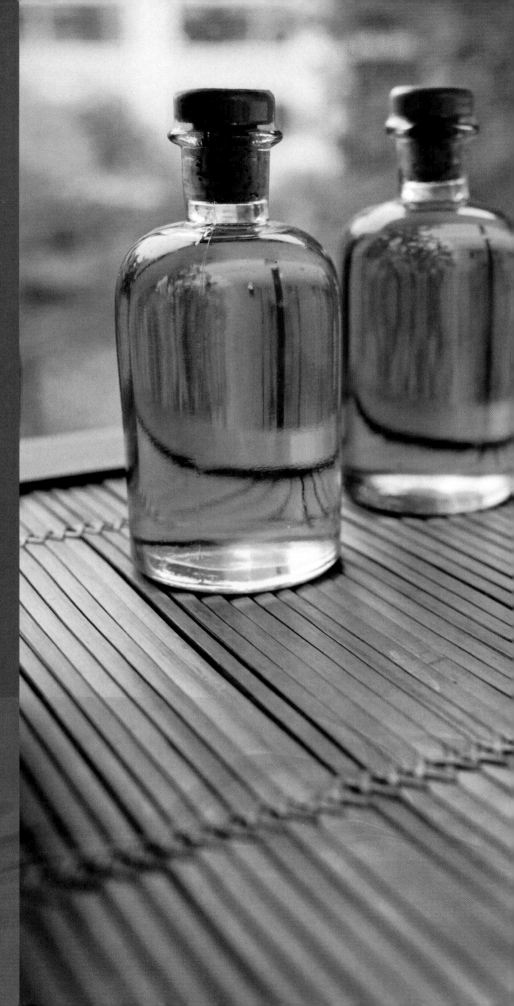

LEARNING OBJECTIVES

After completing this chapter, you will be able to:

- List the basic principles of selling products and services in the salon.

- Explain the purpose of marketing and promotions.

- Name several methods of advertising to promote sales in the salon.

- Explain the importance of understanding client value in selling products and services.

- List the most effective ways to build a clientele.

- Discuss the importance of closing the sale.

KEY TERMS

Selling products and services is critical to the financial success of a skin care salon or spa. Sales keep business flowing and revenues coming in. A confident esthetician, who is comfortable with selling, is a valuable asset to any salon or spa and is likely to increase his or her income. However, the esthetician should not forget that the products and services he or she sells benefit the consumer. Those who place the client's best interests at the forefront of any sale can also take pride in basing the sale on ethical practices. As you review this chapter, keep an open mind. The rewards of selling may surprise you, both personally and financially.

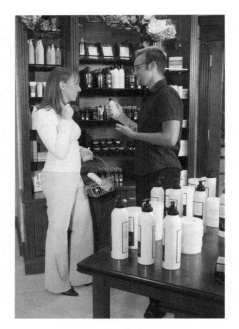

Figure 22-1 Recommending products is a professional responsibility.

SELLING IN THE SKIN CARE SALON

Selling products and services is a fundamental objective in the esthetics business. Unfortunately, many estheticians fail to make the connection between selling and skin care. In many cases, this disconnect stems from negative associations that portray sales agents as pushy or aggressive people who are interested only in making money. To move beyond this negative connotation, estheticians must learn to recognize the value in selling, viewing it as a reputable endeavor that supplies salon and spa goers with certain valued benefits.

To frame the concept of sales positively, the esthetician must first accept that recommending and providing clients with quality skin care products and services is a professional responsibility. Esthetics is a personal service business that promotes beautiful, healthy skin. When estheticians sell treatments and products that are in alignment with this goal, they are also promoting the client's best interest (Figure 22-1).

Principles of Selling

Once you have accepted selling as a necessary and reputable part of your work as an esthetician, you can begin to work on developing principles that promote ethical sales practices.

To be successful selling products and services, you must first be motivated and committed to their value. You will also need to develop the client's trust in your competence and credibility. Looking the part and practicing your own philosophies is a good way to advertise the benefits of healthy skin care. Placing the client's needs and wants at the forefront is another important way of assuring your clients that you have their best interests in mind.

Consultative Selling

Because you are an expert on skin care, clients place their trust in your professionalism. They expect you to have the answers to their skin care concerns and will look to you for guidance in recommending the best treatments and products for their use. From this perspective, you are not simply selling—you are advising or consulting—to clients (Figure 22–2). This practice is known as **consultative selling.** If you begin by recommending only those products and services that meet the client's needs and goals, you will be perceived as a knowledgeable and caring practitioner interested in nurturing skin health. This ultimately builds trust and raises the level of the client–practitioner relationship, creating a "sales" concept the esthetician can be proud of.

Adapting your sales technique to accommodate the client's style is another technique that will help you to sell in a professional manner. Some clients respond best to a "soft sell," in which you inform them about which products are best for them without stressing that they purchase it. Others will prefer a "hard sell" that focuses emphatically on why they should buy the product. As you develop experience, you will learn which approach works best for each client.

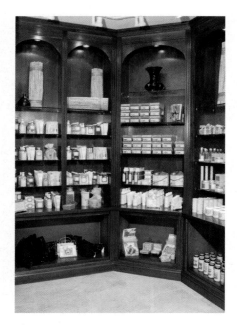

Figure 22-2 Retailing products in the salon benefits everyone.

FOCUS ON . . .

MEETING THE CLIENT'S NEEDS AND GOALS

The following are basic principles of consultative selling.

- Know the benefits and features of your products and services.
- Recommend only those products and services that will benefit the individual client.
- Whenever possible, demonstrate the use of products and treatments.
- Personalize your approach to meet the needs and personality of each client.
- Present a confident, helpful, and pleasant attitude when recommending products and services.
- Find out what your clients want and/or need, and make every effort to fulfill their needs.
- Never make false or unrealistic claims about products or services. This will only lead to client disappointment and will ultimately destroy your credibility.
- Respect your client's intelligence, and acknowledge her efforts to advocate for herself.
- Know when to close the sale without overselling once the client has decided to purchase a product or service.

The Psychology of Selling

What makes people buy? Understanding the consumer's motivation for purchasing products or services will help you refine your sales approach and directly meet client needs. In your work as an esthetician, you will encounter many different personalities with various skin care concerns. Some clients

FOCUS ON . . .

PROFESSIONALISM

In the relationship between esthetician and client, there must be a balance between what the client is asking for and what the professional knows is in the client's best interest. After all, one reason clients patronize professionals is to be advised of what is best for them. This is a delicate communication, but it is vital to satisfying the client. If it appears that the client does not fully realize that her choice will not benefit her, it is your obligation to find a tactful way to let her know.

may come to you to correct a particular skin condition or problem; others may want to feel better about the way they look; while some may simply have issues of vanity. Sometimes the client may be unsure about which product or service will best suit his or her needs. Whatever circumstances the client presents, the esthetician must always remember to keep the client's best interests in mind. It is your job to help him or her resolve the issues presented in the most productive way.

KNOW YOUR PRODUCTS AND SERVICES

It is important to have an extensive and thorough understanding of the products and services offered by your salon. Increased knowledge makes it easier to educate clients and increase retail sales.

Promoting Retail Sales

Clients will rightfully assume that you, as the expert on skin care, are recommending the right products for their skin care needs. This makes **retailing** products, the act of recommending and selling products to clients for at-home use, a major part of the esthetician's training.

However, sorting through the huge number of products available on the market today can be a challenge. To instill client confidence, the esthetician should develop a broad-based knowledge of chemical ingredients, their properties, and their effects on skin. And of course, the esthetician must be familiar with the specific benefits and features of the retail products available for sale in the salon (Figure 22–3).

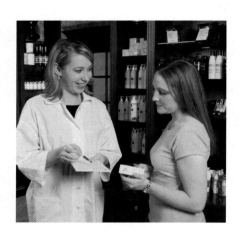

Figure 22–3 Product knowledge is crucial to the success of retail sales.

Recommending Products

It takes time to develop confidence in recommending products. With so many sophisticated new products boasting fantastic technology, the novice esthetician can be easily intimidated. How do you explain such phenomena as *free radicals, liposomes,* and *cosmeceuticals* to clients if you have difficulty understanding these concepts yourself?

Breaking down product knowledge into more manageable categories is a good way to begin sorting through the overwhelming amount of information about products that exists today. The first step is to find out as much as you can about the manufacturer's philosophy. For example, is the manufacturer a proponent of natural ingredients, or does the company support the use of synthetic or chemical sources? Does the company conduct clinical studies, publicize the source of key ingredients, or test products on animals? This information can be easily accessed through promotional materials, such as brochures, pamphlets, the company's Web site, or advertisements in trade publications.

Once you have defined a company's philosophy, you can assess the quality of its products and methods of research and development. Most companies provide literature explaining the theory behind their products and techniques. This may come in the form of marketing materials, instruction booklets, or procedural guides. After reading the manufacturer's literature, conduct your own research using unbiased sources to substantiate the data. Finding out more about key ingredients and the technology used in creating a product will help you understand and explain how it works.

Vendor Education

Many manufacturers and distributors offer seminars to attract new business and educate professionals about their products. Take advantage of these classes whenever possible. This is an excellent opportunity to have technical questions answered by a knowledgeable individual in a give-and-take format. It will also give you a chance to speak with other professionals who are using the product. Learning firsthand about the results other professionals are getting is a good way to assess the credibility of a product. Furthermore, manufacturers who promote this type of exchange realize the benefit of educated salespeople and demonstrate an investment in your success.

Although your personal knowledge is paramount in recommending products, you should also find out what is available from the manufacturer to enhance the client's understanding. Estheticians often need help in explaining a product's advantages and contraindications. Look for companies that supply a simple format for explaining the benefits and features of a product and that address frequently asked questions associated with its use. Using this information as a basis for discussion may help to alleviate some of the pressure you feel as you begin to recommend products to clients.

All of these suggestions will help you to recommend products with ease and confidence. However, it is important to note that the best marketing materials and educational support are no substitute for your professional endorsement. To promote a product successfully, you must first believe in it yourself. Take time to conduct your own trials by testing products that are appropriate for your skin type and condition. You might also consider asking other members of the salon team to try products that are likely to benefit their skin type. Clients will have a greater appreciation of the benefits of a product if they know you are genuinely supporting its use.

Upselling

While the esthetician is the primary person responsible for recommending skin care products and services in a skin care salon or spa, it is also important for other members of the salon team to be knowledgeable about the different products and treatments available (Figure 22–4). In the salon, selling is everyone's business (Figure 22–5). Suggesting a client try something new, or **upselling services** (the practice of recommending or selling additional services to clients that may be performed by you or other practitioners in the salon), keeps business running smoothly.

FOCUS ON . . .

RETAILING

For quick reference, keep these five points in mind when selling.
1. Establish rapport with the client.
2. Determine the client's needs.
3. Recommend products and services based on those needs.
4. Emphasize benefits.
5. Close the sale.

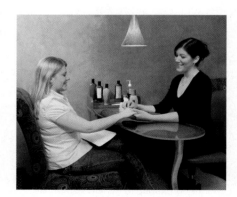

Figure 22–4 Recommending other services to clients keeps business flowing smoothly.

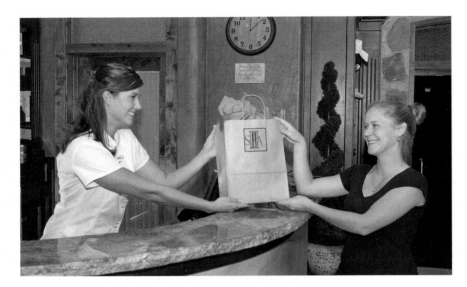

Figure 22–5 In the salon, selling is everyone's business.

CLIENT VALUE

You can have the right approach and the right intention, but the ultimate product sales test is whether your clients want or need it. To successfully market products and services to clients, you must first determine if a product is something that clients are likely to buy. Discovering that a company's philosophy is not in sync with clients' values or skin care needs, or that clients are unwilling to spend $70 on a facial moisturizer, will ultimately shortchange sales efforts.

Collecting Client Information

As you learned in Chapter 3, good communication skills are a critical part of client relations. The 10-step consultation method recommended in Chapter 3 sets the tone for a positive client interaction that will help you to improve communication and better understand the needs and wants of your clients, factors that will ultimately help you to increase sales.

The Questionnaire

The **questionnaire** or *intake form* is an important tool that allows the esthetician to learn about the client's overall skin condition (Figure 22–6). This form documents the client's health history and gives the practitioner a way to open dialogue, discuss client goals, and determine the best products and treatments for meeting these objectives safely and effectively. As you gain experience using this form, you will begin to develop your own interviewing style. You may also adapt the client intake interview to gather additional information that supports your sales efforts.

Client Record Keeping

Client records serve a distinct purpose in building the client relationship, and they should not be confused with the intake questionnaire. **Client record keeping** refers to a method of taking personal notes that helps the esthetician to remember important data and serve client needs better.

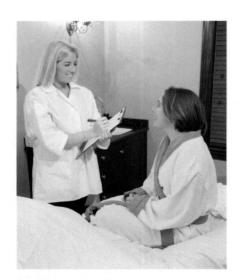

Figure 22–6 The intake questionnaire supplies the esthetician with valuable information about the client's skin care habits and goals.

Every client wants to feel special. However, the truth is that, unless the esthetician has a photographic memory, he or she will have a hard time maintaining a detailed mental account of each client's history. To establish a caring and nurturing bond with the client, the esthetician must find a way to recollect client information easily.

Each salon will have its own method for recording important client data. Some salons utilize computer technology, while others may use a paper file. If the salon you work in does not offer either, it is a good idea to create a system of your own. You should always record the client's

- name.
- address.
- telephone number.
- date of treatment.
- services performed.
- products used.
- treatment results.

Additional information that identifies a client's particular preferences, what products she or he uses at home, special anniversary dates, and personal anecdotes will also help to develop rapport and assure the client's comfort during subsequent visits. Smart estheticians will get in the habit of reviewing this information at a convenient time before the client's visit. This will improve client relations and ultimately increase satisfaction.

Client Education

It seems that most people suffer from information overload these days. This is also true in skin care. With so much data available, it is nearly impossible for the average person to digest it all. That is why clients seek the advice of the esthetician.

FOCUS ON . . .

DEVELOPING GOOD COMMUNICATION

It is a good idea to keep track of what your clients like and dislike, and of important events in their lives. Your awareness of these details will make them feel important. Include the following information on client records:

- client's birthday
- new baby
- upcoming wedding
- job held and job promotions

Also include whatever else you think matters most to that client . . . within reason. Estheticians must exercise caution when it comes to documenting very personal information that could be construed as privileged or might embarrass a client. As a general rule, limit your personal anecdotes to general information that would be part of any casual, polite conversation.

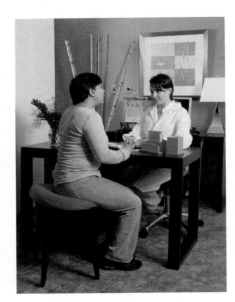

Figure 22–7 It is best to educate clients when you have their full attention.

As a licensed professional, you will be expected to be knowledgeable about the many different products and techniques that are currently on the market. While it is humanly impossible to be an expert on every cosmetic brand and skin care technique, the esthetician can support the client in finding the correct treatments and products for her or his particular needs. But before you inundate the client with a lot of detailed or unnecessary information, consider the following suggestions.

- *Find out what the client already knows about her or his own skin.* What products is the client now using, and what other treatments has she already tried? Some clients may be quite happy with their current regime and products. If so, you should introduce them to any new products or treatments slowly. Developing rapport is an important prerequisite to clients being open to your suggestions.

- *Provide information when you have the client's full attention.* Often, estheticians make the mistake of supplying clients with too much information during the treatment process. While it is important to let clients know what to expect, it is ultimately in the client's best interest to relax and enjoy the treatment. Save explanations for a time when you have the client's full attention; for example, during the skin analysis or closing consultation. The latter is also an ideal time to review product recommendations, prepare a home-care program for the client to follow, and provide any additional literature on other treatment options (Figure 22–7).

- *Be honest about what you do not know.* There may be times when a client requests information about a product or procedure that is not offered at your salon or about which you know very little. Do not be alarmed at such requests. When this happens, it is perfectly acceptable to tell the client you are unfamiliar with the product or procedure and would be happy to find out more about it. On the positive side, this may ultimately give you the incentive to introduce a new treatment option.

MARKETING

Most salon and spa owners understand the value of a good marketing program to stimulate business. **Marketing** provides a strategy for how goods and services are bought and sold, or exchanged. This is an involved process that goes beyond the scope of this text, but it is important for estheticians to realize that marketing is more than a sales technique.

To market skin care products and services successfully, you must first recognize that marketing serves both buyers and sellers. Framing marketing within the context of skin care, we can see that consumers have certain needs and wants when it comes to solving their skin care problems. As businesses looking to satisfy consumers, salons and spas provide certain products and services to help resolve their concerns. What estheticians should remember is that the whole concept is based on an exchange that ultimately benefits both the client and the service provider (Figure 22–8).

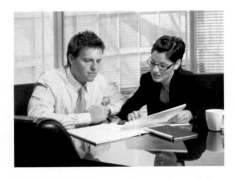

Figure 22–8 Some salons and spas hire freelance marketing consultants or agencies to help them with marketing.

Promotion

All marketing programs involve some form of promotion. **Promotion** is aimed at getting the consumer's attention, with the goal of increasing business. Several different methods of promotion can be employed to market products and services, such as *advertising, public relations, publicity, direct marketing, personal selling,* and *sales promotions.* Most marketing programs incorporate several of these techniques, using a variety of media such as newspapers, magazines, television, and direct mail to create a broad-based campaign.

The following are just a few examples of promotions salons and spas typically use to create excitement and increase sales. They can be applied using a variety of media and techniques.

- Use seasonal themes and holidays to promote packages at special prices.
- Endorse frequent-buyer programs or series savings discounts.
- Reward clients who refer new customers with a gift certificate or free service.
- Introduce new customers to services with a special introductory offer.
- Demonstrate customer appreciation by giving clients a discount or complimentary service during their birthday month.
- Add value to an existing treatment. For example, tie product discounts to the purchase of a related skin care treatment or add on to a service.
- Limit sales promotions to a certain time frame. For example, a winter escape package may be offered only during the months of January and February.
- Introduce new products with trial size samples and a gift certificate that can be applied toward the client's first purchase.
- Offer discounts or add value to services on slower days.
- Host special events to launch a new product or service.
- Team up with other professionals to cross-merchandise.

Advertising

Advertising is one of the more familiar and popular methods of promotion. In the broad sense of the word, advertising encompasses any activity that promotes the salon or spa favorably. For example, engaging in a charity event can be a good way to advertise a salon's services. Most of us can also identify with the popular phrase, "the best form of advertising is a satisfied customer." However, when it comes to marketing, **advertising** typically refers to promotional efforts that are paid for and are directly intended to increase business.

Some of the more popular methods of paid advertising used by salons include *classified, newspaper, magazine, radio* or *television, the Internet,* and *direct mail* (Figure 22–9). If you work at a salon or spa that employs a variety of advertising strategies, consider yourself lucky. Advertising helps to build business and increase sales. A good esthetician will take advantage of these efforts by becoming knowledgeable about special promotions and bringing them to the attention of clients.

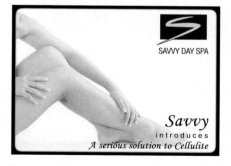

Figure 22–9 A sample direct mail piece.

BUILDING A CLIENTELE

There are any number of reasons for a client's first visit to the salon. Perhaps he or she received a gift certificate, responded to an ad in the newspaper, or noticed that the salon is conveniently located on the route home from work. In any case, a client's initial visit should be considered the salon's first opportunity to make a good first impression and build a lasting relationship. To accomplish this goal, the salon must ensure that the client leaves with two important reasons for returning. First, the client must be happy with the results of treatment and feel he or she derived some benefit from these services. Second, he or she must have confidence in the professional's expertise.

The successful salon owner knows that repeat clients keep the business going. He or she also knows that developing a bond with clients has a great deal to do with whether they will continue to come back. The esthetician is instrumental in this process and should be considered a major partner in building a salon's clientele.

To be successful in developing a clientele, the esthetician must make every effort to provide good service *each* and *every* time a client visits the salon. Frequently, the esthetician will work hard at first to impress a client with her skills, only to fall short of the client's expectations once she becomes accustomed to his or her rebooking. A client's business should never be taken for granted. The goal of every treatment should be to provide the highest-quality service.

CLIENT RETENTION

Salons employ a variety of marketing efforts to support a steady stream of business. However, one simple strategy supersedes all others in the service industry: personal attention. We live in an impersonal world where consumers are often starved for a personal connection. In fact, many clients may visit spas for just that reason. Of course, estheticians would be naïve to think that clients are uninterested in their professional expertise or the benefit they derive from quality skin care treatments. To satisfy the need for both, estheticians are encouraged to adopt the following standards:

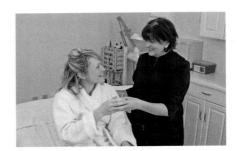

Figure 22–10 To keep clients satisfied and loyal, the esthetician must continually provide quality service.

- *Continually provide quality service.* Once you have won a customer over, it is easy to become complacent. To avoid this common pitfall, estheticians must work hard to maintain their skills and provide excellent service *all the time* (Figure 22–10).
- *Understand what the client wants, and provide it to her or him.* Never forget that each client has a unique agenda. Always set aside time to update information and address client concerns. This lets clients know you are genuinely interested in understanding and fulfilling their individual skin care needs.
- *Give each client your personal, undivided attention.* Again, everyone wants to feel special. Get in the habit of treating clients as if they are special guests. Be warm, welcoming, and cordial. Offer refreshments and practice proper salon etiquette.
- *Develop good listening skills.* There is no substitute for the genuine respect that comes from actively listening to another person. A professional, yet friendly and confidential manner will encourage clients to share their

concerns openly. This will enable the esthetician to provide a more effective treatment plan.

- *Give clients incentives to rebook appointments.* Most salons specifically train the front desk staff to rebook clients. Without the esthetician's support, however, clients may view this as just another sales tactic. Encouraging clients to book their next appointment is a good way to let them know you are dedicated to improving the condition of their skin. Keeping them informed of any special offers or programs that can save them money is also a good way to show that you have their best interests at heart.

Client Referrals

Marketing-savvy salon owners know that word of mouth is one of the best forms of advertising. They make every effort to promote their business through networking and public speaking opportunities. Estheticians should be willing to do their part as well.

Getting clients, coworkers, and other people to refer clients to you is an excellent way to enhance an existing clientele and increase business. Keeping your coworkers abreast of new products and treatments will help to create a buzz about your services. Whenever possible, offer to provide your colleagues with a treatment or new service.

Widening your circle of contacts to include other beauty and allied health professionals is another way estheticians can help spread the word. Beauty professionals, such as nail technicians and hairdressers, who do not offer additional skin care treatments can be an excellent source of referrals. Likewise, broadening this base to include allied health professionals such as massage therapists, fitness instructors, personal trainers, chiropractors, dermatologists, plastic surgeons, and nutritionists can be another mutually beneficial way to increase your clientele.

Community organizations such as the local women's or garden club, church or parent groups, sports teams, and the chamber of commerce or small business association are other good contacts. Many times, such organizations have a need for speakers, or they may be willing to distribute literature for members of their organization. If you are involved with or have contacts in these types of organizations, be sure to give them an ample supply of business cards and the salon's brochures.

Current clients are always a primary source of referrals and one of the best methods of advertising for a salon. A satisfied client is a vote of confidence in your abilities and should always be rewarded in some tangible way. Many salons implement reward programs to purposely encourage client referrals. Others simply reward clients with a free facial, gift certificate, discount on products or services, or special gift when they learn a client has been referred (Figure 22–11). If the salon you work at does not offer these types of rewards, do not hesitate to suggest them; it is always a good policy to let clients know you value their recommendation.

On a final note, it cannot hurt to be prepared with business cards wherever you go. We already know that getting involved in the community and generating positive publicity are good ways to inform the public about your

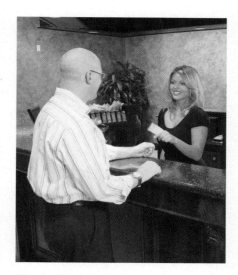

Figure 22–11 Rewarding clients who refer new customers with a complimentary service or added value is a good way to build your client base.

services. However, the esthetician should also learn to be spontaneous. Practicing a nonthreatening introduction that can be used at social or business gatherings will help you to make the most of everyday situations that could eventually result in a new client.

CLOSING THE SALE

One of the most important parts of the esthetician's job actually occurs after the treatment is complete. The **closing consultation** gives the esthetician and client a valuable opportunity to review client concerns and discuss an appropriate home-care program (Figure 22–12). This should be considered a natural part of an effective marketing program that helps clients to derive the most benefit from salon treatments.

Estheticians are fortunate because they are able to work one-on-one with clients. However, when consulting with clients, the esthetician must be sure to communicate his or her recommendations clearly and effectively. The closing consultation is a time to educate clients about their options and listen to their concerns. At times, clients may be overwhelmed by the mention of sophisticated product ingredients and technology. Elaborate explanations may cause further confusion. It is the esthetician's job to motivate and reassure clients and provide them with an individual program that they can follow each day.

Many salons supply estheticians with a worksheet or prescriptive-type memo for use in summarizing product recommendations and explaining proper home usage. This is an excellent way to communicate specific directions about when and how to use products. Clients may have questions about whether a product is best used in the morning or at night. They may also be confused about whether special treatments should be applied before or after a moisturizer or sun protection. Writing down this information is a convenient way to help clients remember exactly what to do when they get home (Figure 22–13). If the salon you work for does not provide a model, consider creating one of your own. A simple format that utilizes generic headings such as *cleanser, toner, moisturizer, specialty treatments,* and so forth, followed by brief instructions and a reminder of when to use the product (for example, day or night) can also be a great reference tool for clients when making future purchases.

Here's a Tip

Sometimes clients may not be interested in purchasing all of the products the esthetician recommends. If this happens, the esthetician should not be too assertive. Perhaps the client is happy with his or her current skin care products—or, because of the cost, would like to ease into a new program gradually as he or she runs out of the products currently being used. It is always best for the esthetician to build the client's trust first. Once this is established, the client may be more open to modifying his or her home-care program.

Skin Care Management Program for _____

Months 1–3	Months 4–6	Months 7–9	Months 10–12
Date _____	Date _____	Date _____	Date _____

Concerns—Conditions	Concerns—Conditions	Concerns—Conditions	Concerns—Conditions
1. _____	1. _____	1. _____	1. _____
2. _____	2. _____	2. _____	2. _____
3. _____	3. _____	3. _____	3. _____

Home regimen	Home regimen	Home regimen	Home regimen
Cleanse _____	Cleanse _____	Cleanse _____	Cleanse _____
Tone _____	Tone _____	Tone _____	Tone _____
Correct _____	Correct _____	Correct _____	Correct _____
Correct _____	Correct _____	Correct _____	Correct _____
Correct _____	Correct _____	Correct _____	Correct _____
Moisten _____	Moisten _____	Moisten _____	Moisten _____
SPF _____	SPF _____	SPF _____	SPF _____

Detail of in-salon program	Detail of in-salon program	Detail of in-salon program	Detail of in-salon program
1. _____	1. _____	1. _____	1. _____
2. _____	2. _____	2. _____	2. _____
3. _____	3. _____	3. _____	3. _____
4. _____	4. _____	4. _____	4. _____

Areas of concern	Areas of concern/ improvement	Areas of concern/ improvement	Areas of concern/ improvement

Figure 22–12 A good skin care management program helps keep the esthetician focused on the client's long-term goals.

Your logo

Date _____

A customized skin care program for _____

Cleanser

1. Cleanse the face with_____by applying about a teaspoon of cleanser, massaging the hands together and massaging both hands over the entire face. Massage in circles for about 30 seconds and rinse with warm water.

Toner

2. Apply_____freshener on moist sponges and wipe the entire face well, turning sponges until all traces of dirt, oil, and makeup have been removed. Apply_____ freshener again by spraying or by using the fingertips and patting the skin.

Moisturizer

3. In the morning, apply a peanut size amount of_____day cream on a clean, toned (after freshener) face, and massage in well. Wait until dry before applying makeup.

4. At night before going to bed, apply_____night cream on a cleansed and toned (after freshener) face and neck. Massage it in well. The skin should feel slightly moist but not too greasy. Allow the cream to nourish the skin during sleep.

Specialty Treatments

5. Apply the_____mask_____times per week on cleansed and toned skin. When applied with the fingertips, the mask should be the thickness of a dime. Do not allow the skin to show through the mask. Rest _____minutes and rinse with warm water. Follow with freshener and a night cream.

If you have any questions, please contact your esthetician immediately at _____.

Figure 22–13 A home-care guide.

Follow-Up

After earning the client's trust, the esthetician will need to work hard to keep it. There is a great deal of competition in the esthetics market today, making it necessary to go that extra mile to let clients know you care. A simple follow-up phone call can make all the difference in maintaining a positive working relationship with the client.

Calling clients takes a considerable amount of time and organization. However, many salons and spas realize it can substantially affect client loyalty. These salons are implementing specific call-back times for estheticans to follow up with clients.

Generally speaking, the esthetician should call clients back anywhere from 24 hours to one week after their salon visit, depending on the type of treatment they received and their skin care program. It is a good idea to call clients who receive more aggressive treatments within 24 hours. Clients starting a new home-care regime should be called within 48 hours. All others should be called within one week. The esthetician may also wish to designate a special call-in hour to address client concerns. Some estheticians also choose to drop clients a note or send a message via the Internet. However the esthetician chooses to follow up with clients, the time is sure to be well spent.

TRACKING YOUR SUCCESS

At first it may be difficult to think of sales as a meaningful part of the esthetician's work. However, once you realize the benefit to the client and the success it brings to the salon, you will probably look forward to assessing your own contribution.

Sales are a significant source of a salon's revenue and a great way for estheticians to increase their profitability. In some salons, the owner or manager may install a sales quota system to stimulate growth. A **quota** system is a method for gauging the amount of sales and targeting production levels. This is a great way to help individuals become more productive, and it can also be a great way to encourage team efforts. Therefore, many managers not only set individual objectives but also provide incentive for meeting team goals. If such a system is not in place at the salon where you work, it is a good idea to formulate your own sales objectives.

As you become comfortable with the idea of setting sales goals, keeping track of the number of salon services you perform and products you sell on a weekly and monthly basis will help you to evaluate your own personal success rate. Numbers allow you to take an honest and objective look at your performance. They can also motivate you to do your job better. Occasionally, sales may be higher or lower, depending on market conditions, promotional efforts, or your personal selling technique. Take all of these factors into consideration, and seek guidance when necessary. Your manager or supervisor and other, more experienced colleagues can be valuable sources of information and inspiration that can help you to reach your goals. Pay attention to their advice, and learn to work with them to make the most of promotions and boost your productivity level. Whenever possible, enroll in classes that help you to educate clients better. At some point, you may find that others will seek your opinion. When this happens, you will know you have met with success.

REVIEW QUESTIONS

1. Define the term *consultative selling,* and discuss how this approach differs from other methods of selling.

2. List the basic principles involved in selling products and services ethically.

3. Why are retail sales important to the salon or spa business?

4. Develop an outline for gathering information about a product line.

5. Discuss how the client's needs and wants (client value) influence the marketing process.

REVIEW QUESTIONS

6. What is the best approach to educating clients?

7. Explain the difference between the *questionnaire* or *intake form* and *client record keeping*.

8. Discuss the esthetician's role in client retention.

9. List several different methods a salon can use to promote business, and provide examples of each.

10. Name several of the more popular forms of advertising used by salons and spas.

11. Describe several methods that can be used to build a clientele.

12. Name several ways you can reward clients who refer other clients.

13. Discuss the best approach to closing the sale.

14. Explain the importance of recommending products and encouraging clients to comply with a home-care program.

15. Why is follow-up with clients important in esthetics? Describe the method of follow-up you are most comfortable with.

CHAPTER GLOSSARY

advertising: promotional efforts that are paid for and are directly intended to increase business.

client record keeping: a method of taking personal notes that helps the esthetician to remember important data and serve client needs better.

closing consultation: an opportunity at the end of a treatment session to review product recommendations, prepare a home-care program for the client to follow, and provide any additional literature on other treatment options that the client may be interested in.

consultative selling: a method of advising or consulting to clients and recommending the best treatments and products for their use.

marketing: a strategy for how goods and services are bought, sold, or exchanged.

promotion: the process of getting the consumer's attention, with the goal of increasing business.

questionnaire: form that provides the esthetician with a complete client profile,

including important information about a client's skin care habits and health.

quota: a method for gauging the amount of sales and targeting production levels.

retailing: the act of recommending and selling products to clients for at-home use.

upselling services: the practice of recommending or selling additional services to clients that may be performed by you or other practitioners in the salon.

A

abdominoplasty: procedure that removes excessive fat deposits and loose skin from the abdomen to tuck and tighten the area.

absorption: the transport of fully digested food into the circulatory system to feed the tissues and cells.

acid-alkali neutralization reactions: when an acid is mixed with an alkali, also called a base, in equal proportions to neutralize each other and form water (H_2O) and a salt.

acid mantle: protective lipids and secretions on top of the skin.

acids: substances that have a pH below 7.0, taste sour, and turn litmus paper from blue to red.

acne: a chronic inflammatory skin disorder of the sebaceous glands that is characterized by comedones and blemishes; also known as acne simplex or acne vulgaris.

acne excoriee: a disorder where clients purposely scrape off acne lesions, causing scarring and discoloration.

acquired immunity: immunity developed after the body overcomes a disease, or through inoculation.

actinic: damage or condition caused by sun exposure.

actinic keratoses: pink or flesh-colored precancerous lesions that feel sharp or rough, usually as the result of sun damage.

active electrode: electrode used on the area to be treated.

adenosine triphosphate (ATP): the substance that provides energy to cells and converts oxygen to carbon dioxide, a waste product we breathe out.

adipose (fat) tissue: a protective cushion that gives contour and smoothness to the body.

advertising: promotional efforts that are paid for and are directly intended to increase business.

AHAs (alpha hydroxy acids): AHAs are naturally-occuring mild acids; glycolic, lactic, malic, and tartaric acid. AHAs exfoliate by loosening the bonds between dead corneum cells and dissolve the intercellular cement. Acids also stimulate cell renewal.

AIDS (acquired immune deficiency syndrome): a disease caused by the HIV virus that breaks down the body's immune system.

air: the gaseous mixture that makes up the earth's atmosphere. It is odorless, colorless, and generally consists of about 1 part oxygen and 4 parts nitrogen by volume.

albinism: the absence of melanin pigment in the body, including skin, hair, and eyes; the technical term for albinism is *congenital leukoderma*.

alcohol: antiseptic and solvent used in perfumes, lotions, and astringents. SD alcohol is a special denatured ethyl alcohol, also known as ethanol.

algae: derived from minerals and phytohormones; remineralize and revitalize the skin.

alipidic: lack of oil.

alkalies: also called bases; have a pH above 7.0, taste bitter, and turn litmus paper from red to blue.

allantoin: used in cold cream, hand lotion, hair lotion, aftershave, and other skin-soothing cosmetics because of its ability to help heal wounds and skin ulcers and to stimulate the growth of healthy tissue.

aloe vera: the most popular botanical used in cosmetic formulations; emollient and film-forming gum resin with hydrating, softening, healing, antimicrobial, and anti-inflammatory properties.

alternating current (AC): rapid and interrupted current, flowing first in one direction and then in the opposite direction.

alum: compound made of aluminum, potassium, or ammonium sulfate with strong astringent action.

amino acid: organic acids that form the building blocks of protein.

amp (A): unit that measures the amount of an electric current (quantity of electrons flowing through a conductor).

ampoules: small, sealed vials containing a single application of highly concentrated extracts in a water or oil base.

anabolism: constructive metabolism; the process of building up larger molecules from smaller ones.

anagen: first stage of hair growth, during which new hair is produced.

anaphoresis: process of desincrustation or forcing negative liquids into the tissues from the negative toward the positive pole; an alkaline, stimulating reaction.

anatomy: the study of the structure of the body that can be seen with the naked eye and what it is made up of; the science of the structure of organisms or of their parts.

angular artery: artery that supplies blood to the side of the nose.

anhidrosis: a deficiency in perspiration, often a result of a fever or skin disease, that requires medical treatment.

anhydrous: describes products that do not contain any water.

anode: positive electrode.

anterior auricular artery: artery that supplies blood to the front part of the ear.

antioxidants: free radical scavengers, vitamins, and ingredients. Antioxidants also inhibit oxidation. They are used both to help the condition of the skin and to stop the oxidation that causes products to turn rancid and spoil.

antiseptics: agents that may kill, retard, or prevent the growth of bacteria.

apocrine glands: coiled structures attached to hair follicles found in the underarm and genital areas.

aponeurosis: tendon that connects the occipitalis and the frontalis.

aromatherapy: the therapeutic use of plant aromas and essential oils for beauty and health treatment purposes.

arrector pili muscle: located in the hair follicle; when it contracts, the hair stands straight up, causing goose bumps.

arteries: thick-walled muscular and flexible tubes that carry oxygenated blood from the heart to the capillaries throughout the body.

arteriosclerosis: clogging and hardening of the arteries.

aseptic procedure: process of properly handling sterilized and disinfected equipment and supplies so that they do not become contaminated by microorganisms until they are used on a client.

asteatosis: dry, scaly skin from sebum deficiency, which can be due to aging, body disorders, alkalies of harsh soaps, or cold exposure.

astringents: liquids that help remove excess oil on the skin.

asymptomatic: showing no symptoms or signs of infection.

atoms: the smallest particle of an element that still retains the properties of that element.

atopic dermatitis: dermatitis is genetically related to overreactive immune systems and is prevalent in people with nasal allergies and asthma.

atrium: one of the two upper chambers of the heart through which blood is pumped to the ventricles (plural: atria).

auricularis anterior: muscle in front of the ear that draws the ear forward.

auricularis posterior: muscle behind the ear that draws the ear backward.

auricularis superior: muscle above the ear that draws the ear upward.

auriculotemporal nerve: nerve that affects the external ear and skin above the temple, up to the top of the skull.

autoclave: apparatus for sterilization by steam under pressure.

autonomic nervous system: the part of the nervous system that controls the involuntary muscles; regulates the action of the smooth muscles, glands, blood vessels, and heart.

axon: the process, or extension, of a neuron by which impulses are sent away from the body of the cell.

ayurvedic: Indian philosophy of balancing life and the body through various methods ranging from massage to eating habits. It is based on three *doshas,* or mind and body types.

azulene: derived from the chamomile plant and characterized by its deep blue color; has anti-inflammatory and soothing properties.

B

bacilli (singular: bacillus): short, rod-shaped bacteria; the most common bacteria; produce diseases such as tetanus (lockjaw), typhoid fever, tuberculosis, and diphtheria.

bacteria: one-celled microorganisms with both plant and animal characteristics; also known as microbes.

bacterial conjunctivitis: pinkeye; very contagious.

bactericidal: capable of destroying bacteria.

balneotherapy: body treatments that use mud or fango, dead sea salt, seaweed, enzymes, or peat baths.

band lashes: eyelash hairs on a strip that are applied with adhesive to the natural lash line.

barbae folliculitis: hair is trapped under the skin, causing a bacterial infection; from improper shaving.

barrier function: lipid matrix that protects the skin's surface.

basal cell carcinoma: the most common and the least severe type of skin cancer, which often appears as light, pearly nodules.

belly (muscle): middle part of a muscle.

benzyl peroxide: drying ingredient with antibacterial properties; commonly used for blemishes and acne.

beta-glucans: ingredients used in antiaging cosmetics to help reduce the appearance of fine lines and wrinkles by stimulating the formation of collagen.

BHAs (beta hydroxy acids): BHAs are exfoliating organic acids; salicylic and citric acids. BHAs are milder than AHAs. BHAs dissolve oil and are beneficial for oily skin.

biceps: muscle producing the contour of the front and inner side of the upper arm.

binders: substances such as glycerin that bind, or hold, products together.

bioflavonoids: biologically active flavonoids; also called vitamin P; considered an aid to healthy skin and found most abundantly in citrus fruits.

blepharoplasty: an eye lift. It removes the fat and skin from the upper and lower lids.

blood: nutritive fluid circulating through the circulatory system (heart, veins, arteries, and capillaries).

bloodborne pathogens: disease-causing bacteria or viruses that are carried through the body in the blood or body fluids.

blue light: therapeutic light that should be used only on oily skin that is bare; contains few heat rays, is the least penetrating, and has some germicidal and chemical benefits.

body masks: remineralize and detoxify the body using clay, mud, gel, or seaweed mixtures.

body scrubs: use of friction to exfoliate, hydrate, increase circulation, and nourish the skin.

body wraps: remineralize, hydrate, stimulate, or promote relaxation by using aloe, gels, lotions, oils, seaweed, herbs, clay, or mud.

booth rental: an arrangement in which the esthetician is required to pay the owner a set rental fee, along with payment of utilities as agreed upon, to operate in a specific space within the owner's establishment.

botanicals: ingredients derived from plants.

Botox®: neuromuscular-blocking serum (botulinum toxin) that paralyzes nerve cells on the muscle when this serum is injected into it.

brain: part of the central nervous system contained in the cranium; largest and most complex nerve tissue; controls sensation, muscles, glandular activity, and the power to think and feel.

brain stem: structure that connects the spinal cord to the brain.

bromhidrosis: foul-smelling perspiration, usually in the armpits or on the feet.

buccal nerve: nerve that affects the muscles of the mouth.

buccinator: thin, flat muscle of the cheek between the upper and lower jaw that compresses the cheeks and expels air between the lips.

bulla (plural: bullae): a large blister containing watery fluid; similar to a vesicle, but larger.

business plan: a strategy for understanding key elements in developing business; also serves as a guide to making informed business decisions.

B vitamins: these water-soluble vitamins interact with other water-soluble vitamins and act as coenzymes (catalysts) by facilitating enzymatic reactions. B vitamins include niacin, riboflavin, thiamine, pyridoxine, folacin, biotin, cobalamine, and pantothenic acid.

C

cake (pancake) makeup: shaped, solid mass; heavy coverage.

calendula: anti-inflammatory plant extract.

calories: a measure of heat units; measures food energy for the body.

capillaries: thin-walled blood vessels that connect the smaller arteries to the veins.

capital: the money needed to start a business.

carbohydrates: compounds that break down the basic chemical sugars and supply energy for the body.

carbomers: ingredients used to thicken creams; frequently used in gel products.

carbuncle: a large circumscribed inflammation of the subcutaneous tissue caused by staphylococci; similar to a furuncle (boil) but larger.

cardiac muscle: the involuntary muscle that makes up the heart.

carpus: the wrist; flexible joint composed of a group of eight small, irregular bones held together by ligaments.

carrot: rich in vitamin A, this essential oil is also used as coloring.

catabolism: the phase of metabolism that involves the breaking down of complex compounds within the cells into smaller ones, often resulting in the release of energy to perform functions such as muscular efforts, secretions, or digestion.

catagen: second transition stage of hair growth; in the catagen stage, the hair shaft grows upward and detaches itself from the bulb.

cataphoresis: process of forcing positive, acidic substances into deeper tissues using galvanic current from the positive toward the negative pole; tightens and calms the skin.

cathode: negative electrode.

cell renewal factor (CRF): cell turnover rate.

cell membrane: part of the cell that encloses the protoplasm and permits soluble substances to enter and leave the cell.

cell mitosis: cell division; occurs continuously in the basal cell layer.

cells: basic unit of all living things; minute mass of protoplasm capable of performing all the fundamental functions of life.

cellulite: gel-like lumps of fat, water, and residues of toxic substances beneath the skin, usually around the hips and thighs of overweight people.

central nervous (cerebrospinal) system: cerebrospinal nervous system; consists of the brain, spinal cord, spinal nerves, and cranial nerves.

ceramides: lipid materials that are a natural part of the intercellular cement.

cerebellum: lies at the base of the cerebrum and is attached to the brain stem; this term is Latin for "little brain."

cerebrum: makes up the bulk of the brain and is located in the front, upper part of the cranium.

certified colors: inorganic color agents also known as metal salts; listed on ingredient labels as D&C (drug and cosmetic).

cervical cutaneous nerve: nerve located at the side of the neck that affects the front and sides of the neck as far down as the breastbone.

cervical nerves: nerves that originate at the spinal cord, whose branches supply the muscles and scalp at the back of the head and neck.

cervical vertebrae: the seven bones of the top part of the vertebral column, located in the neck region.

chamomile: plant extract with calming and soothing properties.

chelating agent: a chemical added to cosmetics to improve the efficiency of the preservative.

chemical change: change in the chemical composition of a substance, in which a new substance or substances are formed and have properties different from the original.

chemical compounds: combination of two or more atoms of different elements united chemically with a fixed chemical composition, definite proportions, and distinct properties.

chemical exfoliation: chemical agent that dissolves dead skin cells.

chemical properties: those characteristics that can be determined only with a chemical reaction and that cause a chemical change in the identity of the substance.

chemistry: science that deals with the composition, structures, and properties of matter and with how matter changes under different conditions.

chloasma: increased pigmentation; liver spots.

cilia: hairlike extensions that protrude from cells and help to sweep away fluids and particles.

circuit breaker: switch that automatically interrupts or shuts off an electric circuit at the first indication of overload.

circulation: general circulation.

circulatory system: system that controls the steady circulation of the blood through the body by means of the heart and blood vessels.

clavicle: collarbone; bone joining the sternum and scapula.

clay masks: masks that draw impurities to the surface of the skin as they dry and tighten.

cleansers: soaps and detergents that clean the skin. Alkalines and fatty acids of oils or soaps are combined to make soaps.

client consultation: verbal communication with a client to determine desired results.

client record keeping: a method of taking personal notes that helps the esthetician to remember important data and serve client needs better.

closing consultation: an opportunity at the end of a treatment session to review product recommendations, prepare a home-care program for the client to follow, and provide any additional literature on other treatment options that the client may be interested in.

cocci: round bacteria that appear alone or in groups.

coenzyme Q10: powerful antioxidant that protects and revitalizes skin cells.

collagen: fibrous, connective tissue made from protein; found in the reticular layer of the dermis; gives skin its firmness. Typically, a large, long-chain molecular protein that lies on the top of the skin and binds water; derived from the placentas of cows or other sources.

colorants: substances such as vegetable, pigment, or mineral dyes that give products color.

combustion: rapid oxidation of any substance, accompanied by the production of heat and light.

comedogenic: a tendency to clog follicles and cause a buildup of dead skin cells, resulting in comedones.

comedogenicity: tendency of any topical substance to cause or to worsen a buildup in the follicle, leading to the development of a comedo (blackhead).

comedone: an open comedo or blackhead; a mass of hardened sebum and skin cells in a hair follicle. When the follicle is filled with an excess of oil, a blackhead forms. It is dark because it is exposed to oxygen and oxidizes. Closed comedones do not have a follicular opening and are called *milia* or *whiteheads*.

commission: a method of compensation that is percentage-based and is directly related to the employee's performance; for example, the employee earns a certain percentage of whatever services he or she performs and/or a certain percentage of the amount of product he or she sells.

common carotid arteries: arteries that supply blood to the face, head, and neck.

communicable: when a disease spreads from one person to another by contact.

communication: the act of accurately sharing information between two people, or groups of people.

complementary colors: primary and secondary colors opposite one another on the color wheel.

complementary foods: combinations of two incomplete foods; complementary proteins eaten together provide all the essential amino acids and make a complete protein.

complete circuit: the path of an electric current from the generating source through conductors and back to its original source.

compound molecules: chemical combinations of two or more atoms of different elements.

concealers: cosmetics used to cover blemishes and discolorations; may be applied before or after foundation.

conductor: any substance, material, or medium that easily transmits electricity.

connective tissue: fibrous tissue that binds together, protects, and supports the various parts of the body such as bone, cartilage, and tendons.

consultative selling: a method of advising or consulting to clients and recommending the best treatments and products for their use.

consumption supplies: items used to conduct daily business operations.

contact dermatitis: an inflammatory skin condition caused by contact with a substance or chemical. Occupational disorders from ingredients in cosmetics and chemical solutions can cause contact dermatitis, or *dermatitis venenata*.

contagious: communicable or transmittable by contact.

contaminants: substances that can cause contamination.

contaminated: when an object or product has microorganisms in or on it.

contraindications: a factor that prohibits a treatment due to a condition; treatments could cause harmful or negative side effects to those who have specific medical or skin conditions.

converter: apparatus that changes direct current to alternating current.

cool colors: colors with a blue undertone that suggest coolness and are dominated by blues, greens, violets, and blue-reds.

corporation: form of business ownership whereby one or more stockholders share ownership; the corporation is considered an independent legal entity separate and distinct from its owners with its own rights, privileges, and liabilities.

corrugator muscle: facial muscle that draws eyebrows down and wrinkles the forehead vertically.

cosmeceuticals: products intended to improve the skin's health and appearance.

cosmetic (esthetic) surgery: elective surgery for improving and altering the appearance.

cosmetics: as defined by the FDA, "articles that are intended to be rubbed, poured, sprinkled or otherwise applied to the human body or any part thereof for cleansing, beautifying, promoting attractiveness or altering the appearance."

couperose skin redness; distended capillaries caused by weakening of the capillary walls.

cranium: oval, bony case that protects the brain.

cross-contamination: contamination that occurs when you touch an object, such as the skin, and then touch an object or product with the same hand or utensil.

crust: dead cells form over a wound or blemish while it is healing, resulting in an accumulation of sebum and pus, sometimes mixed with epidermal material. An example is the scab on a sore.

cyst: a closed, abnormally developed sac containing fluid, infection, or other matter above or below the skin.

cytoplasm: all the protoplasm of a cell except that which is in the nucleus; the watery fluid containing food material necessary for cell growth, reproduction, and self-repair.

D

decontamination: removal of pathogens and other substances from tools and surfaces.

deductive reasoning: the process of reaching logical conclusions by employing logical reasoning.

defecation: elimination of foods from the body.

dehydration: lack of water.

delivery systems: chemical systems that deliver ingredients to specific tissues of the epidermis.

deltoid: large, triangular muscle covering the shoulder joint that allows the arm to extend outward and to the side of the body.

demographics: particular identifying characteristics of an area or population, such as the specific size, age, sex, or ethnicity of its residents; average income; and buying habits.

dendrites: tree-like branching of nerve fibers extending from a nerve cell; short nerve fibers that carry impulses toward the cell.

deoxyribonucleic acid (DNA): the blueprint material of genetic information; contains all the information that controls the function of every living cell.

depilatory: substance, usually a caustic alkali preparation, used for temporarily removing superfluous hair by dissolving it at the skin level.

depressor labii inferioris: muscle surrounding the lower lip; depresses the lower lip and draws it to one side; also known as *quadratus labii inferioris*.

dermabrasion: a medical procedure; strong exfoliation method using a mechanical brush to physically remove tissue down to the dermis.

dermal fillers: products used to fill lines, wrinkles, and other facial imperfections.

dermal papillae: membranes of ridges and grooves that attach to the epidermis.

dermatitis: any inflammatory condition of the skin. Various forms of lesions, such as eczema, vesicles, or papules.

dermatologist: physician who treats skin disorders and diseases.

dermatology: branch of science that studies and treats the skin and its disorders.

dermatophytes: a type of fungi that cause skin, nail, and hair infections.

dermis: live layer of connective tissue below the epidermis.

desincrustation: process used to soften and emulsify grease deposits (oil) and blackheads in the hair follicles.

desmosomes: the structures that assist in holding cells together.

detergents: type of surfactant used as cleansers in skin care products.

diaphragm: muscular wall that separates the thorax from the abdominal region and helps control breathing.

diencephalon: located in the uppermost part of the midbrain; consists of two main parts, the thalamus and the hypothalamus.

digestion: breakdown of food by mechanical and chemical means.

digestive enzymes: chemicals that change certain kinds of food into a form that can be used by the body.

digestive system: the mouth, stomach, intestines, and salivary and gastric glands that change food into nutrients and wastes.

digital nerve: nerve that, with its branches, supplies the fingers and toes.

diplococci: spherical bacteria that grow in pairs and cause diseases such as pneumonia.

direct current (DC): constant, even-flowing current that travels in one direction only.

disincrustation: see *desincrustation*.

disinfectants: chemical agents used to destroy most bacteria, fungi, and viruses and to disinfect implements and surfaces.

disinfection: second-highest level of decontamination, nearly as effective as sterilization but does not kill bacterial spores; used on hard, nonporous surfaces.

dispensary: a room used for mixing products and storing supplies.

disaccharides: sugars made up of two simple sugars such as lactose and sucrose.

DMAE (dimethylaminoethanol): antioxidant that stabilizes cell membranes and boosts the effect of other antioxidants.

Dr. Jacquet movement: beneficial for oily skin; it helps move sebum out of the follicles and up to the skin's surface by kneading.

E

eccrine glands: sweat glands found all over the body; not attached to hair follicles, do not produce an offensive odor.

echinacea (purple coneflower): prevents infection and has healing properties. Used internally to support the immune system.

eczema: an inflammatory, painful itching disease of the skin, acute or chronic in nature, with dry or moist lesions. This condition should be referred to a physician. Seborrheic dermatitis, mainly affecting oily areas, is a common form of eczema.

edema: swelling caused by a response to injury or infection.

efficacy: effectiveness.

effleurage: a soft, continuous stroking movement applied with the fingers and palms in a slow and rhythmic manner.

elastin: protein fiber found in the dermis; gives skin its elasticity and firmness.

electric current: flow of electricity along a conductor.

electricity: form of energy that, when in motion, exhibits magnetic, chemical, or thermal effects; a flow of electrons.

electrode: applicator for directing the electric current from the machine to the client's skin.

electrolysis: removal of hair by means of an electric current that destroys the hair root.

electromagnetic radiation: energy in the form of electromagnetic waves; also called radiant energy because it carries, or radiates, energy through space on waves.

electrotherapy: the use of electrical devices for therapeutic benefits.

element: the simplest form of matter; cannot be broken down into a simpler substance without loss of identity.

elemental molecules: chemical combinations of two or more atoms of the same element.

eleventh cranial nerve (accessory): a type of motor nerve that controls the motion of the neck muscles.

emollients: ingredients that lubricate, moisturize, and prevent water loss.

employee manual: a handbook or guide for employees; contains important general information about salon operations, such as the number of sick days or vacation time allowed, holiday closings, how to call in late or sick, and the appropriate dress code for estheticians.

emulsifiers: surfactants that cause oil and water to mix and form an emulsion.

emulsions: an unstable mixture of two or more immiscible substances united with the aid of an emulsifier.

endermology: a treatment for cellulite.

endocrine (ductless) glands: ductless glands that release hormonal secretions directly into the bloodstream.

endocrine system: group of specialized glands that affect the growth, development, sexual activities, and health of the entire body.

enzyme peels: enzyme products that dissolve keratin proteins (dead skin cells) and exfoliate the skin.

enzymes: catalysts that break down complex food molecules to utilize extracted energy.

epicranius: broad muscle that covers the top of the skull; also called occipitofrontalis.

epidermis: the outermost layer of skin; a thin, protective layer with many nerve endings.

epilation: removes hairs from the follicles; waxing or tweezing.

epithelial tissue: protective covering on body surfaces, such as the skin, mucous membranes, and lining of the heart; digestive and respiratory organs; and glands.

ergonomically correct: furniture and body positions healthy for the body and spine.

ergonomics: the study of adapting work conditions to suit the worker.

erythema: redness caused by inflammation; a red lesion is erythmatous.

essential oils: oils derived from herbs; have many different properties and effects on the skin and psyche.

esthetician (or aesthetician): person devoted to, or professionally occupied with, skin health and beauty.

esthetics (or aesthetics): branch of anatomical science that deals with the overall health and well-being of the skin, the largest organ of the human body; from the Greek word *aesthetikos*, meaning "perceptible to the senses."

ethics: principles of good character, proper conduct, and moral judgment, expressed through personality, human relations skills, and professional image.

ethmoid bone: light, spongy bone between the eye sockets that forms part of the nasal cavities.

excoriation: a skin sore or abrasion produced by scratching or scraping.

excretory system: group of organs—including the kidneys, liver, skin, large intestine, and lungs—that purify the body by elimination of waste matter.

exfoliants: mechanical and chemical products or processes used to exfoliate the skin.

exfoliation: the peeling or sloughing of the outer layer of skin.

exocrine (duct) glands: duct glands that produce a substance that travels through small tubelike ducts, such as the sudoriferous (sweat) glands and the sebaceous (oil) glands.

exposure incident: specific contact of a client's blood or other potentially infectious materials (OPIM) with the esthetician's eyes, mouth, or other mucous membranes as a result of performing services and duties.

extensors: muscles that straighten the wrist, hand, and fingers to form a straight line.

external carotid artery: artery that supplies blood to the anterior parts of the scalp, ear, face, neck, and side of the head.

external jugular vein: vein located on the side of the neck that carries blood returning to the heart from the head, face, and neck.

extractions: the manual removal of impurities and comedones.

eye tabbing: procedure in which individual synthetic eyelashes are attached directly to a client's own lashes at their base.

F

facial: a professional service designed to improve and rejuvenate the skin.

facial artery: artery that supplies blood to the lower region of the face, mouth, and nose; also called external maxillary artery.

faradic current: alternating and interrupted current that produces a mechanical reaction without a chemical effect. Used for muscle contraction.

fats (lipids): macronutrients used to produce energy in the body; the materials in the sebaceous glands that lubricate the skin.

fatty acids: lubricant ingredients derived from plant oils or animal fats.

fatty alcohols: fatty acids that have been exposed to hydrogen.

fatty esters: emollients produced from fatty acids and alcohols.

fibroblasts: cells that produce amino acids and collagen.

fifth cranial nerve: chief sensory nerve of the face; controls chewing; also known as trifacial or trigeminal nerve.

fissure: a crack in the skin that penetrates the dermis. Chapped lips or hands are fissures.

Fitzpatrick Scale: a scale used to measure the skin type's ability to tolerate sun exposure.

fixed costs: those operating costs that are constant, for example, rent and loan payments.

flagella (singular: flagellum): long threads attached to the cell to help it move.

flexors: extensor muscles of the wrist, involved in flexing the wrist.

follicles: hair follicles, and sebaceous follicles are tubelike depressions in the skin.

folliculitis: inflammation of the hair follicles.

foot reflexology: treatment of the body through reflex points located on the bottom of the feet.

fragrances: these give products their scent.

franchised salon or spa: a salon owned by an individual(s) who pays a certain fee to use the company name and is part of a larger organization or chain of salons. The franchise operates according to a specified business plan and set protocols.

free radicals: "super" oxidizers that cause an oxidation reaction and produce a new free radical in the process; are created by highly reactive atoms or molecules (often oxygen) having an unpaired number of electrons. Free radicals are unstable and can damage DNA, causing inflammation and disease in the body.

fresheners: skin-freshening lotions with a low alcohol content.

friction: a rubbing movement; pressure is maintained on the skin to create friction. Chucking, rolling, and wringing are variations of friction.

frontal artery: artery that supplies blood to the forehead and upper eyelids.

frontal bone: bone forming the forehead.

frontalis: anterior or front portion of the epicranium; muscle of the scalp.

fulling: a form of petrissage in which the tissue is grasped, gently lifted, and spread out.

functional ingredients: ingredients in cosmetic products that allow the products to spread, give them body and texture, and give them a specific form such as a lotion, cream, or gel.

fungi (singular: fungus): vegetable (plant) parasites, including molds, mildews, and yeasts.

fungicidal: capable of destroying fungi.

furuncle: a subcutaneous abscess filled with pus; also called boils, furuncles are caused by bacteria in the glands or hair follicles.

fuse: special device that prevents excessive current from passing through a circuit.

G

galvanic current: a constant and direct current, it uses a positive and negative pole to produce chemical reactions (desincrustation) and ionic reactions (iontophoresis).

general infection: infection that results when the bloodstream carries pathogens and their toxins (poisons) to all parts of the body.

glands: a cell or group of cells that produce and release substances used nearby or in another part of the body.

glycerin: formed by a decomposition of oils or fats; excellent skin softener and humectant; very strong water binder.

glycosaminoglycans: a water-binding substance between the fibers of the dermis.

glycoproteins: yeast cell derivatives that enhance cellular metabolism, which boosts oxygen uptake in the cell.

gommage: peeling cream that is rubbed off the skin.

grapeseed extract: powerful antioxidant with soothing properties.

greasepaint: heavy makeup used for theatrical purposes.

greater auricular nerve: nerve at the sides of the neck affecting the face, ears, neck, and parotid gland.

greater occipital nerve: nerve located in the back of the head, affecting the scalp.

green tea: powerful antioxidant and soothing agent. Antibacterial, anti-inflammatory, and a stimulant. Helpful for couperose skin.

H

hair bulb: the swelling at the base of the follicle that provides the hair with nourishment; it is a thick, club-shaped structure that forms the lower part of the hair root.

hair follicle: the tubular shield that surrounds the hair shaft; the "pore" where hairs grow.

hair papillae: cone-shaped elevations at the base of the follicle that fits into the bulb. The papillae are filled with tissue that contains the blood vessels and cells necessary for hair growth and follicle nourishment.

hair root: part of the hair that lies within the follicle at its base, where the hair grows.

hair shaft: portion of the hair that extends or projects beyond the skin, consisting of the outer layer (cuticle), inner layer (medulla), and middle layer (cortex). Color changes happen in the cortex.

healing agents: substances such as chamomile or aloe that help to heal the skin.

heart: muscular cone-shaped organ that keeps the blood moving within the circulatory system.

hemoglobin: iron-containing protein in red blood cells that binds to oxygen.

henna: dye obtained from the powdered leaves and shoots of the mignonette tree; used as a reddish hair dye and in tattooing.

hepatitis: disease marked by inflammation of the liver and caused by a blood-borne virus.

herbs: along with plant extracts, herbs contain phytohormones. Hundreds of different herbs are used in skin care products and cosmetics; they heal, stimulate, soothe, and moisturize.

herpes simplex virus 1: this strain of the herpes virus causes fever blisters or cold sores; it is a recurring, contagious viral infection consisting of a vesicle or group of vesicles on a red, swollen base. The blisters usually appear on the lips or nostrils.

herpes simplex virus 2: this strain of the herpes virus infects the genitals.

herpes zoster: shingles, a painful skin condition from the chickenpox virus characterized by groups of blisters that form a rash.

high-frequency machine: apparatus that utilizes alternating or sinusoidal current to produce a mild to strong heat effect. High frequency is a Tesla current, sometimes called the *violet ray*.

hirsutism: growth of an unusual amount of hair on parts of the body normally bearing only downy hair, such as the face, arms, and legs of women or the backs of men.

histology: study of the structure and composition of tissue.

HIV: human immunodeficiency virus; virus that causes AIDS.

hormones: secretions produced by one of the endocrine glands and carried by the bloodstream or body fluid to another part of the body, or a body organ, to stimulate functional activity or secretion; the internal messengers for most of the body's systems.

horsechestnut: extract containing bioflavonoids; also known as vitamin P. Helps strengthen capillary walls; used for couperose areas or telangiectasia.

humectants: ingredients that attract water. Humectants draw moisture to the skin and soften its surface, diminishing lines caused by dryness. Glycerin is a humectant used in creams and lotions.

humerus: uppermost and largest bone in the arm, extending from the elbow to the shoulder.

hyaluronic acid: hydrating fluids found in the skin; hydrophilic agent with water-binding properties.

hydrators: ingredients that attract water to the skin's surface; also known as *humectants* or *hydrophilic agents*.

hydrogen: colorless, odorless, tasteless gas; the lightest element known.

hydrogen peroxide: chemical compound of hydrogen and oxygen; a colorless liquid with a characteristic odor and a slightly acid taste.

hydrophilic: capable of combining with or attracting water.

hydrotherapy: spa treatments that use water.

hyoid bone: u-shaped bone at the base of the tongue that supports the tongue and its muscles.

hyperhidrosis: excessive perspiration caused by heat or body weakness. Medical treatment is required.

hyperkeratosis: a thickening of the skin caused by a mass of keratinized cells (keratinocytes).

hyperpigmentation: overproduction of pigment.

hypertrichosis: excessive hair growth where hair does not normally grow.

hypertrophy: an abnormal growth; many are benign, or harmless.

hypoglycemia: a condition in which blood glucose or blood sugar drops too low; caused by either too much insulin or low food intake.

hypopigmentation: lack of pigment.

I

immiscible: not capable of being mixed.

immune or lymphatic system: body system made up of lymph, lymph nodes, the thymus gland, the spleen, and lymph vessels. Functions protect the body from disease by developing immunities and destroying disease-causing microorganisms as well as draining the tissue spaces of excess interstitial fluids to the blood. It carries waste and impurities away from the cells.

immunity: Ability of the body to resist infection and destroy pathogens that have infected the body.

impetigo: a contagious bacterial infection often occurring in children; characterized by clusters of small blisters.

implements: tools used by estheticians.

inactive electrode: opposite pole from the active electrode.

individual lashes: separate artificial eyelashes that are applied on top of the lashes one at a time.

infection: the invasion of body tissues by disease-causing pathogenic bacteria.

information interview: a scheduled meeting or conversation whose sole purpose is to gather information.

infraorbital artery: artery that originates from the internal maxillary artery and supplies blood to the eye muscles.

infraorbital nerve: nerve that affects the skin of the lower eyelid, side of the nose, upper lip, and mouth.

infrared rays: invisible rays that have longer wavelengths, penetrate deeper, and produce more heat than visible light does.

infratrochlear nerve: nerve that affects the membrane and skin of the nose.

ingestion: eating or taking food into the body.

injectable fillers: substances used in nonsurgical procedures to fill in or plump up areas of the skin. Botox® and dermal fillers are injectables.

inorganic chemistry: study of substances that do not contain carbon.

insertion: the point where the skeletal muscle is attached to a bone or other more movable body part.

insulator (nonconductor): substance that does not easily transmit electricity.

integumentary system: the skin and its extensions, such as the hair, nails, and glands.

intense pulsed light (IPL): a photo-epilation hair-reduction method using flashes of light and different wavelengths; an intense pulse of electromagnetic radiation.

intercellular cement: lipid substances between corneum cells that protect the cells from water loss and irritation.

internal carotid artery: artery that supplies blood to the brain, eyes, eyelids, forehead, nose, and internal ear.

internal jugular vein: vein located at the side of the neck to collect blood from the brain and parts of the face and neck.

interstitial: the fluid in spaces between the tissue cells.

ion: an atom or molecule that carries an electrical charge.

ionization: the separating of a substance into ions.

iontophoresis (ionization): process of introducing ions of water-soluble products into the skin by using an electric current such as the positive and negative poles of a galvanic machine.

J

Jessner's peel: a light to medium peel of lactic acid, salicylic acid, and resorcinol in an ethanol solvent.

job descriptions: specified list of duties and responsibilities that are required of an employee in the performance of his or her job.

joint: connection between two or more bones of the skeleton.

jojoba: oil widely used in cosmetics; extracted from the beanlike seeds of the desert shrub. Used as a lubricant and non-comedogenic emollient and moisturizer.

K

keloid: a thick scar resulting from excessive growth of fibrous tissue (collagen).

keratin: fiber protein found in skin, hair, and nails; provides resiliency and protection to the skin.

keratinocytes: cells composed of keratin.

keratoma: an acquired, thickened patch of epidermis. A callus caused by pressure or friction is a keratoma.

keratoses: abnormally thick buildups of cells.

keratosis pilaris: redness and bumpiness in the cheeks or upper arms; caused by blocked follicles.

kilowatt (K): 1,000 watts.

kojic acid: skin-brightening agent.

L

lacrimal bones: small, thin bones located in the anterior medial wall of the orbits (eye sockets).

lakes: the common term for certified colors.

lanolin: emollient with moisturizing properties; also an emulsifier with high water absorption capabilities.

lanugo: the hair on a fetus; soft and downy hair covering most of the body.

laser hair removal: a photoepilation hair reduction treatment in which a laser beam is pulsed on the skin using one wavelength at a time, impairing the hair growth; an intense pulse of electromagnetic radiation.

laser resurfacing: procedure used to smooth wrinkles or lighten acne scars. Collagen remodeling stimulates the growth of new collagen in the dermis.

lasers: acronym for "light amplification stimulation emission of radiation"; medical devices using electromagnetic radiation for hair removal and skin treatments.

latissimus dorsi: broad, flat, superficial muscle covering the back of the neck and upper and middle region of the back; controls the shoulder blade and the swinging movements of the arm.

lavender: all-purpose oil having many properties. Anti-allergenic, anti-inflammatory, antiseptic, antibacterial, balancing, energizing, soothing, healing, and, conversely, stimulating.

lentigo/lentigenes: freckles; small yellow-brown colored spots. Lentigenes that result from sunlight exposure are actinic, or solar, lentigenes. Patches are referred to as *large macules*.

lesions: structural changes in tissues caused by damage or injury.

leukoderma: light, abnormal patches caused by a burn or congenital disease that destroys the pigment-producing cells. Vitiligo and albinism are leukodermas.

levator anguli oris: muscle that raises the angle of the mouth and draws it inward.

levator labii superioris: muscle surrounding the upper lip; elevates the upper lip and dilates the nostrils, as in expressing distaste.

licorice: anti-irritant used for sensitive skin.

light therapy: the application of light rays to the skin for the treatment of wrinkles, capillaries, pigmentation, or hair removal.

linoleic acid: omega-6, an essential fatty acid used to make important hormones; also part of the skin's lipid barrier.

lipids: fats or fatlike substances. Lipids help repair and protect the barrier function of the skin.

lipophilic: having an affinity or attraction to fat and oils.

liposomes: closed lipid bilayer spheres that encapsulate ingredients, target their delivery to specific tissues of the skin, and control their release.

liposuction: procedure that surgically removes pockets of fat.

local infection: infection that is confined to a particular part of the body and is indicated by a lesion containing pus.

logarithmic scale: a method of displaying data in multiples of 10.

lubricants: coat the skin and reduce friction. Mineral oil is a lubricant.

Lucas sprayer: atomizer designed to apply plant extracts and other ingredients to the skin.

lungs: spongy tissues composed of microscopic cells in which inhaled air is exchanged for carbon dioxide during one respiratory cycle.

lymph: clear, yellowish fluid that circulates in the lymph spaces (lymphatic) of the body; carries waste and impurities away from the cells.

lymphatic or immune system: body system made up of lymph, lymph nodes, the thymus gland, the spleen, and lymph vessels. Functions to protect the body from disease by developing immunities and destroying disease-causing microorganisms as well as draining the tissue spaces of excess interstitial fluids to the blood. It carries waste and impurities away from the cells.

lymph capillaries: lymphatic vessels that occur in clusters and are distributed throughout most of the body.

lymph nodes: glandlike bodies in the lymphatic vessels that filter lymph products.

lymph vascular system: body system that acts as an aid to the blood system and consists of the lymph spaces, lymph vessels, and lymph glands.

lymph vessels: located in the dermis, these supply nourishment within the skin and remove waste.

M

macronutrients: nutrients that make up the largest part of the nutrition we take in; the three basic food groups: protein, carbohydrates, and fats.

macule: a flat spot or discoloration on the skin, such as a freckle. Macules are neither raised nor sunken.

malignant melanoma: the most serious form of skin cancer. Black or dark patches on the skin are usually uneven in texture, jagged, or raised.

mammoplasty: breast surgery.

mandible: lower jawbone; largest and strongest bone of the face.

mandibular nerve: branch of the fifth cranial nerve that supplies the muscles and skin of the lower part of the face; also, nerve that affects the muscles of the chin and lower lip.

manual lymph drainage (MLD): stimulates lymph fluid to flow through the lymphatic vessels. This light massage technique helps to cleanse and detoxify the body.

marketing: a strategy for how goods and services are bought, sold, or exchanged.

mask: ingredients such as herbs, vitamins, and oils combined with clay, seaweed, or hydrating bases that treat the skin.

massage: a manual or mechanical manipulation by rubbing, kneading, or other methods that stimulate metabolism and circulation.

masseter: one of the muscles of the jaw used in mastication (chewing).

Material Safety Data Sheet (MSDS): Material Safety Data Sheet; information compiled by a manufacturer about its product, ranging from ingredient content and associated hazards to combustion levels and storage requirements.

matte: dull; not shiny.

matter: any substance that occupies space and has mass (weight).

maxillary bones: form the upper jaw.

maxillary nerve: branch of the fifth cranial nerve that supplies the upper part of the face.

mechanical exfoliation: method of rubbing dead cells off of the skin.

median nerve: nerve, smaller than the ulnar and radial nerves, that supplies the arm and hand.

medical esthetics: integration of surgical procedures and esthetic treatments.

melanin: skin pigment; a defense mechanism to protect skin from the sun.

melanocytes: cells that produce pigment granules in the basal layer.

melanosome: pigment granules of melanocyte cells that produce melanin in the basal layer.

melasma: a condition of the skin that is triggered by hormones; causes darker pigmentation in areas such as on the upper lip and around the eyes and cheeks.

mental nerve: nerve that affects the skin of the lower lip and chin.

mentalis: muscle that elevates the lower lip and raises and wrinkles the skin of the chin.

metabolism: chemical process taking place in living organisms whereby the cells are nourished and carry out their activities.

metacarpus: bones of the palm of the hand; parts of the hand containing five bones between the carpus and phalanges.

Methicillin-Resistant Staphylococcus Aureus (MRSA): a highly resistant form of staph infection that can be caused by the overuse of antibiotics.

methyl paraben: one of the most frequently used preservatives because of its very low sensitizing potential. Combats bacteria and molds; non-comedogenic.

microcurrent: a device that mimics the body's natural electrical energy to reeducate and tone facial muscles; improves circulation and increases collagen and elastin production.

microdermabrasion: a form of mechanical exfoliation.

micronutrients: vitamins and substances that have no calories or nutritional value, yet are essential for body functions.

microorganism: any organism of microscopic to submicroscopic size.

middle temporal artery: artery that supplies blood to the temples.

milia: also called whiteheads, milia are whitish, pearl-like masses of sebum and dead cells under the skin. Milia are more common in dry skin types and may form after skin trauma, such as a laser resurfacing.

miliaria rubra: prickly heat; acute inflammatory disorder of the sweat glands resulting in the eruption of red vesicles and burning, itching skin from excessive heat exposure.

milliampere one-thousandth of an ampere.

mineral oil: a lubricant derived from petroleum.

minerals: inorganic materials required for many reactions of the cells and body.

miscible: capable of being mixed with another liquid in any proportion without separating.

mitosis: cells dividing into two new cells (daughter cells); the usual process of cell reproduction of human tissues.

modalities: currents used in electrical facial and scalp treatments.

modelage masks: thermal heat masks.

moisturizers: products formulated to add moisture to the skin.

mole: a brownish spot ranging in color from tan to bluish black. Some are flat, resembling freckles; others are raised and darker.

molecule: a chemical combination of two or more atoms.

monosaccharides: carbohydrates made up of one basic sugar unit.

motility: cell motility refers to single-celled organisms and their ability to move in their environment.

motor (efferent) nerves: nerves that carry impulses from the brain to the muscles.

mucopolysaccharides: carbohydrate-lipid complexes that are also good water binders.

muscular system: body system that covers, shapes, and supports the skeleton tissue; contracts and moves various parts of the body.

muscular tissue: tissue that contracts and moves various parts of the body.

N

nanotechnology: manipulation of materials on an atomic or molecular scale, or the "micronization" of ingredients.

nasal bones: bones that form the bridge of the nose.

nasal nerve: nerve that affects the point and lower sides of the nose.

natural immunity: an inherent resistance to disease.

nerve tissue: tissue that controls and coordinates all body functions.

nerves: whitish cords made up of bundles of nerve fibers held together by connective tissue, through which impulses are transmitted.

nervous system: body system composed of the brain, spinal cord, and nerves; controls and coordinates all other systems and makes them work harmoniously and efficiently.

networking: a method of increasing contacts and building relationships to further one's career.

neuron: nerve cell; basic unit of the nervous system, consisting of a cell body, nucleus, dendrites, and axon.

nevus: a birthmark or mole; malformation of the skin due to abnormal pigmentation or dilated capillaries.

nitrile gloves: gloves made from synthetic rubbers known as acrylonitrile and butadiene; these gloves are resistant to tears, punctures, chemicals, and solvents.

nitrogen: colorless, gaseous element that makes up four-fifths of the air in the atmosphere.

nodules: also referred to as tumors, but these are smaller bumps caused by conditions such as scar tissue, fatty deposits, or infections.

nonablative: procedure that does not remove tissue. Wrinkle treatments that bypass the epidermis to stimulate collagen in the dermis for wrinkle reduction are nonablative.

noncertified colors: colors that are organic, meaning they come from animal or plant extracts; they can also be natural mineral pigments.

nonessential amino acids: amino acids that can be synthesized by the body and do not have to be obtained from the diet.

nonpathogenic: not harmful; not disease-producing.

nonstriated muscles: also called involuntary, visceral, or smooth muscles; muscles that function automatically, without conscious will.

nucleoplasm: a fluid within the nucleus of the cell that contains proteins and DNA; determines our genetic makeup.

nucleus: dense, active protoplasm found in the center of the cell; plays an important part in cell reproduction and metabolism.

O

occipital artery: artery that supplies blood to the skin and muscles of the scalp and back of the head up to the crown.

occipital bone: hindmost bone of the skull, located below the parietal bones.

occipitalis: back of the epicranius; muscle that draws the scalp backward.

occlusive: products that reduce transepidermal water loss (TEWL) to help hold in moisture and protect the skin's top barrier layer.

ohm (0): unit that measures the resistance of an electric current.

oil soluble: compatible with oil.

oil-in-water (O/W) emulsion: oil droplets dispersed in a water with the aid of an emulsifying agent.

olfactory system: gives us our sense of smell, which is the strongest of the five senses.

omega-3 fatty acids: alpha-linoleic acid; a type of "good" polyunsaturated fat that may decrease cardiovascular diseases. It is also an anti-inflammatory and beneficial for skin.

ophthalmic nerve: branch of the fifth cranial nerve that supplies the skin of the forehead, upper eyelids, and interior portion of the scalp, orbit, eyeball, and nasal passage.

orbicularis oculi: the ring muscle of the eye socket; closes the eyelid.

orbicularis oris: flat band around the upper and lower lips that compresses, contracts, puckers, and wrinkles the lips.

organic chemistry: study of substances that contain carbon.

organs: structures composed of specialized tissues and performing specific functions.

origin: part of the muscle that does not move; it is attached to the skeleton and is usually part of a skeletal muscle.

osteoporosis: a thinning of bones, leaving them fragile and prone to fractures; caused by the reabsorption of calcium into the blood.

oxidation: chemical reaction that combines a substance with oxygen to produce an oxide.

oxidation-reduction (redox) reactions: one of the most common types of chemical reactions; prevalent in all areas of chemistry. When oxygen is added to a substance, the substance is oxidized; for example, rust forms when oxygen is added to iron.

oxidize: to combine or cause a substance to combine with oxygen.

oxygen: the most abundant element on earth.

P

packs: cream masks or gel masks that nourish rather than deep-cleanse the skin.

palatine bones: the two bones that form the hard palate of the mouth.

papaya: natural enzyme used in enzyme peels.

papillary layer: the top layer of the dermis next to the epidermis.

papule: a pimple; small elevation on the skin that contains no fluid but may develop pus.

parabens: one of the most commonly used groups of preservatives in the cosmetic, pharmaceutical, and food industries; provide bacteriostatic and fungistatic activity against a diverse number of organisms.

paraffin wax masks: mask used to warm the skin and promote penetration of ingredients deeper into the skin through the heat trapped under the surface of the paraffin.

parasite: organism that lives in or on another organism and draws its nourishment from that organism.

parasympathetic division: as part of the autonomic nervous system, it operates under normal nonstressful situations, such as resting. It also helps to restore calm and balance to the body after a stressful event.

parietal artery: artery that supplies blood to the side and crown of the head.

parietal bones: bones that form the sides and top of the cranium.

partnership: form of business ownership in which two or more people share ownership, although this does not necessarily mean an equal arrangement. In a partnership, each partner assumes the other's unlimited liability for debt. Profits are shared among partners.

pathogenic: causing disease; harmful.

pectoralis major and minor: muscles of the chest that assist the swinging movements of the arm.

pediculosis: skin disease caused by infestation with head lice.

peptides: chains of amino acids used to treat wrinkles and elasticity.

performance ingredients: ingredients in cosmetic products that cause the actual changes in the appearance of the skin.

pericardium: double-layered membranous sac enclosing the heart.

perioral dermatitis: an acne-like condition around the mouth. These are mainly small clusters of papules that could be caused by toothpaste or products used on the face.

peripheral nervous system: system of nerves and ganglia that connects the peripheral parts of the body to the central nervous system; has both sensory and motor nerves.

peristalsis: moving food along the digestive tract.

personal hygiene: daily maintenance of cleanliness and healthfulness through certain sanitary practices.

personnel: employees; staff.

petrissage: a kneading movement that stimulates the underlying tissues.

petroleum jelly: an occlusive agent that restores the barrier layer by holding in water. Used after laser surgery to protect the skin while healing.

pH: relative degree of acidity and alkalinity of a substance.

pH adjusters: acids or alkalis (bases) used to adjust the pH of products.

phalanges: bones of the fingers or toes (singular: phalanx).

phenol: carbolic acid; a caustic poison; used for peels and to sanitize metallic implements.

photoepilation: hair reduction methods using lasers and intense pulsed light (IPL).

phototherapy: phototherapy (light therapy), is a form of treatment used for various skin conditions using artificial light wavelengths from the ultraviolet (blue light) part of the sun's spectrum.

photothermolysis: process by which light from a laser is turned into heat.

physical change: change in the form or physical properties of a substance without a chemical reaction or the formation of a new substance.

physical mixture: combination of two or more substances united physically, not chemically, without a fixed composition and in any proportions.

physical presentation: a person's physical posture, walk, and movements.

physical properties: characteristics that can be determined without a chemical reaction and that do not cause a chemical change in the identity of the substance.

physiology: study of the functions or activities performed by the body's structures.

phytotherapy: the use of plant extracts for therapeutic benefits.

plasma: fluid part of the blood and lymph that carries food and secretions to the cells and carbon dioxide from the cells.

platelets: blood cells that aid in the forming of clots.

platysma: broad muscle extending from the chest and shoulder muscles to the side of the chin; responsible for depressing the lower jaw and lip.

plug: two- or three-prong connector at the end of an electrical cord that connects an apparatus to an electrical outlet.

polarity: negative or positive pole of an electric current.

polyglucans: ingredients derived from yeast cells that help strengthen the immune system and stimulate the metabolism; they are also hydrophilic and help preserve and protect collagen and elastin.

polymers: chemical compounds formed by a number of small molecules; advanced vehicles that release substances onto the skin's surface at a microscopically controlled rate.

polysaccharides: carbohydrates that contain three or more simple carbohydrate molecules.

pores: a tubelike opening for sweat glands on the epidermis.

posterior auricular artery: artery that supplies blood to the scalp, behind and above the ear.

posterior auricular nerve: nerve that affects the muscles behind the ear at the base of the skull.

potassium hydroxide: a strong alkali used in soaps and creams.

preservatives: chemical agents that inhibit the growth of microorganisms in cosmetic formulations. These kill bacteria and prevent products from spoiling.

primary colors: yellow, red, and blue; fundamental colors that cannot be obtained from a mixture.

primary lesions: primary lesions are characterized by flat, non-palpable changes in skin color such as macules or patches, or an elevation formed by fluid in a cavity, such as vesicles, bullae, or pustules.

procedural guide: manual or set of instructions designed to standardize operations; supplies specific protocols for conducting individual services, such as the expected method for performing a glycolic or microdermabrasion treatment.

procerus: muscle that covers the bridge of the nose, depresses the eyebrows, and causes wrinkles across the bridge of the nose.

professional image: the impression projected by a person engaged in any profession, consisting of outward appearance and conduct exhibited in the workplace.

profit: amount of money available after all expenses are subtracted from all revenues.

promotion: the process of getting the consumer's attention, with the goal of increasing business.

pronators: muscles that turn the hand inward so that the palm faces downward.

propylene glycol: a humectant often used in dry or sensitive skin moisturizers.

proteins: chains of amino acid molecules used in all cell functions and body growth.

protoplasm: colorless, jellylike substance in cells; contains food elements such as protein, fats, carbohydrates, mineral salts, and water.

protozoa: single-celled parasites with the ability to move; they can divide and grow only when inside a host.

pruitis: the medical term for itching.

pseudofolliculitis: often referred to as "razor bumps"; resembles folliculitis without the infection.

pseudomonacidal: capable of destroying *Pseudomonas* bacteria.

psoriasis: a skin disease characterized by red patches covered with white-silver scales. It is caused by an overproliferation of skin cells that replicate too fast. Immune dysfunction could be the cause. Psoriasis is usually found in patches on the scalp, elbows, knees, chest, and lower back.

public relations (PR): the planning and developing of relationships to achieve a certain desired behavior.

pulmonary circulation: process of blood circulation from the heart to the lungs to be purified.

pus: fluid product of inflammation that contains white blood cells and the debris of dead cells, tissue elements, and bacteria.

pustule: an inflamed papule with a white or yellow center containing pus, a fluid consisting of white blood cells, bacteria, and other debris produced from an infection.

Q

quaternary ammonium compounds (quats): disinfectants that are considered nontoxic, odorless, and fast acting.

quaternium 15: an all-purpose preservative active against bacteria, mold, and yeast. It is probably the greatest formaldehyde releaser among cosmetic preservatives, causing dermatitis and allergies.

questionnaire: form that provides the esthetician with a complete client profile, including important information about a client's skin care habits and health.

quota: a method for gauging the amount of sales and targeting production levels.

R

radial artery: artery that supplies blood to the thumb side of the arm and the back of the hand.

radial nerve: nerve that, with its branches, supplies the thumb side of the arm and back of the hand.

radius: smaller bone in the forearm on the same side as the thumb.

reconstructive surgery: defined as "restoring a bodily function." It is necessary surgery for accident survivors and those with congenital disfigurements or other diseases.

rectifier: apparatus that changes alternating current to direct current.

red blood cells: also called red corpuscles; blood cells that carry oxygen from the lungs to the body cells.

red light: therapeutic light used on dry skin in combination with oils and creams; penetrates the deepest and produces the most heat.

redox: acronym for *reduction-oxidation;* chemical reaction in which the oxidizing agent is reduced and the reducing agent is oxidized.

redox reactions: oxidation and reduction happening at the same time.

reduction: the loss of oxygen from a substance.

reflective listening: listening to the client and then repeating, in your own words, what you think the client is telling you.

reflex: automatic nerve reaction to a stimulus; involves the movement of an impulse from a sensory receptor along the afferent nerve to the spinal cord, and a responsive impulse along an efferent neuron to a muscle, causing a reaction.

reproductive system: body system responsible for processes by which plants and animals produce offspring.

respiratory system: body system consisting of the lungs and air passages; enables breathing, which supplies the body with oxygen and eliminates carbon dioxide as a waste product.

resume: a summary of education and work experience that highlights relevant accomplishments and achievements.

retail supplies: items available for sale to clients.

retailing: the act of recommending and selling products to clients for at-home use.

retention hyperkeratosis: hereditary factor in which dead skin cells do not shed from the follicles as they do on normal skin.

reticular layer: the deeper layer of the dermis, containing proteins that give the skin its strength and elasticity.

retinoic acid: a vitamin A derivative. It has demonstrated an ability to alter collagen synthesis and is used to treat acne and visible signs of aging. Side effects are irritation, photosensitivity, skin dryness, redness, and peeling.

retinol: a natural form of vitamin A, stimulates cell repair and helps to normalize skin cells by generating new cells.

revenue: income generated from selling services and products; money taken in.

rhinoplasty: nose surgery that makes a nose smaller or changes its appearance.

rhytidectomy: a face lift. This procedure removes excess fat at the jawline; tightens loose, atrophic muscles; and removes sagging skin.

risorius: muscle of the mouth that draws the corner of the mouth out and back, as in grinning.

role model: a person whose behavior and success are worthy of emulation.

rosacea: inflammation of the skin; chronic congestion primarily on the cheeks and nose. Characterized by redness, dilation of blood vessels, and in severe cases, the formation of papules and pustules.

rose: credited with moisturizing, astringent, tonic, and deodorant properties; found in the forms of rose extracts, oil, or water.

rotary brush: machine used to lightly exfoliate and stimulate the skin; also helps soften excess oil, dirt, and cell buildup.

S

salary: a method of compensation that specifies a certain amount of pay based on either a flat or hourly rate.

salicylic acid: a beta hydroxy acid with exfoliating and antiseptic properties; natural sources include sweet birch, willow bark, and wintergreen.

sanitary maintenance area (SMA): an area kept clean for setup of procedure implements and supplies; for example, an SMA can be a towel (paper or cloth) on the workstation.

sanitation: third level of decontamination; significantly reduces the number of pathogens or disease-producing organisms found on a surface.

sanitizer: an ultraviolet (UV), wet, or dry sanitizer is used for disinfecting tools and equipment. An autoclave is a sterilizer.

saponification: chemical reaction during desincrustation where the current transforms the sebum into soap.

scabies: contagious skin disease caused by an itch mite burrowing under the skin.

scale: flaky skin cells; any thin plate of epidermal flakes, dry or oily. An example is abnormal or excessive dandruff.

scapula: one of a pair of shoulder blades; large, flat triangular bone of the shoulder.

scar: light-colored, slightly raised mark on the skin formed after an injury or lesion of the skin has healed up. The tissue hardens to heal the injury. Elevated scars are hypertrophic; a keloid is a hypertrophic (abnormal) scar.

sclerotherapy: procedure that minimizes varicose veins (dilated blood vessels) and other varicosities by injecting chemical agents into the affected areas or by laser treatments.

seaweed: seaweed derivatives such as algae have many nourishing properties. Specifically, seaweed is known for its humectant and moisturizing properties, vitamin content, metabolism stimulation and detoxification, and aiding skin firmness.

sebaceous filaments: similar to open comedones, these are mainly solidified impactions of oil without the cell matter.

sebaceous glands: sebaceous glands are connected to the hair follicles in the reticular layer; these produce sebum, which protects the surface of the skin.

sebaceous hyperplasia: benign lesions frequently seen in oilier areas of the face.

An overgrowth of the sebaceous gland, they appear similar to open comedones; often doughnut-shaped, with sebaceous material in the center.

seborrhea: severe oiliness of the skin; an abnormal secretion from the sebaceous glands.

seborrheic dermatitis: a common form of eczema.

sebum: provides protection for the epidermis from external factors and lubricates both the skin and hair.

secondary colors: colors obtained by mixing equal parts of two primary colors.

secondary lesions: skin damage, developed in the later stages of disease, that changes the structure of tissues or organs.

sensory (afferent) nerves: nerves that carry impulses or messages from the sense organs to the brain, where sensations of touch, cold, heat, sight, hearing, taste, smell, pain, and pressure are experienced.

serratus anterior: muscle of the chest that assists in breathing and in raising the arm.

serums: concentrated liquid ingredients for the skin designed to penetrate and treat various skin conditions.

seventh (facial) cranial nerve: chief motor nerve of the face, emerging near the lower part of the ear.

sharps container: plastic biohazard containers for disposable needles and anything sharp. The container is red and puncture-proof and must be disposed of as medical waste.

shiatsu: a form of acupressure.

silicones: a group of oils that are chemically combined with silicon and oxygen and leave a non-comedogenic, protective film on the surface of the skin.

sinusoidal current: alternating current similar to faradic current; produces mechanical contractions and is used during scalp and facial manipulations.

skeletal system: physical foundation of the body, composed of the bones and movable and immovable joints.

skin tag: small outgrowths or extensions of the skin that look like flaps. They are benign and are common under the arms or on the neck.

skin types: classification describing a person's genetic skin type.

smaller (lesser) occipital nerve: nerve located at the base of the skull, affecting the scalp and muscles behind the ear.

sodium bicarbonate: baking soda; an inorganic salt used as a buffering agent and a pH adjuster. It is alkaline.

sole proprietorship: form of business ownership in which an individual acts as sole owner and manager and is responsible for determining all policies and making all of the necessary decisions associated with running a business.

solute: a substance that is dissolved by a solvent to form a solution.

solutions: a uniform mixture of two or more mutually miscible substances.

solvent/s: a substance or substances that dissolves another substance to form a solution.

sorbitol: Humectant that absorbs moisture from the air to prevent skin dryness.

sphenoid bone: bone that joins all the bones of the cranium together.

sphingolipids: ceramides, or lipid material, that are a natural part of the intercellular cement. Glycosphingolipids and phospholipids are also natural lipids found in the barrier layer.

spinal cord: portion of the central nervous system that originates in the brain, extends down to the lower extremity of the trunk, and is protected by the spinal column.

spirilla: spiral or corkscrew-shaped bacteria that cause syphilis, Lyme disease, and other diseases.

spray machine: spray misting device.

squalene: originally from shark-liver oil; occurs in small amounts in olive oil, wheat germ oil, and rice bran oil; also found in human sebum. A lubricant and perfume fixative.

squamous cell carcinoma: more serious than basal cell carcinoma; characterized by scaly red papules or nodules.

stain: brown or wine-colored discoloration. Stains occur after certain diseases, or after moles, freckles, or liver spots disappear. A port wine stain is a birthmark, which is a vascular type of nevus.

staphylococci: pus-forming bacteria that grow in clusters like a bunch of grapes; cause abscesses, pustules, and boils.

steatoma: a sebaceous cyst or subcutaneous tumor filled with sebum; ranges in size from a pea to an orange. It usually appears on the scalp, neck, and back; also called a *wen*.

sterilization: highest level of decontamination; completely kills every organism on a nonporous surface.

sternocleidomastoideus: muscle of the neck that depresses and rotates the head.

sternum: the flat bone, or breastbone, that forms the ventral support of the ribs.

stone massage: the use of hot stones and cold stones in massage or in other treatments.

stratum corneum: outermost layer of the epidermis; also called the horny layer.

stratum germinativum: first layer of the epidermis above the papillary layer of the dermis; also known as basal layer.

stratum granulosum: layer of the epidermis composed of cells filled with keratin that resembles granules; replaces cells shed from the stratum corneum.

stratum lucidum: clear layer of epidermis under the stratum corneum; found only on the palms of hands and soles of feet.

stratum spinosum: spiny layer of epidermis above the basal layer.

streptococci: pus-forming bacteria arranged in curved lines resembling a string of beads; cause infections such as strep throat and blood poisoning.

striated muscles: also called voluntary or skeletal muscles; muscles that are controlled by the will.

subcutaneous layer: subcutaneous adipose tissue located beneath the dermis.

subcutis tissue: subcutaneous tissue located beneath the dermis.

submental artery: artery that supplies blood to the chin and lower lip.

sudoriferous or sweat glands: excrete perspiration and detoxify the body by excreting excess salt and unwanted chemicals.

sugaring: an ancient method of hair removal, dating back to the Egyptians. The original recipe is a mixture of sugar, lemon juice, and water that is heated to form syrup, molded into a ball and pressed onto the skin, and then quickly stripped away.

sulfur: sulfur reduces oil-gland activity and dissolves the skin's surface layer of dry, dead cells. This ingredient is commonly used in acne products. It can cause allergic skin reactions in some sensitive people.

superficial temporal artery: artery that supplies blood to the muscles of the front, side, and top of the head.

superior labial artery: artery that supplies blood to the upper lip and region of the nose.

supinator: muscle of the forearm that rotates the radius outward and the palm upward.

supraorbital artery: artery that supplies blood to the upper eyelid and forehead.

supraorbital nerve: nerve that affects the skin of the forehead, scalp, eyebrow, and upper eyelid.

supratrochlear nerve: nerve that affects the skin between the eyes and upper side of the nose.

surfactants: surface active agents that reduce surface tension between the skin and the product to increase product spreadability; also allow oil and water to mix; detergents and emulsifiers.

suspensions: state in which solid particles are distributed throughout a liquid medium.

sympathetic division: part of the autonomic nervous system that stimulates or speeds up activity and prepares the body for stressful situations, such as in running from a dangerous situation or competing in a sports event.

systemic (general) circulation: circulation of blood from the heart throughout the body and back again to the heart; also called *general circulation*.

T

tan: an increase in pigmentation due to the melanin production that results from exposure to UV rays. Melanin is designed to help protect the skin from the sun's UV rays.

tapotement: fast tapping, slapping, and hacking movements.

tea tree: soothing and antiseptic; antifungal properties. Used in many products.

telangiectasia: describes capillaries that have been damaged and are now larger, or distended blood vessels. Commonly called *couperose skin*.

telogen: final hair-growth stage, the resting stage.

temporal bones: bones forming the sides of the head in the ear region.

temporal nerve: nerve affecting the muscles of the temple, side of the forehead, eyebrow, eyelid, and upper part of the cheek.

temporalis: temporal muscle; one of the muscles involved in mastication (chewing).

tertiary colors: colors formed by mixing equal amounts of secondary color and its neighboring primary color.

Tesla high-frequency current: thermal or heat-producing current with a high rate of oscillation or vibration; also called violet ray.

test-wise: refers to a student who begins to prepare for taking a test by practicing good study habits and time management as part of an effective study program.

thermolysis: a heat effect; used for permanent hair removal.

thorax: the chest; elastic, bony cage that serves as a protective framework for the heart, lungs, and other internal organs.

tinea: a fungal infection.

tinea corporis: a contagious infection that forms a ringed, red pattern with elevated edges. Also called *ringworm*.

tinea versicolor: yeast infection that inhibits melanin production.

tissue: collection of similar cells that perform a particular function.

tissue respiratory factor (TRF): ingredient derived from yeast cells that functions as an anti-inflammatory and moisturizing ingredient.

titanium dioxide: an inorganic physical sunscreen that reflects UVA rays.

toners: liquids that tone and tighten the skin.

transconjunctival blepharoplasty: procedure performed inside the lower eyelid to remove bulging fat pads, which are often congenital.

transepidermal water loss (TEWL): water loss caused by evaporation on the skin's surface.

transferable skills: those abilities, such as sales training or administrative skills, that were mastered at other jobs and can be applied to a new position.

transverse facial artery: artery that supplies blood to the skin and the masseter.

trapezius: muscle that covers the back of the neck and upper and middle region of the back; stabilizes the scapula and shrugs the shoulders.

triangularis: muscle extending alongside the chin that pulls down the corner of the mouth.

triceps: large muscle that covers the entire back of the upper arm and extends the forearm.

trichloroacetic acid (TCA) peels: a strong peel used to diminish sun damage and wrinkles.

trichology: the scientific study of hair and its diseases.

tubercle: an abnormal rounded, solid lump; larger than a papule.

tuberculocidal: capable of destroying the bacteria that cause tuberculosis.

tuberculosis: a bacterial disease that usually affects the lungs.

tumor: a large nodule; an abnormal cell mass resulting from excessive cell multiplication and varying in size, shape, and color.

turbinal bones: thin layers of spongy bone on either of the outer walls of the nasal depression.

T-zone: the center area of the face; corresponds to the shape formed by forehead, nose, and chin.

U

ulcer: an open lesion on the skin or mucous membrane of the body, accompanied by pus and loss of skin depth. A deep erosion; a depression in the skin, normally due to infection or cancer.

ulna: inner and larger bone of the forearm, attached to the wrist on the side of the little finger.

ulnar artery: artery that supplies blood to the muscle of the little-finger side of the arm and palm of the hand.

ulnar nerve: nerve that affects the little-finger side of the arm and palm of the hand.

ultraviolet (UV) rays: invisible rays that have short wavelengths, are the least penetrating rays, produce chemical effects, and kill germs; also called cold rays or actinic rays.

Universal Precautions: set of guidelines and controls, published by OSHA, that require the employer and the employee to assume that all human blood and specified human body fluids are infectious for HIV, hepatitis B virus, and other blood-borne pathogens.

upselling services: the practice of recommending or selling additional services to clients that may be performed by you or other practitioners in the salon.

urea: properties include enhancing the penetration abilities of other substances. Anti-inflammatory, antiseptic, and deodorizing action allow urea to protect the skin's surface and help maintain healthy skin. Does not induce photoallergy, phototoxicity, or sensitization.

urticaria: hives.

UVA rays: longer, aging rays that penetrate deeper into the skin than UVB rays.

UVB rays: shorter, burning rays that are stronger than UVA rays.

V

vacuum (suction) machine: device that vacuums/suctions the skin to remove impurities and stimulate circulation.

valves: structures that temporarily close a passage or permit flow in one direction only.

variable costs: business expenses that fluctuate, such as utilities, supplies, and advertising.

vasoconstricting: vascular constriction of capillaries and blood flow.

vasodilation: vascular dilation of blood vessels.

vascular system: see *circulatory system*.

vehicles: spreading agents and ingredients that carry or deliver other ingredients into the skin and make them more effective.

veins: thin-walled blood vessels that are less elastic than arteries; they contain cuplike valves to prevent backflow and carry impure blood from the various capillaries back to the heart and lungs.

vellus hair: very fine, soft, downy hair covering most of the body.

ventricle: the lower, thick-walled chamber of the heart.

verruca: a wart; hypertrophy of the papillae and epidermis caused by a virus. It is infectious and contagious.

vesicles: a small blister or sac containing clear fluid. Poison ivy and poison oak produce vesicles.

vibration: a rapid shaking movement in which the technician uses the body and shoulders, not just the fingertips, to create the movement.

virucidal: capable of destroying viruses.

virus: microorganism that can invade plants and animals, including bacteria.

visible light: the primary source of light used in facial and scalp treatments.

vitamin A (retinol): an antioxidant that aids in the functioning and repair of skin cells.

vitamin C (ascorbic acid): an antioxidant vitamin needed for proper repair of the skin and tissues.

vitamin D: fat-soluble vitamin sometimes called the "sunshine vitamin" because the skin synthesizes vitamin D from cholesterol when exposed to sunlight. Essential for growth and development.

vitamin E (tocopherol): primarily an antioxidant; helps protect the skin from the harmful effects of the sun's rays.

vitamin K: vitamin responsible for the synthesis of factors necessary for blood coagulation.

vitiligo: white spots or areas on the skin from lack of pigment cells; sunlight makes it worse.

volt (V): unit that measures the pressure or force that pushes the flow of electrons forward through a conductor.

vomer: a flat, thin bone that forms part of the nasal septum.

W

warm colors: the range of colors with yellow undertones; from yellow and gold through oranges, red-oranges, most reds, and even some yellow-greens.

water: most abundant of all substances, comprising about 75 percent of the earth's surface and about 65 percent of the human body.

water soluble: mixable with water.

water-in-oil (W/O) emulsion: droplets of water dispersed in an oil.

watt (W): measurement of how much electric energy is being used in one second.

wavelength: distance between two successive peaks of electromagnetic waves.

wheal: an itchy, swollen lesion caused by a blow, insect bite, skin allergy reaction, or stings. Hives and mosquito bites are wheals. Hives (urticaria) can be caused by exposure to allergens used in products.

white blood cells: blood cells that perform the function of destroying disease-causing germs; also called white corpuscles or leukocytes.

white light: referred to as combination light because it is a combination of all the visible rays of the spectrum.

witch hazel: extracted from the bark of the hamanelis shrub; can be a soothing agent or, in higher concentrations, an astringent.

Wood's lamp: filtered black light that is used to illuminate skin disorders, fungi, bacterial disorders, and pigmentation.

Z

zinc oxide: an inorganic physical sunscreen that reflects UVA rays. Also used to protect, soothe, and heal the skin; is somewhat astringent, antiseptic, and anti-bacterial.

zygomatic nerve: nerve that affects the skin of the temple, side of the forehead, and upper part of the cheek.

zygomatic or malar bones: bones that form the prominence of the cheeks; the cheekbones.

zygomaticus major and minor: muscles extending from the zygomatic bone to the angle of the mouth; they elevate the lip, as in laughing.

Index

Note: Page numbers referencing figures are italicized and followed by an "f". Page numbers referencing tables are italicized and followed by a "t". Page numbers referencing definitions of terms are in bold.

A

A (amps), **148**, *149f*, **160**
ABCDE Cancer Checklist, 224
abdominoplasty, **463**, **465**
abducent nerve, *111f*
absorption, **119**, **121**, 194–95
AC (alternating current), **148**, **160**, 390
accessibility, *575f*
accessory nerve, *111f*, **112**–13, **122**
accutane, *229t*, *245t*
acid mantle, **135**, **141**, **192**, **208**
acid-alkali neutralization reactions, **135**, **141**
acids, **134**, **141**, 447–48
acne
  causes of, 226–27
  chocolate and, 182
  defined, **216**, **230**
  facials, 351–54
  grades of, 228, *229f*, *229t*
  medications for, *229t*
  overview, 225–26
  treating, 229, 353
  triggers, 227–28
acne excoriee, **216**, **230**
acnegenic products, 228
acquired immune deficiency syndrome (AIDS), **67**, **88**
acquired immunity, **70**, **88**
actinic, **241**, **251**
actinic keratoses, **222**, **230**, *242t*
action plans, 574–76
active electrodes, **151**, **160**
acupressure, 366
adapalene, *229t*, *245t*
adenosine triphosphate (ATP), **168**, **184**
adipose tissue, **198**, **208**
administrative duties, 558–59
adrenal glands, 118
adult acne, *242t*
advertising, **609**, **616**
aesthetic surgery, **462**–63, **465**
aestheticians, **10**, **17**
aesthetics, **17**
afferent nerves, 110, 125, 193–94, *195f*, 200
afferent peripheral system, 108
African esthetics, 6, *7f*
Age of Extravagance esthetics, 7
age spots, 241
aging, *242t*, 406. *See also* mature skin
AHAs. *See* alpha hydroxy acids
AIDS (acquired immune deficiency syndrome), **67**, **88**
air, **134**, **141**
air systems, 71
airbrush makeup, 522
airlines, 13
albinism, **221**, **230**
alcohol, 204, **268**, *268t*, **290**
algae, **270**, *270t*, **290**
algae masks, 282
alipidic skin, **237**–38, **251**
alkalies, **134**, **141**, 447–48

allantoin, *270t*, **290**
allergic contact dermatitis, 218–20
allergies, *64t*, 172, *245t*, 267, 272, 282
almond meal, *270t*
aloe vera, *270t*, **290**
alpha hydroxy acids (AHAs)
  acne treatment, 352, 354
  defined, **245**, **251**, **263**, **290**
  peels, 447, 449
alpha lipoic acid, 275
alpha-linolenic fatty acids, **170**–71, **185**
alternating current (AC), **148**, **160**, 390
alum, **268**, *268t*, **290**
amber light, 452
American Cancer Society, 224
amino acids, **167**–68, **184**
ampoules, **283**, **290**
amps (A), **148**, *149f*, **160**
anabolism, **97**, **121**
anaerobic bacteria, 226
anagen stage, **403**–4, **441**
anaphoresis, **152**, **160**, **386**, **388**, *389t*, **396**
anatomy
  body systems, 97, *98t*
  cells, 95–97
  circulatory system, 113–16
  defined, **95**, **121**
  digestive system, 118–19
  endocrine system, 117–18
  excretory system, 119
  immune system, 117
  integumentary system, 120
  muscular system, 102–7
  nervous system, 107–13
  organs, 97, *98t*
  reasons for studying, 95
  reproductive system, 120
  respiratory system, 119–20
  skeletal system, 99–102
  tissues, 97
androgens, 227–28
angle brushes, 479
angular artery, *115f*, **116**, **121**
anhidrosis, **217**, **230**
anhydrous products, **257**, **290**
anodes, **151**, **160**
ANS (autonomic nervous system), **108**, **121**
anterior auricular artery, *115f*, **116**, **121**
antioxidants
  defined, **136**, **141**, **245**, **251**, **262**, **264**, **290**
  skin care products, 265, 275
antiseptics, **71**, **88**, 273
Antoinette, Marie, 7
apocrine glands, **202**, **208**
aponeurosis, **103**, *104f*, **121**
appearance, personal, 21–23, *547f*, 553
applicators, 79, 413, 498
aqueous calcium, 462
arms
  blood supply of, 116
  bones of, 102
  muscles of, 106–7
  nerves of, 113
arnica, *270t*
aromatherapy, **261**, **273**–74, **290**, 366
aromatic properties, 273